OFFICIAL
ANTI-
AGING
REVOLUTION

STOP THE CLOCK
TIME IS ON YOUR SIDE
FOR A YOUNGER, STRONGER, HAPPIER YOU

RONALD KLATZ, MD, DO

ROBERT GOLDMAN, MD, PhD, DO, FAASP

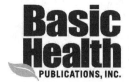

Basic Health
Health
PUBLICATIONS, INC.

Important—Please Read

The content in this book is for educational purposes only, and is not intended to prevent, diagnose, treat, or cure disease or illness. While potentially therapeutic nutraceuticals (dietary supplements such as vitamins, minerals, herbal products, hormone supplementation, and similar preparations) and interventions (processes such as lifestyle changes, dietary modifications, bodywork, prescription medications, and others) are mentioned in the course of this book, you are urged to seek the advice of a medical professional to make the appropriate selection for your particular medical situation.

With nutraceuticals, dosing is highly variable. Proper dosing is based on parameters including sex, age, whether you are well or ill, and whether your illness is chronic or acute. Additionally, efficiency of absorption of a particular type of product and the quality of its individual ingredients are two major considerations for choosing appropriate specific agents for your medical situation.

Just because a product is natural doesn't mean it's safe for you. A small portion of the general population may react adversely to components in nutraceuticals, especially herbal products. Make your physician aware of any and all "natural" interventions you use regularly, and seek medical consultation before starting any others.

Neither the publisher nor the authors advocate the use of any particular health-care protocol, but believe that the information in this book should be available to the public. The publisher and authors are not responsible for any adverse effects or consequences resulting from the use of any of the suggestions, preparations, or procedures discussed in this book. Should the reader have any questions concerning the appropriateness of any procedure or preparation mentioned, the publisher and authors strongly suggest consulting a professional health-care advisor.

Always consult your physician prior to beginning any new healthcare intervention, whether it be nutritional, fitness, medication, hormonal, herbal, or otherwise. Do not change the dosing or cease the intervention without discussing with your physician first.

Basic Health Publications, Inc.

28812 Top of the World Drive • Laguna Beach, CA 92651

949-715-7327 • www.basichealthpub.com

Library of Congress Cataloging-in-Publication Data

Klatz, Ronald.
  The official anti-aging revolution : stop the clock: time is on your side for a younger, stronger, happier you / Ronald Klatz, Robert Goldman. — 4th ed.
      p. cm.
  Includes bibliographical references and index.
  ISBN 978-1-59120-200-4
  1. Longevity. 2. Dietary supplements. 3. Hormone therapy.
I. Goldman, Bob II. Title.

  RA776.75.K53   2007
  613—dc22

                                        2007025380

Revised and updated by Catherine Cebula and Lindsay Steel, under the guidance of Dr. Ronald Klatz and Dr. Robert Goldman.

Editors: Cheryl Hirsch and Carol Rosenberg • Typesetting and book design: Gary A. Rosenberg
Cover design: Robert Buzek Designs Inc.

Printed in the United States of America

10   9   8   7   6   5   4   3   2   1

Contents

The E Factor (William Morrow)

Death in the Locker Room: Steroid & Sports (Icarus Press)

Death in the Locker Room: Drugs and Sports
(The Body Press, HP Books)

Death In the Locker Room: Steroids, Cocaine & Sports
(Price Stern Sloan)

Death in the Locker Room II (ESM)

*Oligomeric Proanthocyanidins (OPCs):
Harvesting Nature's Anti-Aging Bounty* (ESM)

*Cellular Phones/RF Radiation: Medical Menaces
of a Modern Day Convenience* (ESM)

Sleep: Essential for Optimal Health (ESM)

*HGF Human Growth Factors: Advanced Anti-Aging
Science Optimizes Your Peak Performance* (ESM)

Dedication

This book is dedicated to the tireless and selfless efforts of the 20,000-plus physician, health practitioner, and scientist members of the American Academy of Anti-Aging Medicine (A4M), who are poised at the forefront of science and research to prolong the healthy human life span and without whom our pursuit of innovative medical science would be unobtainable.

As a global population, we are experiencing leaps in life expectancy, decreases in death rates from the leading causes of death (heart disease, cancer, and stroke), and, in the United States, we are seeing a decrease in the use of nursing home care. Most important, the accessibility of quality medical care is improving. Clearly, anti-aging medicine has made a distinct impression on the evolution of health care to the betterment of the public at large.

As German physicist and Nobel Laureate Max Planck once remarked:

An important scientific innovation rarely makes its way
by gradually winning over and converting its opponents . . .
its opponents gradually die out and the growing generation
is familiar with the idea from the beginning.

Now celebrating its fifteen-year anniversary, the science of anti-aging medicine continues to experience remarkable continued growth. Over this past decade, in the main streets and back roads of every major nation on this planet, anti-aging medicine is taking hold. Today, the anti-aging clinical specialty continues to flourish in the United States, achieving the support of prestigious public policy groups, and it spreads worldwide as governmental agencies acknowledge the real potential for anti-aging medicine to alleviate the mounting social, political, and economic woes otherwise anticipated to arrive with the swelling aging global population.

We congratulate you on reading *The Official Anti-Aging Revolution.* By doing so, you become part of an elite future-forward group of consumers taking their first steps toward attaining their personal best in productivity and vitality. Soon, we will live in a world in which empowered patients take charge of their own health destinies. Watch with us as we see this bright future unfold.

Acknowledgments

The authors would like to thank the following individuals who provided support for the book: Chief Researcher and Editor Catherine Cebula, Informational Research Assistant Lindsay Steel, John Abdo, Mark Abrahms, Alicia Valaquez, Dr. Tom Allen, Joe Partipillo, Stewart Grannen, Stedman Grahm, Oprah Winfrey, Anthony Barone, Goldie & Jerry Klatz, Sid Bobb, Billy Levenson, Richard Furer, Barry Datloff, Ali Berman, Dr. Saroja Bharati, Paul & Sandy Bernstein, Lloyd Blankfein, Bobbie Jandristis, Bob Brahm, Dr. Eric Braverman, Phil Broxham, Perris Calderon, Lorne Caplan, Neil Cauliffe, Simon Chan, Chan Boon Yong, George Chow, Chris Wakeford, Christina Kamm, Paul Chua, Dr. Gerard Chuah, Leslie Cohen, June Colbert, Sam Lamensdorf, Steve Sotiri, Milt Copulos, Mike Crohn, Angie Daniels, Darrryll Burleigh, Jo Chua, Dato Harnam, Todd Dawes, Bob Dee, Bob Delmontique, Wayne Demelia, Denie Walters, Dr. Nick DeNubulie, Dr. Eduardo DeRose, Dr. Tom Deters, Dion Friedland, Tom Marinovic, Cory & Allen Dropkin, Dr. Ken Dychwald, Adam Eilenberg, Dr. Wade Exum, Fara Lazzara, Alfreda Green, Dr. Perry Gerard, GK Goh, Arnold & Alice Goldman, Paul & Carole Grahm, Mark & Paul Goldman, Dr. Brad Grant, Susan Greenbaum, Lynn Gu, Midred Bonner, Pam Cunningham, Guy Jonkman, Byron Klein, Dr. Harold Hakes, Dr. Lord Hanno Soth, Lee Harris, Warren Price, Dr. Arthur Heath, Tom Heidke, Judy Heifitz, Jack Balani, Dr. Vernon Howard, Andy Hydanto, Mike Interator, Irena Yundov, Susanne Archer, Jana Berentson, Dr. Marcelo Suarez, Gabriela Marinescu, Joni Pitcock, Dr. Fumihiko Umezawa, Dr. Seung-Yup Ku, Dr. M Watabe, Julian Grech, Peter Julian, Pam Kagan, Eric Weider, Ben & Joe Weider, Chuck Kaplan, Dr. Mike Katz, Georgia & Sumner Katz, Mitch Kaufman, Dr.Michael Klentze, Dr. Arkady Koltun, Tommy Konig, David Kravitz, Dr. Mitch Kurk, Andy & Bill Lane, Larry Emdur, Dr. Ron Lawrence, Dr. Sherrie Lechner, Lee Labrada, Lee Felix, Leon Wah Kneong, Dr. Howard Levine, Dr. Marty Levine, Dr. Ed Lichten, Jim Lidhtee, Dr. Shari Lieberman, Tony Little, Jim Lorimer, William Louey, Ross Love, Joe Hing Lowe, Dr. Sidney Malet,

Jon Mangion, Jim & Debbie Manion, Mark Brun, Titus & Vicki Marincas, George & Maria Iusco, U. Tin Maug Swee, Mauricio Fernendez, Tim McKeon, Dr. Joe Mercola, Rick Merner, Tom Merridith, Gary Mezei, Dr. Maurice Modavi, Edmund Murphy, Dr. Art Nahas, Neil Spruce, Mike Clark, Irene Nathan, Dan Neidermyer, Surya Joshi, O.Ben Seng, Ralph Sesso, Richard Ornstein, Dr. Don Owen, Vic Padillino, Giovanna Breu, David Peppin, Dr. Lee Perry, Dr. Peter Kalish, Kevin Philips, Dr. Lynn Pirie, Jeff Plitt, Glen Pollock, Javier Pollock, Ben Posner, Will & Norm Dabish, Tom Purvis, Grahm & Karthyn, Linda Lisahapanya, Curtis Schroeder, Dr. Anongnuth Chiangpradit, Pat Downing, Putnam & Kathryn Grahm, Dr. Rafael Santonja, Sandy Ranilli, Rano Rahmat, Sharon Ringer, Mel Rich, Steve Stern, Jim Rittenberg, Arlene Robbins, Dr. Jerry Rodos, Dr. Tom Rosandich, Dr. Phil Santiago, Larry & Warren Schiffer, Joe Schultz, Steve Schussler, Arnold Schwarzenegger, Barbi Adler, Dr. Marshall Segal, Dr. Uri Schaffer, Brian Sherr, Abby Silverberg, Simon Reynolds, Marty & Tracy Silverberg, Dr. Steve Sinatra, Donald Teo, Eugene Hong, Dr. Y. M. Wong, Janifer Yeo, Dr. SK Tan, Amy Sklar, Ann Sobel, Steve Sokol, Steven Speigle, Greg Stavish, Jake Steinfeld, Russ Stewart, John Stokack, Gary Strauch, Larry Stickler, Christy Morgan, Dr. James Stoxen, Mario Azodina,Dr. Barry Halliway, Fran Saavedra, Sukuma Sudiarsana, Alan & Linda Tamshen, Erica Clark, Dr. Thierry Hertoghe, Dr. Robert Tien, Stephen Tjandra, Drs. Terry & Jan Todd, Mike Tomzak, Dr. Richard Penfil, T.T. Durai, Jay Tuerk, Tim Tyrrell, Victor Vazquez, Gary Vogel, Heather Bird, Bob Voy, David Waite, Wanna Aung, Carole Weidman, Meredith Nussbaum, Cliff Wertheim, Bettie & Joseph Whittaker, Dr. Lumina Love, Brenda Winkle, Kenny Wong, Philip Yeo, Prithpal Singh, Dr. Lynette Yong, Dr. Richard Yong, Dr. Nantapat Supapannachart.

Additionally, the authors would like to acknowledge the thousands of members worldwide of the American Academy of Anti-Aging Medicine (A4M; www.worldhealth.net), a non-profit medical organization dedicated to the advancement of technology to detect, prevent, and treat aging-related disease and to promote research into methods to retard and optimize the human aging process. A4M is also dedicated to educating physicians, scientists, and members of the public on anti-aging issues. A4M believes that the disabilities associated with normal aging are caused by physiological dysfunction, which in many cases are ameliorable to medical treatment, such that the human life span can be increased, and the quality of one's life improved as one grows chronologically older. A4M seeks to disseminate information concerning innovative science and research as well as treatment modalities designed to prolong the human life span. Anti-Aging Medicine is based on the scientific principles of responsible medical care consistent with those of other healthcare specialties.

The Anti-Aging Revolution

In 1992, a meeting of a group of a dozen physicians convened by Dr. Ronald Klatz and Dr. Robert Goldman forever changed the course of preventive medicine to follow. Recognizing that scientific research was quickly making discoveries to identify the mechanisms of deterioration and vulnerability to age-related diseases, Drs. Klatz and Goldman proposed a new definition of aging itself. In this new perspective, the frailties and physical and mental failures associated with normal aging are caused by physiological dysfunctions that, in many cases, can be altered by appropriate medical interventions. As an extension of this redefinition, Drs. Klatz and Goldman described an innovative model for health care that focused on the application of advanced scientific and medical technologies for the early detection, prevention, treatment, and reversal of age-related dysfunction, disorders, and diseases. "Anti-aging medicine" was born.

In the fifteen years that since followed, anti-aging medicine has achieved international recognition. Anti-aging medicine is now practiced by thousands of physicians in private medical offices, as well as in some of the most prestigious teaching hospitals around the world. Many medical schools now include anti-aging in their programs, and physicians have clocked hundreds of thousands of hours of advanced medical education to train in this new medical specialty. Acknowledging the social, economic, and medical dilemmas anticipated to arrive with a rapidly growing aging population worldwide, anti-aging medicine has also garnered important recognition from leading public policy groups and members of academia. Universally, those involved in health care or those whose fields of expertise intersect with healthcare issues support anti-aging medicine as a healthcare model promoting innovative science and research to prolong the healthy life span in humans.

Are you one of the thousands of people who are starting to notice life's first signs of age? Signs of aging are noticeable in our mirrors, on our bath scales, in our bedrooms, and in the job market. A Baby Boomer turns fifty every thirty seconds, and many of them are experiencing an expanding waistline, a receding hairline, a waning sex life, or trouble recalling names and events. As a result, a barrage of "anti-aging" health and beauty products now vie for our attention. Turn the pages of your daily newspaper or weekly magazine, or stroll the aisles of your local drugstore or favorite department store, and you're likely to see dozens of products labeled as "anti-aging." Yet, anti-aging is much more than skin deep. You can't achieve anti-aging through a skin cream, a piece of fitness equipment, or even a vitamin pill (not yet, at least). Anti-aging medical care involves a regimen incorporating multiple elements of scientifically based age-reversal medical interventions administered under the guidance of a trained anti-aging physician or health professional.

To start making sense of the anti-aging phenomenon, we encourage you to read *The Official Anti-Aging Revolution.* Authored by Drs. Klatz and Goldman, founders of the science of anti-aging medicine, this book provides an introduction to this new medical specialty. From nutritional supplementation to hormone replacement therapy, exercise to diet, *The Official Anti-Aging Revolution* explains the basics involved in the anti-aging lifestyle. Once you understand all of the diverse options available to help you look, feel, and act younger, you are able to wisely choose a physician or health professional who will craft a customized program that fits your medical needs.

Anti-aging medicine is a clinical specialty that extends the concept of preventive health care to embrace the very early detection, prevention, and reversal of aging-related diseases, coupled with the aggressive yet gentle disease treatment. Anti-aging medicine has accelerated the pace of advancements in health promotion and prevention, and is the most important new model for health care for this new millennium. You owe it to yourself and your loved ones to take full advantage of all that the anti-aging medical revolution can offer.

Frequent the A4M's educational website, The World Health Network, at **www.worldhealth.net**, to keep updated on the latest advancements that can help you and your customers lead productive, extended lives. At www.worldhealth.net, you are invited to sign up to receive our free Biotech E-Newsletter, an assortment of breaking longevity news you can use.

The Anti-Aging Marketplace

• The consumer public has voted with their wallets overwhelmingly in favor of the anti-aging healthcare model. The anti-aging marketplace is one that is demographics-driven: people around the world are getting older. The anti-aging industry is presently (2006) valued at $55 Billion. With an average annual growth rate (AAGR) of 9.5%, the anti-aging industry is projected to reach $72 Billion by 2009. [Business Communications Company, 2005.]

• Sixty percent (60%) of Americans age 65+ are pursuing anti-aging interventions–including hormone replacement therapies and dietary supplementation. (MSNBC, Jan. 28, 2002)

• Dietary supplement sales in 2000 were $17 billion. (*Nutrition Business Journal,* Nov. 2001) Of these, $1.657 billion were attributed to anti-aging supplements. (*Progressive Grocer,* Vol. 79 No. 8, June 2001)

• According to the Robert Wood Foundation, we are witnessing the emergence of the new "top-tier healthcare consumer"—consumers who are, as a group—college graduates, computer literate, and drawing a household income of $50,000 or more. This group of highly educated, high earners is expected to "have the greatest ability to effect change." (Morgan CM, Levy DL. *Marketing to the Mindset of Boomers and Their Elders,* 2002) They are responsible for reshaping a new healthcare landscape—creating a world in which we all enjoy prolonged life spans, absent of disease and disability, and full of productivity and vitality. This is the new reality that A4M first introduced fifteen years ago.

A4M unites physicians, health practitioners, scientists, academics, and the general public in a spirit to promote cooperative research and application that will yield a scientifically validated, safe, effective, whole-body approach to aging intervention. A4M presently numbers 20,000-plus, hailing from more than 100 nations. By joining the A4M, you open countless opportunities to capitalize on this tremendous marketplace. In doing so, you'll make a real and substantial difference in the quality and quantity of your clients' lives. You'll also be among the first to learn how to improve your life and that of your loved ones.

Welcome to the Anti-Aging Revolution

AGING AND LONGEVITY

It is said that we begin the process of dying at the moment of birth; that, from that miraculous moment onward, we are breathing a finite number of breaths, beating a finite number of heartbeats.

But this is an oversimplification of the truth. From the moment of birth, we begin a process of growth and development that continues into the years of reproduction. These are times, for most of us, of freedom and health, as we experience cognitive and sensory clarity, muscular development, and fluid strength. It is only after these years, during which Nature dictates that we ourselves create new life, that we begin to see our selves and the processes of our bodies decline; that we begin to gain weight and lose muscle tone, sensory acuity, and the graceful motions of youth.

Modern medicine and technology, however, now give lie to the accepted truth that life is finite, that decline is inevitable. Modern medicine now offers not only the possibility, but also the option of maintaining our youth far past the chronological year by which, in ages past, an elderly decline had taken hold.

Thus, we have called this book *The Official Anti-Aging Revolution*. In this book, we will introduce you to a new way of thinking. In this chapter, we submit that the chronological clock by which we have traditionally gauged our "age" is outmoded. To fully understand this innovative thinking, we must first understand some terms and their changing meanings.

MODERN DEFINITIONS

What Is Aging?

We live in a technological age. The computer that fifty years ago took a large, dust-free room to contain now sits smartly on our desktops, and soon to reside compactly on a palm-sized, fully mobile, personal data assistant. And that computer has changed out lives in return. It has given us the opportunity to write books, to run small businesses, and to create works of art, from graphics to videos, all from our homes. And, perhaps more important, through the creation of the World Wide Web, it has given us the opportunity to communicate with and learn from other people all over the world from the comfort of our own homes.

Modern technology has freed us to live our lives more creatively, more intelligently. And this technology has had a profound impact on our culture. We need to look no further than our own changing language to see the far-reaching effects technology has had.

Not only have personal computers created a new set of jargon—who among us had heard of a *byte* or a *modem* twenty years ago—but our evolving technology has also brought about an evolution in the meanings of some very basic terms.

Take "aging" for example. Webster's *New World Dictionary* defines "aging" as "the process of growing old or showing signs of growing old." While this definition may have sufficed for the nineteenth century in which Mr. Webster was still alive, new medical discoveries and biotechnological advancements have made the Webster definition of "aging" totally outmoded.

Indeed, aging may be divided into two very different concepts: *chronological age* and *biological age.* In celebrating a birthday (which is a celebration of chronological age), it is often true that the performance of an individual's body systems—from mental function to sexual performance to physical strength—are better or worse than would be expected when compared with same-aged colleagues (this being an example of biological age). Most of us know at least one individual whose driver's license states that he or she is seventy, but we can observe that person carrying on in their daily life with the vibrancy expected of someone twenty to thirty years younger. Conversely, you may know someone with the chronological age of forty who fails to go about life with the energy expected for that age, who seems far older than his or her years.

Today, scientists know much more about the deterioration and vulnerability to disease that typifies the aging process. As such, "aging" gains a new definition. *Aging is not inevitable.* A modern approach submits that the disabilities associated with normal aging are caused by physiological dysfunctions that, in many cases, are ameliorable to medical treatment. By systematically revitalizing the biological processes involved in aging, the human life span can be increased while the quality of life is maintained or improved.

What Is Longevity?

Webster's defines "longevity" as "long life; the great duration of individual life," and, "research in longevity." It is this last phrase that is the very heart of this book. In a profound way, this book is not at all about aging, although we must take a look at the way in which most of us age, and the biological processes that begin to decline in middle age with the ticking of the clock, in order to truly understand this. Rather, this is a book about longevity. It is about the research into the process of aging that is now offering millions of people the world over the option of living a longer, healthier life.

Thus, as you look through the table of contents, you will see that the word "longevity" begins the title of the majority of the sections into which this book is divided. The first section alone begins with the word "aging." That section gives the reader not only a general understanding of the aging process, but also an up-to-the-minute gathering of modern medicine's theories of aging and mortality.

From here, this book is divided into three sections on the topic of longevity. Each explores an area of human life that has a profound impact on the length and quality of life for each of us. Thus, these sections explore longevity and nutrition, longevity and exercise—diet and nutrition being key factors in living long and living healthy—and a special section on human hormones and how they affect maximum peak performance and longevity. This section explores the endocrine system of ductless glands, the hormones secreted by each, and the impact of these hormones on the length and quality of human life.

What Is Anti-Aging Medicine?

Every day, consumers flock to their doctors' offices in search of ways to erase life's little signs of age: an expanding waistline, a receding hairline, a G-rated sex life, forgetting whether the stove was turned off after making a midnight snack, and the list goes on.

About 77 percent of all Americans now living were born after 1939—and many of these folks are noticing these signs of aging in their mirrors, on their scales, and in the job market. Anti-aging medicine—the application of any therapy or modality that delivers very early detection, prevention, treatment, or reversal of aging-related dysfunction and disease, thus enhancing the quality, and extending the quantity, of the human life span—is the most important new model for health care for this new millennium.

The leading causes of death have undergone a profound shift: due to improvements in sanitation and infection control since the turn of the twentieth century, Americans are now losing their health and lives to heart disease (31.4 percent), cancer (23.3 percent), and stroke (6.9 percent). These three diseases, known collectively as the degenerative diseases of aging, swallow 50 percent of the U.S. healthcare budget. One hundred million Americans are currently being treated for one or another degenerative disease at a health care cost of more than $700 billion per year.

All diseases fall into four categories; the first three—inherited genetic disease, infectious disease, and trauma—account for only 10 percent of the cost for treating all disease in America. Ninety percent of all health-care dollars are spent on extraordinary care in the last two to three years of life.

If we really want to make an impact on health care in this country and throughout the world, we must focus on preventing the degenerative diseases of aging. Today in the United States, the federal government spends $350 billion, or 3.5 percent of Gross Domestic Product (GDP), on health care for the elderly population. That will double in just two decades. Within forty years, Washington will be spending 50 percent more on health care than on Social Security. By 2075, experts are estimating the expenditure to double and stand at 14.5 percent of GDP. Actuaries project that by 2010, per-capita spending on health care for Americans age sixty-five and over will be $10,000. With the widespread adoption of anti-aging medicine, more of the nation's population will receive early screenings to detect illness. This is expected to cut the treatment side of disease by reducing the costs of having to treat full-blown illness in a greater segment of the population. Early detection and treatment will also lead to extended healthy life spans absent of debilitating or disabling medical conditions.

Indeed, if we are to save public programs for seniors, an integral focus must be on adoption of anti-aging medicine in the preventive healthcare setting. By cutting the spending on health care, there will be more funds to appropriate to other public programs. Remarks an article in *U.S. News & World Report:*

> While politicians are debating how to ration healthcare, scientists are focused on a more promising endeavor alleviating the diseases that commonly come with old age. . . . [W]hile there will be many more elderly people, there will not be an increase in chronically disabled elderly. Dying old is generally cheaper than dying young. A 70-year old

consumes almost three times as much health care in the last two years of life as a 101-year old receives. What is expensive is older people living through years of chronic dependence. . . . [Government]-funded programs will reap these savings and reduce their tab.

That's just it—the anti-aging medical model seeks to find solutions to eliminate or, at least, to alleviate the disorders that lead to chronic dependence and disability.

The ultimate accomplishment for the science of anti-aging medicine will be the achievement of *practical immortality,* in which we live vital life spans of 120 years or more. Practical immortality is based on the notion that the exponential expansion of medical knowledge, doubling every 3.5 years or less, will yield biotechnological discoveries that will permit scientists to alter the course and concept of aging. We predict that, by the year 2029, advancements in stem cell research, therapeutic cloning, and nanotechnology (science and technology of building miniscule devices for manipulating single atoms and molecules) will be harnessed into applications that improve and extend the human life span. In this manner, anti-aging medicine is anticipated to have a profound and permanent impact on the future of preventive health care.

How to Use This Book

The Official Anti-Aging Revolution: Stop the Clock: Time Is On Your Side—For a Younger, Stronger, Happier You is a consumer guide to living a longer, healthier life. It is a resource book for lay persons who want to learn how their bodies work, how they age, and what they can do about it.

The first iteration of this book was published in 1996, and, from the first, there was great demand for the information it contained. But now, eleven years have passed since the original publication, and the pace of biotechnology, together with the vast amounts of information uncovered in these past few years, created a need for a new, updated edition.

What you hold in your hands is that new edition. It contains the most up-to-date information available in print today on the subject of longevity and anti-aging medicine. In addition, it gives practical information on diet and exercise, identifying the nutrients that can increase the length and quality of life, and the exercises that increase strength, flexibility and mental acuity. A full-range of information on lifestyle and its impact on longevity, with tips for a long and healthy life has also been included.

Perhaps most important, the new edition of this book gives a complete look at the human endocrine system of ductless glands and the hormones produced by each. As these hormones greatly affect the development and decline of the human system, the information contained in these chapters offers the reader and his or her physician a myriad of options that may retard aging and promote longevity.

As it is the belief of the authors that the proper use of biotechnology, in combination with appropriate changes in nutrition and exercise, offer a vital life span nearly double that now enjoyed by the average American, it is our hope that *The Official Anti-Aging Revolution* will find its way into the hands of those millions who now, in middle age, find themselves facing the decline of age.

To those persons, we say this: "Take the information in this book to heart. Put it to use. It will change your life."

SECTION ONE

On Aging

Health is the first of all liberties.

—HENRI AMIEL (1821–1881)

CHAPTER 1

Who Wants to Live to Be 150?

The banquet hall was filled with 1,400 of the world's most respected scientific minds in medicine and biotechnology. They had assembled at the 3rd Annual International Conference on Anti-Aging Medicine and Biomedical Technology in Las Vegas on December 10, 1995. Dr. Marvin Minsky of the Massachusetts Institute of Technology, the person credited with the invention of artificial intelligence, posed this question to the audience: "Who here wishes to live to the ripe age of 150?" Eighty percent of hands in the room rose with little hesitation. "Well," said Minsky, "now at last we're ready for the next millennium."

"Aging is not inevitable! The war on aging has begun!" So says the official slogan of the American Academy of Anti-Aging Medicine (A4M), founded in 1992 by a small group of physicians and scientists dedicated to slowing, and eventually halting, the aging process. The science of anti-aging medicine is creating a new paradigm of health care and is taking a new approach to aging and to medicine, showing us a new reality for humankind, an adulthood free from the fear of disease, infirmity, and lingering death in old age. In one decade, A4M has become the world's leading non-profit medical and scientific society dedicated to clinical anti-aging medicine, representing the interests of more than 20,000 specialists from over 100 countries worldwide.

To understand the concept of anti-aging medicine, realize that, with the exception of infection and some childhood disorders, the vast majority of degenerative disease shares but one common characteristic: aging itself. Alzheimer's disease, most cancers, heart disease, non-insulin dependent diabetes, osteoporosis, autoimmune disorders, stroke, death by pneumonia and influenza, arthritis, Parkinson's disease, and the myriad of maladies linked to advancing age commonly afflict only those over age forty—the age of lost youth and the "portal to seniority."

AGING "AIN'T WHAT IT USED TO BE"

Even without research directed at aging itself, humanity has, in the past two centuries, realized an unrecognized benefit through advances in sanitation, nutrition, and early detection and treatment of infectious diseases—an increase in average life span of almost fifty years!

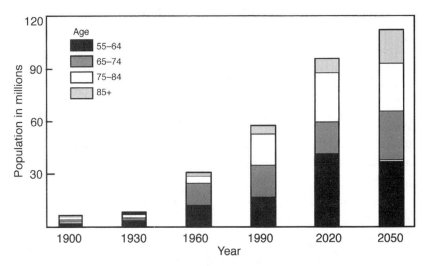

FIGURE 1.1. Actual and projected growth of U.S. population ages 55+, 1900–2050

The very definition of what is *old* is changing daily. New treatments that are giving so many people added years of life are the interventions and therapeutics of *anti-aging medicine*—a combination of hormone replacement therapy, nutritional supplements, high-dose antioxidants and vitamins, and a custom-designed exercise/rehabilitation program. In addition to these tools, patients are asked, for their part, to seek a revolution in their personal attitude.

Contrary to a commonly held misconception, the purpose of anti-aging medicine is not to extend life in order to live a longer period of time as an "older" person, but rather to delay the onset of the aging process and give everyone a greater number of those middle, healthy years. Who wouldn't want to be as fit and vital at age seventy-five as he or she was at forty-five?

> The silent revolution of anti-aging medicine is so gradual yet pervasive that many of us have not even noticed that aging "ain't what it used to be."
> • In 1796, the average life span was twenty-five years.
> • In 1896, the average life span almost doubled to forty-eight years.

- In 2006, a healthy, productive average life span was almost eighty years for most Americans, with many reputable anti-aging scientists predicting average life spans of 120–150 years before 2050.

We have entered an era when older people make up the greatest percentage of America's population. When the first U.S. Census was taken in 1790, half the population was under age sixteen. In 1990, less than one-fourth the population was under age sixteen. The median age had doubled in 200 years! In fact, the U.S. Census Bureau predicts that by the year 2025, there will be two sixty-five year olds for every teenager!

Living to sixty-five used to be a big deal—that's why the government thought that Social Security was a bargain in the 1930s. Only one in ten Americans ever saw their first Social Security check. Not today, when fully 75 percent of the population will sail past sixty-five without a care.

The percentage of Americans over age sixty-five today has tripled from 1900 to 1990 from 4 percent to 12.5 percent, while the total number has increased tenfold, from 3 million to 31.6 million. The fastest-growing segment of the population is over age eighty-five. Other senior populations are also growing quickly, however. If we compare 1900 to 1991, the sixty-five to seventy-four age group had become eight times larger, the seventy-four to eighty-five group thirteen times larger, and the over eighty-five group twenty-five times larger.

Every day in 1990, some 6,000 people celebrated their sixty-fifth birthdays. Almost everybody who turned sixty-five in 1990 was expected to live an average of 17.3 years more. In 1900, it was unusual to reach sixty-five in the first place, and those who did could expect to live only an average of eleven years more.

Americans aged eighty years and older can expect to live up to a year longer than their counterparts in England, France, Japan, and Sweden.

Look around today. It's not uncommon to see people who are still healthy and vibrant in their eighties and nineties. It used to be miraculous for a person to reach their hundredth birthday (a centenarian) while healthy, vital and intact. This is no longer true. Most people reading this can now fully expect life spans of one hundred plus years. From a historical standard, we are rapidly approaching a state of practical immortality for the human race!

In 2000, the US was home to 81,000 centenarians. The US Census Bureau projects this number to rise, to reach to 214,000 in 2020. By the year 2050, conservative estimates by longevity experts predict well over one million centenarians to reside in the US.

AGING IS A TREATABLE MEDICAL CONDITION

The baby-boomer generation (those born between 1946 and 1964, now turning sixty), are to be congratulated for demanding a new approach to aging and the modern-day reality of longevity and rejuvenation. For the first time in recorded history, an entire generation has decided it has better things to do than sit around and get old. The proven benefits of exercise and a balanced diet have been embraced. From the "Boomers" came the fitness movement, which history will record as being the forerunner of anti-aging medicine. They have made the commitment to be very good at what they do—and they want to keep active for as long as possible.

Boomers believe that age is irrelevant; that it is function and ability that matter, and they expect to live practically forever. Boomers have an innate desire to stay healthy, fit, and mentally alert because they know that their lives will not only be fuller and more enjoyable because of it, but also longer and filled with greater opportunity. This is the generation that has said "yes" to anti-aging medicine.

Many political analysts have raised disturbing questions about the demographics of the progressively elderly U.S. population. They point out that traditionally people over age sixty-five have required far higher levels of social services than their younger counterparts. Particularly as they enter their eighties, they may need assistance with transportation, shopping, home maintenance, and other basic life tasks. Older people also tend to require ever-increasing levels of health care, since old age almost always brings with it a lowered immune system and a greater vulnerability to a variety of diseases.

Who then, the politicians ask, will pay for these increased services? Traditionally, the younger portion of the population has supported the elderly, whether directly, through family care, or indirectly, through publicly funded services. Indeed, some commentators have noted that to the extent that we have elderly relatives, we all benefit from Social Security, Medicare, and other programs that serve senior citizens; individuals do not have to assume so great a burden for their own relatives as they did in the past.

But many analysts fear that as the percentage of elderly increases, society will become less willing or able to provide needed services. On the other hand, successful anti-aging medical therapies resulting in an extended and enhanced life span will have a profound impact on the economics of health care in many startling new ways.

For example, when anti-aging medicine is able to delay admission to nursing homes by just one month, the U.S. health-care system will see $3 billion in savings a year! The National Institute on Aging recently reported that if the onset of Alzheimer's disease could be delayed by five years, the nation would save $40 billion per year! As the following statistics show, the savings in disease-related costs of anti-aging medicine are clear. In the United States alone, eliminating the number of deaths from just six diseases would result in hundreds of billions of dollars returned to the economy.

Disease	Savings
Cancer	$46.5 trillion
Heart disease	$48.5 trillion
Stroke	$7.7 trillion
Circulatory disease	$5.8 trillion
Influenza	$3.5 trillion
AIDS	$7.6 trillion

Not only will longevity research pay off in great dividends, but also fears of the graying of America simply will not materialize, thanks to the anti-aging advances already proven to work in the lab. These advances will forever alter our very notion of age, life, disease, and death. Modern medical science has already demonstrated advances that would have been fictional material for science-fiction writers a few short decades ago.

The U.S. Center for Health Statistics reported that 47,000 people under age forty-four had heart attacks in 1993, and only 17 percent of those who died of heart disease in hospitals were under age sixty-five.

The future of anti-aging medicine promises the elimination of the disability, deformity, pain, disease, suffering and sorrow of old age. In a few decades, the traditional enfeebled, ailing elderly person will be but a grotesque memory of a barbaric past, just as we sadly recall the millions who suffered horrible deaths to the then non-treatable diseases such as tuberculosis, smallpox, whooping cough, and dysentery.

Three Leading Causes of Death in the United States
- 1899—influenza, diarrhea, and pneumonia
- 2006—heart disease, cancer, and stroke
- 2050—suicide, homicide, and aerospace accident (predicted)

Just as computer technology is accelerating so that every eighteen months the power and speed of machines doubles, making supercomputers compact and affordable enough for every college student to own, so, too, is biomedical information doubling approximately every three and a half years. For instance, who in 1942, just sixty-five years ago, would have believed it possible to implant neural tissue into the brains of patients suffering from Alzheimer's and Parkinson's disease in order to rebuild lost brain and nervous system tissue? Who would have believed it would be possible to construct artificial hearts, ears, pancreases, and kidneys?

Near-term advances in biotechnology have already demonstrated that spinal cord injuries in animals can be repaired with cell-grafting techniques, and we can expect human spinal-cord injuries to be totally repairable in the near future as well. We are regrowing damaged knee cartilage to reverse arthritis in athletes and it's working today. Therapies are currently being used to repair and rebuild immune systems in the elderly, preventing the onset of the many diseases of aging: cancer, autoimmune diseases, diabetes, and deadly infections.

Research has shown that scientists have already succeeded in producing human-equivalent life spans of 150 to 180 years in animals. Technologies will almost certainly be available to enable everyone to enjoy an added thirty to fifty, even one hundred years of a healthy, youthful life span. Thus, it is not unreasonable that by the year 2028, just twenty-one years from now, we will know sixty-four times more about aging and how to reverse it!

It isn't necessary to wait decades for the benefits of anti-aging medicine, however. It is improving the lives and health of thousands of people right now. In later chapters, you'll read about the latest developments in the new science of anti-aging medicine. You'll learn about hormone treatments, nutritional supplements, diet, and exercise programs that can help prolong the pleasures of youth. There are multitudes of seventy year olds performing, thinking, and feeling every bit as well as when they were fifty-five. If you follow the suggestions outlined in this book you, too, can expect one or more of the following benefits:

- an enhanced immune system

- improved memory and cognitive function

- remodeling of body musculature and reduction of total body fat

- enhanced sexual function

BIOTECHNOLOGICAL APPLICATIONS IN MEDICINE

EYE: Today—Scientists have created the artificial retina.

Future—In January 2002, Japanese scientists announced successfully growing artificial eyeballs and transplanting into a tadpole, connecting to the optic nerve. Future application to enable people to regain vision. [reported by Reuters, Jan. 5, 2002]

BREAST: Today—Reconstruction with saline implants.

Future—Research is underway to grow breast cells in the lab, mix them with polymer scaffolding material, and implant then to form new breast tissue.

STOMACH: Today—Feeding tubes for those with diabetic neuropathy affecting the GI system.

Future—Gastric pacemaker aids digestion by sending signals to electrodes in the stomach wall.

KIDNEY: Today—Dialysis is commonplace and transplants readily achievable.

Future—In January 2002, scientists announce constructing miniature kidneys from an embryo clone. The grown kidneys appear to function similar to genuine organs, capable of producing urine. [reported by Associated Press, Jan. 30, 2002]

PANCREAS: Today—Pancreas transplants are performed now.

Future—Transplants of pancreatic beta-cells, which produce insulin, are in development stage for treating diabetes.

HIP: Today—Replacing the ball-and-socket joint with metal substitute now routine.

HAND: Today—Mechanical prosthetic hands are now available. Success rate for reattachment of severed hands is improving.

Future—First human hand transplants (from cadaver) appear promising.

BLOOD VESSELS: Today—Mechanical means for opening arteries (angioplasty).

Future—Researchers are growing small-diameter arteries on polymer scaffolds lined with two layers of cells. Could replace diseased arteries.

SKIN: Today—Synthetic skin substitutes and sheets of material containing living skin cells are now used to treat burns and severe skin ulcers.

Future—Wide-scale applications to reduce the potential for wounds to increase mortality.

BRAIN: Today—Implants of human or animal nerve tissue into brain are being tried for Parkinson's Disease.

Future—Researchers from US National Institute of Aging state that "Stem cell research suggests methods for replacing damaged or lost brain cells in an array of neurological disorders." [Mattson MP, "Emerging neuropro-tective strategies for Alzheimer's disease: dietary restriction, telomerase activation, and stem cell therapy." Exp Gerontol. 2000 Jul; 35(4); 489-502]

EAR: Today—Electronic cochlear implants can reduce damaged inner-ear tissues.

Future—Scientists have shaped lab-grown cartilage to resemble the outer ear, with pending application in people.

HEART: Today—Human transplants are routine but limited by organ supply. Heart valves can be replaced by mechanical devices. First mechanical heart replacement, conducted in 2001, successful.

Future—Living Implants From Engineering (LIFE) consortium, created in June 1998, seeks to create a "heart in a box," a transplantable heart that could be stored at hospitals until needed. [Stover D, "Growing Hearts from Scratch," Popular Science, April 2000]

LIVER: Today—Transplants now common.

Future—Researchers have grown tissues with some liver functions, and are working on creating an entire, functional liver.

BLADDER: Today—Tissue-engineered bladders have been placed in infants with congenital defects.

Future—Cartilage to reduce incontinence is grown in the lab.

FINGER JOINT: Today—Knuckles can be replaced with metal joints.

Future—Tissue engineering can form a finger joint, implantation in patients in future.

SPINE: Today—In June 2001, researchers in Israel announced success at repairing severed spinal cords and restoring movement in paralyzed people. Into patients' spinal cords, the team injected macrophages—normally scarce in the central nervous system—which the body then used to regenerate spinal tissue. [Reported by Reuters, June 14, 2001] In the February 2002 issue of Spinal Cord, researchers announce they restored walking ability in a quadriplegic through an implanted device that stimulates the spinal cord [Reported by MSNBC, January 31, 2001]

Future—Efforts underway to transplant stem cells into spinal cord, to repair or replace damaged neurons; development of antibodies to encourage nerve regrowth; retraining spinal cord after injury, shifting tasks to undamaged nerves [Arnst C., "Rebuilding the Spinal Cord," Business Week, Dec. 11, 2000]

NERVES: Today—Nerves in the limbs can be repaired and can regenerate.

Future—Electricity-conducting polymer nerve replacements are in research. [Based on Saltus R, "The big fix," The Boston Globe Magazine, May 23, 1999]

- an increased rate of wound healing

- increased aerobic capacity

Does all of this sound too good to be true? It may, but these goals are well within your reach. The physicians and scientists of anti-aging medicine believe not only in longer lives but also in better lives. We stress that old age need not be the gateway to degenerated health and diminished vigor, but rather a time of renewed opportunity, a time of renaissance when we have the energy to make use of a lifetime of accumulated wisdom and experience.

If you're willing to make some simple lifestyle changes, to work with a doctor who can prescribe appropriate anti-aging treatments, and to commit yourself to a longer and healthier life, you too can stop the clock. Read on to find out how. Your very life depends on it!

Who will want to live to be 150? You will . . . the day after you celebrate your 149th birthday!

RULES FOR "IMMORTALITY"

To help you reach that landmark day on which you will blow out the whole 150 candles on your birthday cake, it is important to begin right now—whoever you are, wherever you are and whatever age you are—to change the way you think and the way you live your life. Anti-aging medicine is an important tool in increasing your longevity. But you, yourself, are your most important tool— you, your mind, and your body.

With this in mind, consider the following three rules for "Immortality":

1. DON'T DIE!

2. DON'T GET SICK!

3. DON'T GET OLD BIOLOGICALLY! Every day that you stay healthy and alive is another day medical science comes closer to finding the ultimate cure for aging.

While these rules may seem facetious, consider the following simple steps you can take to help ensure a longer life span:

- Drive a big car (2,800 pounds or more). The survivability in a potentially fatal accident between the largest and the smallest automobiles can differ tenfold.

- Avoid stress and depression. They are major causes for premature aging.

- Exercise at least 30 minutes daily. It is your number-one defense against the infirmities of old age.

- Limit harmful fats such as saturated fats and trans fatty acids in your diet. They are directly associated with an increased risk of both heart disease and cancer.

- Sleep seven to eight hours a night. Quality sleep is essential for rejuvenation and repair. If you're like the 20 million Americans who suffer from insomnia or other sleeping problems—get help!

- Consume little or no alcohol. It is neurotoxic.

- Don't smoke. Not only does it stain your teeth and smell bad, it also kills more Americans than all foreign wars combined. With every minute you smoke, a minute of your life is taken away.

- Try to keep your weight at, or even 5 percent below, ideal body weight (IBW). Mortality increases significantly at 20 percent or more above IBW and 10 percent or more below IBW. (To determine your IBW, see chart on page 381.)

- Maintain optimum antioxidant vitamin blood levels. Animal studies indicate a 20 percent increase in longevity with optimum nutrient supplementation.

- Early detection is the key to a cure for both heart disease and cancer—get blood tests and comprehensive anti-aging physical exams yearly.

- If age fifty-five or older, consider hormone replacement therapy, if needed, administered by a knowledgeable physician.

- Drink eight to ten 8-ounce glasses of purified or bottled water. As much as 70 percent of municipal water systems surveyed were polluted with potentially toxic amounts of flourine and chlorine. According to recent Environmental Protection Agency reports, these chemicals have been associated with an increased risk of urinary tract cancers.

- Think young. Aging is as much a state of mind as it is a state of physiology. Lie about your age (especially to yourself). Keep young-feeling friends around to remind yourself what "youth" feels and thinks like.

- Do not accept "just getting old." Fight tooth and nail to remain youthful and vigorous. At least forty anti-aging drugs now exist, and hundreds more are under development, for everything from bone loss and Alzheimer's treatments, to wrinkle reduction and gray hair. It is the whole point of this book to help you in your fight for longevity. In the pages that follow, we will offer insights into every part of your life—how you can live it longer, better, and healthier.

Before continuing on to the next chapter, take a moment and reread the three rules of "Immortality" on page 16. Then take the time to reread and reconsider the simple suggestions for increased longevity. Take some time and personalize the list. See what other ideas you can come up with yourself— ideas for living a longer and healthier life.

Take the state-of-the-art Cyber Longevity Test to see how many more years you can live: www.mylonglife.com

---

CHAPTER 2

Theories on Aging

We are forever in search of the cure for old age. Dozens of theories have been proposed, yet science has not produced a universal theory of aging. Generally, scientists believe that aging is a mechanism installed in the human body to insure the continued survival of the species. From the species' point of view, the most important time of our lives is our period of fertility, the years during which we're able to create new life. While it's socially functional for some people to live longer than that, to pass on the accumulated wisdom that might help the young survive, from nature's point of view, we are not that useful after around age forty. As a result, many bodily functions begin to decline, with ever-accelerated losses of function continuing in each succeeding decade.

Why do we age? Current theories of aging at the cellular and molecular level generally revolve around two themes: aging is programmed and aging is accidental. Programmed aging theories are based on the idea that from conception to death, human development is governed by a biological "clock." This clock sets the appropriate times for various changes to take place. The changes in vision, loss of calcium in the bones, decreasing hearing acuity, and lowered vital capacity of the lungs all are examples of programmed aging. Accidental theories of aging rely on chance—the notion that organisms get older by a series of random events. An example is DNA damage from free radicals or just the wear and tear of daily life.

ASSUMPTIONS ABOUT AGING

Before we embark on these different theories of aging, it is important to recognize the underlying assumptions that theoretic gerontology (the study of aging) uses for the basis of aging:

- *Aging Is Developmental:* As we age, we become more mature adults, growing older developmentally, not chronologically. A chronologically sixty-year-old person may have the physiological age of a forty-five-year-old person, or a 50-year-old person may have the diseases and ill health paralleling the physiological decline of an eighty-year-old person.

- *Normal Aging and Pathologic Aging Are Different:* Pathologic aging, which is the aging process that is brought on by the presence of disease, such as adult-onset diabetes or arthritis, which may later bring on cardiovascular disease or osteoporosis, is not considered "normal" aging. These conditions are due to heredity or lifestyle. However, developing cataracts is considered "normal" aging, because if you live long enough, you will develop them.

- *Longer Life Spans Are the Result of Modern Science and Technology:* The discoveries of vaccinations, insulin, antibiotics, new surgical techniques, hormone replacement therapies, and treatments for life-threatening diseases all contribute to staying younger longer.

COMMONLY HELD THEORIES OF AGING

Here are the four principal theories of aging. While none fully expresses the hows and whys for the process of aging, each accounts for some aspects of the process.

The "Wear and Tear" Theory

Dr. August Weismann, a German biologist, first introduced this theory in 1882. He believed that the body and its cells were damaged by overuse and abuse. The organs—liver, stomach, kidneys, skin, and so on—are worn down by toxins in the diet and in the environment; by the excess consumption of fat, sugar, caffeine, alcohol, and nicotine; by the ultraviolet rays of the sun; and by the many other physical and emotional stresses to which we subject our bodies. Wear and tear is not confined to our organs, however; it also takes place on the cellular level.

Of course, even if you've never touched a cigarette or had a glass of wine, if you've stayed out of the sun and have eaten only natural foods, simply using the organs in your body is ultimately going to wear them out. By abusing them, you will only wear them out more quickly. Therefore, as your body ages, your very cells feel the effect, no matter how healthy your lifestyle.

When you're young, your body's own maintenance and repair systems keep compensating for the effects of both normal and excessive wear and tear.

(That's why young people can more easily get away with a night of heavy drinking or a binge of pizza or sweets.) With age, your body loses its ability to repair damage—whether caused by diet, environmental toxins, bacteria, or viruses. Thus, many elderly people die of diseases that they could have resisted when they were younger.

This theory also holds that nutritional supplements and other treatments (many of which will be covered later in this book) can help reverse the aging process by stimulating the body's own ability to repair and maintain its organs and cells. The concept of "wear and tear" therefore may be said to differ from person to person, depending upon the lifestyle of each and the methods used to reverse the wear and tear.

The Neuroendocrine Theory

This theory, developed by Vladimir Dilman, Ph.D., elaborates on the wear and tear theory by focusing on the *neuroendocrine system,* which is a complicated network of biochemicals that governs the release of hormones and other vital bodily elements. When you're young, your hormones work together to regulate many bodily functions, including your responses to heat and cold, your experiences, and your level of sexual activity. Different organs release various hormones, all under the governance of the hypothalamus, a walnut-sized gland located within the brain.

The hypothalamus sets off various chain reactions, in which an organ releases a hormone, which in turn stimulates the release of another hormone, which in turn stimulates yet another bodily response. The hypothalamus responds to the body's hormone levels as its guide for how to regulate hormonal activity.

When you're young, your hormone levels tend to be high, accounting for, among other things, menstruation in women and high libido in both sexes. But, as you age, your body produces lower levels of hormones, which can have disastrous effects on your functioning. The growth hormones that helped you form muscle mass, human growth hormone (HGH), testosterone, and thyroid hormone, for example, will drop dramatically as you age, so much so, that, even if you as an elderly person have not gained weight, you will undoubtedly have increased your ratio of fat to muscle.

Hormones are vital for repairing and regulating your bodily functions, and when aging causes a drop in hormone production, it causes a decline in your body's ability to repair and regulate itself as well. Moreover, hormone production is highly interactive: the drop in production of any one hormone is likely to have a feedback effect on the whole mechanism, signaling other organs to release lower levels of other hormones, which will cause other body parts to release lower levels of yet other hormones.

Thus, hormone replacement therapy—a frequent component of any anti-aging treatment—helps to reset the body's hormonal clock and so can reverse or delay the effects of aging. If your hormones are being produced at youthful levels, in a very real sense the cells of your body are stimulated to be metabolically active, and thus, you stay young.

The Genetic Control Theory

This planned-obsolescence theory focuses on the genetic programming encoded within your DNA. You were born with a unique genetic code, a predetermined tendency to certain types of physical and mental functioning. And that genetic inheritance has a great deal to say about how quickly you age and how long you will live. To use a macabre analogy, it's as though each of us comes into the world as a machine that is pre-programmed to self-destruct. Each of us has a biological clock ticking away, set to go off at a particular time, give or take a few years. And when that clock goes off, it signals our bodies first to age and then to die.

However, as with all aspects of our genetic inheritance, the timing on this genetic clock is subject to enormous variation, depending on what happens to each of us as we grow up and on how we actually live (the old "nature versus nurture" debate).

Anti-aging medicine addresses this issue by augmenting the basic building blocks of DNA within each of our cells, preventing damage to and increasing repair of DNA. In this way, we believe, anti-aging treatment can help us escape our genetic destinies, at least to some extent.

The Free-Radical Theory

This exciting development in anti-aging research was first introduced by R. Gerschman in 1954, but was developed by Dr. Denham Harman of the University of Nebraska College of Medicine. "Free radical" is a term used to describe any molecule that differs from conventional molecules in that it possesses a free electron, a property that makes it react with other molecules in highly volatile and destructive ways.

In a conventional molecule, the electrical charge is balanced. Electrons come in pairs, so that their electrical energies cancel each other out. Atoms that are missing electrons combine with atoms that have extra electrons, creating a stable molecule with evenly paired electrons and a neutral electrical charge.

The free radical, on the other hand, has an extra electron, creating an extra negative charge. This unbalanced electrical energy makes the free radical tend to attach itself to other molecules, as it tries to steal a matching electron and attain electrical equilibrium. Some scientists speak of these free radicals as "promiscuous," breaking up the happy marriages of paired electrons in neighboring molecules in order to steal an electron "partner" for themselves. In doing so, they create new free radicals—and extensive bodily damage.

Of course, free-radical activity within the body is not only or even primarily negative. Without free-radical activity—that is, without biochemical electricity—we would not be able to produce energy, maintain immunity, transmit nerve impulses, synthesize hormones, or even contract our muscles. The body's electricity enables us to perform these functions, and that electricity comes from the unbalanced electron activity of free radicals.

But free radicals also attack the structure of our cell membranes, creating metabolic waste products, including substances known as *lipofuscins*. An excess of lipofuscins in the body is shown as a darkening of the skin in certain areas, so-called "age spots" that indicate an excess of metabolic waste resulting from cellular destruction. Lipofuscins in turn interfere with our cells' ability to repair and reproduce themselves. They disturb DNA and RNA synthesis, interfere with synthesis of protein (thus lowering our energy levels and preventing our bodies from building muscle mass), and destroy cellular enzymes, which are needed for vital chemical processes.

This type of free-radical damage begins at birth and continues until we die. In your youth, its effects were relatively minor since the body has extensive repair and replacement mechanisms that in healthy young people function to keep cells and organs in working order. With age, however, the accumulated effects of free-radical damage begin to take their toll. Free-radical disruption of cell metabolism is part of what ages our cells. It may also create mutant cells, leading ultimately to cancer and death.

Moreover, free radicals attack collagen and elastin, the substances that keep our skin moist, smooth, flexible, and elastic. These vital tissues fray and break under the assaults of free radicals, a process particularly noticeable in the face, where folds of skin and deep-cut wrinkles are testaments to the long-term effect of free-radical attacks.

Another way of looking at free-radical damage is to think of it as oxidation, the process of adding oxygen to a substance. Another word for oxidation, of course, is rust, and in a sense, your aging process is analogous to the rusting away of a once-intact piece of metal. Because forms of oxygen itself are free radicals, our very breathing, and our otherwise healthy aerobic exercise, generate free radicals that help promote the aging process.

Hence, substances that prevent the harmful effects of oxidation are known as antioxidants. Natural antioxidants include vitamin C, vitamin E, and beta-carotene (the substance that your body uses to produce vitamin A). Oligomeric proanthocyanidin complexes (OPCs) are a specialized type of antioxidants, of the category known as flavonoids. They occur naturally in plants and offer them defense against invasions from fungi, toxins, and environmental stress. Animals—including humans—cannot produce flavonoids, but we are able to absorb and use plant flavonoids including OPCs. OPCs' ability to fight cell-damaging free radicals means that they could be useful for the prevention of any disease where oxidative stress is involved.

OLIGOMERIC PROANTHOCYANIDIN COMPLEXES (OPCs)	
Nutrient	**Reviewed on**
Grape seed extract	page 333
Pine bark extract	page 333
Red wine extract	page 332
Bilberry	page 283

Specialists in anti-aging medicine often prescribe a host of natural and manufactured antioxidants to help combat the effects of aging.

Another substance that combats free-radical damage is known as a free-radical scavenger. Free-radical scavengers actually seek out free radicals and harmlessly bind them before they can attach themselves to other molecules and/or cause cross-linking. As we'll see in subsequent chapters, many vitamins, minerals, and other substances fight aging by acting as free-radical scavengers.

OTHER THEORIES OF AGING

While the four theories described above may be the most important to our present-day understanding of the process of aging, there are many other theories that have been put forth to give insight into the process.

Waste Accumulation Theory

In the course of their life spans, cells produce more waste than they can properly dispose of. This waste can include various toxins, which, when accumulated to a certain level, can interfere with normal cell function, ultimately killing the cell.

Evidence supporting this theory is the presence of the waste product lipofuscin. The cells most commonly found to contain lipofuscin are nerve and heart muscle cells—both critical to life. Lipofuscin is formed by a complex reaction that binds fat in the cells to proteins. This waste accumulates in the cells as small granules and increases in size as the body ages. Because lipofuscin builds up over time, it has been described as "the ashes of our dwindling metabolic fires."

Limited Number of Cell Divisions Theory

The number of cell divisions is directly affected by the accumulation of the cell's waste products. The more waste we accumulate over time, the faster cells degenerate.

Although an ordinary chicken does not live anywhere near twenty years, French surgeon Dr. Alexis Carrel was able to keep pieces of a chicken heart alive in a saline solution that contained minerals in the same proportion as chicken blood for twenty-eight years. He believed that he had achieved this by disposing of the waste products daily.

Although Carrel's theory was eventually overturned by cell biologist Dr. Leonard Hayflick, when it was found that fresh cells had inadvertently been added to the cultures, making the chicken cells seem "immortal," the experiment helped explain why cells from older people with more waste divided fewer times than cells from embryos, which divided the most often.

Hayflick Limit Theory

In 1961 Dr. Hayflick and cell biologist Dr. Moorehead, made a significant contribution to the history of cellular biology, demonstrating the senescence of cultured human cells. Hayflick theorized that the aging process was controlled by a biological clock contained within each living cell. The 1961 studies concluded that human fibroblast cells (lung, skin, muscle, and heart) have a limited life span. They divided approximately fifty times over a period of years and then suddenly stopped. Nutrition seemed to have an effect on the rate of cell division: overfed cells made up to fifty divisions in a year, while underfed cells took up to three times as long as normal cells to make the divisions. Alterations and degenerations occurred within some cells before they reached their growth limit; the most evident changes took place in the cell organelles, membranes, and genetic material. This improper functioning of cells and loss of cells in organs and tissues may be responsible for the effects of aging.

The Hayflick Limit Theory is being surpassed by the emerging Telomerase Theory of Aging (see page 30). Advancements in stem cell research, therapeutic cloning, and nanotechnology have also compromised Hayflick's theory.

Death Hormone Theory

Unlike other cells, brain cells or neurons do not replicate. You were born with roughly 12 billion of them and over a lifetime about 10 percent perish.

Dr. Donner Denckla, an endocrinologist formerly at Harvard University was convinced that the "death hormone" or DECO ("DECreasing Oxygen consumption hormone") released by the pituitary gland may contribute to the loss of neurons. When he removed the pituitary glands of rats, their immune systems revitalized, the rate of cross-linking in cells reduced, and cardiovascular function was restored to the levels of youth. Denckla speculated that as we age, the pituitary begins to release DECO, which inhibits the ability of cells to use thyroxine, a hormone produced by the thyroid that governs basal metabolism, the rate at which cells convert food to energy. The resulting changes in metabolic rate bring on and accelerate the process of aging.

Thymic-Stimulating Theory

"The thymus is the master gland of the immune system," says Dr. Alan Goldstein, chairman of the biochemistry department at George Washington University. The size of this gland reduces from 200 to 250 grams at birth to around three grams by age sixty. Scientists are investigating whether the shrinkage of the thymus contributes to the aging process by weakening the body's immune system.

Studies have shown that thymic factors are helpful in restoring the immune systems of children born without thymus glands as well as rejuvenating the poorly functioning immune systems of the elderly. Thymic hormones may also play a role in stimulating and controlling the production of neurotransmitters and brain and endocrine system hormones, which means they may be the pacemakers of aging itself as well as key regulators responsible for immunity.

Mitochondrial Theory

The free-radical theory is supported by direct experimental observations of *mitochondrial* aging. Mitochondria are the energy-producing organelles in the cells that are responsible for producing ATP, our primary source of energy. They produce cell energy by a process that leads to the formation of potentially damaging free radicals. Mitochondria are also one of the easiest targets of free-radical injury because they lack most of the defenses found in other parts of the cell. Evidence points to various kinds of accumulated DNA damage over time to be a contributing factor to disease, and new research in mitochondrial repair could play an important part in the fight against aging.

Errors and Repairs Theory

In 1963, Dr. Leslie Orgel of the Salk Institute suggested that because the "machinery for making protein in cells is so essential to life, an error in that machinery could be catastrophic." The production of proteins and the reproduction of DNA sometimes is not carried out with accuracy. The body's DNA is so vital that natural repair processes kick in when an error is made. But the system is incapable of making perfect repairs on these molecules every time, and therefore the accumulation of these flawed molecules can cause diseases and other age-related changes to occur. If DNA repair processes didn't exist, scientists estimate that enough damage would accumulate in cells in one year to make them nonfunctional.

Redundant DNA Theory

Like the errors and repairs theory, the redundant DNA theory blames errors accumulating in genes for age changes. But as these errors accumulate, this theory also blames reserve genetic sequences of identical DNA that take over until the system is worn out. Dr. Zhores Medvedev of the National Institute of Medical Research in London proposed that different species' life spans may be a function of the degree of these repeated gene sequences.

Cross-Linkage Theory

Developmental aging and cross-linking were first proposed in 1942 by Johan Bjorksten. He applied this theory to aging diseases such as sclerosis, a declining immune system and the most obvious example of cross-linking, loss of elasticity in the skin. One of the most common proteins found in the skin, tendons, ligaments, bone, and cartilage is collagen. The collagen protein can be compared to the legs of a ladder with very few rungs. Each protein is connected to its neighbors by other rungs, forming a cross-link. In young people, there are few cross-links and the ladders are free to move up and down. The collagen stays soft and pliable. With age, however, the number of cross-links increases, causing the skin to shrink and become less soft and pliable. It is thought that these cross-links begin to obstruct the passage of nutrients and waste between cells.

Cross-linking also appears to occur when older immune systems are incapable of cleaning out excess glucose, or sugar, molecules in the blood. These sugar molecules react with proteins, causing cross-links and the formation of destructive free radicals. Scientists once thought inflexibility of the body with age was due to cross-linking of tendon, bone, and muscle tissue. However, people who lead a more active lifestyle and follow a good diet seem to inhibit or delay the cross-linking process.

Autoimmune Theory

The immune system is the most important line of defense against foreign substances that enter the body. With age, the system's ability to produce necessary antibodies that fight disease declines, as does its ability to distinguish antibodies from proteins. In a sense, the immune system becomes self-destructive and reacts against itself. Examples of autoimmune diseases are lupus, scleroderma, and adult-onset diabetes (type II).

Calorie Restriction Theory

Calorie restriction, or energy restriction, is a theory proposed by respected gerontologist Dr. Roy Walford of the UCLA Medical School. After years of animal experiments and research on longevity, Walford has developed a high-nutrient, low-calorie diet, which, when followed, demonstrates that "undernutrition without malnutrition" can dramatically retard the functional if not the chronological aging process. An individual on this program would lose the necessary weight gradually until a point of metabolic efficiency was obtained for maximum health and life span. Walford stresses the importance of not only the high-low diet, but also moderate vitamin and mineral supplements coupled with regular exercise.

Gene Mutation and DNA Damage Theories

In the 1940s scientists investigated the role of mutations in aging. Mutations are changes that occur in the genes that are fundamental to the creation of life. Evidence supporting this idea came from experiments with radiation. It was observed that radiation not only increased the gene mutation rate in animals but accelerated their aging process as well. However, later studies showed the radiation-induced changes were only mimicking age-related changes. This hypothesis further diminished in validity when experiments with moderate amounts of radiation actually *increased* the life span of rats!

In April 2002, Dr. deBoer of Erasmus University in Rotterdam and colleagues announced findings that suggest damage to the body's DNA is responsible for aging. We now know that molecules called *reactive oxygen species*, by-products of normal metabolic processes, cause harm to DNA and are suspected of contributing to diseases such as cancer and heart disease.

Dr. deBoer's team identified a defect in a gene involved in DNA repair that causes lab mice to age prematurely. The gene, known as XPD, is responsible for transcribing instructions from DNA to make proteins and repair damage to DNA. Errors in this gene caused mice to age more quickly upon reaching adulthood. Mice that had double-mutations of this gene experienced greater accelerations in aging, thought to be the result of a greater sensitivity to oxidative damage to DNA.

Rate of Living Theory

German physiologist Max Rubner, who discovered the relationship between metabolic rate, body size, and longevity, first introduced this theory in 1908. It simply states that we are each born with a limited amount of energy. If we use this energy slowly, then our rate of aging is slowed. If our energy is consumed quickly, aging is hastened. Other "rate of living" theories focus on limiting factors such as the amount of oxygen breathed or the number of heartbeats spent.

Order to Disorder Theory

From the time of conception to sexual maturation, your body is undergoing a system of orderliness. You are, as Dr. Leonard Hayflick states, "directing most of your energies to fulfilling a genetically determined plan for the orderly production and arrangement of an enormous number and variety of molecules." After sexual maturation, however, these same energies start to diminish in efficiency. Disorder occurs in molecules, in turn causing other molecules to produce errors and so on. These chaotic changes in our cells, tissues, and organs is what causes aging. Disorderliness varies from individual to individual, and this may be the reason why human tissues and organs deteriorate at different rates.

Telomerase Theory of Aging

A new theory of aging that holds many promising possibilities for the field of anti-aging medicine is the *telomerase* theory of aging. This theory was born from the surge of technological breakthroughs in genetics and genetic engineering. First discovered by a group of scientists at the Geron Corporation in Menlo Park, California, telomeres are sequences of nucleic acids extending from the ends of chromosomes. Telomeres act to maintain the integrity of chromosomes. Every time your cells divide, telomeres are shortened, leading to cellular damage and cellular death associated with aging.

Scientists discovered that the key element in rebuilding your disappearing telomeres is the "immortalizing" enzyme telomerase—an enzyme found only in germ cells and cancer cells. Telomerase appears to repair and replace telomeres, manipulating the "clocking" mechanism that controls the life span of dividing cells. Future development of a telomerase inhibitor may be able to cease cancer cells from dividing and presumably convert them back into normal cells.

A4M'S TECHNODEMOGRAPHY THEORY ON AGING

A number of academicians, most notably demographers and gerontologists who are not involved in the clinical care of the aging patient, suggest that the maximum life span of humans stands—and will remain—at eighty-five years. It is A4M's position that human life expectancy is not predetermined, finite, or immutable. As documentation of this position, A4M submits a study conducted by demographers J. R. Wilmoth and L. J. Deegan of the University of California–Berkeley along with H. Lundström, and S. Horiuchi and appearing in a recent issue of *Science*. In this report, the team finds that in Sweden, the maximum age at death has risen from 100 years during the 1860s to about 108 years during the 1990s. The team cites "an intensification of efforts . . . to prevent or even cure ailments such as coronary heart disease, stroke, and cancer" has profoundly contributed to "the more rapid rise in the maximum age since 1969." Gerontologists have long been mired by calculating maximum human longevity by solely focusing on mortality rates. The Gompertz mortality model, in which maximal longevity is based on constants reflecting solely the variables of population sizes and mortality rate, and other similar linear models, completely ignore the enormous potential for technology to function as the quantum leap accelerating the extent and achievement of scientific discovery leading to practical human immortality. It is time to incorporate the variable of technological knowledge in order to shed the very small, linear perspective of the potential human life span that scientists have held steadfastly for the past 100 years.

Thus, it is the position of A4M that life expectancy projections based on past-cast models will be quickly abandoned in favor of a new forecasting projection of longevity. In an innovative model known as technodemography crafted by A4M, five near-term biotechnological interventions could bridge the timeframe for many Baby Boomers of today to capitalize on the biomedical advancements of tomorrow (see Chapter 23). By living to reap the benefits of the future's biomedical achievements, the human species will achieve a maximum life span of 150 to 200 years. This new model for human longevity is represented by The Longevity Link:

$$\lambda \propto \sum_{k=1}^{5} T_k^{\frac{\tau}{3.5}}$$

where: λ = human longevity

$T_k = \{$

   genetic engineering and stem cell research, advancements to allow scientists to alter genetic makeup to eradicate disease and permit development of a supply source for human cells, tissues, and organs for use in acute emergency care as well as treatment of chronic, debilitating disease

cloning, a technique holding tremendous promise in producing consistent organs, tissues, and proteins for biomedical use in humans

nanotechnology, enabling scientists to use tiny tools to manipulate human biology at its most basic levels

artificial organs, making replacement body parts available

nerve-impulse continuity, in which machine enhancements may help individuals with serious medical conditions that cause the brain to fail to communicate properly with the rest of the body to regain control over their trunk and limbs

$\}$ technological knowledge

and τ = year (after 2000 A.D.), where the exponent $\frac{\tau}{3.5}$ represents the doubling time of medical knowledge and technology every 3.5 years.

As advanced by A4M starting in 1995, the Technodemography Theory culminates with the achievement of practical immortality—healthy life spans of 120 years and more. This is a direct result of applications of biotechnology to medicine, within the grasp of men and women living today.

Frequent the A4M's educational website, The World Health Network, at **www.worldhealth.net**, to keep updated on the latest advancements that can help you and your customers lead productive, extended lives. At www.worldhealth.net, you are invited to sign up to receive our free Biotech E-Newsletter, an assortment of breaking longevity news you can use.

CHAPTER 3

The Ticking Clock: Top Ten Biological Processes That Decline in Aging

As we age, changes take place in our body systems. Cellular processes slow down, and our organs and tissues become less robust in performing their tasks and functions.

From head to toe, and beginning as early as the second decade of life, our body systems begin to demonstrate *senescence*—signs of old age. An understanding of these age-related declines enables us to better grasp the potential for contemporary medical discoveries and applications of biomedical technology to retard or reverse the otherwise inevitable process of senescence. In other words, we will, in this chapter, obtain an idea of just how we age if we choose to sit back and do nothing about it, if we let the process of aging engulf and, ultimately, end our lives long before necessary.

Therefore, let us take a look at ten key systems in the body and how each ages. Let us also see how the aging process of one system intertwines with that of another, as senescence descends.

1. THE ENDOCRINE SYSTEM

The endocrine system is made up of a number of glands including the adrenals, ovaries, testes, thyroid, parathyroid, and pituitary. They are known as the "ductless" glands. Each of these secretes a hormone or hormones—chemical messengers that influence the function of organs throughout your body. Too much or too little of any of these hormones will cause an imbalance that can have serious consequences to your overall system.

The health of your endocrine system is also intimately tied to your "biological age." When your endocrine system is in peak condition, you are likely to feel good, look good, and successfully defend yourself against almost all infection and chronic disease.

Lots of internal signals and external factors—called *modulators* or *dis-*

rupters—can impact or even short-circuit the endocrine communications system. Today's 24/7 lifestyle is a major culprit that undermines the endocrine system. Lack of exercise, poor quality or insufficient sleep, inadequate nutrition, prescription and over-the-counter medications, and environmental toxins all negatively impact endocrine function.

In 1990, Dr. Meites at Michigan State University observed three distinct aspects of endocrine control over body functions in aging:

- First, correlating to a decline in reproductive functions;

- Second, correlating to a reduction of growth hormone secretion;

- Third, indicating a decrease in thymic functional activity, which results in an altered relationship between endocrine and immune systems.

Dr. Meites found that an age-related decrease in production of the neurotransmitters dopamine and noradrenaline by the hypothalamus region in the brain changes the endocrine control of the three systems bulleted above.

According to Dr. Meites, the age-related decrease in functions of the hypothalamus is apparently caused by the damaging effect of free radicals and toxins, ultimately resulting in a "wearing out" of the endocrine system and organs and tissues that the system controls. In contrast, antioxidants can help to combat the accumulation of free radicals and toxins, and perhaps hold off the onset of endocrine decline.

2. THE IMMUNE SYSTEM

As the human race ages, the death and disability rates due to disease tend to increase. The reduced efficiency of the immune system is a major contributor to the pathology of old age. Cofactors such as age-related diseases and nutritional deficiencies worsen the effect of compromises in immune function.

Physicians generally agree that risk assessment and preventive measures to slow the decline of immune functions are the best approaches to improve immune functions in aging patients.

In 2000, Dr. Burns at the Medical College of Wisconsin observed from data both *in vitro* and *in vivo* on both animal and human studies that clear age-related alterations occur in the immune system. They submit that the decline in immune function leads to an accumulation of cellular and DNA mutations that may actually make the body more susceptible to developing cancerous malignancies and cell death.

The foundation of our immune systems is based on the responses of three categories of white blood cells, each of which has a specific action when the body is challenged by infection or disease:

- *Neutrophils,* a type of white blood cell that patrols the body at all times, are the first to arrive at any trouble site. Neutrophils send distress signals and block the spread of the disease agents. In 2001, Dr. Lord at Birmingham University Medical School in the United Kingdom observed that age-related changes in neutrophil responses cause decline in the immune system's ability to operate at the optimal response level.

- *Macrophages,* cells stationed at strategic points all over the body, are next on the scene. They start engulfing the invader and send out chemical messengers called *cytokines* that activate still more immune cells. Macrophages also support the function of helper T cells that arrive later in the immune response.

- White blood cells called *lymphocytes* or *T cells* and *B cells* produce and secrete antibodies. B cells focus on only one antigen, bind with the antigen, and morph into large plasma cells that produce antibodies called immunoglobulins. These immunoglobulins patrol the body like smart bombs searching for specific targets.

There are several different kinds of T cells, each with a specific duty:

- *Helper T cells* dispatch and coordinate other T cells. They also direct B cells to make antibodies. Helper T cells can live a long time. And, perhaps most important, they actually remember the invaders they've encountered. They learn which invaders are more dangerous than others. They can help the immune system to react even faster in a repeat attack.

- Some Helper T cells (TH1) deal with the immune response to bacteria, viruses, and parasites; others (TH2) focus on allergic reactions and antibody responses. Research indicates that poor diet, high stress, and exposure to environmental toxins can suppress TH1 activity. It's the nature of the system that when TH1 activity decreases, TH2 activity is increased. When this happens, TH2 cells secrete chronically high amounts of compounds that stimulate inflammation and fever. This reaction, when stimulated inappropriately or chronically, leads to inflammatory diseases such as arthritis and autoimmune conditions such as asthma, lupus, multiple sclerosis, and chronic fatigue.

- *Killer T cells,* also called *NK,* or *Natural Killer* cells, have special receptors on their surfaces that recognize certain antigens, or invaders. When a cell is infected with a virus, for example, the cell presents a fragment of the virus on its surface. The Killer T cell latches on to this fragment, recognizes it as "non-self," and injects a chemical called a *cytokine* into the cell to destroy the virus. NK cells demonstrate an ability to inject a lethal substance to cause the cell to explode.

Age-associated modifications occur in NK cells. In 2001, Dr. Mariani and researchers at University of Bologna in Italy determined that T lymphocytes and NK cells spontaneously produced detectable amounts of interleukin-8 (IL-8)—responsible for mobilizing neutrophils and lymphocytes in an immune reaction. Stimulation of T lymphocytes significantly increased IL-8 production. The team reports that the decreased production of IL-8 can be involved in the defective functional activity of NK cells in older people.

In a study of 229 subjects conducted in 1998 by Dr. McNerlan and researchers at Queen's University of Belfast in Northern Ireland, the team found a significant increase with age in the NK-cell populations. Evidence also showed that these cells remained activated for prolonged periods of time, suggestive of a role of chronic disease. The researchers suggest that the increase in NK cells is the body's attempt to compensate for age-related declines in T and B cells.

- *Suppressor T cells* are the immune system's "cease fire" switch, keeping B cells and Helper T cells under control.

Thymic Function

Immunological functions peak at around puberty and gradually decline with advancing age. This immunological decline mainly occurs in the T cell-dependent immune system and is generally associated with an increase in not only susceptibility to infections but also incidence of autoimmune diseases. Scientists have now determined that age-related changes in our T cell-dependent immune functions can be largely attributed to the shrinkage of the thymus.

The thymus gland, located in the chest, is a primary organ of the immune system. The thymus produces T lymphocytes, T cells essential for resistance to infection and protection against development of cancer and autoimmune disorders, including allergies and rheumatoid arthritis. The thymus gland releases hormones (*thymosin, thymopoietin,* and *serum thymic factor*), low levels of which are associated with depressed immunity and increased susceptibility to infection.

At puberty, our immune system reaches its zenith, allowing the highest resistance we will ever have not only to disease, but also to aging. This is also the time at which the thymus grows to its largest size.

After the teen years, the thymus begins to shrink (a process known as *involution*), until by age forty it is a shriveled shadow of its former self; by age sixty it is difficult to locate. The shrinking of the thymus coincides with a rise in the diseases associated with aging, including cancer, autoimmune diseases, and infectious diseases. At the same time, T cells, along with immune factors such as interleukin-2 (IL-2)—a substance responsible for triggering production of T- and B-lymphocytes—decline. In a sense, then, aging is a degenerative disease in and of itself.

Scientists have speculated that the immune system would return to the potency of youth if the thymus were made to grow during adulthood. In 1985, Dr. Keith Kelley, a research immunologist at the University of Illinois at Urbana-Champaign, showed that injections of cells that secrete human growth hormone (HGH) could regrow the shriveled thymus gland in old rats so that it was as large and robust as that of young rats. Kelley's work has been confirmed by Israeli scientists. They used bovine growth hormone to reverse thymus shrinking in mice, and similar results have been shown in dogs.

Dr. Hirokawa from Tokyo Metropolitan Institute of Gerontology in Japan observed in 1992 that the age-related decline of immunological function primarily occurs in the T cell-dependent immune system and is generally associated with increase in susceptibility to infections, as well as in incidence of autoimmune disease in the elderly. Dr. Hirokawa attributes the age-related change in T cell-dependent immune functions to the decline of the thymus. He found that the thymic capacity to promote quantity and quality of T-cell differentiation actually changes in the teen years. This ultimately causes an alteration of T-cell functions in aging. These researchers suggest that the restoration of immunological functions in aging may be beneficial for the prevention of disease. They also suggest that the process of thymic decline may be explained by further understanding of the relationship between the endocrine and the immune systems.

In subsequent research released in 1994, Dr. Hirokawa's group determined that it is alterations in the thymus itself that ultimately affect the number and type of T cells circulating in the lymphatic system. Promoting factors present in the thymic environment that are responsible for proliferating *thymocytes—*

the cells that become T lymphocytes—decrease with age, while inhibitory factors increase with age. Fortunately, the team also determined that various endocrine hormones can function as important factors influencing the thymic function. In fact, the shrinking of the thymus itself can be halted by manipulation of the endocrine system, sometimes resulting in rejuvenation of immune functions to a certain extent.

3. THE METABOLIC SYSTEM

It is generally accepted that aging is associated with impaired glucose handling. Although the relationship between advancing age and insulin resistance is widely known, the causes of this association are less well understood.

Age-related changes in *anthropometric characteristics* (body composition) and environmental factors (diet habits and physical activity) have been hypothesized as being among the main causes for this association. More recently, the role of plasma Insulin-like Growth Factor 1 (IGF-1), dehydroepiandrosterone sulphate (DHEA-S, a form of the adrenal hormone DHEA, most commonly used in testing as its level is less subject to variation), as well as the degree of oxidative stress have also been evaluated. As far as the anthropometric changes are concerned, a decline in lean body mass and an increase in fat mass are common findings in aged individuals.

Potential Causes of Insulin Resistance

Dr. Paolisso from the University of Naples in Italy observed that changes in lean body mass are combined with a decline in plasma DHEA-S and IGF-1 concentration and a rise in plasma TNF-alpha concentrations (tumor necrosis factor α, a marker of macrophage activity) and oxidative stress, which, as a result, may interact with the anthropometric changes—thereby triggering a worsening of insulin-mediated glucose uptake. The researchers report that age-related environmental factors—specifically, changes in diet quality and decline in the degree of physical activity—may be common causes that hasten the changes in insulin and insulin-resistance that may develop as people age.

In 1999, Dr. Paolisso released findings of a study on the predictive role that low plasma IGF-1 concentration may have on insulin-mediated glucose uptake in older persons. Fifty-eight healthy subjects, ages sixty to eighty, were studied. The researchers found that the predictive role of plasma IGF-1 on age-related decline in whole body glucose uptake was independent of age, sex, body fat, waist/hip ratio. The team determined that low plasma IGF-1 concentration predicts a decline in whole body glucose uptake. Thus, plasma IGF-1 concentration may have a modulating role on insulin action in older people. The researchers suggest that IGF-1 administration may be of benefit in insulin sensitivity in older adults.

In previous studies investigating the occurrence and the degree of insulin resistance in healthy centenarians (people 100 years of age and older), there is no basis for an age-related cause. In actuality, healthy centenarians have a preserved insulin action compared with younger individuals. Dr. Barbieri and colleagues from the University of Naples explain that, according to the remodeling theory of age, the preserved insulin action in centenarians might be the net result of the continuous adaptation of the body to the deleterious changes that occur over time. Such adaptive metabolic changes lend a positive health status in aging.

Changes in the Body's Chemical Messengers

The consequences of changes in the body's composition of lean versus fat mass may include decreased strength and physical activity, altered energy metabolism, and impaired resistance to infection.

Dr. Roubenoff from the Human Nutrition Research Center on Aging at Tufts University has suggested that the mechanism behind these age-related events may involve changes in some of the hormonal and cytokine mediators (chemical messengers) that seem to regulate body composition. Dr. Roubenoff and his researchers suggest that endocrine and immune modulators of metabolism have distinct impact during aging, especially in regard to inflammation-based diseases such as arthritis.

Higher Percentages of Body Fat

Increasing levels of total and central body fat with advancing age contribute to the development of cardiovascular and metabolic disease.

In 1995, Dr. Poehlman at the Baltimore Veterans Affairs Medical Center in Maryland examined gender-related differences and physiological predictors of the rate of increase in total and central body fat in 427 men and women. Controlling for these variables reduced the increase in fat mass from 17 to 3 percent per decade in men and from 26 to 5 percent per decade in women. Dr. Poehlman's team found that the increase in waist circumference with age was greater in women than in men, and was most strongly associated with declines in VO2 and leisure-time physical activity. Control for these variables reduced the age-related increase in waist circumference from 2 to 1 percent per decade in men and from 4 to 1 percent per decade in women. Their findings suggest that:

- Age-related increase in fat mass and waist circumference is greater in women than in men;

- Changes in physiology with age reflect a decline in physical activity-related energy expenditure—an important predictor of total and central body fat;

- Most important, the team concludes that lifestyle changes which increase the level of physical activity may be advantageous in retarding age-related increases in fat.

Leptin

Leptin is a molecule made in adipose (fat) cells. Leptin is important in the feedback regulation of energy expenditure, in food intake, and in the creation of fat.

In a study of 76 men and women in 2000, Dr. Soares at the Curtin University of Technology in Australia studied the interrelationship of circulating leptin concentrations, basal metabolic rates (BMR), and respiratory quotients in younger versus older adults. The researchers observed older subjects to have significantly higher percentages of body fat, fat mass, and waist-to-hip ratio.

However, older subjects demonstrated significantly lower fat-free mass and BMR. Additionally, absolute leptin concentrations were found to be 60 percent higher in older subjects. These results are confirmed by a study conducted by Dr. Neuhauser-Berthold at Justus-Liebig-University in Germany. Dr. Neuhauser-Berthold's team found that leptin was an accurate predictor of fat mass in aging of both sexes.

Slower Metabolism

In 1998, Dr. Piers at Monash Medical Centre in Australia found evidence of an age-related reduction in metabolic rate. As compared with young subjects, older subjects were found to demonstrate lower basal metabolic rate and lean tissue mass in the extremities, along with higher fat mass. Adjusted for differences in other measurements, BMR in older subjects was found to be 644 kiliJoules (a measurement of calories burned at rest) per day lower than in younger subjects. Additional analysis demonstrated that older subjects experienced a reduction in the quantity, as well as the quality, of metabolic activity of lean tissue mass.

4. THE CARDIOVASCULAR SYSTEM

In most healthy older individuals, the cardiovascular system is adequate to meet the body's need for both the pressure and flow of blood. The resting heart rate is unchanged, and heart size remains essentially unchanged throughout life.

Understanding the impact of aging on the cardiovascular system first requires an understanding of those effects pertaining specifically to any disease processes and lifestyle changes that are typical in aging. Once these specific disease factors are removed from the equation, a picture of the aging cardiovascular system appears.

The following are now recognized as age-related changes in the cardiovascular system:

- Stiffening of the arteries which increases *systolic blood pressure* (amount of pressure against the arterial walls), imposing a greater load on the heart;

- Decline in peripheral circulatory factors, including a decrease in muscle mass with age during exercise, a decreased ability to direct blood flow to muscles, and a decreased ability of muscle to utilize oxygen;

- Decline in aerobic exercise capacity, whether measured as total work performance or maximal oxygen consumption. In older people who maintain a high level of physical activity, however, the decline appears to be approximately half of the 10 percent per decade decrease seen in sedentary persons;

- Decline in maximal exercise heart rate is universally found as an age-related occurrence.

It is important to note that age-related changes in the cardiovascular system are highly nonuniform. Some functions undergo a definite impairment while others tend naturally to be much better preserved. And some are even enhanced. Thus, aging is by no means associated with a generalized decline in cardiovascular functions. It should instead be viewed as a complex, highly selective, and individualized process.

Dr. Bild at the National Heart, Lung, and Blood Institute studied a group of 5,200 subjects age sixty-five and older to observe for signs of *subclinical* cardiovascular disease. (Subclinical disease of any kind is that which exhibits some or all of the positive findings of a specific disease, but does not necessarily meet the minimum measurement levels considered relevant to make the diagnosis for that disease.) Their findings include:

- In women, the prevalence of cardiovascular disease and other chronic conditions increased with age, and the highest rates occurred among those eighty-five years and older;

- In men, prevalence rates increased between the two younger groups, but the oldest group had lower than expected rates for coronary heart disease, cerebrovascular disease, hypertension, and chronic lung disease;

- In contrast, there were strong age-related linear trends in most of the sub-clinical measures of blood pressure, atherosclerosis and pulmonary function, and in virtually all measures of functional status in both gender groups across the age range.

The team concludes that subclinical disease appears to increase and functional status to decline in men and women ages sixty-five and over, regardless of the presence of cardiovascular disease. This finding is important in determining appropriate cardiovascular disease prevention and management in the older population.

5. THE GASTROINTESTINAL SYSTEM

A wide array of changes occur in the function of the gastrointestinal (GI) system throughout life. With aging, there is a decline in the actual form of the intestines. Scientists have observed alterations in the structure of the intestines, and in the membrane composition of the intestine. This causes declines in the absorption of some nutrients, such as fatty acids and cholesterol.

In additional, consider the following changes common in the GI system during aging:

- Decreased ability of the intestinal walls to hold and absorb nutrients makes older people highly sensitive to minor bodily insults;

- Drugs appreciably affect taste sensation and thereby appetite;

- Malabsorption can be caused by low levels of gastric acids, possibly compounded by gastric hypochlorrhydria with small bowel bacterial overgrowth;

- Lowered gastrointestinal movement including incontinence may occur.

Age-related changes in gastrointestinal-associated mucosal immune response also occur.

In 2001, Dr. Beharka from the USDA Human Nutrition Research Center on Aging at Tufts University found that serum levels of immunoglobuin-A (IgA)—a type of antibody responsible for immune response—increased with age. Additionally, older subjects were less able to produce interleukin-2 (IL-2).

In 2001, Dr. Gill from Massey University in New Zealand published findings that recommend dietary supplementation as a method to safely and effectively counter the physiological changes of the GI system with age. The researchers suggest that doing so strengthens important immune and GI functions.

6. THE REPRODUCTIVE SYSTEM

Deterioration of reproductive function is one of the most striking alterations that occurs during aging. All sex hormone levels decline with age. In women, estrogen is steadily produced from puberty to midlife, with its levels dropping abruptly at menopause. Production of *androgens* starts to decline around age thirty, causing men to experience a slow and gradual decline of their sexual interest and performance—a condition referred to as *andropause.*

The perfect hormonal balance in each sex requires complementary levels of androgens from the opposite sex: women need a bit of testosterone, and men need a bit of estrogen. Additionally, *pregnenolone,* as a precursor hormone from which many of the sex steroids are produced, is critical to both sexes.

The pituitary gland is responsible for releasing a set of hormones that promotes the ovaries in women and testes in men to produce sex hormones. Deterioration is attributable to a complex interplay of factors. Alterations occurring within the reproductive system and the pituitary gland, located in the brain, act to disrupt the normal release of *gonadotrophins,* or hormones related to the reproductive system. Age-related impairment in growth hormone secretion—*hyposomatotropism*—is linked to a progressive defect in growth hormone releasing hormone-producing neurons in the hypothalamus of the brain.

Also implicated in aging of the reproductive system are alterations of *somatostatin*-producing neurons. Dr. Cocchi at the University of Bari in Italy suggests that compounds aimed at restoring the physiologic function of the hypothalamus may be effective restorers of the failing endocrine system in aging individuals.

Menopause

Menopause is the point in a woman's life when menstruation stops permanently, signifying the end of her ability to have children. Known as the "change of life," menopause is the last stage of a gradual biological process in which the ovaries reduce their production of female sex hormones—a process that begins about three to five years before the final menstrual period. This transitional phase is called the climacteric, or *perimenopause*. Menopause is considered complete when a woman has been without periods for one year. On average, this occurs at about age fifty. But like the beginning of menstruation in adolescence, timing varies from person to person.

More than one-third of the women in the United States today, about 36 million, have been through menopause. With a life expectancy of about eighty-one years, a fifty-year-old woman can expect to live more than one-third of her life after menopause. Scientific research is just beginning to address some of the unanswered questions about these years.

After menopause, women cease to release egg cells from the ovaries. A decrease in the production of the hormones estrogen and progesterone cause a thinning and shrinking of tissues in the female reproductive tract. Ovarian hormones also affect all other tissues, including the breasts, vagina, bones, blood vessels, gastrointestinal tract, urinary tract, and skin. Typically, the ovaries begin to decline in hormone production during the mid-thirties. When a woman is in her late forties, the process accelerates and hormones fluctuate even more, causing irregular menstrual cycles and unpredictable episodes of heavy bleeding. By her early to mid-fifties, a woman's periods finally end altogether. However, estrogen production does not completely stop. The ovaries decrease their output significantly, but still may produce a small amount. And another form of estrogen is produced in fat tissue with help from the adrenal glands. And although this form of estrogen is weaker than that produced by the ovaries, it increases with age and with the amount of fat tissue.

Osteoporosis

One of the most important health issues for middle-aged women is the threat of osteoporosis, a condition in which bones become thin, fragile, and highly prone to fracture. Numerous studies over the past ten years have linked estrogen insufficiency to this gradual, yet debilitating disease. In fact, osteoporosis is more closely related to menopause than to a woman's chronological age.

Bones are not inert. They are made up of healthy, living tissue that continuously performs two processes: breakdown and formation of new bone tissue. The two are closely linked. If breakdown exceeds formation, bone tissue is lost and bones become thin and brittle. Gradually and without discomfort, bone loss leads to a weakened skeleton incapable of supporting normal daily activities.

Each year about 500,000 American women will fracture a vertebra—one of the bony segments that make up the spine. And about 300,000 will fracture a hip. Nationwide, treatment for these fractures costs up to $10 billion per year, with hip fractures being the most expensive. Vertebral fractures lead to curvature of the spine, loss of height, and pain. A severe hip fracture is painful and recovery may involve a long period of bed rest. Between 12 and 20 percent of those who suffer a hip fracture do not survive the six months after the fracture. At least half of those who do survive require help in performing daily living activities, and 15 to 25 percent will need to enter a long-term care facility. Older patients are rarely given the chance for full rehabilitation after a fall. However, with adequate time and care provided in rehabilitation, many people can regain their independence and return to their previous activities.

In dealing with osteoporosis, researchers believe that an ounce of prevention is worth a pound of cure.

The condition of an older woman's skeleton depends on two things: the peak amount of bone attained before menopause and the rate of the bone loss thereafter. Hereditary factors are important in determining peak bone mass. For instance, studies show that black women attain a greater spinal mass and therefore have fewer osteoporotic fractures than white women.

Other factors that help increase bone mass include adequate intake of dietary calcium and vitamin D, particularly in children prior to puberty; exposure to sunlight; and physical exercise. These elements also help slow the rate of bone loss. Certain other physiological stresses can quicken bone loss, such as pregnancy, nursing, and immobility. The biggest culprit in the process of bone loss is estrogen deficiency. Bone loss quickens during perimenopause, the transitional phase when estrogen levels drop significantly.

The most effective therapy against osteoporosis available today for postmenopausal women is estrogen replacement therapy (ERT). Estrogen saves more bone tissue than even very large daily doses of calcium.

Today, many doctors prescribe hormone replacement therapy (HRT) for postmenopausal women, placing them on a combination of estrogen plus progesterone. Although the hormonal combination more closely mimics the body prior to menopause, it greatly reduces the risk of endometrial cancer associated with using estrogen alone, but it may also reduce some of the benefits of estrogen on the heart. But taking estrogen in combination with progesterone is still more favorable for the heart than not taking any hormones.

In July 1999, the prestigious International Clinical Synthesis Panel on Hormone Replacement Therapy issued its affirmation of the value of HRT for postmenopausal women. The panel found that:

- For the symptoms of menopause, HRT is "the treatment of choice"—no other treatment is as effective;

- For osteoporosis, benefits are "very well founded";

- In cardiovascular disease, the "overwhelming observational data" suggests cardioprotection;

- In dementia, "there may be long-term beneficial effect";

- For colorectal cancer, a possible 50 percent protective role.

A 1995 study conducted by Annalia Paganini-Hill, Ph.D., of the University of Southern California at Los Angeles found that elderly women between seventy-five and seventy-nine years of age were 19 percent less likely to wear dentures and 36 percent less likely to have no teeth if they were on HRT. HRT has also been found effective at preventing bone loss in the spine and hip up to a very old age. Findings from a 2001 study conducted at the University of Bochum in Germany suggest HRT may be capable of halving the incidence of vertebral and hip fractures in postmenopausal women.

Interestingly, the bone-sparing effect of ERT, as well as other aspects of age-reversal benefits such as the skin's ability to maintain its thickness and moisture, may be due to its stimulation of human growth hormone (HGH). According to a 1987 article by a team of researchers headed by Dr. Michael Thorner at the University of Virginia in Charlottesville, there is help for the aging process.

He writes, "Some investigators have hypothesized that restoration of pulsatile HGH secretion in the elderly may reverse many of these involutional (shrinking) processes of aging. Indeed, it is possible that the positive effect of estrogen on postmenopausal bone metabolism is in part mediated by activation of HGH secretion."

Heart Disease

Heart disease is the number one killer of American women and is responsible for half of all the deaths of women over age fifty.

Ironically, in past years women were rarely included in clinical heart studies, but finally physicians have realized that it is as much a woman's disease as a man's. Postmenopausal women face at least fifteen times the risk of dying of heart disease than of an estrogen-dependent cancer. In 1993, Dr. Zubialde found that women who began hormone replacement therapy at age 50 years showed benefits ranging from 0.3 years of additional life for those at low risk of developing coronary artery disease, to 2.3 years for those at high risk. In 2001, researchers at the Chinese University of Hong Kong found that women with coronary heart disease who were taking estrogen and progesterone experienced significantly fewer ischemic events during the sixteen-week study than women who were receiving a placebo.

Menopause brings changes in the level of fats in a woman's blood. These fats, called *lipids,* are used as a source of fuel for all cells. The amount of lipids per unit of blood determines a person's cholesterol count. There are two components of cholesterol: high-density lipoprotein (HDL) cholesterol, which is associated with a beneficial, cleansing effect in the bloodstream, and low-density lipoprotein (LDL) cholesterol, which encourages fat to accumulate on the walls of arteries and eventually clog them. LDL cholesterol appears to increase while HDL decreases in postmenopausal women as a direct result of estrogen deficiency. Elevated LDL and total cholesterol can lead to stroke, heart attack, and death.

Estrogen is also beneficial for women who are at great risk for stroke or hypertension because it raises the HDL cholesterol level and lowers the LDL cholesterol, decreases the risk of heart attack, and does not elevate blood pressure. A 2002 study conducted at the University of Baskent in Turkey found that estrogen also reduces homocysteine levels. Elevated levels of homocysteine, an amino acid formed when other amino acids in the blood are broken down by normal metabolic processes, are considered a major risk factor for heart disease.

Cognitive Changes

One of the most common complaints of menopause relates to its effect on the mind, causing symptoms such as mood swings, memory lapses, and difficulty concentrating. Estrogen can improve all of these.

Women who took estrogen supplements after surgical removal of their ovaries were able to learn and recall pairs of words more easily than the control group. In other studies, estrogen replacement therapy in older women improved their recall ability on a number of different tests, including proper names. This familiar memory lapse is seen even in middle-aged people and illustrates the ability of HRT to improve failing memory and cognitive function. In addition, women on ERT had less depression and a better quality of life. There is evidence that estrogen may prevent Alzheimer's disease and benefit those who are afflicted. Two studies show that women on estrogen are far less likely to develop Alzheimer's. The first, a study of a group of 143 women with Alzheimer's disease by Victor Henderson and associates, found that only 7 percent of them were on ERT, while 18 percent of the non-Alzheimer's group used estrogen postmenopausally.

The second study on estrogen and Alzheimer's disease, conducted on 9,000 women living in a retirement community in southern California, found that those on ERT had a 30 to 40 percent lowered risk of developing Alzheimer's compared with those not receiving ERT.

Henderson and his colleagues also found that women who had Alzheimer's and were receiving estrogen did better on a test for mental function than the women who had Alzheimer's and were not on estrogen. A 2001 study by researchers at the Geriatric Research, Education, and Clinical Center in Tacoma, Washington, found that estrogen significantly improved attention, and verbal and visual memory in postmenopausal women with Alzheimer's compared to patients with the disease who took only a placebo.

Dr. Howard Fillit, a geriatrician at Mount Sinai Medical Center in New York City, found that after only three weeks of daily treatment with estrogen, women with mild to moderate Alzheimer's symptoms were suddenly able to recall the day and month of the year, even though they had been previously unable to do so. The women were also more alert, ate and slept better, and were more sociable.

These studies have compelled the National Institutes of Health (NIH) to fund an unprecedented comprehensive study of the effects of hormone replacement therapy (HRT) on Alzheimer's disease. The five-year study will examine 4,500 women age seventy-five and older who belong to the Kaiser Permanente Medical Group in southern California. It includes women who are on long-term HRT, short-term HRT, and those who have never had HRT. "This will be the first large-scale study of whether HRT can prevent Alzheimer's in women genetically predisposed to the disease," says Dr. Diana Petitti, one of the lead researchers.

Patients with Parkinson's disease have a higher incidence of dementia, but it was not known whether HRT benefited women with Parkinson's as well as those with Alzheimer's. New research reveals that HRT may slow the progression of Parkinson's disease in postmenopausal women who are not taking L-dopa, a prescription drug for the disease. Postmenopausal women who have taken HRT have less severe disease and a slower progression during the two-year period of the study than a similar group of women not on HRT. The non-HRT users tend to be older when they got Parkinson's, but their disease was more severe when it occurred.

Long-Term Benefits of HRT

One of the most startling clinical studies ever conducted was a 1996 survey examining the benefits of ERT on 454 women born between the years of 1900 and 1915 who were members of the Kaiser Permanente Medical Care Program in Oakland, California. About half the group, 232 women, used ERT for a least a year, starting in 1969, while the rest, 222 age-matched women did not. This is what Dr. Bruce Ettinger and his colleagues found when they compared the estrogen users versus the nonusers:

- Overall mortality from all causes were reduced 46 percent (fifty-three deaths for estrogen-takers versus eighty-seven for nonusers);

- Coronary heart disease deaths were reduced 60 percent;

- Stroke deaths were reduced 70 percent;

- Cancer deaths were approximately the same in both groups, with the estrogen users having a slightly higher death rate from breast cancer and a slightly lower death rate from lung cancer.

The study concluded, "The overall benefit of long-term estrogen use is large and positive," noting that women who use this "relatively inexpensive drug can substantially reduce their overall risk of dying prematurely."

Ultimately, the risk of death in women from heart disease is almost 10 times greater than premature death from breast cancer. Given the significant improvements in the early detection and prevention of breast cancer, with modern detection such as mammography and full-body CAT scans, ERT should be viewed as a big net win in the life extension equation.

Andropause

In contrast to the rapid decline in ovarian function in women at menopause, at *andropause*—the male version of menopause—men experience a gradual decline in testicular function and testosterone production. At andropause, various physiological and psychological changes occur with the age-related decline in male reproductive function. Between their late forties and early seventies, men experience a gradual drop in testosterone of about 50 percent.

In fact, about 20 percent of men over age sixty have levels below normal. Stress, illness, medications, obesity, malnutrition, and psychiatric conditions may compound the reduction of testosterone production.

Many men older than age fifty have experienced *frailty syndrome,* which includes decrease of libido, easy fatigue, mood disturbance including depression, accelerated osteoporosis, and decreased muscle strength. Additionally, reduced testosterone production results in an increase in upper and central body fat, decreased muscle mass, diminished libido, and erectile dysfunction. Cognitive impairment may also occur. This clinical picture closely resembles the features of primary or secondary *hypogonadism*—the condition of abnormally low levels of testosterone.

Testosterone is the more convenient hormone for substitution therapy in classic hypogonadism as well as in age-related *hypoandrogenism.* Indeed, testosterone replacement is now considered to be highly valuable in treating andropause.

Testosterone is somewhat misunderstood. Testosterone replacement therapy (TRT) in men who are deficient in male hormones appears to be as potent in its anti-aging effect as the counterparts, estrogen and progesterone replacement, for women. It renews strength, improves balance, raises red blood cell count, increases libido and bone density, and lowers LDL cholesterol. Recent studies demonstrate a clear beneficial effect of testosterone replacement in aging men:

- Testosterone levels rise in response to aggressive behavior, rather than the other way around. Rises in testosterone levels do not automatically lead to aggression, and violent behavior cannot be attributed to testosterone alone.

- Men with higher levels of testosterone have less accumulation of fatty plaque in their coronary arteries, and have higher levels of HDL (good) cholesterol.

- Muscle mass and strength increases, while central fat decreases, in men receiving testosterone injections.

- Testosterone is important to behavioral functions including sexual arousal, emotional state, and cognition. Evidence is mounting for a link between waning testosterone levels and major depression in men.

- Men lose about 25 percent of their bone mass by age eighty-five and experience a significant number of hip fractures. Men with osteoporosis may benefit from testosterone replacement therapy to increase the bone mineral density.

- Illnesses such as diabetes, kidney failure, and AIDS can lead to testosterone deficiency.

- Testosterone supplementation reverses the damage to skeletal and soft tissues caused by long-term use of the glucocorticosteroid class of asthma medications.

Muscle Mass

Weekly injections of 500 mg of testosterone added an average of more than one pound of lean body mass a week to male weight lifters who were pumping iron compared with fellow weight lifters who received placebo injections, according to an article in *The New England Journal of Medicine*. Testosterone supplementation increased strength and power-lifting performance. It also bulged the triceps and quadriceps of a second group of men who received testosterone but did not exercise.

Heart Disease

Until recently, high testosterone levels were assumed to be the reason why men develop heart disease at a younger age than do women. A recent study at Columbia University College of Physicians and Surgeons indicates that it is far from the whole story. The male sex hormone may actually help protect the heart. When the researchers looked at fifty-five men undergoing x-ray exams of their coronary arteries, they found that the men with higher levels of testosterone had higher levels of protective HDL cholesterol, while those with low testosterone had higher degrees of heart disease as shown by their coronary clogging. Testosterone supplementation may also lower the bad LDL cholesterol and total cholesterol. Low testosterone is also correlated with hypertension, obesity, and increased waist-to-hip ratio—all heart attack risk factors.

Osteoporosis

Bone loss and osteoporosis is not only a female problem. Men after age sixty have a dramatic rise in hip fractures, with the rate doubling every decade. Hypogonadal males (those producing less than adequate amounts of testosterone) are six times more likely to break a hip during a fall than are those with normal testosterone levels. According to studies of TRT in both young hypogonadal men and older men with low testosterone levels, TRT increased bone density, bone formation, and bone minerals.

Autoimmune Disease

Testosterone benefits age-related autoimmune disease. Giving male hormones to men with autoimmune conditions, such as rheumatoid arthritis or systemic lupus erythematosus, improved their condition. Testosterone, like estrogen, also heightens mood and sense of well-being and increases some mental functions, particularly visual-spatial ability.

Long-term Benefits of TRT

The major benefits of testosterone replacement therapy for men are:

- promotes libido and aggressiveness;
- stimulates the growth and repair of muscles and the heart and immune system;
- helps build muscle, skin, and bone;
- stimulates sperm production;
- nourishes the male urinary and reproductive system;
- regulates prostaglandin production, which may keep prostate growth under control.

Two side effects to watch out for with TRT are a rise in prostate-specific antigen (PSA) levels and a rise in *hematocrit*—a measure of blood volume.

7. THE NERVOUS SYSTEM

Aging exerts a profound influence on the *peripheral nervous system* (PNS). Scientists have documented a loss, along with abnormalities of functional features, in myelinated (coated) and unmyelinated (noncoated) nerve fibers in older subjects. The deterioration of the protective myelin sheaths during aging may be due to a decrease in the expression of the major myelin proteins.

In 2000, Dr. Verdu from the Universitat Autonoma de Barcelona in Spain observed that aging also affects functional and electrophysiologic properties of the PNS, including a decline in nerve conduction speed, muscle strength, sensory discrimination, autonomic responses, and blood flow within the nerves themselves.

The age-related decline in nerve regeneration after injury may be attributed to changes in responses of both nervous and immune cells. In fact, as we age, the interaction between nerve cells takes longer, as levels of transmission-producing factors decline. Regeneration of nerve fibers slows, and the density of regenerating fibers decreases with age.

Age-related biological changes in neurons and skeletal muscle commonly affect neuromuscular function and strongly influence the expression of neuromuscular disease. Dr. Flanigan at the University of Utah observed that, with age, entire motor units of nerve cells die off, compromising the skeletal muscle in which these units are contained. Dr. Flanigan's team also reports that other age-related neurological decline includes loss of sensory neurons (see "The Sensory System" on page 56), along with mutations of mitochondrial DNA in muscle. They report that decline for most of these begins in early life and proceeds steadily as we age.

In 2000, Dr. Chan at the University of Alberta in Canada reported on a study of the relative contributions from the muscle and the central nervous system to muscle fatigue resistance in aging. He found that greater fatigue resistance was accounted for by increased fatigue resistance at the muscle level as well as in the central nervous system. This demonstrates the interaction between the nervous and muscular systems that persists throughout the aging process.

Numerous normal age-related changes occur in the nervous system of older individuals. Dr. Biedert from Psychiatrisches Landeskrankenhaus Wiesloch in Germany observed that:

- Changes in the cranial nerve examination correlate to decline in sensory functions, especially of vision and hearing, and to a restriction in the range of eye movements, especially vertically;

- Progressive decrease in the bulk and strength of muscles and in the speed and coordination of movements;

- Posture and gait show conspicuous changes, partially correlating with diminished sensation in the legs and/or with a change in gait;

- Reflexes are depressed due to degeneration of sensory nerves.

8. BRAIN FUNCTION

Perhaps the most feared aspect of the aging process has nothing to do with weight gain and loss of muscle tone or natural immunity to disease, but, instead, has to do with proper brain function. Who among us does not fear loss of mental acuity, memory, or, at the very worst, dementia?

Cognitive Ability

In analysis of data from the Italian Longitudinal Study on Aging, in 2000 Dr. Di Carlo and colleagues found that cognitive impairment without dementia increases with age, and is more prevalent in women.

Similarly, in the same year, Dr. Capurso and researchers at the University of Bari in Italy observed that age-related decline of cognitive functions causes a mild deterioration in memory performance, executive functions, and speed of cognitive processing.

This aging-associated cognitive decline may be preventable, suggests Dr. Capurso. Avoidance of cardiovascular and other chronic diseases, attaining a high-level education, and maintenance of vision and hearing have been identified as protective factors.

To the contrary, hypertension, effects of altered metabolism of steroid hormones, smoking, low-complexity occupation, crowded living conditions, and low level of physical activity have been identified as risk factors. Dr. Capurso's team suggests that dietary antioxidants, specific nutrients, estrogens, and anti-inflammatory drugs may act synergistically with other protective factors, opening new therapeutic interventions for cognitive decline.

Interestingly, some relatively common diseases of the elderly may aggravate the age-related decline in cognitive ability. In 1998, Dr. van Boxtel at Maastricht University in the Netherlands found that insulin-dependent and non-insulin-dependent diabetes negatively affected all cognitive measures.

Additionally, a specific association was found between chronic bronchitis and a decline in performance, speed, and memory. Similarly, earlier work by Dr. Lal and team at the Texas College of Osteopathic Medicine found that autoimmune disease is directly correlated to age-associated cognitive dysfunction. In Lal's study with accelerated autoimmunity, mice were found to show accelerated age-related declines in learning capacity. Dr. Lal suggests that the immune system could be an important target for the development of intervention strategies aimed at extending the intellectually competent period of life.

Memory

The age-related decline in growth hormone (GH) is one of the most robust endocrine markers of biological aging and has been hypothesized to contribute to the physiological deficits observed in aged animals.

Dr. Thornton at Wake Forest University in North Carolina studied the impact of GH decline on brain aging. His team administered growth hormone-releasing hormone (GHRH) to animals for twenty-one months to study memory. Results indicated that spatial memory decreased with age and that chronic GHRH prevented this age-related decrement. Additionally, GHRH attenuated the age-related decline in plasma concentrations of insulin-like growth factor 1 (IGF-1). The researchers suggest that GH and IGF-1 have important effects on brain function. Specifically, the decline in GH and IGF-1, with age, contributes to impairments in reference memory. Most important, the study shows that these changes can be reversed by the administration of GHRH.

Vision

Dr. Fahle and researchers at the University Eye Clinic in Germany studied visual memory and learning. They found that older subjects were less able to reproduce more complex geometrical material that exceeded short-term memory capacities than young subjects. Visual memory functions showed a significant age-associated decline during adulthood. However, they found that short-term retention of visual stimuli remained comparable in the different age groups.

9. THE MUSCULAR SYSTEM

Muscle strength is a critical component of the ability to walk and to avoid falls and fractures. Reduced muscle strength as we age is a major cause for an increased prevalence of disability.

Advancing adult age is associated with profound changes in body composition, the principal component of which is a decrease in skeletal muscle mass. This age-related loss in skeletal muscle is referred to as *sarcopenia*. Age-related reduction in muscle is a direct cause of the age-related decrease in muscle strength.

Dr. Evans and researchers from Pennsylvania State University report that muscle mass—not function—appears to be the major determinant of the age- and sex-related differences in strength. Additionally, they observe that this relationship is independent of muscle location and function.

Further, daily energy expenditure declines progressively throughout adult life. In sedentary individuals, the main determinant of energy expenditure is fat-free mass, which declines by about 15 percent between the third and eighth decade of life, contributing to a lower basal metabolic rate in the elderly. Dr. Evans reports the preservation of muscle mass and prevention of sarcopenia can help prevent the decrease in metabolic rate. He also suggests that age-related decline in skeletal muscle may contribute to such age-associated changes as reduction in bone density, insulin sensitivity, and aerobic capacity.

Dr. Proctor from the Mayo Clinic in Minnesota reports that, along with the aging process, there also occurs a decline in the synthesis rate of certain proteins that make up muscle. The declining ability of the body to remodel these important muscle proteins may, therefore, play a role in the development of muscle wasting, metabolic abnormalities, and impaired physical functioning seen in old age. Reduction in muscle protein production results with decrements in muscle strength and aerobic exercise tolerance. Dr. Proctor's team found that these changes are related to the decline in insulin-like growth factor 1 (IGF-1), testosterone, and dehydroepiandrosterone sulfate (DHEA-S).

10. THE SENSORY SYSTEM

The aging process typically is associated with decline in function for the various senses. All aspects of sensory function—touch, taste, smell, sight, and hearing—diminish with age, resulting in modest sensory changes in older people. Sensory decline can lead to adverse changes in quality of life.

Declines in sensory function often reflect the combined effect of age-related changes in both the sensory organ and the central nervous system processing of sensory information. Combinations of defects in several sensory modalities are often found in older individuals.

With regard to touch, Dr. Shimokata at Hiroshima University in Japan studied age-related changes in two-point discrimination—a test administered with an instrument making light skin contact on the palm of the hand.

The team found an age-related decline in the ability to discriminate two points with no significant differences in ability between men and women. The minimal distance of discrimination on the hand increased almost linearly between ten and sixty years of age. The results of the two-point discrimination test of the skin were independent of those of visual accommodation tests and hearing loss of high-frequency sound.

With regard to the senses of taste and smell, The National Geographic Society in 1987 found that 1 percent of their 1.2 million respondents could not smell three or more of six odors using a "scratch and sniff" test. Age was an important factor, with a decline beginning in the second decade of life. No comparable data have been available for taste, although it has been suggested that the sense of taste remains more robust than smell with age.

In 1993, the National Institute on Deafness and Other Communication Disorders (NIDCD), a branch of the National Institutes of Health (NIH), began collaborating with the National Center for Health Statistics (NCHS) in 1993 to acquire information on the prevalence of smell/taste problems. They administered a survey to 42,000 randomly selected households (representing about 80,000 adults over eighteen years of age) in 1994. Adjusted national estimates derived from this survey showed a prevalence of 2.7 million (1.4 percent) American adults with a smell problem. Also, 1.1 million (0.6 percent) adults reported a taste problem. When smell or taste problems were combined, 3.2 million (1.65 percent) adults indicated a chronic chemosensory problem. The prevalence rates increased exponentially with age. Almost 40 percent with a chemosensory problem (1.5 million) were sixty-five years of age or older.

In a multivariate analysis, the individual's overall health status, other sensory impairments, functional limitations (including difficulty standing or bending), depression, phobia, and several other health-related characteristics were associated with an increase in the rate of chemosensory disorders.

Dr. Murphy at San Diego State University in California found an underlying central nervous system activity to be responsible for age-related changes in olfactory (smell) functions. The olfactory event-related potential (OERP) shows reduced amplitude and longer latency in elderly subjects, with these findings most pronounced in men. They reported that the significantly longer latency begins in middle age. The team's study demonstrates that the aged brain shows smaller responses to odors, is less able to focus attention-directed resources, and slows in its olfactory cognitive processing.

Dr. Chauhan at University of Alberta in Canada reports that changes in the taste system with age may be related to nutrient intake, which in turn can be influenced by taste. Vitamins A, thiamin, B_6, B_{12}, folic acid, zinc, and copper are thought to influence taste function. Moreover, adequate intake of these nutrients is of concern in the aged.

Visual aging is generally associated with a decline in spatial vision for stationary stimuli, especially those of high spatial frequency. Dr. Kline at the University of Notre Dame in Canada observed that some, but probably not all, of this loss can be attributed to age-related changes in the ocular media responsible for attenuating and scattering incident light. He also suggests that a loss in the temporal resolving capacity of the aging visual system contributes to loss of spatial vision.

Additionally, the degeneration of the eye's rods and cones—responsible for acquisition of visual signals—contributes to age-related vision decline. A decrease in the number of rods by 30 percent takes place over the course of adulthood, while the number of cones is stable. The vulnerability of rods corresponds to a decrease in visual sensitivity. Dr. Curcio at the University of Alabama at Birmingham suggests that deficiency of function in the retina due to aging is partly to blame.

THREE KEY WAYS TO SLOW THE TICKING CLOCK

With age, scientists have observed a variety of declining performance in the body's ten leading body systems. These changes, although they may have, until now, been considered "natural," no longer need to be considered inevitable.

In the chapters ahead, we will turn our attention to how three modes of treatment—nutrition, lifestyle, and hormone therapy—may both expand the number of years that comprise the human life span, while, at the same time, enhance the quality of that human life.

SECTION TWO

Longevity Through Hormone Therapy

Die, my dear doctor?
That is the last thing I shall do.

—LORD PALMERSTON (1784–1865)

IMPORTANT—PLEASE READ

The content in this book is for educational purposes only, and is not intended to prevent, diagnose, treat, or cure disease or illness. While potentially therapeutic nutraceuticals (dietary supplements such as vitamins, minerals, herbal products, hormone supplementation, and similar preparations) and interventions (processes such as lifestyle changes, dietary modifications, bodywork, prescription medications, and others) are mentioned in the course of this book, you are urged to seek the advice of a medical professional to make the appropriate selection for your particular medical situation.

With nutraceuticals, dosing is highly variable. Proper dosing is based on parameters including sex, age, whether you are well or ill, and whether your illness is chronic or acute. Additionally, efficiency of absorption of a particular type of product and the quality of its individual ingredients are two major considerations for choosing appropriate specific agents for your medical situation.

Just because a product is natural doesn't mean it's safe for you. A small portion of the general population may react adversely to components in nutraceuticals, especially herbal products. Make your physician aware of any and all "natural" interventions you use regularly, and seek medical consultation before starting any others.

Neither the publisher nor the authors advocate the use of any particular health-care protocol, but believe that the information in this book should be available to the public. The publisher and authors are not responsible for any adverse effects or consequences resulting from the use of any of the suggestions, preparations, or procedures discussed in this book. Should the reader have any questions concerning the appropriateness of any procedure or preparation mentioned, the publisher and authors strongly suggest consulting a professional health-care advisor.

Always consult your physician prior to beginning any new healthcare intervention, whether it be nutritional, fitness, medication, hormonal, herbal, or otherwise. Do not change the dosing or cease the intervention without discussing with your physician first.

CHAPTER 4

The "Fountain of Youth": Human Growth Hormone

A sixty-year-old man becomes Mr. Physical Fitness USA.

*A fifty-year-old college instructor
regains the face and figure of her modeling days.*

*A senior citizen recovers his interest in sex—
and reports that his penis size has increased by 20 percent.*

These are only some of the reports of the aging people who claim to have been helped by supplemental doses of human growth hormone (HGH). HGH is a hormone that is naturally present in the human body when we're young, but tends to disappear as we age. People who have taken supplemental HGH have found it to produce striking improvements in their health, energy levels, and sense of well-being. The list of benefits seems to grow with each new study.

MASTER HORMONE OF YOUTH

Most people think of HGH as the miraculous treatment for children doomed to dwarfism, which over the past thirty years has saved tens of thousands from this fate. The next great benefit of HGH therapy appears to be in the aging population. People with age-related deficiency of HGH become overweight, flabby, frail, and lethargic; lose interest in sex; have trouble sleeping, concentrating, and remembering things; tire easily; and in general, lose their zest for life. With HGH, all these so-called signs of aging can be reversed.

Indeed, nearly 20,000 clinical studies conducted around the world document the broad benefits of pharmacological HGH therapy. These studies suggest a wide range of effects when HGH is replaced:

- reduced body fat

- increased muscle mass

- higher energy levels

- enhanced sexual performance

- regrowth of vital organs

- restoration of youthful immune function

- stronger bones

- lower cholesterol and blood pressure

- faster wound healing

- smoother, firmer skin

- regrowth of hair

- sharper vision

- elevated mood

- improved cognition

HOW HUMAN GROWTH HORMONE IS MADE

Hormones are chemical messengers that are made in one part of the body and tell other parts of the body what to do. Once a hormone reaches its destination, it binds to a special docking place on the cell called a *receptor,* where it stimulates a specific metabolic activity. Hormones are involved in every aspect of human function from sex and reproduction, growth and development, to metabolism and mood. A well-known example of a hormone is *insulin.* Insulin is produced by endocrine cells in the pancreas in response to elevated levels of glucose in the blood. This hormone then helps regulate the speed at which cells absorb sugar from the bloodstream.

HGH is made by the pituitary gland, which is located in the center of the brain. Pituitary cells (called *somatotropes*) make HGH, which is also known as *somatotropin*—from the Greek, meaning "turning towards the body." Fifty percent of the cells of the pituitary are somatotropes, making HGH the most abundant hormone produced by the pituitary gland.

Researchers have long noticed that peak HGH production coincides with the rapid growth phase of adolescence, hence the hormone's name. Most HGH secretion occurs in brief bursts, or pulses, which take place during the early hours of the deepest sleep. Indeed, the old adage that "you grow during your sleep" appears to have a basis in fact.

HGH remains active in the bloodstream for only a few minutes, but that is long enough to stimulate its uptake to the liver where it is converted into growth factors. The most important of these is insulin-like growth factor 1 (IGF-1), also known as somatomedin C. IGF-1 is directly responsible for many of the positive benefits of HGH. Most clinicians prefer to test the level of HGH indirectly by measuring the level of IGF-1, since the level of HGH can vary widely throughout a twenty-four-hour period.

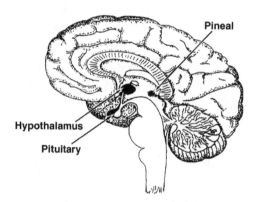

FIGURE 4.1. The most abundant neurohormone produced by the brain is HGH, which is secreted by the anterior pituitary gland. The pineal gland is the site for production of the hormone melatonin.

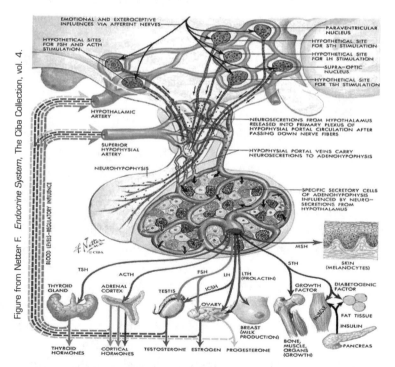

FIGURE 4.2. The complex cycle of HGH. HGH is converted by the liver into IGF-1. It can then be utilized by muscle or proceed by a feedback loop to become somatostatin. Or HGH can also directly stimulate bone building.

Synthetic Production of HGH

HGH is an FDA-approved drug. In August 1996, the FDA approved HGH for use in adult patients. Before this, it was authorized only for use to promote growth in HGH-deficient children. The new indication is somatotropin (growth hormone) deficiency syndrome (SDS), resulting from pituitary disease, hypothalamic disease, surgery, radiation therapy, or injury.

In effect, the FDA approval covers the use of HGH for anti-aging purposes since low levels of HGH or IGF-1 indicate a failure of the pituitary to release adequate amounts of this vital substance. In addition, the signs of SDS, such as decreased physical mobility, lower energy, and higher risk of cardiovascular disease, are exactly the same as those seen in aging adults with low HGH levels. The FDA approval for HGH in adults means that any physician may now prescribe it to their HGH-deficient aging patients without fear of practicing outside of conventional orthodox mainstream medicine.

Today, HGH is made in the laboratory by genetic engineering methods, generating an identical protein to the one made naturally in the human body. For this reason, allergic reactions to the drug are rare, and it is extremely safe for human use. The injections are similar to that of insulin—very small needles deliver HGH *subcutaneously* (under the skin). Most people find it easy to do and even less painful than a pinprick. While different doctors use different dose regimens, the usual recommendation is between 2 and 8 IUs per week (1 milligram equals 3 IUs, or international units).

Many specialists in anti-aging endocrinology are now dividing daily doses into two per day, one in the morning and one at night, to more closely approximate the way HGH is released in the body. The idea is to raise the levels of IGF-1 (IGF-1, a byproduct of HGH, is the substance often analyzed to determine correct dosage of HGH supplementation) to about where it was at age thirty to forty, which for most people is in the high 200s to low 300s.

In June 2000, Genetech, Inc. and Alkermes, Inc. announced availability of the first long-acting dosage form of recombinant human growth hormone. It began shipment to the pediatric endocrine community in the United States after receiving FDA approval on December 23, 1999. The long-acting form of HGH is produced by embedding growth hormone in biocompatible, biodegradable microspheres of polyactive co-glycolide (PLG) microspheres, which allow the HGH to be manufactured in a biologically active form. Following subcutaneous injection, bioactive growth hormone is released from the microspheres into the subcutaneous environment initially by diffusion, followed by both polymer degradation and diffusion. This form of HGH increases patient con-

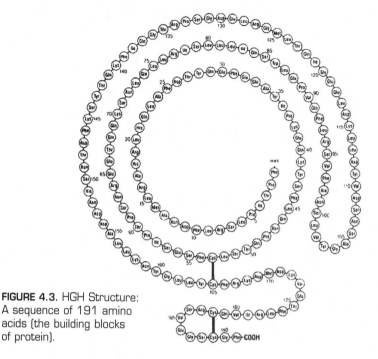

FIGURE 4.3. HGH Structure: A sequence of 191 amino acids (the building blocks of protein).

venience as well as compliance by decreasing the number of injections required for growth hormone therapy. Genetech, Inc. reports that it is pursuing FDA approval for use of this product in the treatment of growth hormone deficiency in adults.

HOW HGH DECLINE MIMICS AGING

On July 5, 1990, Daniel Rudman, M.D., a pioneer researcher in the use of HGH, and his colleagues at the Medical College of Wisconsin made medical history with an article in the prestigious *New England Journal of Medicine*. It was the first clinical trial of elderly men on HGH. They compared the effects of six months' of HGH injections on twelve men, ages sixty-one to eighty-one, with an age-matched control group. The result made headlines all over the world. Those taking the hormone injections gained an average of 8.8 percent in lean body mass and lost 14 percent in fat, without diets or exercise. Their skin became thicker and firmer and the lumbar bones of the spine increased.

In other words, HGH had virtually turned their flabby, frail, fat-bulging bodies into their sleeker, stronger, younger selves. In language rarely used in conservative medical journals, the researchers wrote: "The effects of six months of human growth hormone on lean body mass and adipose-tissue mass were equivalent in magnitude to the changes incurred during 10 to 20 years of aging."

HGH declines with age in every animal species that has been evaluated to date. In humans, the amount of HGH after ages twenty-one to thirty-one falls about 14 percent per decade, so that the total twenty-four-hour HGH production rate is reduced in half by age sixty. In numerical values, on a daily basis we produce about 500 mcg (micrograms) at age twenty, 200 mcg at age forty, and 25 mcg at age eighty. The fall in IGF-1 with an increase in age mirrors that of HGH.

Dr. Rudman considered plasma IGF-1 levels under 350 evidence of a deficiency. Between the ages of twenty and forty years, fewer than 5 percent of healthy men have IGF-1 levels lower than 350. But after age sixty, 30 percent of apparently healthy men have this low amount. And after age sixty-five, about half the population is partially or wholly deficient in HGH.

Why does HGH decline with age? The answer to this question still eludes scientists and physicians. Studies have shown that the aging pituitary somatotrope cell is still able to release as much HGH as the young cell if it is adequately stimulated. This implies that the fault must lie somewhere in the factors that regulate hormone release. Some researchers believe that the problem lies with somatostatin, the natural inhibitor of HGH. It has been found to increase with age and may act to block the secretion of HGH. When researchers knocked out the action of somatostatin in old rats, they had HGH

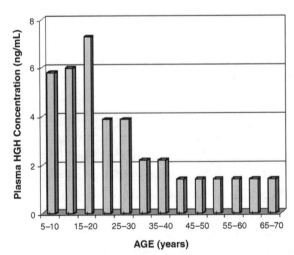

FIGURE 4.4. A study involving 173 subjects demonstrated a highly significant decline in plasma growth hormone concentrations after the second decade of life. After age sixty-five, deficiency is common. *(Adapted from Sadik et al., 1985)*

pulses that were as large as those of young rats. Other researchers believe that the precursor hormone, growth hormone releasing hormone (GHRH), which stimulates the release of HGH, becomes less sensitive to feedback signals.

It may be also be possible that both these problems occur as we age. The latest thinking is that not only does the amount of HGH available to the tissues decline with age, but also our tissues become more resistant to the action of the HGH that is there. In this view, aging can be seen as a disease of HGH resistance in the same way that adult-onset diabetes (type II) is not caused by the failure of the pancreas to produce adequate insulin; rather, it is a disease of insulin resistance.

The most recent research shows that despite what aging does to cause the decline of HGH, it is not irreparable and it is not permanent. William Sonntag, professor of physiology at Bowman Gray School of Medicine in Winston-Salem, North Carolina, and his colleagues conducted an experiment that clearly shows the decline in HGH secretion with age is reversible. Like old rats, older people experience a decline in the bursts of HGH that are secreted. But when Sonntag and his colleagues restricted the caloric intake of old rats (age twenty-six months), HGH secretion was restored after two months.

The take-home message is that the decline of HGH with age can be reversed. Even if the activity of growth hormone releasing hormone (GHRH) declines, somatostatin increases, or the receptors become less responsive to the effect of HGH. The administration of either HGH or GHRH can produce a correction of the decline.

Affects Psychological and Physical Well-Being

People who produce little or no HGH as a result of pituitary tumors, disease, or removal of the pituitary gland often seem like doddering old people. In studies, such patients show a consistent pattern of mental and physical characteristics associated with aging. The psychological and emotional symptoms include a reduced sense of well-being; low energy, vitality, and capacity for work; and emotional liability, including mood swings, anxiety, depression, and increased social isolation. Important physical signs are increased body fat, especially around the waist (apple-shape rather than pear-shape), decreased muscle mass, and thin, wrinkled, or prematurely aged skin.

As Silvio Inzucchi of Yale University wrote in the January 15, 1997 issue of Hospital Practice, "Growth hormone deficiency is now formally recognized as a specific clinical syndrome, typified by decreased muscle mass, increased body fat (predominantly at intra-abdominal sites), decreased exercise capacity, osteopenia (a loss of bone mass), abnormal lipid profiles, and diminished feelings of well-being. The critical reader will recognize that most, if not all, of these signs and symptoms are common in an aging patient population."

Shortens Life Span

Bengt-Ake Bengtsson, M.D., and his colleagues at Salgrenska Hospital in Goteburg, Sweden, studied 333 patients who had been diagnosed with pituitary insufficiency in a thirty-year period between 1956 and 1987. All these patients had been treated with pituitary hormone replacement, including cortisone, thyroid hormones, and sex hormones. The one hormone that was not replaced was HGH. The HGH-deficient patients died at twice the expected rate—107 deaths compared with 57 in the overall population matched for age and sex. The primary cause of death was cardiovascular disease, which showed an almost twofold increase with 60 deaths versus 31 in the general population.

Improves Quality of Life

Three pioneering studies in Sweden, Denmark, and England found that four to six months of HGH replacement in adults who had low levels due to pituitary insufficiency experienced beneficial effects on body composition, cardiac function, exercise capacity, renal function, and quality of life. Bengtsson also showed that after twelve to eighteen months of HGH therapy, bone-mineral density increased.

Some of the most striking effects were in the area broadly defined as quality of life. Before treatment, the scores of these patients on the Nottingham Health Profile, a questionnaire, indicated that many of them were struggling with problems of low self-esteem, anxiety, and depression. Bengtsson characterized some of these patients as "Zombies, who moved in slow motion." But within a short time on HGH therapy, the difference was like night and day.

"We called it the Lazarus effect," he says. "We woke them up. With some patients it was like giving them a kick in the butt. Their lives changed within a few weeks." The treatment went on to change the lives of all that participated in the program, according to Dr. Lena Wiren, a psychologist who evaluated the patients. "Nobody wants to stop treatment," she says. "Sometimes it is not even the patient who notices the difference it is making. Rather it is their wives or children or friends at work." In Bengtsson's opinion, the effects of six months of HGH therapy on lean body mass and fatty tissue was equivalent to reversing the aging process ten to twenty years.

In 1987, Douglas Crist and colleagues at the University of New Mexico

School of Medicine worked with eight healthy, athletic, young people—five men and three women, all between ages twenty-two and twenty-three. After six weeks of HGH injections three times per week, these young adults, already in good shape, had gained an average of close to three pounds of muscle while losing an average of 1.5 percent of body fat. Their overall ratio of muscle to fat (a key sign of being well conditioned) improved by an average of close to 25 percent.

Even before Crist, Dr. Robert Kerr had been administering HGH to healthy adult athletes. Kerr, a family physician in San Gabriel, California, had prescribed HGH for some 8,000 athletes in the course of his practice.

Kerr said his patients took HGH for only three to six weeks. In that short period, bodybuilders claimed their results lasted up to twelve months. According to Dr. Kerr, some athletes claimed to have gained up to forty pounds in six weeks while reducing their body fat. Others claimed to have gained appreciably in height. Of his first 150 patients to take HGH, ages twenty-nine to fifty-two, one in six gained from three-quarters to one inch of height. Subsequent patients in their twenties claimed to have gained even more. Kerr reported that many patients found relief from chronic lower back pain with this increased height. Although they did not always retain the additional inches, most did retain freedom from chronic back pain, said Kerr.

Dr. Julian Whitaker of Newport Beach, California, has been prescribing HGH to his elderly patients, and has taken it himself. He states, "In the 20 years I have practiced nutritional and rejuvenative medicine, I have not seen anything that even comes close to the restorative power of HGH supplementation." In Whitaker's opinion, HGH is most effective in combating the effects of chronic diseases that involve muscle wasting: stroke, chronic obstructive pulmonary disease, and AIDS. He thinks it can also be useful in treating severe burns and in helping patients recover from surgery—both instances in which the skin and other organs must be regenerated and restored.

HOW HGH FIGHTS AGING

HGH therapy may prevent or reverse many of the most common diseases and conditions of aging. In fact, it appears that a program of hormone replacement therapy (HRT), including HGH stimulation, may provide one of the most effective means of maintaining health and vigor into one's eighties, nineties, and beyond.

HGH rejuvenates the immune system. The thymus gland, located in the chest, is a primary organ of the immune system. It matures the T-cell lymphocytes, the same cells that when dangerously low make AIDS patients vulnerable to the diseases that finally kill them.

At puberty, the immune system reaches its zenith, allowing the highest resistance to age-related changes that we will ever have. Then the thymus begins to shrink. By age forty, it is a shriveled shadow of its former self, and by age sixty, it is difficult to find. The shrinking of the thymus coincides with a rise in the diseases associated with aging, including cancer, autoimmune diseases, and infectious diseases.

At the same time, there is also a decline in the T cells as well as in immune factors such as interleukin 2 (IL-2). In a sense, aging is like a slow form of AIDS. What would happen if the thymus could be made to grow again? Would our immune resistance return to that of a twelve year old?

In 1985, Dr. Keith Kelley, a research immunologist at the University of Illinois at Urbana-Champaign, showed that injections of cells that secrete HGH could cause the shriveled thymus gland in old rats to regrow so that it was as large and robust as that of young rats. Kelley's work has now been confirmed by Israeli scientists, who used bovine growth hormone to reverse thymus shrinking in mice, and similar results have been shown in dogs.

Immune activities that HGH improves include:

- manufacture of new antibodies

- increased production of T cells and IL-2

- greater proliferation and activity of disease-fighting white blood cells

- greater activity of anticancer NK cells

- stimulation of bacteria-fighting macrophages

- increased maturation of neutrophils

- increased production of new red blood cells

The latest study showed that HGH promoted the rate of new red and white blood cells after bone marrow transplantation in mice. The researchers from the National Cancer Institute conclude that HGH may help cancer victims grow new cells after bone marrow transplants.

Helps the Heart

HGH replacement therapy improves cardiac function and protects against cardiovascular disease in a number of ways. It reduces body fat particularly in the abdominal (belly) region, which has been shown to be associated with an increased risk of heart attack. In studies of HGH-deficient adults, HGH improves blood cholesterol profiles—raising HDL cholesterol (the "good" kind) while lowering the LDL cholesterol (the "bad" kind), and reduces the diastolic blood pressure by about 10 percent (without change to the systolic pressure).

Treatment with HGH also reversed heart failure in several studies. In a 1996 *New England Journal of Medicine* article, seven patients treated with HGH (five men and two women) who had moderate to severe heart failure were said to have experienced increased thickness of the left ventricular wall; enhanced ability of the heart to contract and pump out blood; reduced oxygen requirement of the heart; and improved exercise capacity, clinical systems, and quality of life.

In April 2002, a team from The Christie Hospital, Manchester (UK), administered a low-dose GH regimen to sixty-seven GH-deficient adults. They found:

- Significant improvements in total cholesterol, LDL, triglycerides, and ratio of total cholesterol to HDL.

- Greatest improvements seen in patients with the most adverse lipid profiles at the start of GH treatment.

As a result, the scientists commented that "Growth hormone deficiency in adult life is associated with a number of adverse biological changes . . . Most of these changes can be reversed by growth hormone replacement therapy."

In June 2002, researchers from University of Toronto (Canada) administered HGH for a six-month treatment period to sixty-seven men and forty-eight women who were found to be GH deficient at the start of the study. As a result of the therapy:

- Lean body mass increased by an average of 2.1 kg.

- Fat mass decreased by 2.8 kg.

- Greatly improved left ventricular systolic function.

- Significantly restored ejection fraction ("approaching normalcy").

The team concluded that "GH replacement therapy in adults demonstrated beneficial effects on lean body mass composition [and] . . . cardiac function improvement." Furthermore, they stated that there was "no apparent relationship between IGF-I levels and the occurrence or severity of adverse events."

Restores Lung Function

HGH injections have been shown to benefit heart-lung function by increasing the ability to exercise, raise maximum oxygen uptake, and increase the stroke volume and cardiac output (the quantity of blood the heart has the capacity to pump). It also improved forced-expiratory volume (FEV1), the ability to force the air from the lungs in one second. Dr. David Clemmons, chief of endocrinology at the University of North Carolina School of Medicine in Chapel Hill, found that three weeks of HGH injections in patients in the later stages of chronic obstructive pulmonary disease significantly raised the maximum inspiratory force by 10 to 12 mm Hg (millimeters of mercury) on average, and increased their maximum expiratory force (the ability of lungs to move air). Dr. Clemmons believes that HGH is a promising treatment for emphysema and other chronic obstructive pulmonary diseases.

Builds Bones

A Swedish study of forty-four men and women between the ages of twenty-three and sixty-six, who were severely deficient in HGH, found that two years of HGH treatment caused significant increases in the density of the bones that form the hip joint and the vertebrae of the lower spine. There were increases in calcium, osteocalcin, and two types of collagen, which are markers of bone formation. The researchers estimate that they have reduced the possibility of fracture so that it now equals that of healthy individuals in the control group.

Improves Brain and Nerve Conditions

HGH replacement raises energy levels, improves slow-wave (REM) sleep, and elevates mood. Three years ago, a team of Swedish scientists discovered why HGH replacement makes so many people feel good. It acts in the brain exactly like an antidepressant, raising the level of the neurotransmitter B-endorphin, which has been called the brain's own opiate, and lowers the level of dopamine, which is associated with feelings of agitation. In other reports, it appears to reduce stress, improve focus and concentration, and build self-esteem and self-confidence. It may also play a role in depression, as shown by a 1998 report that depressed men have a marked decrease in HGH secretion during the first three hours of sleep when compared with non-depressed individuals.

HGH can reverse decline in memory and cognitive performance. A Dutch study found that HGH deficiency was directly related to impairments in iconic memory (the ability to process a flash of information), short-term memory, long-term memory, and perceptual motor skills such as hand-eye coordination.

Other benefits of HGH therapy on the brain include a restoration of slow-wave sleep, a particular problem among the elderly, and anecdotal reports of improved vision, both near and far, as well as night vision.

HGH, IGF-1, and nerve growth factors in the brain show promise in the treatment of neurodegenerative disease and injury. IGF-1, which is also available in recombinant drug form, has been shown to repair and reconnect severed nerve endings of up to a distance of six millimeters, a feat previously unheard of, and it has increased motor neuron activity in spinal cord cells grown in the laboratory.

Some of the diseases for which IGF-1 may be useful are amyotrophic lateral sclerosis (ALS) and peripheral neuropathies, such as Charcot-Marie-Tooth syndrome. It may also allow more aggressive chemotherapy of certain cancers, since drugs like Vincristine and Cisplatin can cause nerve problems at the higher dosages needed to control the cancer.

HGH normalizes the impaired motor activity of dwarfed mice, suggesting that it may be of value in treating people with Parkinson's disease. It also helps motor activity by stimulating the growth of myelin sheath on nerve cells, making it a potential treatment for multiple sclerosis (MS).

With Alzheimer's disease, there is a loss in a number of neurotransmitters, particularly acetylcholine and noradrenaline, which stimulate HGH. A number of investigators have suggested that HGH may be useful for the treatment of this disease.

Enhances Sexual Function

The decline of male potency parallels the decline of HGH release in the body. HGH levels and sexual potency peak during puberty and steadily decrease throughout manhood until, by age eighty, 75 percent of men are incapable of having or sustaining erections. Although there are no clinical studies that specifically look at HGH and its effect on sexual function, people who are HGH deficient due to pituitary disease have decreased libido and sexual function. After treatment with HGH replacement, they experience increased sexual drive and function, according to their responses on the Nottingham Health Profile.

In a clinical study conducted at the Medical College of Wisconsin in Milwaukee with 320 aging adults on HGH, investigators found that 76 percent of the men reported improvement in sexual potency and frequency, and 62 percent had longer lasting erections. In fact, in interviews with people who have used HGH for anti-aging purposes, almost everyone, male and female, reports improvements in libido and sexual function.

Rejuvenates Skin

HGH is the only anti-aging treatment known to actually make people look younger. The skin of older people tends to become papery thin and lose its firm texture. However, in Dr. Rudman's pioneering six-month study of HGH replacement in elderly men, skin thickness actually increased 7.1 percent. And in a self-evaluation of 202 people who took HGH for six months, more than 66 percent reported improvement in skin texture, skin thickness, and skin elasticity, while 61 percent observed fewer wrinkles and 38 percent reported new hair growth. Patients usually started noticing changes within a few weeks of treatment. Fine lines vanished, deeper wrinkles receded, and facial fat decreased so that puffs of fat under the eyes diminished, while the facial muscles that lift and hold the skin became stronger.

HGH also increased the synthesis of new proteins that lie underneath skin structure. In animal experiments, it increased the strength and collagen content of the skin. Collagen and elastin are the underlying foundation of the epidermis. HGH restored the turgor, or bounciness, that is characteristic of young skin, so the skin bounced back more readily on a pinch test, became better toned, and sagged less.

Resculpts the Body

HGH does something no weight-loss regimen does—it recontours the body, melting away fat and building muscle. In many cases, people look like they've shed years, along with the body fat. Even better, the greatest loss occurs in the deep belly fat, the area that is not only the bane of aging men and women but is also a marker of increased risk of heart attack. In every study of HGH in pituitary-deficient adults, as well as aging "normal" people, HGH replacement reduced body fat and increased lean body mass.

In a six-month placebo-controlled study of twenty-four adults with HGH deficiency at Thomas Hospital in London, the hormone-treated group had no net change in weight but they had lost an average of 12.5 pounds of fat and gained an average of 12.1 pounds of lean body mass.

Rudman's study on elderly men between ages sixty and eighty-one found that after six months of treatment, the treated group gained an average of 8.8 percent in lean body mass and lost an average of 14.4 percent in fat mass. The lean body mass included an increase in the bone density of the lumbar spine

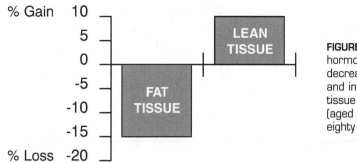

FIGURE 4.5. Growth hormone therapy decreases fat tissue and increases lean tissue in the elderly (aged sixty-one to eighty years).

by 1.6 percent and the liver and spleen grew by 19 percent and 17 percent respectively.

In a follow-up study, the same trends held after twelve months of treatment, with lean body mass increasing by 6 percent, fat decreasing by 15 percent, skin thickness up by 4 percent, an 8 percent growth of liver, and a 23 percent growth of spleen. All this was happening while the untreated control group was losing an average of 2.5 to 4.5 percent in their lean body mass per year.

HGH therapy may be one of the most effective fat-loss regimens ever discovered. In a double-blind, placebo-controlled, crossover study of overweight women, HGH therapy caused an average loss of more than 4.6 pounds of body fat, most of this in the abdomen. Most diets cause loss of muscle along with the fat, but in this study, the women's lean body mass increased by 6.6 pounds.

In two double-blind, placebo-controlled studies by Dr. David Clemmons, of the University of North Carolina in Chapel Hill, HGH, in combination with dieting, accelerated weight loss. All of the people participating in the study exceeded their ideal body weight by 35 to 60 percent. In the studies, lasting either six or eleven weeks, HGH combined with diet caused a 25 percent acceleration in the rate of fat loss above and beyond the effects of diet alone. In the eleven-week period, the HGH-treated subjects lost thirty to thirty-two pounds, compared with twenty to twenty-five pounds in the control subjects. Moreover, while the control subjects lost muscle along with fat, the treated group retained their body tone.

Controls Obesity

It is well known in human physiology that muscle and fat tissue metabolism are directly influenced by the interplay between HGH, amino acids, exercise, insulin, stress hormones, proteins, and fats. Little, if any, fat burning can take place in the presence of high insulin levels, such as those found commonly after eating a meal high in fat or carbohydrates. During fasting, insulin levels are at their lowest. Insulin is an inhibitor of HGH, so it is very important to fast for a minimum of two hours before taking HGH, or its precursors, at bedtime.

Obesity is also a strong inhibitor of HGH secretion. Body fat is the largest public health problem in America. According to the American Obesity Association, 120 million American adults are overweight or obese, that is, thirty or more pounds overweight (about sixty-nine million are overweight and fifty-one million are obese). The number of adults who are overweight or obese has been rising steadily.

Being fat is not a benign lifestyle choice. The excess body fat is like a huge magnet that attracts such diseases as adult-onset diabetes (type II), heart disease, high blood pressure, and some forms of cancer. The American Heart Association has now upgraded obesity from a risk factor to a contributing factor for heart attack. But for most people, taking weight off and keeping it off is about as easy as falling up. About 90 percent or more dieters gain back all the pounds they lose. HGH may well prove to be the answer not only in reducing body fat, but also for many of the problems that accompany obesity.

A group of healthy older men who were administered low-dose HGH injections for nine months lost an average of 9.2 percent total body fat, 6.1 percent of abdominal fat, and an astounding 18.1 percent of the deep layer of central body fat. These results were accomplished without dieting or exercise. The 1997 study, which was carried out by Johannson, Bengtsson, and their colleagues at Salgrenska University hospital, was a randomized double-blind study involving thirty men between ages forty-eight and sixty-six. Not only did the treated group lose a significant portion of their belly fat (the placebo group actually put on fat during that period), they had improved glucose metabolism, lower blood cholesterol and triglycerides, and lower blood pressure.

How was HGH able to do all these things? The Swedish scientists suggest that the low HGH secretion in obese people who carry their weight mostly in the belly is a sign that the neuroendocrine system is off kilter, particularly when it comes to regulating HGH and IGF-1. When you fix this defect by providing the body with HGH, the other benefits follow, such as lower total cholesterol and triglycerides, decreased LDL cholesterol (the "bad" kind), increased HDL cholesterol (the "good" kind), and lowered blood pressure.

In addition to all these benefits, HGH improved glucose metabolism. Type II diabetes is now reaching epidemic proportions in the United States. Overall, there are 17 million Americans suffering from diabetes. The chances of contracting this disease are directly related to obesity. The more overweight you are, the greater your risk for developing this form of diabetes.

The major defect in this form of diabetes is insulin resistance, the inability of the cells to use the insulin that is there. Central belly fat appears to be the major culprit in producing insulin resistance. By eliminating this form of fat, HGH improves insulin sensitivity and allows the body to manage blood sugar more efficiently. While some early studies showed increased blood sugar and insulin resistance among HGH-treated individuals, later studies showed that after six months of treatment, insulin sensitivity returned to baseline. While it is yet to be proven, it seems reasonable to assume that over the long run, stimulation of HGH by getting rid of abdominal fat could prevent type II diabetes or even reverse the disease process.

Independent Living

In November 2001, an important study conducted by the KIGS/KIMS Outcomes Research Group (Stockholm, Sweden) involved a pharmacoepidemiological survey of 304 GH-deficient adults treated with GH for one year. The researchers found that visits to the doctor, number of days in the hospital, and the amount of sick leave all decreased significantly. Patients needed less assistance with daily activities (dressing, grooming, bathing, mobility). The researchers concluded that "GH replacement therapy, in adults with growth hormone deficiency, produces significant decreases in the use of healthcare resources, which are correlated with improvements in quality of life."

HGH: THE SILVER BULLET OF LIFE EXTENSION?

HGH appears to be the silver bullet of life extension. The most consistent extension of life span comes from experiments in which animals are put on a restricted diet. In well-carried out experiments, animals on a calorie-restricted diet have enjoyed a maximum life span that was more than twice the average life span for that species. In human life expectancy, this would be equivalent to a life span of about 160 years.

Dr. William Sonntag at the Bowman Gray School of Medicine at Wake Forest University in Winston-Salem, North Carolina, has examined what happens to HGH and IGF-1 secretion in diet-restricted animals. Normally, when we age, the amount of HGH and IGF-1 decreases along with protein synthesis. Nevertheless, Sonntag and his associates found just the opposite happened in these animals. Young rats on a moderate food restricted diet actually experienced a reduction of their growth hormone secretion, but by the time they reached twenty-six months (old age for a rat), their growth hormone pulses were the same as that of a young rat.

Could a significant factor in these animals' ability to delay death be growth hormone? More growth hormone meant higher rates of making new proteins needed by the cell. While the rates of protein synthesis went down in old control rats, the age-restricted rats had 70 percent increase of new protein in the heart and 30 percent in the diaphragm compared with the unrestricted animals.

With all these amazing benefits, HGH—which vanquished dwarfism over the past thirty years in children—may yet again prove to be the wonder drug of the next decade; this time, for adults seeking the benefits of anti-aging medicine.

The largest clinical study of HGH replacement therapy in "normal" older people shows that it "appears to improve several attributes believed by many to be associated with performance, quality of life, and longevity," says Dr. L. Cass Terry, Chairman and Professor of Neurology at the Medical College of Wisconsin in Milwaukee. Terry reported his findings at the Fifth Scientific Conference of the American Academy of Anti-Aging Medicine in December 1996.

According to Terry, the largest effects were seen among those who were most deficient in HGH. The study was based on the analysis of 320 responses to self-assessment questionnaires drawn from a group of more than 900 patients, 200 of which were physicians. The patients, who were between ages thirty-nine and seventy-four, had been treated an average of 191 days. Terry analyzed the data before and after treatment so that each person served as his or her own control.

Dr. Terry found total cholesterol and triglycerides dropped significantly in both men and women. There were striking changes in muscles and body fat: 88 percent reported improvements in muscle strength, muscle size, and exercise endurance, and 72 percent reported a loss of body fat. IGF-1 levels increased by 61 percent from an average of 239 before treatment, to an average of 385 after treatment. In addition, 76 percent reported an increase in sexual potency and frequency; 84 percent reported higher energy levels; 80 percent reported an improved attitude toward life; 73 percent reported increased resistance to common illness; 73 percent reported improved skin elasticity; 67 percent reported enhanced emotional stability; and 64 percent reported having a better memory.

There were no serious side effects. The most common complaint was fluid retention, joint pains, and five instances of carpal tunnel symptoms, which disappeared when the dosage was lowered. Terry attributes the low incidence of side effects to the low-dose, high-frequency treatment regimen with 4 to 8 IU per week of HGH in divided doses given twice daily, in the mornings and at night, compared with 16.5 IU per week, given once every other day, in previous clinical studies. This dose, which is about one-quarter to one-half of the weekly dosage used by Dr. Rudman in his studies, is safe, well tolerated and virtually free of side effects, yet it is equally effective. Terry believes the regimen used in his study more closely mimics the normal physiologic pulsating-like pattern of HGH release.

HGH THERAPY: RISK VERSUS BENEFIT

Although HGH is a drug that can be prescribed only by a physician, it is important to remember that like many hormonal treatments, the long-term effects are unknown. Proponents of HGH stress that negative effects can occur, but generally only when the patient is taking more than the physiologic dose for a long period. Some of these effects have included carpal tunnel syndrome, arthritis, high blood pressure, vocal cord thickening, excess fluid in the legs, the growth of small breasts in men (gynecomastia), osteoporosis, heat intolerance, impotence, and in supraphysiologic doses acromegaly (the enlargement of the bones in the head, hands, and feet), and diabetes-like symptoms.

Researchers also have expressed concern over the hormone's ability to spur cell growth and how this may promote the growth of cancerous cells present in the body. Recent case-controlled studies have found increases in the serum levels of IGF-1 in subjects who had, or who eventually developed, prostate or premenopausal breast cancers. The concern has been raised regarding its potential role as a cancer initiation factor since growth hormone increases IGF-1 levels.

In May 1998, the British medical journal *The Lancet* published an article that linked elevated levels of GH to a risk of breast cancer seven times higher than the risk in those with low levels of GH. The researcher, Dr. Hankinson, analyzed blood samples of women taken in 1989 to 1990 before any of them were diagnosed with the disease. Over the next five years, the level of IGF-1 was measured in the original blood samples on the 397 women who later developed breast cancer. Among the 76 premenopausal women, those with IGF-1 concentrations in the highest category had three times the risk of those with low levels. The sevenfold increase suggests that the relation between IGF-I and risk of breast cancer may be greater than other established breast cancer risk factors. The study finds an association but it does not speak to whether the higher hormone levels cause the disease.

A 1998 article in *Science* suggested there is an association between men who naturally have high levels of IGF-1 and prostate cancer. In their study, Dr. June Chan and associates at the Harvard School of Public Health found that men with the highest levels of IGF-1 had about four times the risk of men with the lowest levels.

In nature, it would appear that this could not be the case for the simple reason that IGF-1 levels in men markedly decline with age, while the risk of prostate cancer increases with age. Or, as Michael Anchors, a physician with a Ph.D. in biochemistry from Harvard theorizes, "If IGF-1 goes down with normal aging and high IGF-1 is associated with prostate cancer, wouldn't you predict that the risk of prostate cancer would decline with age rather than increase?" Indeed five other reports found that there was no association between IGF-1 and prostate cancer.

Three of these reports (from Stanford University in California, Tel-Aviv University in Israel, and Kolling Institute of Medical Research in Australia) found that patients with prostate cancer had normal levels of IGF-1. In fact, in some cases, the cancer patients had lower-than-average IGF-1 levels. Moreover, Bengtsson of Goteburg University, studying the largest group of HGH-treated adult patients anywhere in the world, has not found any increase in prostate cancer or any other malignancies among several thousand adult patients or in a registry of 20,000 children treated the equivalent of 40 to 50,000 patient years.

Weighing all the evidence, it does not appear that there is any significant reason for concern for those who are *deficient* in HGH in using HGH replacement. With HRT, as with most of the important things in life, having the right balanced amount is the key, as too much or too little can lead to problems. The men who were at greatest risk in the Chan study had unusually high levels of IGF-1. People with acromegaly as a result of abnormally high HGH levels or taking dangerously excessive doses of HGH are known to have a higher risk of cancer. This is why it is important to work with an anti-aging physician who can ensure that your levels of HGH and IGF-1 are neither too high nor too low. Critics of HGH point out how expensive it is to use. A year's treatment could cost as much as $30,000, but recent cost cutting, thanks to several new brands becoming available, has lowered the price of HGH for anti-aging therapeutics to an average of $13,000 a year and even as low as $3,000 a year.

Researchers are also turning to testosterone replacement therapy (TRT) in elderly men as an alternative to HGH. At about $32 for a year's worth of treatment, it is far less expensive than growth hormone. But synthetic HGH costs as little to make as insulin, and because the seven-year monopoly held by Eli Lilly and Genentech on this drug has expired, competition within the industry may eventually drive prices down to even more affordable levels.

NATURAL HGH RELEASERS: HUMAN GROWTH FACTORS

People who are concerned about cost, side effects, and safety, yet want the innumerable benefits of HGH, may consider another option: promoting the enhanced production of the hormone itself.

As we age, changes take place throughout all of our body systems. Cellular processes slow down, and our organs and tissues become less robust in performing their tasks and functions. From head to toe, and beginning as early as the second decade of life, our body systems begin to demonstrate *senescence—* signs of old age. There are ten key biological systems that are susceptible to age-related changes that subsequently cause declining performance of our overall health.

With age, your body reduces its production of HGH. While HGH remains active in the bloodstream for only a few minutes, that is long enough to stimulate its uptake to the liver where it is converted into growth factors. The most important of these is insulin-like growth factor 1 (IGF-1), also known as somatomedin C. IGF-1 is directly responsible for many of the positive benefits of HGH. Innovative anti-aging research now suggests that there are many more types of growth factors.

These newly discovered agents, which we refer to as "Human Growth Factors" (hGf), are chemicals within the human body that help regulate growth modulation and repair such that cells retain their youthful function and metabolism. Anti-aging science suggests that growth factors hold the key to delaying the aging process in two ways:

1. To help modulate cellular metabolism; and

2. To retard the early onset of degenerative diseases.

Human Growth Factors are considered to be responsible for optimizing cellular repair and replacement mechanisms, for keeping metabolism young, active, and efficient in replacing old cells that have lost optimal function. The ability to contribute to cellular repair, regrowth, and rejuvenation is markedly reduced when we experience age-related declines in the production, secretion, and efficacy of utilization of hGf.

Human Growth Factors employs advanced cytokine technology. Cytokines are proteins and peptides with three major functions:

1. to regulate the functional activities of individual cells and tissues

2. to mediate interactions between cells, including processes taking place in the extracellular environment

3. to act as cellular survival factors to prevent programmed cell death

Containing cytokinetic promoting agents, hGf may be considered to be the ultimate twenty-first century natural HGH releaser. A powerful combination of dozens of vitamins, minerals, pro-hormones, and herbs aid in creating a balanced intracellular environment that promotes youthful metabolic and hormonal levels.

In many respects, the biological activities of cytokines resemble those of classical hormones produced in specialized glandular tissues. Some cytokines behave like classic hormones, in that they act at a systemic level to affect biological processes such as wound healing and reactions to shock and trauma.

However, cytokines act on a wider spectrum of target cells than just hormones. Indeed, because cytokines are not produced by specialized cells in specialized glands, there is no one single organ source for these mediators. This is perhaps one of the most important reasons to supplement with cytokinetic-promoting nutrients as we age.

Most cytokines were detected initially by functional tests *in vitro*. Their presence was associated with a range of biochemically undefined activities, or as distinct factors with distinct biological activities. As such, Human Growth Factors can be categorized as a cytokinetic product.

Presently, the relevance of many *in vitro* activities of cytokines to their endogenous (within-the-body) functions within an organism remains to be defined. This may be partially a result of the synergistic effect of cytokinetic agents within the body. While each of the individual nutrients offers rejuvenative effects, it is highly likely that a multiplicative result of taking these agents in combination may yield even greater anti-aging benefits.

Almost all cytokines demonstrate multiple biological activities, and some perform overlapping activities. Often, a single cell frequently interacts with multiple cytokines to yield what appear to be identical responses. This functional overlap further points to the synergy between cytokinetic agents such as those found in Human Growth Factors.

Cytokines play a pivotal role in both extracellular and intracellular functions. Their ubiquitous presence points to a basic biological necessity in the regulation of human physiology—and the process of aging.

Individually, hGf nutrients have documented anti-aging benefits of their own, and are likely to act synergistically to produce a wide spectrum of benefits across target tissue and body functions with prolonged supplementation.

Human Growth Factors is a dietary program that broadly addresses aging-related growth factor deficiencies. The potent effect of Human Growth Factors has been independently established by a study authored by Dr. Suarez and research colleagues. In their study titled "Biometric Analysis of Controlled Clinical Study for Growth Factor Formulation on Multiple Parameters of Aging-Related Dysfunctions," the team enrolled thirty healthy men and women, mean age of fifty-three, in a thirty-day or sixty-day controlled clinical trial of Human Growth Factors. Dr. Suarez reports that "Clinical evidence demonstrates that the replacement significantly reduces symptoms of aging, resulting with:

- higher level of energy
- improved immune response
- thicker and more supple skin
- fewer wrinkles
- increase of positive mood

- better sleep
- decrease body fat 35%
- increase exercise capacity 75%
- promote regular digestion
- promote regular urinary function"

Continuing, Dr. Suarez and colleagues note that 87 percent of subjects reported these benefits in the first ten weeks of hGf supplementation:

- Mean reduction in fat mass of approx. 3.03 Kg, with a significant decrease in abdominal fat

- Enhanced energy level (significant improvement in 78% of subjects)

- Mood improvement (significant improvement in 61% of subjects)

- Improved sleep efficiency, decreased sleep latency, and reduced nighttime awakenings (76% of subjects experienced poor sleep before receiving hGf)

- Increase in sexual potency and frequency

- Skin improvements: improved skin elasticity by 90%; reduced fine lines, coarse facial wrinkling, and tactile roughness

Finally, laboratory testing of hormones at the conclusion of the study term found that testosterone rose by 392 percent (in men), DHEA rose by 502 percent, and serotonin increased by 159 percent—reflecting the capacity of Human Growth Factors to beneficially affect circulating levels of hormones.

For a thorough discussion about this innovative nutritional breakthrough, please read *Human Growth Factors: Advanced Anti-Aging Science Optimizes Your Peak Performance* (Goldman and Klatz, 2003).

Adult hormone replacement is an evolving science, and as such, ongoing research around the world will continue to elucidate the nuances of physician-administered hormone replacement therapy. At the present time, one of the more prudent ways to boost hormone levels that decline with age is to supplement with natural agents that demonstrate the ability to stimulate cellular metabolism, growth, repair, and rejuvenation.

New discoveries from anti-aging research suggests that natural Human Growth Factors help our bodies to regulate growth modulation and repair such that cells retain their youthful function and metabolism. By doing so, Human Growth Factors may delay the aging process by modulating cellular

hGf NUTRITIONALS

Nutrient	Reviewed on	Nutrient	Reviewed on
VITAMINS		Pregnenololone	page 43
Vitamin A	page 174	Melatonin	page 103
Vitamin B$_5$	page 184	**VITAL NUTRIENTS**	
Vitamin B$_{12}$	page 179	Colostrum	page 351
Folic acid	page 188	Alpha-GPC	page 358
Inositol hexanicotinate	page 191	**HERBS AND BOTANICALS**	
MINERALS		*Tribulus terrestris*	page 340
Chromium	page 214	Chrysin	page 290
Zinc	page 232	*Coleus forskohlii*	page 291
Magnesium	page 220	*Griffonia simplicifolia*	page 315
Iodine	page 218	Milk thistle (silymarin)	page 327
AMINO ACIDS		***ADAPTOGENIC HERBS***	
Glutamine	page 245	Panax ginseng	page 307
Carnitine	page 235	Ashwagandha root	page 280
Arginine	page 238	Schisandra berry extract	page 354
GABA	page 243	Astragalus root	page 281
Taurine	page 260	Dong quai	page 295
Lysine	page 252	Wild yam extract	page 347
Ornithine alpha-ketoglutarate	page 255	Lycium berry extract	page 326
HORMONES		Fo-ti root extract	page 301
DHEA	page 87	Red date (jujube) fruit	page 319

metabolism and retarding the early onset of degenerative diseases. Human Growth Factors may help us with optimizing cellular repair and replacement mechanisms, keeping a youthful metabolism, and promoting the replacement of old and tired cells. Human Growth Factors have a low side effect profile and can produce dramatic beneficial effects on how you look, act, and feel.

NATURAL HGH RELEASERS: THE POWER OF EXERCISE

Exercise is an excellent way to increase your body's access to HGH. High-intensity exercise such as weight-lifting or resistance exercises, two to three times per week, will raise your HGH levels. Be sure you are doing only the most strenuous lifting—loads you can only lift six times, rather than the lighter loads that can be hefted fifteen times or more. Lower-body workouts seem to be most effective with regard to HGH, so allot at least half your workout time to leg lifts. Others have found that sprinting or handball two or more times a week also tends to raise HGH levels. Long-distance running doesn't seem as effective; HGH seems to be released in response to particularly intense and strenuous activity. (Check with your doctor before you do any type of exercise.)

Of course, the most powerful combination of all is exercise plus hGf-stimulating supplements (or vitamin supplements that help produce HGH). Likewise, taking HGH supplements (or their equivalents) is no substitute for watching what you eat and reducing fat, and perhaps calories, in your daily diet.

Because of the importance of nutrition and exercise, we have dedicated Sections Three and Four of this book to a hands-on look at how you aim to defy the aging process in your own life. The information contained in Chapters 10 through 21 will help you to make important changes to help "stop the clock" right now. In Chapters 5 through 9, we look at additional hormones, produced naturally by the human body, whose therapeutic use in anti-aging medicine has given us our most powerful tool for living longer and living better. Yet, these tools must be used appropriately.

"Anti-aging has long been equated with trying to live longer, but if we can move the emphasis away from death prevention and toward quality of life, then I don't see anything wrong with that," says George Annas, a Boston University bioethicist. "We all have to age, but the aged should be allowed to age gracefully."

HGH alone is not the antidote to aging, but it may contribute to living more productively for many of the elderly. Used wisely, under a knowledgeable physician's care, physiological hormone replacement therapy of HGH may add more than a few sips from the fountain of youth into our upturned mouths.

CHAPTER 5

The "Grace" Factor: Adrenal Hormone (DHEA)

Hormones and aging have long enjoyed a kind of chicken-and-egg relationship. Does aging result in falling levels of key hormones or does a drop in the levels of key hormones bring on the aging process? Either way, researchers have been impressed that restoring levels of the body's hormones seems not only to halt aging but also to combat a number of debilitating diseases, and possibly even reverse the process of aging for some of the body's organs.

DHEA AT A GLANCE

DHEA has been dubbed the "mother of all hormones." DHEA is the most abundant steroid in the human body and is involved in the manufacture of testosterone, estrogen, progesterone, and corticosterone. The decline of DHEA with age parallels that of HGH, so by age sixty-five, your body makes only 10 to 20 percent of what it did at age twenty.

> By age seventy-five, DHEA levels are only 10 to 20 percent of what they were at age twenty.

WHAT IS DHEA?

DHEA is produced by the adrenal glands. Production of DHEA is high even when the fetus is still developing. Our body's DHEA levels continue to rise up to about age twenty-five, when production drops off sharply. As with melatonin and human growth hormone (HGH), falling levels of DHEA are closely associated with a number of age-related diseases and disabilities. Scientists speculate that if aging men and women can restore their DHEA to youthful levels, their youthful health and vigor will also be restored.

DHEA

General Information	Proponents of DHEA claim that it may be able to enhance immune resistance against infection; reduce risk of age-related diseases, including cancer, coronary artery disease, and osteoporosis; improve blood sugar and help prevent adult-onset diabetes (type II); facilitate weight loss and help convert fat to lean muscle; control Alzheimer's disease, lupus, AIDS, Epstein-Barr, and chronic fatigue syndrome; treat herpes, menopause, depression, and memory and learning problems; and increase life expectancy.
Deficiency Symptoms	Symptoms of DHEA deficiency may include persistent fatigue; depression; anxiety; hypersensitivity to noise; loss of libido; dry eyes, skin, and hair; and loss of head hair, axial (armpit) hair, and pubic hair.
Therapeutic Daily Amount	Exact dosages have not been clearly established. Daily dosages range from 5 to 10 mg to as much as 2,000 mg. Tablets or capsules usually contain 5, 10, 25, or 250 mg of the hormone.
Maximum Safe Level	Not established.
Side Effects/ Contraindications	Children, adolescents, pregnant and nursing women, and people suffering from benign prostatic hyperplasia (BPH), cancer, and endometriosis should not take DHEA. The hormone can interfere with dihydrotestosterone and estrogen levels and large doses can cause liver damage. Women taking doses in excess of 100 mg per day may experience facial hair growth.

According to Dr. Samuel Yen, reproductive endocrinologist and principal investigator of a DHEA study at the University of California at San Diego, DHEA is "a drug that may help people age more gracefully." When taking DHEA, 82 percent of women and 67 percent of men scored higher tests rating their ability to cope with stress, their quality of sleep, and their basic well-being. Only 10 percent of the group not receiving the hormone reported feeling any better.

Small amounts of DHEA were found to lessen amnesia and enhance long-term memory in mice. Even very low levels of DHEA supplementation may increase the number of neurons in the brain as well as prevent neuronal loss and/or damage.

If DHEA decreases with age, increasing our levels later in life may be the answer. Dr. William Regelson, a medical oncologist at Virginia Commonwealth University's medical college, agrees: "If you want to maintain a youthful level of health, then you have to be youthful physiologically and that means maintaining youthful levels of these hormones [DHEA]."

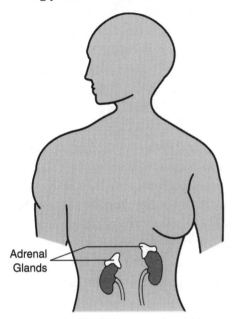

FIGURE 5.1. The adrenal glands

In animal studies, DHEA has been shown to be useful for fighting obesity, diabetes, cancer, autoimmune disease, heart disease, stress, and infectious disease. In other words, it is an all around anti-aging drug. It extends life of laboratory animals by as much as 50 percent. Mice given the hormone look younger and healthier, maintaining the glossiness and coat color of their youth. It may have a life-extending effect in humans as well, although not as great as was originally reported in a study that now spans nearly nineteen years. In 1986, Elizabeth Barrett-Connor and associates at the University of California in San Diego reported a 70 percent drop in mortality from heart disease in men with high DHEA levels. However, a 1995 follow-up study of the same group found only a 20 percent drop in deaths when compared with those who had low DHEA levels. Higher DHEA levels did not protect women at risk of dying from cardiovascular disease.

A 1998 study published in the *Journal of the American Geriatric Society* found that, out of a group of men between ages sixty and eighty, those with the highest levels of DHEA were younger and leaner, more fit, and had higher testosterone levels than those who were lower in DHEA. However, no such differences were found in women of the same age group between those with the highest and lowest levels of DHEA.

HOW DHEA FIGHTS AGING

One of DHEA's key jobs is to help our bodies fight bacterial and viral infection. The immune system is based on the cooperation of several different types of cells, which learn to recognize and then attack infectious viruses and bacteria. Vaccines work on the principle that if the body is "introduced" to a relatively harmless form of an infectious bacteria, it will form antibodies to combat the intruder—antibodies that will then move quickly to attack similar germs when next exposed to them.

In the elderly, however, this process often breaks down. It's not that antibodies can't destroy infectious bacteria, it's that somehow the immune system fails to recognize them. According to Dr. Peter Hornsby of the Huffington Center on Aging in Houston, Texas, the adrenal gland, where DHEA is produced, atrophies significantly as we get older, possibly putting elderly people at an even greater risk for lower immunity. The body doesn't mobilize to fight the disease until the person has already gotten sick.

The *Journal of Clinical Endocrinology and Metabolism* reported that "an enzyme essential for synthesis of DHEA is functionally reduced with aging," resulting possibly in the loss of DHEA as we age. However, whatever the cause of this hormonal decrease, Dr. John Nestler of the New York Academy of Sciences has found that the loss may be at least partially reversible. According to Nestler, "DHEA is one of the most abundant hormones in humans, so it stands to reason that it has some biological effect on us, [and] if I had to guess which of those effects were the strongest, I would say protection against heart disease and boosting immunity."

Indeed, DHEA appears to be a potent immune-system booster. Dr. Raymond Daynes, head of the division of cell biology and immunology at the University of Utah at Salt Lake City, found that it rejuvenated many measurements of immune function in mice, including the production of T cells and other immune factors, which declines with age. In mice with viral encephalitis, DHEA eased some symptoms, reduced the death rate, and postponed both the onset of the disease and death. Older people do not respond as well to vaccines as younger people. However, when Daynes gave old mice vaccines laced with DHEA, their ability to mount defenses to such diseases as hepatitis B, influenza, diphtheria, and tetanus equaled that of a young animal. The animals he placed on DHEA replacement therapy, according to Daynes, also looked "far, far healthier in their later months."

DHEA may also be beneficial in autoimmune diseases, such as lupus, where the body's immune system attacks its own tissue as though it were a foreign invader. In a clinical trial of fifty-seven women with lupus erythematosus, researchers at Stanford University Hospital found that DHEA relieved symptoms, such as skin rashes, joint pain, headaches, and fatigue. Many also reported a higher tolerance for exercise and better concentration.

In humans, low levels of DHEA have been shown to be predictive of heart disease in men, as well as of breast cancer and ovarian cancer in women. It may play a role in maintaining brain cells and protecting against Alzheimer's disease. Brain tissue contains five to six times more DHEA than any other tissue in the body, but people with Alzheimer's have almost 50 percent less DHEA in their blood than those in an age-matched control group, according to several studies. One study of sixty-one men ages fifty-seven to one hundred four, who were confined to a nursing home, found how well they functioned depended on their levels of DHEA—the lower the level, the more dependent the man was and the more difficulty he had carrying out daily activities. DHEA also has antidiabetic action, increasing insulin sensitivity in mice and actually preventing the disease in rats bred to develop diabetes. Some clinicians report that their patients need less insulin when they are on DHEA.

DHEA may have value in treating obesity. In one study, high doses of DHEA (1,600 mg per day) given for four weeks, caused a 31 percent decrease in body fat in four of five subjects with no overall weight change, implying a substantial increase in muscle mass. Their LDL levels also fell by 7.5 percent, showing that DHEA was protecting their hearts as well. The weight-loss potential of the hormone has been explored by Arthur Schwartz, Ph.D., of the Fells Institute for Cancer Research and Molecular Biology at Temple University, a pioneer in DHEA research. He found that animals on the steroid lost weight regardless of how much they ate. When he took mice of normal weight and controlled their activity and diet for four weeks, they reacted exactly like the humans, with four out of five losing 31 percent fat while their overall weight remained the same.

There are a number of explanations for the antiobesity effect. First, DHEA inhibits an enzyme called glucose-6-dehydrogenase, which may block the body's ability to store and produce fat. Second, Schwartz found that it stimulates the hormone cholecystokinin (CCK), which signals the body to feel "full." Third, it may work through IGF-1 to shift the metabolism from producing fat to creating muscle and energy.

While these animal studies are impressive, reports from physicians using replacement levels of DHEA have not seen significant weight reduction in their human patients. Still, they do report elevated levels of testosterone, which is a metabolic product of DHEA, and this appears to help increase lean body mass.

In 1994, Drs. Arlene Morales, Samuel Yen, and their associates at the University of California School of Medicine in San Diego, carried out a double-blind, placebo-controlled, crossover study of DHEA in aging men and women. It involved seventy-one women and thirteen men between the ages of forty to seventy who were on 50 mg of DHEA for three months, and a placebo ("dummy" pill) for three months. When they were on the drug, their levels of DHEA and DHEA-S (a form of DHEA that is most commonly tested for as its level is less subject to variation) rose to that of a young adult. Although the subjects did not know when they were on a placebo or the real thing, 82 percent of the women and 67 percent of the men reported an improved sense of well-being. They attested to their better quality of sleep, increased energy, improved ability to handle stress, and feeling more relaxed. Five of the volunteers also noted improvement in chronic joint pain and mobility. There were no changes in body composition, even though other studies, including a year-long study by Dr. Yen, found that it increased muscle mass in men and women, and that men gained strength and lost fat.

Most intriguing, the San Diego group found that DHEA caused a significant rise in IGF-1, although it did not affect the twenty-four-hour measurement of HGH levels. They speculate that restoring the levels of DHEA may stimulate the liver to produce more IGF-1 or generate more HGH receptors. In other words, we may find that the anti-aging benefits attributed to DHEA may actually be due to the stimulation of the HGH-IGF-1 system.

DHEA and the Brain

Animal studies have also revealed that DHEA supplementation helps to reduce inflammatory processes in the brain. This finding implies that the hormone may have a role in protecting against neurological diseases, such as Alzheimer's disease and Parkinson's disease, whose pathology has been linked to chronic inflammation.

In November 2001, researchers at the University of Pavia (Italy) tested their hypothesis that brain aging in humans causes changes in the mechanisms involving the activity of the calcium-phospholipid-dependent protein kinase C (PKC). PKC-dependent pathways become defective in aging due to reduced levels of the major anchoring protein RACK-1. The team found that DHEA supplementation reversed brain aging by three main mechanisms:

- "regulating neuronal function [by] influenc[ing] transmitter-gated ion channels and gene expression"

- "modulating age-associated impairment of PKC signal transduction"

- "reverting the alteration of RACK-1 anchoring protein expression"

With additional research, these results may demonstrate that DHEA can exert a protective role on the brain.

About DHEA and Cancer

Suggestions that "DHEA causes cancer" are, at present, nothing more than unsupported speculation. Many of the clinical studies investigating DHEA and cancer have been conducted on lab animals in which researchers induce a cancerous state through chemical or genetic means—this experimental setting may not adequately or accurately mimic the way in which human cancers onset and progress. To date, there has been no conclusive study that explicitly implicates DHEA in the onset of cancer in either humans or lab animals. Endocrinologists and hormone researchers worldwide are continuing their study efforts to come to a definitive position on the whether DHEA is, or is not, tumorigenic.

To the contrary, there is an *abundance* of reputable scientific studies that instead suggest that DHEA is critical in *protecting* from cancer.

Recently, a team of researchers at the University of Wisconsin's Institute on Aging, led by Dr. TD Pugh, conducted an experiment that sought to determine the effect of DHEA supplementation on cancer onset in rodents. The researchers separated 300 middle-aged male rats prone to developing cancer into four groups. Of these, in the two groups that were fed a diet that was either calorically restricted or not restricted, and were given DHEA in their drinking water, Dr. Pugh reports that "DHEA administration did not influence cancer . . . at two [different] caloric intake [levels]."

Scientists suspect that a leading mechanism causing cancer to manifest is the failure of the p53 gene to be activated. In cells of lab animals in which the p53 gene is missing or not dormant, mutations of DNA (that subsequently replicate in uncontrolled cell division) occur. Since the mid-1990s, dozens of studies report that DHEA supplementation in these p53-deficient animals staves off cancer. Dr. Hursting and team from the National Cancer Institute spliced out the p53 gene from rats and then supplemented a subgroup with DHEA. The researchers found that "DHEA treated mice experienced a delay in tumorigenesis (particularly lymphomas) and subsequent mortality" as compared to their unsupplemented counterparts." Continuing their report, Dr. Hursting states that "Tumor development in p-53 deficien[cy] can be delayed by DHEA."

Studies presented at an annual meeting of the American Association for Cancer Research indicate that DHEA supplementation may actually be helpful in preventing prostate cancer and benign prostatic hypertrophy (BPH)—noncancerous overgrowth of the prostate. First, DHEA blocked the growth of both human and rat prostate cells in culture in a dose-related fashion—that is, the higher the concentration of DHEA, the greater the inhibition of cancer growth. Second, separate studies at Johns Hopkins University in Baltimore, and Humbuldt University Medical School in Berlin, found that levels of DHEA and DHEA-S were significantly lower in patients with prostate cancer when compared with age-matched healthy controls.

Dr. Rao and colleagues from the IIT Research Institute (Illinois) evaluated the efficacy of DHEA in inhibiting prostate cancer in rats. In the first part of their study, DHEA was supplemented for one week before the researchers induced the cancer state. In the second part, DHEA was administered one week before, twenty weeks after, and forty weeks after the cancer was induced. In both groups, the researchers reported that "DHEA confer[s] significant protection against prostate carcinogenesis." As to the second part of their study, in which the researchers gave DHEA both before and many weeks after cancer was induced, they reported that "The efficacy of delayed administration of DHEA suggests that the compound confers protection against later stages of prostate cancer induction and can suppress the progression of existing precancerous lesions to [become an] invasive disease."

Dr. JE Green and colleagues from the National Cancer Institute (Maryland) studied female mice genetically modified to be prone to developing mammary (the equivalent of the breast in humans) tumors. To a subgroup of female rats in which mammary tumors developed and progressed to invasive carcinoma state, the team administered DHEA. In this group, Dr. Green found that DHEA exerted a dose-dependent reduction in the spread of the cancer. Both the tumor multiplication and tumor burden were reduced by 50 percent by the DHEA. While DHEA also caused serum estradiol levels to increase, no correlated increase in the formation of mammary tumors was observed. The researchers concluded that there is a "tumor inhibitory effect of DHEA on mammary cancer growth [that] . . . inhibit[s] tumor progression."

DHEA is also now regarded as having potent protective activities against skin cancer. Dr. Alberg and colleagues from the Johns Hopkins School of Public Health (Maryland) followed a group of men and women to investigate the impact of DHEA on the risk of developing skin cancers. The researchers first collected and stored blood from a population living in Maryland; twenty-seven years later, several dozen of these men and women developed skin cancers. The team analyzed the collected blood samples from this subgroup. Dr. Alberg did not find any statistically significant difference in the blood concentration of DHEA/DHEA-S in the skin cancer patients versus matched controls, and the risk of developing skin cancer could thus not be correlated to an elevated DHEA level.

These studies suggest that DHEA may have anticarcinogenic properties; and we are hopeful that further research elucidates a safe and effective use for DHEA as a cancer therapeutic.

DHEA has been used by millions of athletes worldwide as a food supplement over the past twenty years without any reported serious, significant adverse effects. In comparison to athletes, DHEA is used for anti-aging purposes in Fractional Physiological Replacement dosages, from which adverse effects are even less likely to result.

DHEA and Cardiovascular Conditions

Another typically age-related disease is atherosclerosis, in which the arteries' inner walls are lined with fat, or "plaque," posing a potential risk of coronary heart disease. One study that extended nearly twenty years found that the DHEA-S levels were far lower in men who died of coronary heart disease than in healthier men. DHEA was also found to be effective in reducing the levels of plaque in rabbits suffering from atherosclerosis: animals with high levels of DHEA were able to reduce plaque by almost 50 percent over those with lower levels. Some scientists believe that DHEA's preventive effect on diseases such as atherosclerosis may relate to its ability to decrease platelet adhesiveness.

> Clinical studies on DHEA show that supplemental oral DHEA can lower cholesterol levels, particularly LDL cholesterol, by an average of 18 percent without modification of lifestyle.

DHEA certainly seems to be a predictor of coronary heart disease. In one study of thirty-two men suffering from myocardial infarction, aged twenty-six to forty, DHEA levels were found to be abnormally low. A 1986 study published in the *New England Journal of Medicine* measured the DHEA levels in 242 men, ages fifty-nine to seventy-nine. (The typical blood level of DHEA in a twenty-year-old ranges from 300 to 500 mcg per deciliter of blood.) It was found that men whose DHEA levels were 140 mcg or higher were less than half as likely to die of heart disease—even when allowing for smoking and high cholesterol levels. This doesn't necessarily indicate that raising DHEA levels would cure or even reduce the men's heart conditions. In fact, there is a sex difference in regard to coronary disease; testosterone appears to protect men against heart diseases, while estrogen appears to protect women. How DHEA plays a role in this gender difference is yet to be discovered.

DHEA levels are an accurate indicator of arterial blockage, LDL cholesterol levels, hypertension, and other risk factors associated with heart disease.

DHEA and Alzheimer's Disease

One of DHEA's key jobs is to maintain the function of our brain cells. It seems that brain tissue contains five to six times more DHEA than any other tissue in the human body. In studies of people with Alzheimer's disease—another condition strongly associated with aging—DHEA levels were found to be abnormally low. Studies have shown that people with Alzheimer's disease have an overwhelming 48 percent less DHEA in their blood than do controls of the same age group! When small amounts of DHEA were added to nerve-cell tissue cultures, not only was the number of neurons increased, but the neurons' ability to establish contacts and connections improved, as well. Therefore, many scientists believe that DHEA may play a key role in improving the function of human brain tissue cells and in reducing the debilitating symptoms of Alzheimer's disease.

A study conducted on sixty-one men, ages fifty-seven to one hundred four, who were confined to nursing homes found that plasma DHEA-S levels were inversely related to the degree of dependence the men had in performing daily activities. In fact, the men confined to the nursing home had 40 percent subnormal DHEA-S levels, as compared with men studied outside of the nursing home who had only 6 percent subnormal levels.

According to Dr. Majewska of the Maryland National Institute on Drug Abuse, DHEA-S may play a role in the GABA theory of aging (gamma-aminobutyric acid is a naturally occurring brain neurotransmitter chemical that acts similarly to Valium), which is linked to Alzheimer's disease. According to this theory, the brain enzyme that manufactures GABA rises as we age and stimulates effects that slow the brain and promote neurodegeneration. DHEA-S would be expected to act as an antagonist to this GABA function.

Furthermore, the excessive GABA we manufacture as we age has been found to lower nerve growth factor in the brain. DHEA, therefore, could logically block GABA's neurodestructive effects and help to promote neuron activity in the aging brain. Majewska also believes that DHEA-S may have fewer side effects than the anti-GABA drugs currently on the market. Such results give scientists hope that eventually DHEA will be beneficial in the treatment or prevention of Alzheimer's disease. In laboratory tests on rodents,

DHEA also seemed to improve short-term and long-term memory and lessen amnesia.

DHEA and Osteoporosis

Most of us are familiar with the term *menopause*—the condition in women in which the ovary stops making estrogen, progesterone, and testosterone, during which menstruation stops, and conception is no longer possible. What researchers are now discovering is that menopause is also associated with low levels of DHEA, and subsequent reduced bone mass in women. When ovarian production of DHEA slows during menopause, the adrenal glands cannot adequately take over, and the resulting DHEA deficiency may be why osteoporosis afflicts so many older women. One study showed the average plasma level, measured in nanograms (1 nanogram equals 1 billionth of a gram) per 100 ml, of DHEA in premenopausal women to be 542, 197 in postmenopausal women, and only 126 in women who had their ovaries surgically removed! The lower a woman's DHEA level, the lower her bone density and the higher her risk for developing osteoporosis will be.

> Women with higher DHEA levels tend to have greater bone mass than those with lower DHEA levels.

DHEA and Lupus

Systemic lupus erythematosus is a chronic inflammatory disease in which a defective immune system causes abnormalities in the blood vessels and connective tissues, as well as damaging the kidneys, nervous system, joints, and skin. The usual treatment for lupus—steroids and chemotherapy—is often more painful and debilitating than the disease itself.

Now scientists are wondering whether DHEA might be a safer and more effective treatment for lupus. Dr. James McGuire, chief of staff at Stanford University Hospital, and Dr. Ronald van Vollenhoven, assistant professor of immunology and rheumatology at Stanford, administered 50 to 200 mg of oral DHEA to fifty-seven women with lupus. Over the three to twelve months that the study lasted, some two-thirds of the patients reported that their symptoms had been relieved, at least to some extent: their skin rashes were less severe and less frequent, and they suffered less from joint pain, headaches, and fatigue. Many also reported a higher tolerance for exercise and better concentration.

DHEA and Diabetes

Another disease frequently associated with aging is adult-onset diabetes (type II). Here, too, DHEA may be an effective preventive treatment. Dr. Nestler, of the Medical College of Virginia at Richmond, hypothesized that the age-related decrease in DHEA and DHEA-S levels may be attributed to the typical age-related rise in insulin levels in the human body. This rise in insulin is a significant phenomenon on its own, as it can lead to obesity, hypertension, and most commonly, diabetes. Nestler observed that certain drugs can reverse the high amount of insulin produced as we age, and thereby restore levels of DHEA in elderly people to what they were in midlife.

One way of understanding diabetes is to think of it as a problem metabolizing carbohydrates. Although a person with a normal metabolism can absorb these nutrients, a person with diabetes needs extra insulin to help the process along.

While some 10 percent of people with diabetes suffer from an insufficient production of insulin, the other 90 percent suffer from a condition known as insulin resistance. That is, their bodies manufacture a normal, or even a high, amount of insulin—but they have difficulty making use of it.

As a result, people with diabetes who have high amounts of (unused) insulin in their bodies tend to have relatively low levels of DHEA. These low levels in turn may contribute to the cardiovascular problems and tendency to be overweight that are typical of diabetics, particularly of those who develop the condition late in life.

In laboratory experiments, Nestler noted that not only did increased levels of insulin drive DHEA levels down, but insulin also interfered with the adrenal activity responsible for DHEA synthesis. Insulin actually stimulated the enzyme that destroys DHEA! In studies of rats genetically predisposed to diabetes, injections of DHEA appeared to reduce their need for insulin and inhibit the onset of the disease.

In studies on both insulin-resistant mice and normally aging mice, DHEA seemed to increase the sensitivity to insulin. It also ameliorated the effects of diabetes in disease-prone mice. Although no full-scale studies have yet been done on the effect of this hormone on humans with diabetes, some physicians report that DHEA treatment reduces the need for insulin in humans.

DHEA, Weight Loss, and Muscle Mass

As we have seen, aging usually brings with it a shift in body composition. The older we become, the greater the proportion of fat in our bodies. Many older people tend to gain weight; others lose muscle mass and gain fat, even if their aggregate weights remain the same.

Many hormones have the effect of restoring muscle mass and reducing fat, and DHEA is no exception. It seems to behave similarly to thyroid hormone in regard to weight loss, by indirectly enhancing thermogenesis, or fat-burning, and energy production at the cellular level.

Various studies have shown low levels of DHEA to be associated with obesity. For example, a 1964 study found that DHEA was completely absent from urine samples of thirty-two elderly, obese people with diabetes. Obese people were also found to excrete less DHEA than people of normal weight.

Many researchers believe that DHEA's antiobesity effects are due to its ability to block a specific enzyme called glucose-6-phosphate-dehydrogenase (G6PD). Scientists believe that by inhibiting G6PD, DHEA actually blocks the body's ability to store and produce fat.

In a yearlong study of fifteen people conducted at the University of California at San Diego, endocrinologist Dr. Yen discovered that DHEA increased muscle mass in men and women, and that men gained strength and lost fat.

> Studies have shown that DHEA works against obesity by encouraging weight loss by raising metabolism and decreasing appetite and fat storage.

Dr. Edmund Chein is a strong supporter of DHEA supplementation and is the founder of the Palm Springs Life Extension Institute. He reported that his patients respond with comments such as "I've never felt this good," and "I can't believe how much weight I've lost." Dr. Chein believes that this weight loss and increase in muscle strength can lead to greater personal independence and freedom as we age.

In a human study conducted in 1988, DHEA was given to five male normal-weight subjects at a dose of 1,600 mg per day. After twenty-eight days of treatment, four out of the five subjects reported an average body fat decrease of 31 percent with no overall weight change; their fat loss had been balanced by a gain in muscle mass! Simultaneously, LDL cholesterol levels dropped by 7.5 percent, thereby protecting against cardiovascular disease. Some researchers hypothesize that DHEA's effect on fat loss and increased muscle mass may be due in part to its ability to help expend energy, rather than store it for future use.

In the 1980s, Dr. Arthur Schwartz of the Fells Institute for Cancer Research and Molecular Biology at Temple University found that administering DHEA to lab animals caused them to lose weight no matter what they ate. DHEA appeared to stimulate the production of cholecytokinin (CCK).

When Dr. Schwartz gave DHEA to five normal-weight male rats over a period of twenty-eight days, controlling their diet and activity, he found that four of them lost an average of 31 percent of their body fat. These animals did not lose weight; rather, their metabolisms had shifted from producing fat to creating muscle and energy. Scientists are now doing research into the possibility of treating obese humans with DHEA.

DHEA and Stress Reduction

Reducing stress, some scientists say, may also help increase depleted levels of DHEA. In a study conducted by the Institute of HeartMath in Boulder Creek, California, it was found that people can raise their levels of DHEA by practicing emotional stress management techniques and listening to relaxing music. In fact, out of the fourteen men and fourteen women, aged twenty-four to fifty-two, who participated in the study, results showed a 100 percent increase in DHEA levels and a 23 percent decrease in the hormone *cortisol*—the "stress hormone." The results of this study were recorded after only one month of practicing the relaxation techniques, and scientists believe that even greater results may be achieved if the techniques are continued over a longer period.

DHEA and the Aging Process

Consider the biological results of growing old: a greater susceptibility to the "aging" diseases of cancer, heart disease, diabetes, and Alzheimer's disease; a tendency to gain weight and a gradually increasing proportion of body fat; and a general weakening of the immune system. DHEA appears to respond to each of these conditions, yet levels of this vital hormone begin falling drastically after age twenty-five. It would seem logical that restoring DHEA levels would help to restore a biological condition of youth.

Moreover, studies have shown that DHEA prolongs life expectancy up to 50 percent in laboratory animals. Although much remains to be learned about the side effects and the limits of DHEA, we're justified in feeling optimistic about this "mother of all hormones".

DHEA and Sex

In August 2001, the University of Vienna (Austria) studied twenty-seven men with erectile dysfunction (ED) of an organic etiology and twenty-eight men with ED of non-organic origin. To both groups, the researchers administered DHEA for six months: after three months, the men with non-organic ED demonstrated statistically significant improvements on the Index of Erectile Function scale. The team concluded that "Oral DHEA treatment may be of benefit to patients with ED who have hypertension or to patients with ED without organic etiology."

TAKING DHEA

In comparison to HGH therapy, DHEA replacement therapy is a much less expensive alternative. However, the anti-aging benefits of DHEA are not yet proven in long-term human studies and the FDA has approved it by prescription only.

Dosage

Medical supervision should always be sought when using DHEA. Common dosages usually range from 25 to 150 mg per day, but it is best to start at the lower end of the spectrum and increase the dosage later if needed. For best results, it is recommended to divide DHEA dosages into three or four smaller doses taken at fixed times over the course of the day. You should also have your DHEA levels measured every two to three months and supplement your diet with additional antioxidants during therapy. Some physicians also recommend that people taking DHEA should have their liver enzymes measured regularly.

Side effects caused by doses at the high end of the recommended daily intake (25–150 mg per day) include acne, increased facial hair, and increased perspiration. Less common side effects reported with DHEA supplementation include: breast tenderness, weight gain, mood alteration, headache, oily skin, and menstrual irregularities.

Warning

Take note that too much DHEA supplementation could suppress the body's natural ability to synthesize it. Therefore, it might be wise to take DHEA every other day, alternating with a DHEA *precursor,* a supplement such as wild yam that causes the body to make DHEA. Scientifically referred to as *Dioscorea,* the wild yam is a plant that grows mainly in China, Japan, and Central America. It's been reported to improve overall health, boost the immune system, increase energy, and help balance the hormonal system.

Men with prostate cancer or women with ovarian cancer should avoid DHEA replacement therapy, as the hormone stimulation associated with

DHEA may aggravate these conditions. Moreover, anyone who is involved in hormone replacement therapy should have his or her biomarkers monitored for early cancer detection at least once a year.

CHAPTER 6

The "Wonder Drug": Melatonin

Imagine a "wonder drug" that extended your life span by 25 percent or more, allowing you to live to be 120 years old. Imagine, too, that this drug not only extended your life, but also maintained your youth, enabling you to enjoy work, sex, and social activities with the same zest and vigor that marked your life as a forty-five year old. Imagine, finally, that this drug had no harmful side effects or known long-term dangers, because it was actually not a drug at all, but a substance that occurred naturally in your body.

The fact is, we don't have to imagine this "wonder drug" at all. It already exists, in every living substance from algae to humans, and its name is *melatonin*.

MELATONIN AT A GLANCE

Melatonin is produced in the dark, while we sleep, and wanes upon daybreak: bright light signals the production cycle to shut down. It is secreted by the pineal gland, a small organ set behind and between the eyes. The pineal is called the "third eye," a reference to our evolutionary heritage—a time when the pineal may have extended the sensory capacities. The pineal gland serves as the timekeeper of the brain, helping to govern the sleep-wake cycle and, in animals, seasonal rhythms of migration, mating, and hibernation. In the human population, melatonin levels are highest in children.

Melatonin is made from an amino acid called tryptophan. Tryptophan is an essential amino acid—we can get it only from the foods that we ingest. The tryptophan we consume during the day is converted into serotonin, a brain chemical involved with mood. Serotonin, in turn, is converted into melatonin.

WHAT MELATONIN DOES

Although research on melatonin has been ongoing since its discovery in 1958,

MELATONIN

General Information	Melatonin, a hormone made by the pineal gland, affects many organs including the thymus, the pituitary, and the hypothalamus. Melatonin plays a major role in setting the body's internal clock.
Deficiency Symptoms	Insomnia and/or frequent waking are symptoms of melatonin deficiency.
Therapeutic Daily Amount	Melatonin is widely available in drugstores and health food stores, both as capsules and in slow-release preparations. Therapeutic doses range from 0.5 to 5 mg per day.
Maximum Safe Level	A safety study carried out in 2000 found that a dose of 10 mg of melatonin daily produced no toxic effects when given to forty healthy males for a period of twenty-eight days. Check with your physician before using long-term.
Side Effects	Melatonin causes sleepiness, so it should be taken only at bedtime. At high doses, it may increase depression and psychosis in people already suffering from these disorders. Women who are pregnant or are trying to become pregnant children, and people with cancer, Hodgkin's disease, leukemia, lymphoma, or multiple myeloma should not take melatonin supplements. It is advised that men who have prostate cancer should not take more than 3 mg of melatonin per night, if at all.

it is only recently it has attracted high interest. Why? Research breakthroughs over the past decade have revealed some startling properties of this amazing substance:

- Studies by immunologist Dr. Walter Pierpaoli of the Biancalana-Masera Foundation for the Aged in Ancona, Italy, and various colleagues have shown that melatonin treatments extended the life span of mice by as much as 25 percent. Moreover, mice that had been treated with melatonin not only lived longer, they also appeared younger, healthier, more vigorous, and sexually rejuvenated.

- Researchers at Tulane University School of Medicine in New Orleans have done studies suggesting that melatonin can stop or retard the growth of human breast cancer cells. Cancer specialists in Milan have added melatonin treatments to chemotherapy and immunotherapy in their treatment of cancer patients. They have found that such patients experienced tumor regression, in addition to living longer and suffering from fewer side effects than patients who received chemotherapy and immunotherapy alone.

- Studies suggest that melatonin may be a kind of "natural" sleeping pill, inducing sleep without suppressing REM (dream) sleep and without producing side effects, such as those caused by sedatives and other artificial sleep aids.

- Travelers have found that by using melatonin they can "reset their biological clocks" after flying across one or more time zones. Numerous studies have confirmed melatonin's efficacy in combating jet lag and restoring restful sleep patterns.

- Melatonin may help to prevent heart disease by lowering blood cholesterol in people with high cholesterol. (Interestingly, melatonin seems to have no such effect on those with normal cholesterol.)

- In a study conducted by the Medical University of Lodz (Poland) in April 2002, women between ages sixty-four and eighty years took melatonin at bedtime for six months, and were found to have a slight but significant increase in IGF-1 and an increased level of DHEA.

- New research suggests that melatonin may be effective in combating, treating, or preventing AIDS, Alzheimer's disease, Parkinson's disease, asthma, cataracts, diabetes, and Down's syndrome. Some scientists also believe that it may be the basis of a new estrogen-free birth control pill that combats breast cancer at the same time that it prevents conception.

Studies conducted by pioneering University of Texas melatonin researcher Dr. Russel Reiter show melatonin to be the most potent scavenger of *free radicals*—unstable molecules that promote cancer and heart disease by damaging DNA, cells, and tissue.

HOW MELATONIN WORKS

To understand more about how melatonin produces its extraordinary effects, we have to consider the aging process itself. Humans are born with the ability to grow, to develop, to mature sexually, and to protect themselves from disease. These functions are carried out via a complicated system whereby various glands secrete a number of different hormones, which in turn stimulate activity elsewhere in the body.

Previously, scientists had viewed the hormonal activity of different systems as relatively discrete. They understood that the endocrine system regulated growth and sexual development, while the immune system protected us from disease. What they didn't realize was that the two systems are interconnected, and that both operate under the direction of the pineal gland.

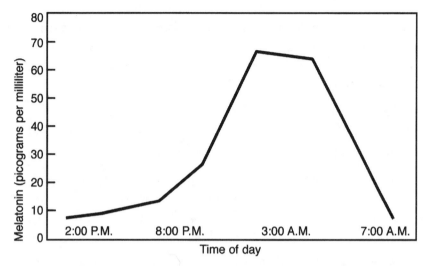

FIGURE 6.1. The twenty-four-hour cycle of melatonin production.

The pineal gland helps govern circadian rhythms, the biological rhythms that take place over a twenty-four-hour day, such as the sleep-wake cycle. This may be one of the reasons why it feels "natural" to sleep at night.

The pineal gland also governs seasonal rhythms that extend over weeks or

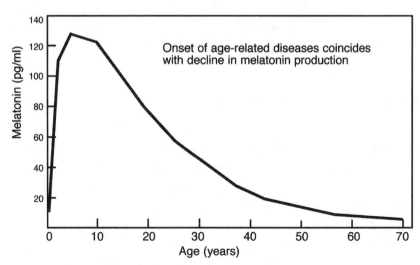

FIGURE 6.2. Melatonin levels through life.

months. By registering changes in the length of each day, for example, the pineal gland helps animals know when the seasons are changing. Animals who mate in the spring are responding to hormonal changes set off by the pineal gland, as are animals that migrate in the fall or hibernate in the winter.

Women who menstruate every twenty-eight days or so are also following a kind of seasonal rhythm, keeping time to the pineal clock. Indeed, researchers have noticed that women's pineal glands are larger than men's, perhaps because women need more internal time cues than men do—that is, to help regulate their menstrual cycles.

Immunologist Dr. Pierpaoli is the pioneer of much of the research into the function of the pineal gland. He sees this organ as a kind of orchestra conductor. Just as an orchestra is composed of many different instruments, so, too, is the human body made up of many different systems. The conductor tells each group of musicians when to start playing, how loudly to play, when to stop, and when to start once again. Likewise, the pineal gland "tells" our endocrine and immune systems when and how to release key substances: growth hormones, sex hormones, and antibodies.

How does the pineal gland "tell" other systems what to do? Dr. Pierpaoli believes that the messenger is melatonin. Changes in our levels of melatonin tell the body to enter puberty and begin sexual development. Melatonin may also be the trigger that sets the menstrual cycle in motion, that puts us to sleep and wakes us up, and that alerts our bodies to produce antibodies to combat disease. The complicated music of these processes is organized by that orchestra conductor, the pineal gland, using melatonin as a kind of baton.

HOW MELATONIN FIGHTS AGING

As we've seen, nature isn't much interested in us after we're too old to reproduce. One system after another starts to go, leaving us with lower levels of sexual functioning and a weakened immune system. This breakdown, too, is governed by the pineal gland, via its output of melatonin.

If we think of the pineal gland as our own internal clock, it "knows" how old we are—and it knows when we're past our reproductive prime. As soon as this gland senses that we're too old to reproduce effectively, sometime around age forty-five, it begins to produce far lower levels of melatonin. This in effect signals all of our other systems that it's time to break down, time for the aging process to begin. (Some scientists speculate that women's larger pineal gland is another reason why women age more slowly than men, and it may be why they live longer.)

What if we could somehow raise our levels of melatonin after they start to fall? What if, at age forty-five, we could duplicate the levels of melatonin that we had in our youth? We would in effect be "tricking" our bodies into believing that they were still young. The pineal gland would continue to give orders appropriate to a young body, calling for higher levels of sex hormones, a well-functioning immune system, and so on. Chronologically, we'd be entering middle and old age; biologically, we'd still be young.

Researchers have found that doses of melatonin do, in fact, help the body to mimic a youthful state. Dr. Pierpaoli and Dr. Vladimir Lesnikov of the Institute of Experimental Medicine in St. Petersburg, Russia, cross-transplanted pineal glands between the brains of young and old mice. Transplanting pineal glands from eighteen-month-old mice into four-month-old mice accelerated the animals' rate of aging. But the reverse procedure allowed the older mice to regain much of their youthfulness, and maintain excellent health throughout their maximum life span. While Bonilla et al. (*Exp Gerontol.* 2002;37: 629–638.) found that daily supplementation of melatonin in fruit flies increased maximum lifespan by 33%, much of the life-extending benefit of melatonin in these cases is suspected to be a result of the potent antioxidant activity of the hormone.

One of the key glands stimulated by melatonin is the thymus, a tiny gland that weighs only one-half ounce at birth, doubles in size by puberty, and then shrinks and all but disappears in adulthood, degenerating over 90 percent by age sixty-five. The thymus plays a pivotal role in the immune system, for it is full of the white blood cells known as T lymphocytes or T cells that fight infection. T cells are originally manufactured in the bone marrow, but when we are still children, our T cells migrate to the thymus, which stores them as they mature and releases them when they're needed.

One of the reasons that we lose our ability to fight disease as we age is that the thymus degenerates and virtually disappears—presumably in response to decreased levels of melatonin released by the pineal gland. When Pierpaoli and his associates added melatonin to the drinking water of older mice, the mice's ability to resist disease significantly improved. At the same time, the weight of their thymus glands increased, and their thymus cells became more active, suggesting that they were more actively producing T cells.

Melatonin and Stress

One of the key causes for the breakdown of our immune systems is stress. Stress causes our adrenal glands to produce corticosterone or cortisol, the so-called "stress hormone," which helps our bodies key up for the fight or flight response. However, corticosterone also suppresses our immune systems, which is why we're so much more likely to get sick when we're under pressure or going through a grueling emotional time.

Melatonin seems to counter the immune-suppressing effects of corticosterone. That may be why younger people seem better able to handle high-pressure jobs or demanding schedules, as well as to bounce back more easily from emotional blows and life difficulties. Restoring melatonin levels may also restore our youthful ability to handle challenging situations with grace and resilience.

A 1995 study conducted by Italian researchers demonstrated that melatonin boosted the immune systems of people under extreme stress. The subjects were twenty-three cancer patients who were undergoing traditional cancer therapy. Not only is the diagnosis of cancer in itself a stressful experience, but the psychological stress coupled with the negative side effects of chemotherapy and radiation severely weaken the immune system.

The patients were put on a program of 10 mg of melatonin nightly. After a month of therapy, they found that melatonin strengthened their immune systems. The production of interferon-gamma and interleukin-2 (IL-2 is a hormone that aids in T-cell production) had increased considerably. Melatonin acted as a stress buffer and also made the patients less likely to succumb to the cancer.

Melatonin and Cancer

A number of researchers have been exploring melatonin's potential role in combating cancer. It has been suggested for the treatment of colon, ovarian, and prostate cancers; for melanoma; and for brain tumors. So far, though, the most exciting possibilities are emerging in the treatment of breast cancer.

According to Dr. Steven Hill, associate professor at Tulane University's School of Medicine's Cancer Center, more than half of all women with breast cancer have lower-than-normal levels of melatonin. Furthermore, in 2001, Kliukiene et al. (*Br J Cancer.* 2001;84:397–399.) reported that the incidence of breast cancer in women who had become blind before the age of 65 was 49% lower than that in normally sighted women. Because melatonin production is high in the blind at all times of the day, the researchers offer this finding as suggestive of the anti-cancer role of melatonin. Tynes et al. (*Cancer Causes Control.* 1996;7:197–204.) found that women who worked in occupations requiring night time work were 1.5 times as likely as daytime workers to be diagnosed with breast cancer. The researchers suspect that the increase in cancer risk may be due to low melatonin levels because exposure to artificial light suppresses production of melatonin, which normally takes place at night. These studies suggest that increasing levels of melatonin might help to prevent or treat breast cancer in women.

Breast cancer in women has been linked to a cumulative exposure to estrogen, the female hormone that is released every month during ovulation. Every time a woman becomes pregnant, she stops ovulating, giving her a "break" from estrogen exposure. That's why women who have few or no children are at an increased risk of breast cancer.

Moreover, according to Dr. Hill, more than half of all women with breast cancer have tumors marked by "estrogen receptors," chemical sites that help the tumor interact with estrogen. Thus, estrogen stimulates the growth of tumors with such receptors.

Melatonin seems to combat these effects of estrogen, stopping the tumors from growing and ultimately getting them to shrink. In a laboratory experiment, Dr. Hill exposed breast cancer cells with estrogen receptors to extremely high levels of melatonin. The number of estrogen receptors markedly decreased.

University of Arizona College of Medicine Professor David Blask found that melatonin directly inhibited the growth of breast cancer tumors grown in lab dishes. Blask also administered melatonin to several hundred lab rats infected with breast cancer, and in half the cases, tumors decreased by 50 to 70 percent. Blask found that melatonin was at least as effective as tamoxifen, a popular new estrogen-inhibiting anticancer drug, which had previously been used to combat estrogen-related breast cancer tumors, yet had far fewer negative side effects.

A study conducted in 1992 by Dr. Paolo Lissoni and his colleagues at San Gerardo Hospital in Monza, Italy, found that melatonin significantly increased the one-year survival rates of people with metastatic lung cancer. When patients were given 10 mg of a nightly melatonin supplement, growth of their tumor cells slowed. Lissoni and his colleagues also found that the melatonin enabled IL-2 to work in smaller doses and seemed to amplify its activity.

Lissoni was involved in another study of 200 cancer patients with advanced solid tumors, for whom "no effective standard therapy was available." All patients had a predicted life expectancy of less than six months, and among them, 90 had been previously treated with chemotherapy. IL-2 was injected subcutaneously at a dose of 3 million IUs a day for six days a week for four consecutive weeks. Melatonin was given orally at a dose of 40 mg every day, starting seven days before the first IL-2 injection. Complete response was achieved in two percent of the patients, partial response in 18 percent, and stability of the disease in 42 percent; progression of the disease occurred in 38 percent. Cancers located in the liver or in the brain were less responsive to the treatment, as were cancers that had metastasized.

Prostate cancer and breast cancer have similar properties—and this may be why melatonin has been shown to inhibit both of them. Both breast and prostate cancer are hormone-dependent in their initial stages of development and can be stopped if detected early. (Breast cancer is stimulated by estrogen and prolactin, and prostate cancer is stimulated by testosterone.)

Studies done by Arizona's David Blask and a group of researchers showed that when prostate cancer cells were incubated with melatonin, cell division decreased by 50 percent. Another similarity in people with breast cancer and prostate cancer is that they have very low levels of melatonin. It is not yet known if these low levels contribute to the disease.

Dr. Roman Rozencweig is a Montreal physician who has treated numerous patients with melatonin for more than eight years. His then seventy-one-year-old father had been diagnosed with prostate cancer through a routine PSA (prostate-specific antigen) test, the results of which were abnormally high. Rozencweig recommended 6 mg of melatonin each night. After six months of treatment, results showed better sleep and a lower PSA count, indicating that the tumor had become less active.

When used in conjunction with, or substituted for, the sex hormones estrogen, testosterone, and progesterone, melatonin may also be used to prevent certain cancers. Endocrinologist Dr. Michael Cohen of Applied Medical Research in Fairfax, Virginia, is testing a drug that substitutes 75 mg of melatonin for the progesterone normally given to postmenopausal women on estrogen replacement therapy (ERT). (In older women, progesterone can promote breast cancer and stimulate risk factors for heart disease.) In addition, Dr. Cohen already has a patent for a male contraceptive that combines melatonin with testosterone. The pill functions by stopping sperm production and reducing the risk of prostate cancer.

Clearly, we've just begun to explore the possibilities of using melatonin to fight cancer. Because melatonin therapy for cancer is not yet clinically proven, patients diagnosed with cancer should not rely on melatonin alone. It may be used in conjunction with other treatments, but cancer is a serious disease that should be treated by a knowledgeable physician. However, the success of melatonin in this area is yet another reason scientists should pursue its research.

Melatonin and Sexual Function

Just as lower levels of melatonin signal our immune systems to shut down, so, too, do they signal our endocrine systems to produce fewer sex hormones. Lower levels of sex hormones in turn may lead to the atrophy of sexual organs in both men and women, as well as a decrease in sexual interest and ability to perform.

When the mice in Pierpaoli's experiments were given melatonin, they seemed to undergo a sexual transformation. Not only did they maintain a sexual interest and vigor characteristic of much younger mice, but also the mice's sexual organs, male and female, actually underwent repair, regeneration, and rejuvenation, making them comparable to those of younger animals.

Melatonin and Free Radicals

Much of the damage that we attribute to aging is the cumulative effect of bombardment by free radicals. One of the key ways that melatonin helps combat cancer is its ability to act as an intercellular antioxidant, preventing and reducing the damage done to the body by these free radicals. Melatonin is perhaps the only antioxidant that is capable of penetrating every cell of the body. Also, it is the most active and effective of all naturally occurring antioxidant compounds.

In 1993, Dr. Russel Reiter of the University of Texas Health Science Center in San Antonio and his colleagues suggested that melatonin might be the most effective antioxidant or scavenger of free radicals. The team conducted a study in which rats were fed carcinogen-laced food designed to damage their DNA by producing oxygen-based free radicals. When melatonin was given to the rats before they ingested the carcinogenic food, they sustained 41 to 99 percent less genetic damage than rats that had not been treated with melatonin. Also, the more melatonin the rats had been given, the greater their protection from damage.

In several other tests, melatonin has continued to perform as well as or better than other *antioxidants,* substances that defuse free radicals, unstable, destructive oxygen molecules. For example, glutathione (GSH) is a valued scavenger for free radicals that travel between cells—yet melatonin proved to be five times more effective. Vitamin E is used to combat oxidants within cells—yet melatonin seems to be at least twice as effective.

Furthermore, most antioxidants work on only one part of the cell, either the lipid-rich membrane or the water-based cell itself. Melatonin is soluble in both fats and water, making it a wider-ranging antioxidant than its vitamin and mineral counterparts.

Melatonin Aids Sleep

About 60 million Americans a year have insomnia frequently or for extended periods of time, which leads to even more serious sleep deficits. Insomnia tends to increase with age and affects about 40 percent of women and 30 percent of men. Research on humans has shown that increasing melatonin levels may bring an end to those restless nights.

> Only half of adults can say they get a good night's sleep a few nights/week or more. Fifty percent (50%) report feeling tired, fatigued or not up to par during wake time at least one day a week.
>
> —*National Sleep Foundation, 2005 Sleep in America poll*

Melatonin production occurs almost entirely at night and is actually stimulated by darkness; bright light suppresses its secretion. The amount of melatonin that is produced is directly linked to how well we sleep, and its chemical structure is important in explaining our body's internal clock.

Recently, scientists discovered the enzyme that turns on melatonin production in the brain. According to David Klein of the National Institute of Child Health and Development, the enzyme's presence in the brain cells suggests that it regulates serotonin. This enzyme is turned on and off by the body's internal clock. In essence, serotonin and melatonin act as our day and night regulators. We get our high energy level from serotonin during the day and our restful state from melatonin at night. Daytime levels of melatonin are very low; nighttime levels may be five to ten times higher.

The National Institute of Mental Health found that subjects who spent fourteen hours a day or more in darkness returned to what amounted to primordial sleep patterns, during which their brains produced high levels of melatonin. These levels decline with age, explaining the common occurrence of age-related insomnia.

A study conducted in Israel found that the quality of sleep in the elderly was proportional to the amount of melatonin secreted by the pineal gland. Elderly people with insomnia have half the amount of melatonin as young people. They may spend more time in bed but less time asleep.

Dr. Steven Novil has been treating patients with melatonin for ten years. One patient, an elderly woman in her eighties, had trouble falling back to sleep after getting up to urinate frequently. She was put on a program of 3 mg of melatonin an hour before bedtime. Within a week, the patient's sleep pattern had changed remarkably. Her need to urinate throughout the night lessened and when she did wake up to use the bathroom, she was able to fall back to sleep without problem. In addition to a more restful night, the patient experienced pleasant, vivid dreams for the first time in many years, and woke up feeling refreshed. The melatonin allowed her to sleep more and sleep better.

Even very small doses of the hormone can shift the body's clock forward. Dr. Richard Wurtman, director of the Massachusetts Institute of Technology's Clinical Research Center, conducted a study in 1994 in which young adults took melatonin or a placebo before a midday nap. While the placebo group took an average of twenty-five minutes to fall asleep, those on melatonin fell asleep within six minutes. The sedative effect was noticeable in those subjects on as little as 0.1 mg of melatonin.

Another study complementing the pilot study done at MIT was conducted in the United Kingdom by a team of researchers led by Dr. Phillip Cowen. The double-blind, placebo-controlled crossover study gave subjects two doses (.3 mg and 1.0 mg) of melatonin and a placebo on three different nights over several weeks. Then the subjects were monitored for the length of time it took

---

Other Sites Where Melatonin Is Found

Recently it was found that the pineal gland is not the only site in the body where melatonin is produced and secreted. Dr. Gerald Huether of the Neurobiologisches Labor, Psychiatrische Universitatsklinik, Gottingen, Germany, reported that melatonin has an extrapineal and gastrointestinal presence.

Melatonin was discovered in the gut when scientists were studying tryptophan metabolism in the body. It was found that administrating tryptophan to the body in turn increased circulating levels of melatonin. It is speculated that the concentration of melatonin present in the endocrine cells lining the gut, believed to act as a protectant for the stomach and intestines, may in fact be higher than in the pineal gland.

Small concentrations of melatonin were also found in the fibers of the retina, which act as a photoprotectant to light sensitivity in the eye. It is thought that the daytime trace levels of melatonin have their origin in the retina. However, the highest levels of melatonin in the plasma occur at night, which accords with pineal rhythms.

them to fall asleep and the quality of their sleep. The researchers found that each of the doses of melatonin reduced the time it took to fall asleep, increased actual sleep time, increased quality of sleep as reflected in deep or "slow-wave" sleep, increased sleep efficiency as measured by the percentage of time in bed spent sleeping, and reduced the number of awakenings after the onset of sleep. The study supported the hypothesis that even at low doses melatonin has hypnotic effects, and unlike most currently available sleep aids, improves the quality of sleep as well.

Melatonin Cures Jet Lag

The dictionary definition of jet lag is a "temporary disruption of bodily rhythm caused by high-speed travel across several time zones . . ." And as millions of long-distance travelers know, it can feel more like a hangover with insomnia and symptoms of the flu. In addition, it can cause a lack of concentration and a feeling of disorientation. Disrupting the body's rhythm brings with it changes in blood pressure, blood sugar, mood, energy level, arousal, and hormonal levels.

Although conventional sleeping pills may help induce sleep in travelers, many times the other symptoms of jet lag are left hanging. Numerous human studies have shown that melatonin has become one of the most effective ways in combating jet lag or nightshift work because it resets the body's biological clock and restores balance. Melatonin is a hormone that is released only at night, and giving it to people in the daytime can successfully trick the body into thinking it is in another time zone.

In Britain, an endocrinology professor at the University of Surrey tested the effects of melatonin on some 400 travelers and noted that those to whom melatonin was administered were able to reduce their jet lag by 50 percent.

Another study was conducted by researchers in France. It involved thirty volunteers who were scheduled to fly from the United States to France. All the volunteers had had difficulty with jet lag in the past. On the day of the flight and for three days thereafter, they took either a placebo or 8 mg of melatonin. The volunteers on melatonin were able to sleep and focus better and experienced fewer mood swings.

Melatonin functions on two levels—it helps you to sleep better and it readjusts your body's clock faster. It may be nature's sleeping pill, but remember "insomnia is a symptom and not a diagnosis," says Dr. David Zeiger. Zeiger was part of a sleep deprivation program at Stanford University, and now practices at Rhema Medical Associates in Chicago, where his patients with sleep disorders are treated with melatonin. He stresses that the causes of insomnia may be physical disorders, psychological difficulties, substance overuse/misuse, inadequate sleep habits, improper sleep environment, or circadian-cycle abnormalities.

Scientists predict a rapidly expanding role for melatonin not only in treating sleep disorders and jet lag but for mental disorders as well. The newly discovered enzyme that turns on melatonin production may, some think, lead to the development of new therapies not only for improving sleep but also for improving alertness and wakefulness. In addition, the enzyme's regulation of the vital brain chemical serotonin, which has been linked to aggressive behavior, depression, and psychosis, indicates that it might be a good candidate for treating mental disorders.

TAKING MELATONIN

The first thing to remember is that sometimes less is more. Although melatonin has an extremely important role in the body, it is present only in tiny amounts, even when we're at our youthful peak. Megadoses of melatonin won't necessarily help us maximize our energy or our health. Rather, we should try to approximate the levels of melatonin that our youthful bodies once knew.

Note: Children *should not* be given melatonin. The highest levels of melatonin in the body occur during childhood; no supplementation is necessary. People who have serious illnesses such as an autoimmune disorder, multiple sclerosis, leukemia, or lymphoma should consult a physician who is familiar with melatonin before usage. Immune-suppressing drugs such as cortisol and cyclosporine may react adversely with melatonin, as may antidepressants. People who have diabetes, experience major depression, have severe allergies, or have a hormonal imbalance should also take caution.

Finally, pregnant or nursing women should avoid melatonin supplements. They are already transmitting melatonin to the fetus or infant via the placenta or their breast milk. It is unknown if increasing melatonin levels might adversely affect the child.

On the other hand, women who are already taking hormone-replacement supplements may take melatonin without fear of any ill effects. Estrogen and melatonin coexist in young women's bodies, so there's no reason why hormones designed to replace estrogen should not coexist with melatonin in the bodies of older women.

Currently the immense popularity of melatonin has brought with it some unbalanced and potentially dangerous views on the hormone. The fact of the matter is that there are no conclusive human studies that guarantee any positive long-term results. We have found through personal experience and communication with multiple physicians who have treated patients with melatonin that its only proven safe use is as a short-term remedy for jet lag and sleep disorders. A note of caution should be raised, as the dosages of 3 to 10 mg recommended here and in many popular books and magazines are many times more than the amount normally made by the body, and could have unforeseen long-term effects.

Beginning Melatonin Supplementation

Melatonin levels drop most sharply at around age forty-five, so consumers who wish to take melatonin to combat aging should probably begin at that time of life. People with a family history of cancer, cardiovascular disease, or heart disease might begin in their late thirties or early forties, as melatonin might help combat their inherited predisposition to these diseases of aging.

Since the goal is to keep melatonin levels constant, starting earlier isn't going to head off aging later. The idea is to start taking melatonin when your levels drop, not before. On the other hand, if you are already past forty-five, you're not too late! You can begin reversing the effects of age no matter when you start taking melatonin supplements.

Remember, take melatonin only at bedtime. Because this substance helps regulate our sleep-wake cycles, it generally makes people very sleepy. If you work at night, take melatonin before your daytime bedtime. And in no case should anyone take melatonin before they need to drive, operate machinery, or otherwise be alert. Although melatonin will not make you feel drugged (for example, you could still respond to an emergency call from a child), it will make you feel drowsy and relaxed.

Availability

Melatonin supplements are currently available in .75 mg, 2 mg, 3 mg, 5 mg, and 10 mg tablets or capsules. Lozenges are available in 2.5 mg and 5 mg. Melatonin is not patented, so a number of companies manufacture and distribute it. However, since melatonin is not regulated by the FDA, its purity cannot be guaranteed. We recommend the synthetic form, rather than animal-derived melatonin, both for standardization of strength and elimination of risk of biological contamination.

Dosage

Each person's physiology is unique and finding the right dosage of melatonin may be trial and error in the beginning. If you find that you're waking up tired and groggy, reduce your dose in increments of .5 mg until you find the amount that's right for you. It is wise to take melatonin every other day, as it is not yet known whether supplementation can inhibit natural production.

Side effects of melatonin use have been minor. Grogginess in the morning is common. Some people find it more difficult to sleep when taking melatonin and experience nightmares. Others report mild headaches, upset stomach, lower sex drive, and depressed feelings. Most side effects occur in people who take high doses of 20 mg or more of melatonin, use it every day, or are on medications. People taking 1 mg or less experience almost no side effects.

Melatonin in the range of .5 mg to 12 mg is usually effective in inducing and maintaining deep sleep. If you do not respond to a low dose, such as 1 or 2 mg, you are more likely to respond to higher doses, such as 5 to 10 mg. If there is no response to the capsules or tablets, lozenges can be tried. Lozenges seem to be more consistently effective than pills, since the melatonin goes directly into the bloodstream from absorption through the mouth.

Melatonin does not seem to be as consistently effective when taken on a full stomach; perhaps it is not absorbed as well, or it is absorbed too slowly. Taking it with a snack or on an empty stomach is more effective. There is a wide variation between people on the best time to take melatonin. But because of its drowsiness-producing effect (most people notice a yawn within thirty minutes of dosing), the best time is half an hour to two hours before going to bed; lozenges dissolved in the mouth should be taken twenty minutes to an hour before going to bed.

Withdrawal symptoms are not common, but for some people melatonin may cause rebound insomnia. Therefore, when deciding to stop taking melatonin (or any sleeping medicine), it is recommended to taper off over a period of one to two weeks. For example, if you have been using 4 mg of melatonin regularly and feel you don't need it anymore, lower the dose to 3 mg for a few nights, then 2 mg for another few nights, and so on. By tapering off melatonin, any rebound sleep disturbances should be avoided.

For more information about melatonin and other nutritional supplements to promote sleep and aid with possible age reversal, please read *Sleep: Essential to Optimum Health* (Goldman and Klatz, 2003).

CHAPTER 7

The "Female's Monitors": Estrogen and Progesterone

The most-often prescribed prescription medication in America is estrogen, the female sex hormone. Some 13 million American women—about 20 percent of those in or past menopause—regularly opt for estrogen replacement therapy (ERT) to help them through the process of menopause. As the baby-boom generation approaches menopause, these numbers are going to sky-rocket.

The multibillion-dollar business in female hormones has generated enormous controversy. Proponents claim that hormone replacement therapy (HRT), where estrogen is given with the hormone progesterone, can help curb menopausal symptoms such as hot flashes, night sweats, vaginal dryness, and aging skin, while also lessening a woman's risk of heart disease, osteoporosis, colon cancer, and mental deterioration.

> Men have more heart attacks than women until women pass the age of menopause. Researchers think the high level of estrogen in pre-menopausal women helps protect them from heart disease.

Skeptics reply that hormone replacement therapy puts women at a higher risk of breast, uterine, and ovarian cancers; that it frequently induces a sense of lethargy or sluggishness; and that diet, exercise, and vitamin and mineral supplements can combat most of the dangers of aging and menopause. If necessary, the skeptics say, women can treat certain symptoms with estrogen creams and/or with natural sources of progesterone, rather than undergoing expensive and potentially dangerous synthetic hormone therapy.

However, more and more research is providing strong evidence that taking estrogen replacement therapy significantly reduces the rate of death from all causes for postmenopausal women, and offers even greater protection against heart attack and stroke. A study evaluated the medical history of 454 healthy women born between 1900 and 1915 and compared the health outcomes of those who started estrogen supplementation with those who did not. About half the group used estrogen for at least a year starting in 1969. Among those women who did not use ERT, there were eighty-seven deaths from all causes compared to fifty-three deaths among the estrogen users—a 46 percent lower overall mortality rate. More specifically, the estrogen group had a 60 percent reduction in mortality for coronary heart disease and a 75 percent reduction for other cardiovascular problems such as stroke. Although there was a slightly higher rate of breast cancer death among estrogen users, this was statistically offset by a slightly lower rate of death from lung cancer.

A new generation of estrogen products that appears to side step the increase in risk for cancer has recently entered the marketplace. Called *SERMs* (*selective* estrogen-*receptor* modulators), these drugs are designed to deliver estrogen to the heart and bones, but not to the uterus and breasts. In February 2002, results from the leading SERM (raloxifene) study of 7,705 post-menopausal women with osteoporosis or history of vertebral fracture were presented in the *Journal of the American Medical Association* (JAMA). Researchers reported that among women at high risk for cardiovascular disease, the use of raloxifene did not result in an initial increase in the number of new events. Moreover, after 4 years there was a reduced incidence of new cardiovascular events. Raloxifene was also found to have beneficial lipid effects. The substance has been shown in other studies to reduce the incidence of vertebral fractures, increase bone mineral density, reduce the risk of breast cancer, and does not stimulate the endometrium.

> On average, women are ten times likelier to die from heart disease than from breast cancer, suggesting that estrogen's benefit in reducing risk of heart disease outweighs a possibly greater risk of breast cancer.

WHAT IS ESTROGEN?

Estrogen is one of the female hormones that help regulates a woman's passage through menstruation, fertility, and menopause. Estrogen is one of the most powerful hormones in the human body. Some 300 different tissues are equipped with estrogen receptors—chemical sites that make the tissues responsive to estrogen. That means that estrogen levels in the body can affect a wide range of tissues and organs, from the brain to the liver and to the bones themselves. The uterus, urinary tract, breasts, skin, and blood vessels depend on estrogen to stay toned and flexible.

Although we are used to thinking of *menarche* (the onset of menstruation and fertility) and *menopause* (the cessation of menstruation and fertility) as single points in life's journey, they are actually more like peaks and valleys. Estrogen levels start to rise well before menarche, as early as age eight in some girls. The hypothalamus is the prime mover in this process, signaling the pituitary to release hormones; the pituitary, in turn, signals the ovaries to produce more estrogen.

For three or four years, estrogen levels continue to rise, and by age eleven or twelve, they are sufficiently high (along with other key hormones) to begin the menstruation process. Estrogen also sets off the development of the breasts and the growth of hair under the arms and in the pubic region. The body often responds to this new hormonal activity with confusion: oily hair, acne, budding sexual interest, mood swings, and, sometimes, painful menstrual cramps.

MENSTRUATION AND PERIMENOPAUSE

Under normal circumstances, a healthy woman will continue to menstruate for many years, from about age twelve until some time in her early fifties. However, just as hormone levels began to rise well before the onset of menstruation, they begin to fall well before the onset of menopause. By their early thirties, most women experience decreased levels of estrogen and progesterone, and a consequent drop in fertility.

Then, sometime in their early forties, most women enter the *climacteric*—a period in which falling hormones begin to have more obvious symptoms. This is known as *perimenopause*—the stage just before menopause. The skin tends to become dryer, hair grows more brittle, and pubic and underarm hair becomes sparser. Some women experience a loss in libido; others suffer mood swings.

In addition, even while women are still menstruating, hormonal fluctuations often play havoc with their systems, especially before and during their periods. Endocrinologist Dr. Lila Nachtigall of New York University explains that falling estrogen levels cause the hypothalamus to send out ever more signals to incite the ovaries to produce more estrogen. The ovaries contain aging eggs that respond rather erratically to the frantic signals from the hypothalamus. These erratic responses result in fluctuating hormone levels that may rise and fall within a single day, "and that can drive you crazy."

According to Dr. David G. Williams, this craziness is not only the result of fluctuating estrogen; it's also the result of insufficient progesterone. Williams cites the work of British physician Dr. Katharina Dalton, who in the early 1950s identified premenstrual syndrome (PMS), the bundle of symptoms that plague many women three to ten days before their periods. Dr. Dalton found that progesterone supplements helped alleviate her own menstrual migraines, and went on to develop progesterone-based treatments that helped thousands of women with PMS.

Ideally, both estrogen and progesterone levels will rise from the time of ovulation until just before the menstrual flow begins. But if estrogen levels alone are rising, the hormonal imbalance may lead to a host of symptoms: salt and fluid retention; low blood-sugar levels; blood clotting; fibroid and tumor development; interference with thyroid hormone function (leading to weight gain and/or feelings of exhaustion); increased cholesterol and triglyceride levels; allergic reaction; increased production of body fat; reduced oxygen levels in the cells (creating a sluggish, low-energy feeling); and a number of adverse mineral reactions, such as retention of copper and loss of zinc.

These symptoms may occur even in relatively young women. However, they tend to intensify—or to appear, intensely, for the first time—in premenopausal women. Women who are still menstruating in their forties and fifties note painful menstrual migraines, hot flashes and night sweats, extreme irritability, and difficulty with bladder control (resulting from loss of uterine tone). They also describe unusually heavy, gushing periods, and periods that last from ten days to six weeks.

MENOPAUSE

An estimated 40 million American women are in or past menopause, with another 20 million due to reach menopause within the next decade. With the increase in life expectancy, many women will be spending one-third or more of their lives in postmenopausal years. Menopause by definition begins after the last spontaneous menstrual period.

Once a woman has gone from six to twelve months without a period, she is considered to have reached menopause. In the United States, the average age for menopause is fifty, although considerable variation certainly exists.

Many people tend to associate menopause with a host of psychological problems, particularly depression, loss of energy, and crying episodes. It isn't clear what amount of these reactions stems from hormonal changes and what may be due to negative images of older women. In any case, many women experience renewed zest and vigor after menopause. Anthropologist Margaret Mead called this period "postmenopausal zest," while author Gail Sheehy commented that postmenopausal women feel "a greater sense of well-being than any other stage of their lives."

> Studies show that women who predict that menopause will be miserable do, in fact, suffer more negative emotional and physical symptoms than women who expect it to be easier.

Hot Flashes

Some 85 percent of all women do experience hot flashes, either during perimenopause or in menopause itself. The physiology of the hot flash is still not understood, but it appears to start in the hypothalamus, "the body's thermostat," in response to a drop in estrogen. During a flash, a woman experiences a severe feeling of heat, especially in the head and neck, often in the entire upper half of the body. Sometimes the face is blotched and ruddy as a result of the dilation of blood vessels on the surface of the skin. In some cases, flashes are accompanied by disruptions in sleep patterns and night sweats.

In the Massachusetts Women's Health Study, the incidence of hot flashes rose from about 10 percent during the perimenopausal stage to about 50 percent just after cessation of menses, and dropped back to about 20 percent four years after menopause.

Flashes usually last for only a few minutes, but may continue for up to an hour. The body will attempt to cool down by beading with perspiration. Hot weather, hot food or drink, stress, and other sources of heat can trigger flashes without warning. Although most women experience them, few—only one in four—find them uncomfortable enough to seek treatment.

> Some studies have shown that as little as 15 to 30 IU of vitamin E daily helps ease hot flashes and vaginal dryness, prevents hysterectomy, and in some cases, eliminates the need for estrogen replacement.

Many women who seek estrogen treatment for their hot flashes do find relief. Yet in all cases, whether treated or not, they will eventually stop as soon as the body adjusts to postmenopausal levels of estrogen.

Lower Sex Drive

Another key symptom of menopause is the atrophy of the reproductive tract.

Estrogen, produced by the ovaries, keeps the uterus, vagina, and base of the bladder moist and supple. When estrogen levels start to fall, these organs start to shrink, and the vaginal walls thin. Generally, blood flow to the area decreases, as does lubrication. Women may have difficulty controlling their bladders under stress, and they're more likely to suffer from vaginal itching, dryness, and sometimes pain during or after intercourse. As a result, some women become less interested in sex. Other women may experience a loss in libido even without these symptoms.

Osteoporosis

This bone disease is another common response to menopause. Up until the mid-thirties, bone mass continues to grow; that is, our bodies use minerals, especially calcium, to strengthen, widen, and perhaps lengthen our bones. By age forty, however, minerals begin to be leeched out of the bones, making them more brittle. The extreme version of this condition is known as osteoporosis, a disease that affects 10 to 15 million Americans and causes some 1.5 million fractures a year. Of these, some 120,000 are elderly women who break their hips—accidents whose complications result in close to 20,000 annual deaths.

BOTANICAL NUTRIENTS THAT MAY EASE MENOPAUSE

Several botanical therapies that are commonly used to alleviate symptoms at the onset of menopause and that may provide comfort include:

Black cohosh and blue cohosh: Used extensively for hot flashes and in regulating the menstrual cycle and bringing on uterine bleeding. Both contain *phytosterols*—plant substances that have estrogen-like activities.

Dong quai: A Chinese herb otherwise known as angelica with anticoagulant properties. It is used to relieve menstrual cramping associated with PMS and to regulate hormonal imbalances in menopausal women. Dong quai has vital estrogen compounds that mimic the body's natural estrogen.

Motherwort: One of the most popular herbs used to combat menopausal symptoms. It has been shown to decrease the frequency, duration, and severity of hot flashes; thickens the vaginal wall; relieves anxiety; and lessens menstrual cramping and stress-related palpitations. May cause a rash in high doses.

Licorice root: Contains flavonoids that have an estrogen-like activity, and saponin, which has progestational-like activity. The root also has anti-inflammatory properties. Note that licorice root promotes potassium loss and sodium retention, can cause hypertension, is dangerous for those taking antihypertensives or diuretics, and can be addictive.

Red raspberry: A uterine wall relaxant and an antispasmodic, used to decrease uterine bleeding.

HOW ESTROGEN FIGHTS AGING

Proponents of estrogen cite both scientific studies and the experiences of numerous women to show that this female hormone can ease or eliminate menopausal woes. Estrogen supplements, which are available as skin patches, topical creams, and long-lasting injections, appear to relieve hot flashes, night sweats, and other discomforts, as well as vaginal dryness and atrophy. Some women find that this hormone helps keep their skin thicker, moister, and more youthful-looking.

Collagen, which is stimulated by estrogen, is the main protein in the dermis. A loss of collagen results in increased wrinkling, bruising, and thinning of the skin. Administering estrogen not only prevents collagen loss but also increases collagen synthesis, which can relieve symptoms of diminished urinary control sometimes experienced by menopausal women. Estrogen moistens the vaginal mucous membranes, which increases lubrication, and also helps maintain flexibility of the connective tissues.

Estrogen and progesterone supplements have also been proven to reduce the bone loss associated with osteoporosis. Women's bones slowly begin to lose minerals and become less dense even before menopause. After menopause, however, the pace accelerates rapidly for five to ten years. Estrogen inhibits bone re-absorption and progesterone stimulates bone formation. Unless a woman is taking these hormones, she has about a one-in-four chance of developing serious osteoporosis.

Osteoporosis increases the risk of bone fractures and all their ensuing complications. One study found that older women who took estrogen were subject to only half the number of bone fractures as those women who avoided the hormone supplement.

A recent analysis by the Postmenopausal Estrogen and Progestin Intervention Trial revealed that estrogen alone and in various combinations with progesterone is equally effective in increasing bone mass in postmenopausal women. Data found that fewer than 3 percent of women on estrogen therapy continued to lose a clinically relevant and measurable fraction of bone density at the spine.

By age seventy, almost 50 percent of women have had at least one osteoporotic fracture, at an estimated cost of $17 billion annually in the United States. A menopause symposium sponsored by the Oregon Health Sciences University School of Medicine concluded that estrogen is the therapy of choice for prevention and treatment of osteoporosis. Although supplemental calcium, diet, and exercise are also beneficial, they don't seem to be as effective as estrogen.

The most important benefit of estrogen replacement therapy is the reported reduction in coronary artery disease—the leading cause of death in postmenopausal women. Some 500,000 women die from coronary artery disease per year—that's twice as many women as those who die each year from cancer. Apparently, the high premenopausal levels of estrogen tend to protect women from heart disease, partly by keeping levels of HDL cholesterol high and LDL cholesterol low.

Without estrogen replacement, a woman's risk of heart attack becomes equal to a man's within fifteen years after menopause. Simply being postmenopausal puts a woman at a higher risk for heart disease, and having just one additional risk factor—smoking, high blood pressure, HDL cholesterol below 35 mg/dl, diabetes, or a family history of heart disease—puts her at an even higher risk. With estrogen, however, the blood vessels dilate slightly, cholesterol balance is maintained, and the risk of heart disease vastly decreases. This can be seen in a report from a ten-year study of some 48,470 nurses from the Nurses Health Study (National Health and Nutrition Examination Survey, or NHANES)—one of the largest studies to date—which found that estrogen use reduced the risk of major coronary disease and fatal cardiovascular disease by half. In addition, researchers at Baskent University (Turkey) found that a six-month combined estrogen-progesterone therapy administered to forty-six postmenopausal women significantly decreased plasma homocysteine levels, a new marker for heart disease.

Dr. Lawrence Brass of Yale University School of Medicine predicts that ERT may soon emerge as one of the most effective therapies for stroke prevention, cutting the risk of stroke in postmenopausal women in half. He believes that because estrogen prevents heart disease by 50 to 70 percent, it may also "plausibly" prevent stroke.

In a Leisure World prospective cohort study, estrogen therapy was associated with a 46 percent overall reduction in the risk of death from stroke, with a 70 percent reduction in recent users. This protection was present in women both with and without hypertension and in both smokers and nonsmokers. In addition, a population-based cohort study in Uppsala, Sweden, documented a 30 percent reduced incidence of stroke in postmenopausal users of estrogen, as well as in women given an estrogen-progestin combination.

However, a large cohort from the Nurses' Health Study produced results in striking contrast, failing to show a protective effect of estrogen against stroke. However, critics have pointed to the fact that the women in the study were too young, where there was little protective effect against stroke.

Although estrogen is primarily a female hormone, men also produce it. In fact, estrogen levels in men can be higher than in postmenopausal women.

In addition to reducing the risk of cardiovascular disease and osteoporosis, postmenopausal hormone replacement therapy may allow more women to retain their teeth as they age. By preventing osteoporosis, estrogen may add the benefit of preventing tooth loss and the need for dentures in older women. A new study of 3,921 women found that those on hormone replacement were 19 percent less likely to have some tooth loss and 36 percent less likely to have no teeth than women who had never taken hormones. Researchers also suggest that because tooth loss provides a measure of skeletal bone health, it may be the first clinical sign of osteoporosis.

Estrogen also seems to reduce the risk of colon cancer—and the longer a woman takes estrogen, the lower her risk. New research has found that estrogen users had a 29 percent lower risk of dying from colon cancer than nonusers; risk for users of ten years or more was 55 percent lower.

The North American Menopause Society suggests that the addition of a low-dose testosterone to oral estrogen therapy may be more effective than estrogen alone in diminishing symptoms of menopause in older women. Hot flashes and vaginal dryness seem to improve, and most significantly, fatigue, insomnia, irritability, and nervousness are relieved.

Estrogen administered transdermally was found by a team at Massachusetts General Hospital/Harvard Medical School (Massachusetts, USA) to promote the remission of depression. Even after a one-month period of not being administered the estrogen, the antidepressant benefit was sustained, treatment was well tolerated, and adverse events were rare. The researchers suggested that transdermal estradiol replacement is an effective treatment of depression for perimenopausal women.

Estrogen also appears to aid in the prevention of skin aging (see Chapter 20) in several ways. Scientists from the University of California San Francisco School of Medicine found that estrogen prevents a decrease in skin collagen in postmenopausal women; topical and systemic estrogen therapy can increase the skin collagen content and therefore maintain skin thickness. In addition, estrogen maintains skin moisture by increasing acid mucopolysaccharides and hyaluronic acid in the skin and possibly maintaining the function and integrity of the stratum corneum, the skin's outermost layer. Sebum levels are higher in postmenopausal women receiving hormone replacement therapy.

Skin wrinkling also may benefit from estrogen as a result of the effects of the hormone on the elastic fibers and collagen. Topical estrogen also was found to accelerate and improve wound healing in elderly men and women.

Researchers from the University of Vermont College of Medicine found that estrogen or replacement therapy, in nondiabetic women, improved parameters that regulate carbohydrate metabolism, including insulin resistance. Therefore, the team suggests that ERT could be of value for women with type II diabetes, not only in relieving menopausal symptoms but also in improving the metabolic abnormalities associated with diabetes and in preventing cardiovascular disease.

In order to get the positive benefits of ERT, doctors believe that it should be taken for at least seven years, although a full 95 percent of the women engaged in hormone replacement therapy continue for only three years or less. According to Dr. John Gallagher, an endocrinologist at Creighton University in Omaha, Nebraska, three years is "not long enough to get any positive effects on their bones."

Estrogen and Alzheimer's Disease

Mounting evidence suggests that estrogen supplements help ease the mental fogginess and memory lapses that many women experience after menopause. Studies have shown that women are three times more likely than men to suffer from Alzheimer's disease. Women's systems produce estrogen only until menopause, while men's bodies continue converting testosterone to estrogen into later life. Researchers believe this may provide men with natural protection against Alzheimer's disease. ERT has been shown to reduce or eliminate some of the symptoms of this disease by supporting the body's production of *acetylcholine,* a chemical that helps transmit nerve signals across synapses, which is abnormally low in people with Alzheimer's disease, and may explain their impaired abilities to learn and remember.

Estrogen plays a large role in the development and maintenance of our brain cells. Scientists now understand that estrogen helps shape the brain during the fetus's earliest stages of development, as both male and female fetuses are exposed to the estrogen in their mother's system. By the twelfth week of gestation, male fetuses are also producing testosterone in their testes, so that some male-female differences in learning and memory may be "hard-wired" very early on. Thus, boys tend to have greater facility with math, while girls have greater facility with language, have slightly superior hearing, and have more talent at interpreting facial expressions.

As children mature, they continue to rely on estrogen to keep their brains functioning at peak level. (Boys convert some testosterone to estrogen in the brain.) Apparently, estrogen increases the number of synapses, or connections, among nerve cells in the hippocampus, the region in the brain where new memories are formed. Research by Catherine Woolley of the University of Washington and Bruce McEwen of Rockefeller University found that removing the ovaries from rats caused the number of synapses in their hippocampuses to decline rapidly—although when the rats were given estrogen supplements, their synapses remained relatively intact.

In a related process, estrogen appears to protect nerve cells that produce acetylcholine. Meharvan Singh and James Simpkins of the University of Florida found that giving estrogen supplements to rats increased the rats' production of an enzyme needed for the production of acetylcholine. Rats that had access to estrogen, either from their own ovaries or from supplements, were twice as successful at learning to avoid an electric shock than were rats that had no ovaries and therefore no estrogen.

Apparently, estrogen helped the rats synthesize a protein known as the nerve-growth factor. Nerve-growth factor, created within the brain itself, promotes the health of cholinergic neurons, the cells that make and use acetylcholine. When rats had their ovaries removed and stopped producing estrogen, nerve-growth factor declined by nearly 45 percent over a period of only three months.

> In a Massachusetts research protocol, women who had undergone surgical menopause (removal of ovaries) were more likely to become depressed than those who went through natural menopause. Researchers speculate that the sudden termination of the body's estrogen supply—rather than a gradual decline—may explain the psychological impact as well as the decline in libido and orgasmic capacity.

Estrogen helps the part of the brain that governs new memory two ways: it creates more connections among nerve cells and helps information travel more easily along those connections. Conversely, a loss of estrogen means our bodies are manufacturing less nerve-growth factor; less nerve-growth factor means that our brains have fewer cholinergic neurons; fewer cholinergic neurons means that there is less acetylcholine in our brains; and less acetylcholine means that we'll have a harder time learning and remembering new things.

Tests of 158 postmenopausal women with either Alzheimer's disease or *ischemic vascular dementia* found that these women were only half as likely to have been on ERT as 148 cognitively normal women of the same age. A lack of estrogen actually doubled the risk of these dementias.

Psychologist Barbara Sherwin of Montreal's McGill University administered estrogen supplements to women whose ovaries had been removed and thus produced very little natural estrogen. Women who took the supplements, she found, could more easily learn and recall pairs of words than those who were given only a placebo. Interestingly, the estrogen seemed to affect only their verbal skills, having no effect on their visual memory.

Moreover, Sherwin found, young women with intact ovaries did better on word-pair memory tests during the phase of their menstrual cycle when estrogen levels were highest, while they did less well during menstruation itself, when estrogen levels had dropped. Sherwin says that the changes are too minor "to have any effect in the real world." Nevertheless, her results suggest the relationship between estrogen and mental functioning, a relationship that has powerful implications for women with Alzheimer's disease.

Dr. Howard Fillit, a geriatrician at Mount Sinai Medical Center in New York City, has given estrogen supplements to women with mild to moderate Alzheimer's disease. After only three weeks of daily hormone treatment, patients who could not remember the month or year were suddenly able to recall those details. The women also seemed more alert, showed improved social behavior, and ate and slept better. (Fillit suspects that male patients will benefit from testosterone supplements in similar ways.)

A larger-scale study at the University of Southern California found that estrogen supplements also helped in preventing Alzheimer's disease. Researchers examined the medical histories of some 2,418 women who had lived at a retirement home over a period of eleven years. Many of the women had been taking estrogen supplements for reasons unrelated to their condition. Statistics showed that women who had taken estrogen were 40 percent less likely to have developed the disease than those who hadn't. And the longer they had taken estrogen, the more their risk was reduced.

In August 2001, the Geriatric Research, Education and Clinical Center of the Veterans Affairs Puget Sound Health Care System (Washington, USA) assessed postmenopausal women with Alzheimer's disease. Those administered estrogen demonstrated clear improvements in scales measuring attention, verbal memory, and visual memory. In addition, women treated with estrogen demonstrated improved performance on a test of semantic (word) memory. The research team suggested that estrogen may enhance attention and memory for postmenopausal women with Alzheimer's disease.

THE ROLE OF PROGESTERONE

When ERT was first put into practice, estrogen was generally prescribed alone. Doctors later discovered that it was more effective and often safer in combination with progesterone.

Progesterone is the gestational hormone that prepares the lining of the uterus for the fertilized ovum and maintains pregnancy. It is derived primarily from the *corpus luteum* that is formed in the ovary from the ruptured follicle. It is also produced in the placenta during pregnancy and in small amounts by the adrenal cortex. Progesterone is a "precursor" hormone. This means that it can be converted by the body into other steroid hormones.

Artificially produced progesterone or *progestins* are synthetic hormones that closely resemble the body's own production of progesterone, but differ in important ways. Both natural and synthetic hormones share the ability to sustain the lining of the vagina and uterus but progestins do not have the full range of biological activity of natural progesterone. Progestin has actually been shown to inhibit biosynthesis of progesterone.

Some doctors now believe that progestin is responsible for a long list of side effects. And since many women who are engaged in hormone replacement therapy are filling their prescriptions with synthetic progesterone, they are exposing themselves to unnecessary risks.

According to Dr. David G. Williams, progestin can cause abnormal menstrual flow or cessation, fluid retention, nausea, insomnia, jaundice, depression, fever, weight fluctuations, allergic reactions, and the development of male characteristics. Natural progesterone, on the other hand, has few side effects: occasionally it may cause a feeling of euphoria, and, for some women, it may alter the timing of their menstrual cycles.

Dr. Williams recommends that women begin by taking vitamin supplements to increase their own production of progesterone. Animal studies suggest that beta-carotene can stimulate the production of this vital hormone. Likewise, a daily dose of 150 IU of vitamin E can raise progesterone levels; however, dosages of 300 to 600 IU of vitamin E can actually lower levels of the hormone.

San Francisco nutritionist Linda Ojeda advocates dietary sources of estrogen and progesterone: soybean products such as tofu, miso, and soymilk. These products contain phytoestrogens, which have different levels of estrogenic activity. Women who are reluctant to take synthetic estrogens may consider phytoestrogens as an alternative therapeutic agent. Ojeda points out that Japanese women experience a very low rate of menopausal complaints, which she attributes to their high consumption of soybeans.

For women who want more, Dr. Williams recommends natural progesterone. Unfortunately, natural hormone supplements are hard to come by, since drug companies cannot patent them and therefore are not interested in selling them commercially. Cream extracted from the Mexican wild yam (*Dioscorea mexicana*) has long been recognized as a natural source of estrogen and progesterone. Dioscorea is not a hormone. It is the food for hormone production in the body, and because of its effect on DHEA, it affects the production of all hormones, not only estrogen and progesterone. Products made from the ovaries of cows may help a woman who still has her ovaries to raise her own progesterone levels. Other alternatives are creams containing plant-derived estrogens and progesterones.

Dr. Julian Whitaker, medical director of the Wellness Institute in Newport Beach, California, also points to the importance of progesterone in treating menopause: "Estrogen slows down the leaching of calcium from the bone, but does not facilitate deposition of calcium in the bone to strengthen it. Progesterone does that, and given by itself, will not only prevent osteoporosis, but will even reverse it."

Like Dr. Williams, Dr. Whitaker recommends natural, topical hormone creams for both progesterone and estrogen supplements. He cites the work of Dr. John Lee, who treated a group of 100 patients over six years with transdermal ("through the skin") natural progesterone only. Lee's patients experienced no significant side effects while enjoying increased bone density and strength.

HRT: RISK VERSUS BENEFIT

Unfortunately, as breast-cancer specialist Dr. Susan Love points out, "there's no free lunch." In addition to estrogen's unquestioned benefits, it also poses a number of proven and suspected dangers, drawbacks that may make it an undesirable treatment for many women.

Estrogen therapy has come under controversy in light of recent studies on its possible link to various cancers, most notably breast cancer. One study demonstrated that patients receiving estrogen (with and without progestin) had a 30 to 40 percent increased risk of breast cancer. Another study, however, reported no increased risk of breast cancer in women who had ever taken combined estrogen-progestin HRT. These conflicting results underscore the continued uncertainty over estrogen's possible role in breast cancer risk.

Breast cancer is more likely to occur in premenopausal women with normal or high estrogen levels and low progesterone levels. This situation may occur in early adult life in a few women but is quite common after age thirty-five. It also occurs after menopause when women are given estrogen supplements without progesterone.

Some researchers estimate that a woman's risk of endometrial cancer is four times greater if she is taking estrogen supplements. A study of 240,000 women sponsored by the American Cancer Society found that women who took estrogen for at least six years had a 40 percent increased risk of contracting ovarian cancer; women who had taken estrogen for eleven or more years faced an increased risk of 70 percent. Again, this risk can be greatly eliminated by the co-administration of progestin.

Other proven risks of ERT include the possible return of menstrual bleeding when taken with progesterone. Women sometimes experience premenstrual symptoms such as fluid retention, tender breasts, irritability, and a possible increase in the growth of benign fibroid tumors in the uterus. Many women also risk abnormal blood clots, weight gain, an increased likelihood of gallstones, and migraine headaches.

For these reasons, ERT is usually not recommended for women at high risk for breast cancer. People who suffer from high blood pressure are also advised not to take estrogen, as the supplement tends to raise levels.

Estrogen/progesterone combined should be avoided in women with any of the following conditions or circumstances: known or suspected pregnancy; known or suspected breast cancer; known or suspected estrogen-dependent neoplasia; undiagnosed abnormal genital bleeding; active or past history of thrombophlebitis, thromboembolic disorders, or stroke; or liver dysfunction or disease. Always consult with your physician before embarking on estrogen/progesterone therapy or any type of hormone replacement therapy.

HRT and Breast Cancer

The relationship between the estrogens and the risk of breast cancer has been studied intensively. Presently, there is no conclusive evidence that the estrogen doses known to protect against osteoporosis and cardiovascular disease increase the risk of breast cancer. However, various studies have suggested that

Clarification Regarding the Women's Health Initiative Study

In the early summer of 2002, the United States of America's National Heart, Lung, and Blood Institute (NHLBI) of the National Institutes of Health (NIH) halted the Women's Health Initiative (WHI). The large multicenter trial administered conjugated equine estrogens with medroxyprogesterone acetate to healthy menopausal women. While the WHI did find "noteworthy benefits of estrogen plus progestin, including fewer cases of hip fractures and colon cancer," reports of the number of cases of invasive breast cancer exceeded the predefined safety boundary, causing the premature termination of the WHI study. The researchers terminated this study because they found an increased risk of invasive breast cancer and coronary heart disease that outweighed the benefits from the hormone replacement therapy. In halting the WHI study, the NHLBI conceded that, over the time of 10,000 personal years of women taking this form of HRT, they would expect that:

- only seven more women would have a heart attack; and
- only eight more cases of invasive breast cancer would be diagnosed;

whereas:

- colon cancer reduced by six cases; and
- hip fractures reduced by five cases

In addition, NHLBI failed to disclose that their researchers used synthetic, not bioidentical, hormones in the treatment protocol of WHI. Bioidentical hormones have the same chemical structure as hormones that are made in the human body. The term "bioidentical" reflects that the chemical structure of the replacement hormone is identical to that of the hormone naturally found in the human body. In order for a replacement hormone to fully replicate the function of hormones that were originally naturally produced and present in the human body, the chemical structure must exactly match the original. Thus, bioidentical replacement therapy (BHRT) is a method by which replaced hormones follow normal metabolic pathways so that the essential active metabolites are formed in response to the treatment. The molecular differences between bioidentical and non-bioidentical may prove to be the defining aspect in terms of hormone replacement therapy safety, and we find NHLBI remiss in making this differentiation and thereby causing undue extra public alarm.

the two hormones increase a woman's risk of breast cancer by as much as 30 percent. Also, studies have found that women whose ovaries were removed early in life have markedly reduced rates of breast cancer, presumably because they lack ovarian estrogen and progesterone. Early menarche and late menopause—an extended period of estrogen production—have also been shown to increase the risk of breast cancer.

In the Nurses' Health Study, Harvard researchers looked at 70,000 healthy women who had reached menopause. Roughly one-third used ERT, and a third of those used a formulation that included synthetic progesterone. Using estrogen for more than five years gave women 1.3 to 1.4 times the risk of developing breast cancer. Therefore, taking hormones continuously from age fifty-five onward gave a woman a 3 percent chance of developing the disease between ages sixty and sixty-five, whereas a woman who chose not to receive ERT would have less than a 2 percent chance. Also, the use of synthetic progesterone neither increased nor decreased the risks found with estrogen alone. The risk rapidly diminished when women stopped taking the hormones altogether.

> Industrial pollutants having potent estrogenic effects called xeno-estrogens are recognized as a pervasive environmental threat and a contributing factor in the incidence of breast cancer. New research shows that plastic dishes, utensils, food cartons, food wrap, and beverage bottles can leach mildly estrogenic agents into foods. At this time, your best choice for kitchenware is glass.

An extended follow-up of participants in the Nurses' Health Study showed that current estrogen users were 32 percent more likely to develop breast cancer, and current users of estrogen and progestin were 41 percent more likely to develop breast cancer than women who had never taken hormones. Women who were currently on estrogen, and had been for more than five years, were 46 percent more likely to develop breast cancer than nonusers. The risk was even greater for older women. A sixty- to sixty-four-year-old woman who had been on estrogen therapy for more than five years was 71 percent more likely to develop breast cancer than a nonuser of the same age.

Doctors are at odds about how seriously to take these reports. "The benefits of [HRT] will outweigh the risks for most people," says Dr. William Andrews, former president of the American College of Obstetrics and Gynecology. "Eight times as many women die of heart attacks as die of breast cancer."

Breast Cancer and Early Detection

Early detection is crucial in the battle against breast cancer. It strikes one out of eight women, nearly 78 percent of cases occurring in women over age fifty. Despite strong evidence that yearly mammograms could cut the number of breast cancer deaths by one-third, a National Cancer Institute study found that in 1990 only 39 percent of women in their fifties, and 36 percent of those sixty and older had a mammogram in the past year. And 40 percent of women over fifty have never had a mammogram!

• In 2002 there will be more than 203,500 new cases of breast cancer in the United States; 20 percent of these cases will be fatal.

• If a malignancy is present in a woman over age fifty, mammography has a 90 percent chance of finding it.

• Women who undergo regular mammography are more likely to be diagnosed early, when the chances of being cured are higher and less radical treatment options are available.

In a study of more than 1,000 women with operable breast cancer, those whose cancers were diagnosed by mammography had tumors that were significantly smaller and more often lymph node-negative (both a result of early diagnosis), compared with women whose malignances were not detected by mammography. If you are over age forty, it is important for a physician to examine your breasts every one to three years. After age forty, the American Cancer Society recommends a screening mammography every one to two years. And if you are fifty or older, it's a good idea to have a mammogram every year.

It is important to realize that breast cancer should not be categorized by age. It does strike women under age forty, some cases even occurring in women in their twenties. Therefore, if you have a history of breast cancer in your family or have any suspicious lumps, do not rule out mammography as a protective measure. The dose of radiation needed to get a clear image of the breast today is one-fourth as high as it was ten years ago. Facilities accredited by the American College of Radiology use equipment that exposes the breast to 0.3 rad (radiation-absorbed dose), which is comparable to the exposure in a dental X-ray.

On the other hand, Dr. Isaac Schiff, chief of obstetrics and gynecology at Massachusetts General Hospital, comments, "Basically, you're presenting women with the possibility of increasing the risk of getting breast cancer at 60 in order to prevent a heart attack at 70 and a hip fracture at age 80. How can you make that decision for a patient?"

It is important to realize that not all estrogens are equivalent in their actions on breast tissue. Natural estrogen actually takes three forms: *estrone, estradiol,* and *estriol.* Estrone is the most stimulating to breast tissue, estradiol is second, and estriol is by far the least. Estradiol has actually been shown to decrease the risk of breast cancer. Synthetic estrogen supplements are composed primarily of estrone and estradiol. On the other hand, natural estrogen is high in estriol.

Women should realize that estrogen alone does not contribute to breast cancer. Many other hormone-related risk factors seem to appear as a woman approaches menopause. For example, postmenopausal obese women have a greater chance of developing breast cancer because fatty tissue produces a form of estrogen. But, interestingly enough, premenopausal obese women enjoy significantly less risk of early breast cancer than leaner women. A woman who gives birth in her late teens or early twenties increases her risk of early breast cancer, as do women who have children after age thirty. Over time, the risk falls, becoming much smaller after menopause.

These are but a few examples that illustrate how complicated the biology of breast cancer really is. Will estrogen therapy increase a woman's chances of developing breast cancer? Conflicting evidence has kept this controversy alive, but the risk appears to be small, weighed against the long-term benefits for heart and bone.

TAKING ESTROGEN

Although many women take estrogen supplements, many also report feeling worried, skeptical, or discouraged about the effects. A 1987 national poll showed that one-fifth of the women given a prescription for estrogen never fill it. Of those who do, one-third stop within nine months, and more than half stop within a year. Still others stop their hormone supplements and then start them again, moving back and forth between the discomforts of being on estrogen and the frustrations of being off it.

Natural supplements, such as those mentioned in this chapter, may be the solution for some of these women. However, nutritional therapies are not nearly as powerful as hormone supplementation. Women may also benefit

Advance in Estrogen Delivery System

ERT took another step forward with the release of Vivelle (estradiol transdermal system). This Ciba Pharmaceuticals product is a medication that is actually embedded in the adhesive of a multipolymer, thin, clear, flexible patch, which is applied to the body twice weekly. This gives the skin direct contact with the medication and allows the skin itself to control the rate of transmission.

from a healthy regimen: not smoking, moderate alcohol intake, regular aerobic exercise (twenty to thirty minutes, three to five times a week), a low-fat, high-fiber diet, and vitamin and mineral supplements. Indeed, many women have reported that their menopausal symptoms eased or disappeared as they paid more attention to diet and exercise.

In addition to having an anticancer effect on cells, soybeans manipulate estrogen by blocking the hormone's ability to stimulate malignant changes in breast tissue. Thus, soybeans should help thwart both the occurrence and spread of breast cancer in both premenopausal and postmenopausal women.

Making a decision about going on HRT can be difficult—but it's a decision that virtually all women over forty have to face sooner or later. Knowing the facts can help. So, too, can coming to terms with your own responses to aging. Women approaching, entering, or living with menopause can derive huge benefits from a holistic approach to easing this stage in their lives, considering hormone therapy, diet and lifestyle, and emotional support as they seek the treatment that is right for them.

CHAPTER 8

The "Male Motor": Testosterone

Just as estrogen and progesterone are the female sex hormones, testosterone is the male sex hormone (although women have testosterone levels one-tenth to one-twelfth those of men). Testosterone is the main hormone produced in the testicles and secreted by the testes.

The major effects of testosterone are:

- promotes libido, aggressiveness, and sexual desire;

- stimulates the growth of certain organs;

- promotes protein anabolism, that is, the use of protein to build muscle, skin, and bone, and militates against protein catabolism, or breakdown;

- stimulates sperm production;

- nourishes all the tissues of the male urinary and reproductive systems;

- regulates the production of prostaglandin, which seems to keep prostate growth under control.

The effects of testosterone are most pronounced during puberty. It brings on the enlarged larynx, thicker vocal cords, new body hair, increased muscle mass, and increased oil-gland secretion by the skin commonly associated with puberty. After puberty, levels of testosterone drop gradually in men, with profound effects on physical health and well-being and particularly on mood and libido.

Some males suffer when their bodies produce insufficient levels of testosterone, resulting in a condition called *hypogonadism*. Hypogonadism can be caused by ailments of the testes, such as testicular injury or infection, Klinefelter's syndrome (a chromosomal abnormality), and/or from disorders of the pituitary and hypothalamus glands.

Dr. Anthony Karpas, director of the Institute for Endocrinology and Reproductive Medicine in Atlanta, believes that the condition is underdiagnosed. He states, "As many as 20 percent of men over age 50 may be hypogonadal."

Some telltale signs of hypogonadism are:

- loss of sex drive/inability to maintain an erection

- fatigue

- irritability

- depressed mood

- aches and pains in the joints

- dry skin

- osteoporosis

- loss of weight

- absence or regression of secondary sexual characteristics, such as muscle development, deep voice, and hair distribution on the chest and face

Testosterone production is affected by a number of external factors, such as illness, medications, psychological state, obesity, exercise, and lifestyle (smoking and excessive alcohol intake). Factors such as reduced activity, nutritional deficiency, diabetes, and growth hormone deficiency can also contribute to lower levels.

> It is estimated that testosterone levels will drop to abnormally low levels in 20 percent of men after age fifty.

ANDROPAUSE: THE MALE MENOPAUSE

The phenomenon termed *andropause*, (known in England as *viropause*) involves the progressive decline of free testosterone levels with age, coupled with an increase in production of a protein called *sex hormone-binding globulin*. Testosterone links with the protein, reducing its availability to the tissues. As a result of these hormonal changes, men as early as age forty can develop impotency or libido problems.

A large-scale epidemiological study of male sexual behavior called The Massachusetts Male Aging Study of 1984–89 looked at a cross-sectional random

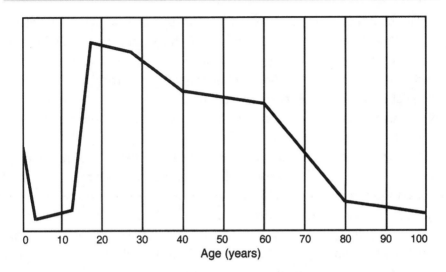

FIGURE 8.1. Testosterone levels by age.

sample of 1,709 men between ages forty and seventy. It was found that mean testosterone levels decline annually by about one percent. Also, 51 percent of normal, healthy males in this age group reported experiencing some degree of impotence. However, Dr. Irwin Goldstein, an organizer of the study, points out that organic factors contribute to impotence in up to 80 percent of men affected. Goldstein cites diabetes, hypertension (medications used), smoking, chronic alcohol use, and high cholesterol as major factors in loss of male potency.

Andropause is not universally understood, and study of the phenomenon is still relatively new. However, scientists do know that it is not analogous to menopause. As we learned in the last chapter, the profound reduction in ovarian function at the time of menopause for women has substantial physiologic consequences, including an accelerated loss of bone mass, sleep and behavioral changes, vaginal atrophy, and the loss of fertility. Andropause can also have profound effects on physical health and well-being in men, particularly on mood and libido, and some men even experience sweating and hot flashes at night. But the difference between the two conditions is that men experience a more gradual and incomplete loss of testicular function with increasing age (many men can sire children well into older age), resulting in reduced testosterone and sperm production.

HOW TESTOSTERONE FIGHTS AGING

Men diagnosed with hypogonadism are good candidates for testosterone replacement therapy (TRT). However, only about 5 percent of the estimated 4 to 5 million American men with hypogonadism currently receive TRT.

Major studies of TRT in hypogonadal men ages fifty to sixty-five were conducted at the University of Utah, Johns Hopkins University, and Karolinska Hospital in Stockholm Sweden. Overall, treatment resulted in normalization of morning testosterone levels in 92 percent of the ninety-four patients who completed the trials.

While most people think of testosterone as the "sex drive" hormone in men, it has a multitude of additional and noteworthy benefits. University of Texas (USA) researchers found that "High endogenous testosterone levels predict better performance on visual spatial tests," noting that "Testosterone replacement in hypogonadic patients improved cognitive functions." The team concludes that "Androgen replacement may be beneficial for treating cognitive decline in some male patients."

In April 2002, researchers from the University at Munster, Germany, conducted a study to compare sixty-one testosterone-treated hypogonadal men with twenty-four untreated hypogonadal men and sixty healthy eugonadal men (men with levels of testosterone consistent with that for their age): The hypogonadal men who did not receive testosterone, and the untreated men, all experienced rising body mass index (BMI; a marker of overweight), and increasing fat mass with age. In contrast, the hypogonadal men who received testosterone supplementation did not experience any age-dependent change in BMI, body fat content, or serum leptin (the hormone scientists suspect is responsible for fat deposits). The German team concludes that "Ageing men should benefit from testosterone substitution as far as body composition is concerned."

The mood of elderly depressed males can benefit from testosterone replacement therapy. Sixteen elderly men were administered testosterone for six weeks. Researchers noticed a 42 percent decrease in responses on the depression rating scale, with men late-onset depression (occurring after forty-five years old) gaining the greatest mood improvement. All totaled, 50 percent of the late-onset depression patients experienced remission of their depressive state thanks to TRT.

As for sexual drive and performance, another eight-week study of twenty-nine patients produced notable improvements in erectile function, libido and mood, and decreases in complaints of fatigue.

Men undergoing andropause have also benefited from TRT. One study of men over age fifty who received the hormone found that it renewed strength, improved balance, increased red blood cell count, increased libido, and lowered LDL cholesterol. In a double-blind, placebo-controlled, crossover study, thirteen healthy elderly men with low testosterone levels were given 100 mg of the hormone a week for three months. Twelve of them experienced behavioral changes such as increased libido and feelings of well-being.

Another study of men ages fifty-seven to seventy-five found that testosterone supplementation likewise increased red blood cell count and lowered LDL cholesterol as well as overall cholesterol levels. Of the thirteen men in the study who were receiving testosterone (as compared with a control group that was receiving a placebo), twelve could predict that they were, in fact, getting the actual supplement, because they felt more aggressive and energetic at work. In addition, the men reported better sexual performance, more frequent initiation of sexual intercourse, and increased ability to maintain an erection.

Dr. Michael Perring, medical director of the Optimal Health Clinic in London, which specializes in hormone replacement therapies, has seen more than 800 patients with symptoms of andropause. Dr. Perring believes that the benefits of TRT in conjunction with other hormone precursors, such as DHEA, are beneficial to men who have demonstrably low testosterone levels for their age. However, he stresses the importance of a full-patient assessment, including a careful history, clinical examination, and endocrine, biochemical, and blood profiles before embarking on therapeutic interventions.

In addition, Dr. Perring points out that an individual's lifestyle, including physical, emotional, and sexual factors, can put strain on the prostate. "The lifestyles of men attending the clinic suggest a high prevalence of stress either in the workplace or at home, with poor communication within the primary relationship. There may be excessive alcohol intake, high cigarette consumption, and a sedentary job with inadequate or inappropriate exercise. The total cholesterol and HDL cholesterol levels may be elevated with a diet that is erratic, and unbalanced by too much saturated fat and insufficient fresh fruit, vegetables and fiber."

Numerous studies have found correlation between low testosterone levels and higher risks of cardiovascular disease. Men who have had heart attacks tend to have low testosterone levels, according to Dr. Gerald Phillips of Columbia University Medical School. Phillips studied fifty-five men undergoing X-ray exams of their arteries and found that those with low testosterone levels had higher degrees of heart disease. He also found that men with higher testosterone levels also had higher protective HDL cholesterol levels.

Another study demonstrating the positive effects of testosterone on heart disease was conducted by Dr. Maurice Lesser. He studied the effect of testosterone injections in 100 people with angina pectoris—caused by a spasm or blockage of arteries in the heart. Ninety-one of the 100 showed "moderate to marked" improvement in chest pain, with both the frequency and severity of heart attacks reduced. Only nine showed no improvement at all.

Advocates of HGH in elderly men are also focusing on TRT because of its comparative cheapness and bone-strengthening qualities. After age sixty, hip fracture rates in men increase dramatically. Short-term studies with testosterone on mildly deficient elderly males have reported beneficial effects on lean body mass and muscle. According to Dr. Fran Kaiser, associate director of geriatric medicine at St. Louis University School of Medicine, hypogonadal males are about six times more likely to break a hip during a fall than are those with normal testosterone levels.

TAKING TESTOSTERONE

Most physicians today prefer to use pure natural testosterone, which may be administered by intramuscular injections, suppositories, a patch attached to the scrotum, a cream applied to the scrotum or elsewhere on the body, oral capsules, or sublingual lozenges. There are also experimental forms that include pellets that are implanted under the skin. Administration of testosterone in the form of a percutaneous gel (absorbed by the skin into the bloodstream) is currently used in Europe and has been shown to be very effective in mimicking the natural mode. In the United States, compounding pharmacies custom formulate testosterone creams to suit an individual's therapeutic needs. The least effective method seems to be via the oral route: studies have shown that testosterone administered this way becomes inactive. Synthetic testosterone such as methyl testosterone is not recommended because of its link to liver damage.

Testosterone for Women

Women's ovaries and adrenal glands do provide a modest amount of testosterone—one-tenth to one-twelfth in the blood. When the ovaries shut down during menopause, the quantity is cut in half. Women who opt for ERT usually notice a lessening of hot flashes and other symptoms. However, a small number of women do not. Researchers believe that these women may be more sensitive to the accompanying loss of testosterone. Dr. John Moran of the Optimal Health Clinic in London has pioneered HRT over the past few years, prescribing testosterone to men as well as to women. He has noticed that many women respond positively when a dash of testosterone is added to their ERT program. Notably, libido and energy seem to be replenished.

However, more research is needed to determine if the benefits outweigh the risks. Possible side effects of TRT in women can range from masculinization, including unnatural body hair growth and deep voice to acne, oily skin, higher blood pressure, and an increased risk of heart disease.

TESTICULAR AND PROSTATE CANCER

While prostate cancer usually hits men after age fifty, testicular cancer is the most common malignancy diagnosed in men between ages twenty and thirty-five. However, this type of cancer is not common, accounting for one percent of cancers in men.

Testicular Cancer

Unlike prostate cancer, testicular cancer is virtually without symptoms. Some men experience a dull ache or a sensation of heaviness in the lower abdomen or groin area. But even if no pain exists, it is important to do a monthly self-exam, as follows:

- Perform the exam after a warm bath or when the scrotal skin is relaxed;

- Massage the surface of the testicle lightly, using both hands. Remember to check both testicles;

- If you experience any pain, feel any lumps or hardness, or notice that one testicle is larger than the other, consult your physician. He may administer blood tests and/or an ultrasound to find the problem.

Diet and exercise don't play much of a role in prevention of testicular cancer. The most important measure a man can take to detect any cancers early is self-examination.

Prostate Cancer

The prostate gland, otherwise known as the "male breast" because of some of its parallels to the mammary gland in women, is about the size of a chestnut and weighs less than an ounce. It contains about 70 percent glandular tissue and 30 percent fibromuscular tissue. It plays a significant role in the male reproductive system. Responsible for the production of semen, the prostate adds fluid to the sperm to power it during ejaculation and increase its mobility. It also provides a potassium-and-enzyme-rich fluid that bathes and nourishes the sperm for good health, and serves as its storage area.

The prostate sits just below the urinary bladder in the bottom of the pelvis, surrounding the urethra. All during a man's life, the prostate continues to grow. At puberty, it reaches adult size; around age twenty-five, it goes through a second stage of growth; and it enlarges again between the ages of forty and fifty. It is in the last stage that the prostate gland may cause problems.

> More than 50 percent of men who have reached age seventy will have an enlarged prostate gland. And by age eighty, the number goes up to 80 percent.

These problems have become so prevalent that cancer of the prostate has become the second most diagnosed malignancy in men. Nearly 180,000 men were diagnosed with prostate cancer in 1999, and close to 50,000 men will die as a result of it. It is the second leading killer of men after heart disease. However, very few of these cases occur in men under age fifty. The risk for African-American men, overall, is substantially higher, perhaps due to a diet higher in saturated fat.

The best way to detect prostate enlargement early is to have a routine physical exam of the prostate (most men have their first exam just after turning age forty) and a PSA blood test (which is discussed in the inset "Detection of Prostate Cancer" on the next page). However, because the first symptoms of prostate cancer are so vague, 90 percent of these cancers go undetected. Therefore, it is important to familiarize yourself with the prostate and signs of abnormality in order to spot cancers before they spread beyond the easily treated stage.

Some symptoms of prostate enlargement include:

- frequent daytime and nighttime urination

- slight pain or a burning sensation during urination

- dribbling and difficulty starting or stopping urine flow

- standing a long time before urination

- leakage of urine

- straining to empty your bladder

- blood in the urine

- inflammation or swelling

- decreased sexual activity/painful intercourse

- back pain

Detection of Prostate Cancer

In addition to the *digital rectal exam* (DRE), where a physician feels the back of the prostate with his fingers, the *prostate specific antigen* (PSA) blood test significantly increases the ability to detect cancers and identify any abnormalities early, even before they can be felt on the exam. A recent study published in the *Journal of the American Medical Association* suggests that "a combination of PSA testing and DRE may nearly double the detection rate for localized prostate cancer . . ."

The PSA is a test of an enzyme produced by normal and cancerous prostate cells. Normally, a small amount of PSA is constantly released into the bloodstream. When the prostate is irritated or damaged, larger amounts of PSA can be detected by the blood test, suggesting an increased possibility of cancer.

The normal range of a healthy PSA level is 0.0 to 4.0. Some PSA tests have the upper limit of normal as 2.5, depending on the type of test administered. Men with prostate cancer usually have PSA levels in the 10s or 20s, and sometimes as high as the hundreds or thousands, indicating that the cancer may have spread to the bones or lymph nodes. However, an elevated PSA level doesn't always indicate cancer. Causes can include inflammation or infection of the prostate, simple enlargement or BPH, prostate stones, a recent urinary procedure, a recent prostate biopsy, or prostate or bladder surgery. Because the test is organ-specific, non-urinary infections such as the flu will not affect PSA level.

Most physicians recommend both the DRE prostate exam and the PSA test once a year after age fifty. For high-risk patients, it is recommended that they have three yearly ultrasounds in addition to a PSA test every six months.

Three of the most common problems associated with the prostate are infection, enlargement, and cancer. The condition known as *benign prostate hyperplasia* (BPH), the medical term for a non-cancerous enlarged prostate, involves an infection that usually starts in some other part of the body and travels to the prostate. BPH can also be caused by an inflammation (*prostatitis*), a benign tumor, or even a dietary or nutritional imbalance. The prostate swells and pinches off urine flow to the urethra, and if not treated immediately, it can completely block the flow of urine. This squeezing of the urethra causes painful constriction and an excess of urine in the bladder. The bladder then becomes infected, passing the infection on to the kidneys. Some researchers believe this enlargement may be caused by a reduced production of testosterone with age, coupled with increased production of testosterone in the form of dihydrotestosterone (DHT). DHT is what causes baldness in men and overproduction of prostate cells and enlargement.

Treatments for Prostate Disorders

The standard treatments for prostate cancers are radical *prostectomy* (total removal of the prostate gland) and radiation therapy. Both treatments can cause serious side effects such as impotence and urinary incontinence. According to a review conducted by the Patient Outcomes Research Team (PORT), 25 percent of men after surgery and six percent of men after radiation suffer from incontinence. In addition, about 85 percent of men after surgery and 40 percent after radiation reported changes in sexual function.

Although radiation and surgery may be the only alternative for advanced prostate disorders, drugs such as Finasteride and Terazosin are available to treat prostate enlargement without an operation.

Finasteride has been shown to shrink the prostate by blocking the activity of an enzyme that converts testosterone into DHT. However, the results, which can take anywhere from three to six months, have been mixed. A study of 895 men conducted at twenty-five medical centers across the United States found that 50 percent of men tested experienced an overall reduction in BPH. Other studies have shown a less than 50 percent reduction rate or no effect—positive or negative—on prostate cancer.

A problem with Finasteride is that it reduces the PSA level, which can complicate an accurate reading on a blood test. According to Dr. Jerome Richie, professor of surgery at Harvard and chief of urology at Brigham and Women's Hospital, if PSA levels have not dropped by one-third to one-half after taking Finasteride for several months, cancer may be present.

Also often prescribed for BPH, Terazosin, an alpha-blocker drug, works by alleviating some of the most troublesome symptoms of BPH by relaxing muscle tissue and ending the constriction of urine flow. Studies have shown that Terazosin can produce results in a few weeks and that the drug doesn't affect PSA levels.

Be aware, however, that the use of these drugs does not represent a permanent cure for BPH. It is common to both drugs that once you stop taking them prostate symptoms return.

Preventing Prostate Problems

Diet and lifestyle play a critical role in the health of the prostate. Research points to a sedentary lifestyle, a diet high in fat and low in fiber with an abundance of sugar and processed foods, and excessive intake of alcohol and caffeine as the main cause of many prostate disorders. Dr. James Balch reported in the *Journal of Longevity Research* that "the evidence that diet and lifestyle are important comes from the observation of health patterns in many underdeveloped countries, where unrefined, high-fiber diets and physical activity typify daily life—and where prostate ailments are extremely rare."

It is imperative that men take a preventive approach toward prostate care. Of course, not smoking and drinking little or no alcohol are obvious initiatives for maintaining overall health. Here are some of the other dietary and lifestyle changes that we recommend:

- *Lower cholesterol.*
  The American Heart Association recommends lowering total blood cholesterol levels to no more than 200 mg/deciliter of blood. Enlarged prostate tissue is high in cholesterol, and lowering levels seems to improve symptoms.

- *Eat less fat.*
  Some researchers believe that fat actually triggers prostate disease and can speed its growth. In particular, red meat, dairy products, and fried foods are red-light areas. Countries with low-fat diets, such as Japan, have a notably lower prostate cancer rate than those of western countries, with their much higher-fat diets. Another major reason for Japan's lower rate may be a high soybean intake, which researchers strongly believe inhibits prostate growth and cancers in general. (High-fat diets appear to be associated only with aggressive, rapidly developing prostate cancer, and not with the much

more common localized, slow-growing form that often remains dormant for years.)

- ***Avoid red meat and dairy foods.***
  Some studies have indicated that the fatty alpha-linolenic acid might be a strong link in stimulating tumor growth. Red meat and dairy foods are high in alpha-linolenic acid and low in linolenic acid, a polyunsaturated fat abundant in corn, safflower, soybean, and sunflower oils. Researchers believe the imbalance of these two fats may contribute to tumor growth.

- ***Eat more vegetables.***
  Cruciferous vegetables, such as broccoli, cabbage, cauliflower, Brussel sprouts, Swiss chard, kale, spinach, beets, carrots, sweet potatoes, and yams, all contain powerful anticancer nutrients. These foods are high in beta-carotene, which has been shown to reduce and/or slow rapid cell growth in cancers. In order to reduce your risk of cancer, it is important to eat five to ten servings of fresh fruit and vegetables a day, every day, not just once in a while.

- ***Get enough zinc.***
  Studies show that men with genitourinary problems tend to be zinc deficient and should be supplementing or eating foods rich in the mineral. In fact, a healthy prostate gland normally contains about ten times more zinc than any other organ in the body! The *Journal of Steroid Biochemistry* reported that zinc prevents the hormonal action that causes prostate enlargement. Furthermore, it has an antibacterial factor that kills organisms causing urinary infections, and, aside from being critical to testosterone synthesis and sperm formation, zinc is essential to healthy prostate functioning. In an article in the *Journal of Nutrition,* Drs. Gary Evans and E. C. Johnson recommend that when zinc is taken orally, it should be taken in conjunction with the nutrient pyridoxine, because pyridoxine is essential in converting zinc to a form that the prostate can readily use.

- ***Exercise, exercise.***
  Men who exercise for at least an hour a day are at significantly less risk for prostate cancer than men who don't. Therefore, it is important that you exercise. (It's also important that you drink a lot of water, preferably steam-distilled. Two to three quarts of water a day stimulates urine flow and helps

prevent retention, cystitis, and kidney infection.) Also, vigorous exercise on a routine basis has proven to maintain free-circulating testosterone in the body.

Other helpful nutrients that can prevent and aid in relieving many of the symptoms of an enlarged and inflamed prostate include:

- **Vitamins A and E**
  Known as "protector nutrients," these two vitamins have an exceptional ability to aid in recovery from prostate ailments. Both vitamins also play a significant role in sustaining and enhancing the immune system.

- **Vitamin B$_6$**
  This B vitamin enhances zinc absorption and helps combat the adverse effects of too much prolactin. Increased prolactin levels in men over age forty can contribute to the development of tumors in the prostate.

- **Selenium**
  Early research points to a relationship between increased selenium intake and a reduced risk for developing prostate cancer. Selenium also fights the noxious effects of cadmium, which have been shown to cause prostate enlargement in males. Cadmium is found in cigarettes; in beverages and foods such as coffee, tea, soft drinks, and seafood; and in the atmosphere from leaks in car batteries.

- **Magnesium**
  This mineral is helpful for benign prostate problems and prostatitis. It improves muscle function, muscle relaxation and contraction, and aids the immune system in fighting off infection. However, it is important to balance high doses of magnesium with vitamin B$_6$.

- **Lycopene**
  This natural substance gives tomatoes their red color. (Watermelon and pink grapefruit have lycopene too, but in much smaller amounts.) It is a very powerful anticancer phytochemical that has been shown to prevent and slow the growth of cancer cells. Specifically, a study indicated that lycopene intake reduced the risk of prostate cancer considerably, the benefit increasing with the number of servings of tomatoes consumed per week. The study found that in addition to tomatoes with the skin on, strawberries, which also contain lycopene, also lowered prostate-cancer risk.

- **Saw palmetto extract (Serenoa repens)**

  Saw palmetto extract can be found in health food stores and has been used in France under the name Permixon since 1982. Studies have shown it to be a valuable nutritional supplement for BPH and prostatitis with no significant side effects. Its effectiveness is in limiting the conversion of testosterone to DHT. The *British Journal of Clinical Pharmacology* reported that saw palmetto contains sterol-like compounds that inhibit the formation of DHT, which contributes to an enlarged prostate. Instead of being used by the body, DHT is broken down and excreted. Saw palmetto is also known as a mild aphrodisiac, which can help restore reduced libidos.

- **Evergreen tree extract (Pygeum africanum)**

  This extract is taken from an evergreen tree that is indigenous to Africa, the bark of which contains anti-inflammatory and antibacterial substances. This remedy has long been used to treat urinary tract disorders. Sold in health food stores, it has shown to be extremely effective when taken in combination with extracts of saw palmetto extract and stinging nettles. It can reduce prostate inflammation and pain and throbbing, increase sperm count, improve urinary flow, help in achieving and sustaining erections, and improve sexual vigor.

- **Others**

  The three amino acids glycine, alanine, and glutamic acid; essential fatty acids such as linseed (flaxseed) oil and omega-3 oils found mainly in fish; panax ginseng; horsetail (*Equisetum arvense*); quercetin; green tea extract; and bee pollen may help to relieve many symptoms of an enlarged and inflamed prostate.

TRT: RISK VERSUS BENEFIT

When contemplating the use of testosterone replacement, the possible risks as well as the benefits must be considered. Although many men experience the positive impact of testosterone on both their prostate and their genitourinary problems, some men have reported adverse side effects. These include atrophying of the testicles with prolonged use; a high red blood cell count; depression; fluid retention; reduced sperm count and volume of semen; and a reduction in HDL cholesterol levels (the "good" cholesterol).

Testosterone supplementation can produce dangerous side effects if administered to men with normal levels. In fact, extra doses will inhibit your own natural production and may contribute to stimulating the growth of pre-existing prostate tumors.

The major concern about testosterone may be its potential to stimulate and/or accelerate the growth of benign or malignant prostate tumors. The popular hypothesis is that the buildup of testosterone in the form of DHT within the prostate is potentially dangerous. However, scientists have not yet concluded if DHT causes prostate disorders. In fact, eliminating or drastically reducing DHT production can be harmful. Some studies have indicated an increase in DHT in the prostate cells of men with BPH, compared with normal prostates of men the same age. But generally, both testosterone and DHT levels decrease with age. Is it the decreasing levels of testosterone and DHT that occur in aging men with an increase in other hormones—estradiol (a female sex hormone), and prolactin, luteinizing hormone (LH) and follicle-stimulating hormone (FSH) from the pituitary gland—that contributes to the risk of prostate disease?

Scientists do not have any definite answers yet. Thus, while the use of testosterone replacement for those with naturally occurring low levels of the hormone in their system is not without controversy, testosterone offers a powerful anti-aging tool to millions of men.

CHAPTER 9

The "Regulator": Thyroid Hormone

All too often in our society, the slowing down of physical or mental functions is accepted as the normal course of old age, rather than being diagnosed as an illness or condition that may be treated with nutrition, hormones, exercise, or lifestyle changes. Perhaps one of the most pernicious "masks" for old age is *hypothyroidism*—an insufficient production or absorption of the thyroid hormone that won't allow our metabolism to function at its peak efficiency.

WHAT IS THE THYROID?

The *thyroid* is a small, butterfly-shaped gland located in the neck, over the trachea, or windpipe, just below the larynx. Despite its tiny stature, the thyroid has tremendous responsibilities, as it is the gland that affects virtually all metabolic processes. It does this by releasing certain hormones, which in turn regulate the body's metabolism, temperature, and heart rate. If the thyroid is not functioning at its optimal level, neither are you.

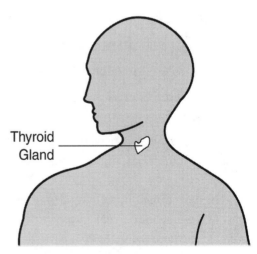

FIGURE 9.1. The thyroid gland.

The following are some of the most common symptoms of thyroid deficiency, also known as hypothyroidism. Many of them will sound to you like physical maladies that are supposed to be expected and tolerated as old age approaches:

- fatigue and general loss of energy; moving more slowly

- weakness

- susceptibility to colds, viruses, and respiratory ailments

- heavy, labored breathing

- muscle cramps

- persistent low back pain

- bruising easily

- mental sluggishness, poor memory

- headache

- emotional instability—crying jags, mood swings, easily upset, temper tantrums, and the like; more easily made nervous or anxious

- getting cold easily, particularly in the hands and feet

- dry, coarse, or leathery skin; pale skin

- coarse hair and/or loss of hair

- brittle nails

- loss of appetite

- stiff joints; mild arthritis

- reduced interest in or energy for sex

- atherosclerosis (arteries clogged with fat, or plaque, leading to other cardiovascular problems)

- decrease in heart contractility; that is, the heart doesn't pump blood with sufficient force, leading to insufficient circulation, particularly to the brain

The detection of hypothyroidism is especially important for older individuals. One study found that in a population of elderly people, ages sixty and over, all of whom belonged to a particular senior citizens' center, 5.9 percent suffered from hypothyroidism. Another study, published in 1993 in the *Journal of Endocrinology and Metabolism,* found a noticeable decrease of thyroid activity and a very low prevalence of thyroid autoantibodies in healthy centenarians (people who are 100 years old or older).

Despite its prevalence in older individuals, hypothyroidism is one of the most overlooked conditions in those sixty and over. In fact, telltale symptoms are diagnosed in as little as 25 percent of elderly hypothyroid patients. In one instance, laboratory confirmations of hypothyroid patients were compared with these individuals' initial clinical examinations. The results? Only 10 percent of people with the disease were properly diagnosed in their primary clinical examination.

> Some studies indicate that as many as 15 percent of people over age sixty have subclinical hypothyroidism. Which is to say, while they are, indeed, victims of hypothyroidism, their symptoms are too vague or too mild to yield a proper diagnosis. Thus, they continue to suffer without appropriate diagnosis or treatment.

Of course, it's possible that these symptoms may be the inevitable outcome of the aging process—but they are far more likely to result from a combination of low thyroid and nutritional deficiencies.

Correcting hypothyroidism can restore your energy, endurance, body heat, sexuality, mental vigor, and emotional resilience. It can boost resistance to colds and other respiratory conditions, protect against heart and arterial disease, and raise your defenses against cancer. Restoring the proper levels of thyroid hormone can even make your hair, skin, and nails smoother, stronger, and healthier.

> The failure of physicians to diagnose underactive thyroid (T4 disease) is at epidemic proportions, and grossly compromises the quality of self-perceived health of those patients. You can learn more about thyroid diagnosis, treatment, and healthy metabolism by visiting www.worldhealth.net and searching our educational area on the thyroid.

HOW YOUR BODY MAKES THYROID HORMONE

In order to be sure you're getting all the thyroid hormone (TH) your body needs, it's helpful to understand how your body makes it. The whole process begins with the hypothalamus—the body's "thermostat," which regulates many hormonal activities. When the hypothalamus determines that blood levels of TH have fallen too low, it sets a chain of activity in motion by discharging thyroid releasing hormone (TRH). TRH signals the pituitary to release a second hormone, thyroid-stimulating hormone (TSH). Finally, TSH tells the thyroid gland to get to work, and the thyroid gland produces TH. When levels of TH have risen high enough for the body to function properly, the pituitary responds by ceasing to release TSH and the process stops—until the hypothalamus determines that it's time to start again.

There are two ways that thyroid hormone levels can become insufficient in the body. One is when the thyroid itself has difficulty producing it. Lack of iodine, a tumor, or some other thyroid problem may result in a gland that doesn't properly carry out the orders given by the hypothalamus and the pituitary. This is known as *primary hypothyroidism.*

The other way that TH levels can fall is when the hypothalamus and/or the pituitary aren't functioning properly. This is known as *secondary hypothyroidism.*

The thyroid itself needs iodine to function. Lack of iodine will cause the thyroid to swell, a condition known as goiter—a visibly enlarged thyroid gland on the front and side of the neck. You need only a very tiny amount of iodine, however. A daily dose of 100 mcg for women and 120 mcg for men is quite sufficient. Most people get that in iodized salt or seafood.

Many people think that if they don't have goiter, their thyroid glands are getting everything they need to function. Unfortunately, that's not the case. Adequate iodine will keep you from getting goiter, but by itself, it's not enough to assure efficient production of TH.

THYROID AND VITAMIN DEFICIENCIES

Thyroid and vitamin deficiencies tend to interact with one another, so that insufficient vitamins keep the body from producing thyroid, while an insufficient thyroid keeps the body from making proper use of vitamins. Sometimes vitamin deficiencies result in either primary or secondary hypothyroidism.

Vitamin A

The thyroid gland has a particularly powerful interactive relationship with vitamin A. On the one hand, if your thyroid is underactive, it can't properly convert beta-carotene into this essential vitamin, and carotene may accumulate in the body. This accumulation can cause the carotene to bind to the cells of the *corpus luteum,* preventing vitamin A from forming the vital hormone progesterone. Some people with hypothyroidism may notice a slight yellowish tinge to their skin, revealing that the beta-carotene they're consuming—in food sources or in daily supplements—is remaining unconverted within their systems.

On the other hand, a body with a low level of vitamin A can't produce TSH. Studies by Dr. Isobel Jennings on cattle and sheep revealed that the basophils of the pituitary gland—the actual cells where TSH is produced—degenerate with insufficient vitamin A. The pituitary's release of TSH is the final step in the thyroid-producing chain, and if the pituitary isn't producing TSH, the thyroid gland won't do its job either.

A deficiency in vitamin A also reduces the ability of the thyroid to absorb iodine. The research of Danish scientist B. Palludan showed that after only two weeks of severe vitamin A deficiency, the thyroid secretion of pigs dropped by 40 to 50 percent. That means that even if you are getting enough iodine in your diet, insufficient levels of vitamin A may be preventing your thyroid from making use of it, causing your thyroid to produce lower levels of TH, and leading to hypothyroidism.

Abnormal thyroid has all the makings of a vicious circle. If your thyroid can't help convert beta-carotene to vitamin A, neither your pituitary nor your thyroid will be getting enough vitamin A to do its job—and your thyroid will become even less able to help your body manufacture the vitamin A that it needs.

B Vitamins

The B vitamins are particularly key to efficient thyroid production. A shortage of vitamin B_2 will depress the function of ovaries and testes and will prevent the thyroid and adrenal glands from secreting necessary hormones.

Vitamin B_3 (niacin) is necessary not only for TH production but also for respiration and for the metabolism of proteins, carbohydrates, and fats.

We don't know whether vitamin B_6 (pyridoxine) is necessary for the thyroid or the pituitary gland, but we do know that without sufficient quantities of it, TH production falls.

On the other hand, TH itself is necessary for your body to make use of vitamin B_{12} (cyanocobalamin). A severe vitamin B_{12} deficiency could result in anemia (possibly fatal), mental illness, neurological disorders, neuralgia, neuritis, or bursitis—all symptoms that might be confused with the "normal" aging process. Since B_{12} can't be produced by the body itself, you have to ingest it in your diet or in vitamin supplements. However, without adequate TH levels, your body can't absorb this essential vitamin, no matter how much you ingest.

Vitamin C

Vitamin C is also a key supplement that can facilitate the production of TH, and vitamin C deficiencies can cause gross disorders in TH production. Guinea pigs, like people, don't manufacture vitamin C in their own bodies. When experimental guinea pigs were deprived of vitamin C, the capillaries in their thyroid glands began to bleed, a condition that worsened as the scurvy—the shortage of C—also got worse.

Long-term deficits in vitamin C can cause *hyperplasia*, in which normal thyroid gland cells begin to multiply at an abnormal rate, producing too much TH, a condition known as *hyperthyroidism*. The pituitary is supposed to regulate the production of TH, monitoring hormone levels in order to tell the thyroid when to start and stop. Insufficient vitamin C, though, seems to interrupt the pituitary's governing function.

On the other hand, as soon as the guinea pigs were given adequate supplies of vitamin C, all the thyroid gland problems disappeared. Taking a vitamin C supplement, then, can benefit your thyroid as well as help your body to perform many other functions.

Vitamin E

Vitamin E deficiencies also affect TH production. In one experiment, rabbits deprived of vitamin E experienced a range of TH problems, including the rapid multiplication of certain thyroid gland cells and insufficient TSH synthesized by the pituitary gland. Rats deprived of vitamin E had a similar response, and in addition, they transmitted hyperplasia to their litters.

HOW THYROID HORMONE FIGHTS AGING

The symptoms of hypothyroidism mimic many of the conditions that people associate with aging. Mental problems that resemble Alzheimer's disease and other degenerative brain diseases may also result from low TH production. In fact, hypothyroidism may be responsible for cases of treatable dementia, and has been related to negative changes in cognitive function in elderly patients. Without adequate TH, your heart pumps less vigorously, sending less blood—and less of the essential nutrients and oxygen that blood carries—into the brain. Many patients find that memory problems, confusion, loss of concentration, and similar symptoms clear up when TH levels are back to normal.

Depression may result from the changes of life that come with growing older. However, hypothyroidism may also produce emotional reactions, including a loss of energy that impedes making positive changes. Crying jags, antisocial behavior, phobias, insomnia, anxiety, and a sense of helpless confusion may result both from hypothyroidism and from *hypoglycemia* (low blood sugar), a related condition. Many people suffering from these symptoms have reported immediate changes in mood and energy levels as soon as they started taking TH supplements.

Diabetes

Proper levels of TH are essential to the body for the maintenance of appropriate levels of blood sugar. Thus, hypothyroidism may be implicated in diabetes, particularly adult-onset diabetes (type II)—a condition in which the body has extreme difficulty regulating blood sugar levels. Essentially, the thyroid allows us to convert glucose into energy. In cases of hypothyroidism, however, glucose cannot be utilized. This results in glucose waste and hypoglycemia. Hypoglycemia then leads to the secretion of adrenaline, which causes toxicity of the circulatory system. These circulatory problems are prevalent in people with diabetes, but they may be reduced or avoided with thyroid supplements. TH supplements have also been shown to reverse other symptoms of diabetes and, in some cases, have reversed adult-onset diabetes itself.

Weight Gain

TH governs your body's metabolism. Therefore, if TH levels are unnaturally low, you will have an unnaturally hard time losing weight and will find yourself gaining weight with unusual ease. The weight gain—or difficulty with weight loss—often associated with aging may be logically due to reduced TH levels, which can be corrected. (Also, weight gain in age often results from a drop in physical activity. So, in addition to checking your TH levels, be sure to read Section Four.)

Heart Disease

Low thyroid levels have been linked to high levels of cholesterol, and an increased risk of heart disease and vascular problems. In fact, elevated cholesterol is a classic symptom of extreme hypothyroidism, and studies show that administering two grains of thyroid can reduce the levels of cholesterol and triglycerides in people with hypothyroidism.

Cancer

Finally, a number of studies have associated hypothyroidism with an increased risk of developing cancer. Dr. J.G.C. Spencer of Frenahay Hospital in Bristol found that the so-called "goiter belts" (regions where goiter is extremely prevalent, due to low levels of iodine in the water and diet) had higher than average cancer rates, a finding that extended over fifteen nations on four continents. According to Dr. Bernard Eskin, director of endocrinology at the Department of Obstetrics and Gynecology at the Medical College of Philadelphia, iodine deficiencies are associated with breast cancer in both rats and humans. As the thyroid gland needs iodine to function, we may infer that thyroid problems are somehow related to the cancer. Moreover, the *Neurology Journal* and the *Southern Medical Journal* have both reported cases in which thyroid supplements actually reversed certain types of cancer.

DETECTING A THYROID PROBLEM

In *Solved: The Riddle of Illness,* Dr. Stephen Langer reports that some 40 percent of the population is deficient in thyroid hormone in some way. Most hypothyroidism isn't clear-cut on standard medical tests, but there is a simple way to find out if you have this condition. Take the *Barnes Basal Temperature Test* by following these steps:

1. Before you go to bed at night, shake down an oral or under-the-arm thermometer and leave it by your bed.

2. As soon as you awaken the next day, place the thermometer in your armpit and leave it there for ten minutes before getting up.

3. Record the temperature. A normal temperature for under the armpit will be 97.8 to 98.2 degrees Fahrenheit. If your temperature is lower than that on two consecutive days, you are very likely suffering from a degree of hypothyroidism. (*Note:* menstruating women should not take this test on the first day of their periods, when temperatures are likely to fluctuate more than usual.)

Another test that does a particularly good job of detecting any malfunctions is a new, highly sensitive thyroid stimulating hormone (TSH) assay. TSH is an excellent indicator of thyroid hormone action at the tissue level, and many doctors believe that these TSH assays will provide the best indication of hypothyroidism.

Serum TSH levels are measured by radioimmunoassay, and many experts believe it is the best available test not only for revealing primary hypothyroidism, but also for distinguishing secondary hypothyroidism. The test is conducted as follows: synthetic thyroid releasing hormone (TRH) is injected intravenously, which causes the release of TSH from the anterior pituitary. TSH levels are measured both before and after the injection of TRH, and by comparing these levels, thyroid function can be monitored. The higher your TSH concentration, the more likely you are to be suffering from primary hypothyroidism; whereas in secondary hypothyroidism, TSH levels are usually low.

Recent widespread use of this highly sensitive TSH assay has not only eliminated the need for TRH stimulation tests in patients with thyroid cancer or goiters, but it has also allowed physicians to better monitor thyroid hormone replacement therapy in their patients so that TH is not over-replaced.

Complications in Treatment for Women

Women may have more reason to measure their TSH levels than men. This is because nearly all women who are diagnosed with high levels of TSH have some form of hypothyroidism. In fact, hypothyroidism is much more common in women than in men. Treatment, however, has certain complications.

Studies have shown that thyroid hormone increases bone mineral re-absorption, increasing the risk of osteoporosis, especially in postmenopausal women. One study found that women being treated with enough thyroxine, prescription thyroid hormone, to suppress TSH for ten years or more had a 9 percent decrease in bone density. Patients with conditions such as goiters or thyroid cancer must receive TSH-suppressive doses of thyroxine and, therefore, are at a particularly high risk for osteoporosis.

Women who want to check the functioning of their thyroid or who are presently taking thyroid replacement hormones—especially older women—should be screened with this highly sensitive TSH assay around age forty-five, and then follow up with a screening every two years. This is to ensure, primarily, that their thyroid is functioning properly, and secondly, that there is no overtreatment with TH, which would increase the risk of osteoporosis.

TAKING THYROID SUPPLEMENTS

If your home self-test suggests that hypothyroidism may be a problem for you, we urge you to see your physician to verify these results and to discuss the possibility of thyroid supplements. It is important that your health-care provider adjust the dose until you've found the level that is right for you. Also, adjust your diet and vitamin supplements in such a way as to support your thyroid needs.

You may be one of the 60 percent of Americans whose thyroid is functioning normally. If you're in the other 40 percent, however, you may be surprised by the extent to which TH supplements seem to restore your youth.

Your first line of defense against hypothyroidism is to take a good multivitamin along with vitamin B complex and vitamin C supplements. Some cases of hypothyroidism may be treated in this way, without the affected person ever having to take thyroid supplements. However, if your thyroid problem is caused by something other than a vitamin deficiency, your body won't be able to make use of the vitamin supplements you are taking. In that case, you may need TH supplementation.

NUTRIENTS FOR A HEALTHY THYROID

The following thyroid hormone cofactors and thyroid gland stimulants have been reported as being helpful in people with hypothyroidism. Consult your physician before beginning any therapy.

Supplement	Suggested Dosage	Comments
Vitamin A, plus beta-carotene	15,000 IU daily.	Included in a multivitamin complex.
Vitamin B complex, including riboflavin (B_2) and B_{12} lozenges	B complex: 100 mg with meals. B_2: 50 mg twice daily. B_{12}: 15 mcg dissolved under the tongue, 3 times daily or as directed.	Improves cellular oxygenation and energy. B_{12} is absorbed better in lozenge form.
Brewer's yeast	As directed on label.	Rich in B vitamins.
Vitamin C	500 mg 4 times daily.	Do not take extremely high doses of vitamin C—this may affect the production of the thyroid hormone.
Vitamin E	400 IU daily.	Avoid larger amounts.
Iron chelate or Floradix formula	As directed on label.	Essential for enzyme and hemoglobin production.
Sea kelp	As directed by physician.	Contains iodine, the basic substance of the thyroid hormone.
Raw thyroid glandular (Armour extract)	As directed by physician.	Available by prescription only. Synthetic thyroid hormones are often ineffective.
Tyrosine (amino acid)	500 mg twice daily on an empty stomach with 25 mg of B_6 (may be taken as part of a B complex).	Low plasma levels have been associated with hypothyroidism.
Unsaturated fatty acids	As directed on label.	For proper functioning of the thyroid gland.
Zinc	50 mg daily.	An immune system stimulant.

Vitamin deficiencies aren't the only factors involved in sabotaging your TH production. Here are some other common causes of this problem:

- environmental pollutants, particularly fluoride in water

- barbiturates and other drugs that contain cyanide

- certain medications, such as sulfa drugs and antidiabetic medications

- prednisone

- supplemental estrogen, found in birth control pills and HRT

- some cough medicines

- amiodarone HCl (Cordarone)

- lithium

- aspirin and other painkillers that contain salicylates

- oil of wintergreen (found in rubbing liniment)

- cigarette smoke, primary and secondary

Even if your TH production has been adequate all your life, the circumstances associated with aging may lead you to take medications that create a thyroid problem, or push an already existing problem into a major deficiency. Unless you and your physician identify this as an easily correctable thyroid condition, you are both likely to mistake it for the "inevitable" process of aging. Arriving at the proper level of thyroid for your system can actually determine how long—and how well—you will live. Note: Regulation of thyroid hormone imbalance can be a complicated medical situation. Find a qualified physician (preferably an A4M member and anti-aging specialist) to be your health-care advisor.

SECTION THREE

Longevity and Nutrition

We should conduct ourselves
not as if we ought to live for the body,
but as if we could not live without it.

—SENECA THE YOUNGER (5 B.C.–A.D. 65)

IMPORTANT—PLEASE READ

The content in this book is for educational purposes only, and is not intended to prevent, diagnose, treat, or cure disease or illness. While potentially therapeutic nutraceuticals (dietary supplements such as vitamins, minerals, herbal products, hormone supplementation, and similar preparations) and interventions (processes such as lifestyle changes, dietary modifications, bodywork, prescription medications, and others) are mentioned in the course of this book, you are urged to seek the advice of a medical professional to make the appropriate selection for your particular medical situation.

With nutraceuticals, dosing is highly variable. Proper dosing is based on parameters including sex, age, whether you are well or ill, and whether your illness is chronic or acute. Additionally, efficiency of absorption of a particular type of product and the quality of its individual ingredients are two major considerations for choosing appropriate specific agents for your medical situation.

Just because a product is natural doesn't mean it's safe for you. A small portion of the general population may react adversely to components in nutraceuticals, especially herbal products. Make your physician aware of any and all "natural" interventions you use regularly, and seek medical consultation before starting any others.

Neither the publisher nor the authors advocate the use of any particular health-care protocol, but believe that the information in this book should be available to the public. The publisher and authors are not responsible for any adverse effects or consequences resulting from the use of any of the suggestions, preparations, or procedures discussed in this book. Should the reader have any questions concerning the appropriateness of any procedure or preparation mentioned, the publisher and authors strongly suggest consulting a professional health-care advisor.

Always consult your physician prior to beginning any new healthcare intervention, whether it be nutritional, fitness, medication, hormonal, herbal, or otherwise. Do not change the dosing or cease the intervention without discussing with your physician first.

CHAPTER 10

Vitamins, Co-Vitamins, and Cofactors

INTRODUCTION TO NUTRITIONAL SUPPLEMENTATION

Sixty percent of Americans aged sixty-five and older are engaging in anti-aging interventions, most notable of which is nutritional supplementation. Also referred to as dietary supplementation, these are naturally occurring substances in pharmaceutical dosage forms with which disease-preventing and health-promoting properties may be associated.

A survey conducted by Roper Starch Worldwide reported that the nation's seniors consume dietary supplements for the following reasons:

- 39 percent to maintain general wellness
- 17 percent to enhance energy levels
- 16 percent to strengthen bone health
- 12 percent to improve stamina
- 11 percent to relieve joint pain and arthritis

With more and more research discovering tangible health benefits of nutritional supplementation, it is becoming evident that nature provides safe and effective ways for each of us to improve our well-being. To maximize your utilization of nutritional supplementation, it is prudent to receive a personalized, specialty anti-aging regimen designed just for you by a qualified medical professional, such as one Board Certified by the A4M (see Anti-Aging Resources– ABAARM Physicians [page 575] and ABAAHP Health Practitioners [page 576]). As you will find by perusing Chapters 10 through 13, we will present a variety of dietary supplements accompanied by reliable scientific documentation.

The Dosing That Is Right for You

The U.S. Department of Agriculture (USDA) Food Guide Pyramid recommends that we eat at least 3–5 servings of vegetables and 2–4 servings of fruit every day. This helps us to achieve the Daily Value (DV) (formerly known as Recommended Daily Allowances; RDA) of vitamins and minerals as established by the National Academy of Sciences. But new science is indicating that getting our daily dose of nutrients by food alone may be insufficient. For example, to neutralize free radicals (see Chapter 2), some scientists suggest that we consume two or three times the USDA's recommendations on vegetables and fruits. This is not practical for many of us. Additionally, the Food Guide Pyramid recommends quantities of nutrients without being specific about the quality. Foods that are processed (frozen vegetables, canned fruits, and so on) lose much of their nutritional values and potencies during manufacture. Refined food also contains unwanted substances such as preservatives and dyes.

DVs have become subject to great scrutiny in light of fast-paced discoveries being made in nutrition and nutritional medicine. The DV estimates the amount of a nutrient needed by an average healthy person to avoid showing signs of deficiency, then adds a margin that increases the dose to levels considered appropriate for avoiding common health problems. For example, the minimum level of vitamin C needed to prevent scurvy, for example, is around 10 mg, so the DV is set at 60 mg to allow for individuals with certain health problems, such as cancer and cardiovascular disease, who may require more vitamin C.

The DV numbers are based upon the amount a person needs to keep from getting sick, plus a margin of error. This may be less than the amount needed to achieve optimum health. Some nutritionists believe that the DV has not kept pace with the latest nutritional research and believe that some of the recommendations may be thirty years out of date. Many scientific studies show that our bodies need the vitamins A, C, E, beta-carotene, lipoic acid, and the antioxidant-helping minerals selenium and zinc in doses that are well in excess of the DV. As a result, some nutritionists believe the DVs for these health-promoting nutrients should be at least two to five times the current values.

So, nutritional supplementation of vitamins, minerals, amino acids, and other nutrients as an adjunct to our diets becomes essential to our wellness. For best results, each of us should, first and foremost, make an effort to consume a daily diet that is as high in fresh, unprocessed fruits and vegetables as possible. Then, we can get extra boosts of nutrients that might benefit our bodies, by supplementing with high-quality, natural dietary supplements, the selection of which should be matched to our individual health needs by a qualified anti-aging physician.

Dietary Supplements as a Potent Public Health Promotion Initiative

There is a long and strong timeline of recent research to support the application of vitamins and minerals as dietary supplements to promote wellness in humans, the highlights of which include:

February 2002 *(American Journal of Clinical Nutrition)*: Dr. Bruce Ames, professor of molecular and cell biology at University of California Berkeley (USA) found that the amino acid acetyl-L-carnitine and the antioxidant alpha-lipoic acid fed to older rats improved memory, boosted overall energy, and increased cellular energy-producing mechanisms. Remarks Dr. Ames, "With the two supplements together, these old rats got up and did the Macarena. Everything we looked at looks more like a young animal." Administration of the nutrient combination for a month triggered increases in levels of antioxidants, including vitamin C. Colleagues of Dr. Ames predicted that similar therapeutic benefits of this combination to "rejuvenate aging humans" would likely be found.

April 12, 2002 *(American Journal of Clinical Nutrition)*: A team of scientists from University of California/Berkeley (USA) conducted a meta-analysis of previous research employing megavitamin treatment—vitamins in amounts at least ten times greater than the United States Recommended Daily Allowance ([RDA], set by the Food and Drug Administration [FDA]). The researchers found that more than fifty genetic diseases could be successfully treated with by megavitamin therapy, which saturates the body in order to overcome a binding defect associated with a genetic mutation in these specific illnesses. Their research also suggested that there may be many more diseases treatable with high-dose vitamins—in particular the B vitamins, which lead researcher Dr. Bruce Ames commented "are sold over the counter in dosages up to 100 times the US RDA and are generally considered safe at such levels." Additionally, "because aging involves similar biochemical deficiencies, megavitamins may help perk up an increasingly older population." The researchers submit that flooding the body with an excess of vitamins creates an ample supply of coenzymes required for optimal metabolic functions that otherwise become deficient with age. To conclude their paper, this research team states that "there is potentially much benefit and possibly little harm in trying high-dose nutrient therapy because of the nominal cost, ease of application, and low level of risk."

June 18, 2002 *(Journal of the American Medical Association)*: Harvard Medical School (Cambridge, MA, USA) researchers recommend that "everybody—regardless of age or health status—take a daily multivitamin." The research team reviewed thirty-six years of scientific literature that investigated the links between vitamin intake and diseases. Across the board, the researchers found numerous benefits and little risks. Warning that vitamin deficiencies can occur in both the elderly and sick, who may not absorb vitamins properly and may follow restrictive diets, and in people who don't follow good nutritional habits, the team comments that "It's rare to find a health-promoter that offers such a substantial benefit with a relatively low cost and low risk of problems. When you have such a thing, you ought to jump on it."

April 3, 2003 *(Annals of Internal Medicine)*: U.S. researchers conducted a one-year-long study of a group of 130 adults over age forty-five, a portion of whom took a multivitamin and mineral supplement daily and another portion of whom took a placebo. The multivitamin contained amounts of vitamins and minerals similar to those found in most commercially available multivitamin and mineral supplements. The researchers found that the group taking the multivitamin and mineral supplement fell ill to an infection far less (43 percent versus 73 percent on placebo), resulting with significantly less infection-related work absenteeism (21 percent versus 57 percent on placebo). The difference in the chances of getting ill was even more pronounced in those with diabetes (type II). Of the fifty-one diabetic participants in the study, 17 percent of those taking the supplement reported contracting an infection—compared to 93 percent of those taking the placebo.

While the concept of vitamin and mineral supplementation is a newcomer to the conservative mainstream medical arena, there is strong evidence (as the above selections demonstrate) that multivitamin and mineral dietary supplementation is perhaps the single most potent preventive health measure that offers the greatest return on the investment. Those "in the know," know. A number of reputable scientists have been personally consuming antioxidants for years. At the U.S. National Institutes of Health, Dr. Trey Sunderland, age fifty, takes vitamin E and anti-inflammatory drugs such as ibuprofen, while he conducts work as the Chief of Geriatric Psychiatry at the Institute of Mental Health into Alzheimer's prevention. At Case Western Reserve University (Cleveland, OH, USA), Dr. Craig Atwood takes vitamin E and drinks blueberry shakes while conducting research commissioned by the Alzheimer's Association to find antioxidant compounds to decrease plaques in brain tissue. Such conduct begs the question: If such nutrients were of no preventive or therapeutic value, why would these experts on aging-related diseases continue to consume them?

Dr. Dean Hamer, Chief of the Gene Structure and Regulation Section, Laboratory of Biochemistry, U.S. National Cancer Institute, remarked at a February 2003 forum that "An ounce of prevention is worth $20,000 of pharmaceuticals." This point is proven by research conducted by Dr. Ranjit Chandra and colleagues from Memorial University (Newfoundland). A supplement containing eighteen vitamins, minerals, and trace elements was given to healthy men and women aged sixty-five and over. Reports the team, "Those who took the supplement showed significant improvement in short-term memory, problem-solving ability, abstract thinking, and attention." Dr. Chandra suggested that nutritional supplementation "may be instrumental in preserving the anatomy and function of neurons and their appendages." As a result, these men and women enhanced their capacities to live independently and without

---

A Reminder

The content presented in Chapters 10 through 13 are published by the American Academy of Anti-Aging Medicine in its annual *Anti-Aging Desk Reference*, a publication that is intended solely for educational purposes. It is not intended to prevent, diagnose, treat, or cure disease or illness. A4M's *Anti-Aging Desk Reference* is not intended to provide medical advice, and is not to be used as a substitute for advice from a physician or health practitioner. Prior to engaging in any of the programs or therapies described in the A4M's *Anti-Aging Desk Reference*, consult a knowledgeable physician or health practitioner. Read the Disclaimer appearing on the copyright page of this book for further details.

major disability. Additionally, the multivitamin, multimineral supplement improved immunity. The numbers of natural killer cells and helper T cells, and the production of interleukin-2, all improved. Further, infection-related illness in those taking the supplement occurred at less than half the rate (twenty-three days per year) compared with those who took placebo (forty-eight days per year). Most compelling was the cost-effectiveness and simplicity of a nutritional supplement to prevent or delay illness and functional decline in the elderly. Dr. Chandra calculated that for every one U.S. dollar spent on the supplement, twenty-eight U.S. dollars would be saved in healthcare costs.

VITAMINS

Vitamin A (Retinol)

GENERAL DESCRIPTION

Vitamin A is a fat-soluble vitamin that participates in numerous biological functions. In nature, vitamin A occurs mainly in the form of fatty acid esters such as retinyl acetate. Vitamin A is only found in animal tissues; although its precursor beta-carotene (provitamin A) can be found in certain fruits and vegetables. Fish liver oils (as in cod liver oil), liver, milk, cream, cheese, butter, and eggs are good natural sources of vitamin A.

ROLE IN ANTI-AGING

Vitamin A is needed for **cells to reproduce properly; it is required for vision and the proper growth and maintenance of the skin, bones, and reproductive organs; and it helps in building resistance to respiratory infections and boosting immunity. Vitamin A may also protect against cancer, and is useful in the treatment of skin conditions such as acne and psoriasis.**

Several studies have shown that vitamin A is a **potent stimulator of growth hormone production.** Researchers believe that vitamin A may directly affect intracellular growth hormone levels and IGF-binding protein 3, which is necessary for the production of growth hormone.

Vitamin A may also help to **promote healthy thyroid function.** In research conducted by Morley, et al. (*Am J Physiol* 1980;238:E174–179), it was found that vitamin A increased the peripheral clearance of thyroxine (T4) and decreased its total circulating levels. Vitamin A did not alter basal thyroid stimulating hormone (TSH) or its response to thyroid releasing hormone. Vitamin A decreased thyroid gland size and enhanced conversion of T4 to T3, the active form of thyroid hormone that is utilized by the body.

Numerous studies point to the value of vitamin A in **boosting immunity**.

Research suggests that retinyl acetate, a form of vitamin A found naturally in food, primes the immune system. Coutsoudis, et al. (*Pediatr Infect Dis J.* 1992;11:203–209) studied the effect of vitamin A supplementation on selected factors of immunity in children with measles. Results showed that children receiving the vitamin were significantly less likely to die and had markedly higher numbers of lymphocytes and IgG antibodies to measles. Vitamin A has also been shown to enhance Th2 (T-helper cell type 2) mediated immune responses, a finding that suggests that it may be useful in treating bacterial and parasitic infections, and mucosal infections.

Finally, there is also some evidence to suggest that vitamin A may offer some **protection against cancer**. Liu, et al. (*Carcinogenesis* 2000;21:2245–2253) found that doses of beta-carotene of approximately 6 mg a day may help **to protect against lung damage induced by cigarette smoke**. Meanwhile, Forni, et al. (*J Natl Cancer Inst* 1986;76:527–533) studied the effect of vitamin A and the growth of transplantable tumors in mice. Results showed that the tumors did not take in the mice given high-dose vitamin A treatment. This protective effect lasted throughout ninety days of supplementation. New research conducted at the University of California in San Francisco suggests that a cream containing a derivative of vitamin A could help to **prevent basal cell carcinoma**—the most common type of skin cancer. Dr. Ervin Epstein, Jr. and his colleagues found that mice that were genetically predisposed to developing skin cancer developed 85 percent less tumors after being exposed to UV radiation if they were treated with the cream. Furthermore, tumors that did develop in treated mice were significantly smaller than those seen in untreated animals.

DEFICIENCY SYMPTOMS
Vitamin A deficiency is associated with night blindness or loss of adaptation to the dark; dry eye disease; sty in the eye; increased susceptibility to infection; sinus and bronchial infections; drying out of skin and mucous membranes; loss of taste and smell, which leads to loss of appetite; loss of vigor; defective teeth and gums; and slowed growth.

People who eat little liver, dairy foods, and beta-carotene-containing vegetables are at risk of developing vitamin A deficiency, although severe deficiencies causing blindness are extremely rare in the Western world. People with diseases causing malabsorption, such as HIV, are also at risk.

THERAPEUTIC DAILY AMOUNT
7,000–10,000 IU. RDA is 3,000 IU (900 mcg) for men, and 2,300 IU (700 mcg) for women. The European RDA is 800 mcg.

MAXIMUM SAFE LEVEL

3,000 mcg (long-term usage), 7,500 mcg (25,000 IU) (short-term usage). People over the age of sixty-five and those with liver disease are advised to take no more than 15,000 IU of vitamin A. Vitamin A toxicity can be serious, thus, it is important to ensure that the recommended dose is not exceeded.

SIDE EFFECTS/CONTRAINDICATIONS

Women who are planning to become pregnant or those who are in the first three months of pregnancy should not eat liver, or take vitamin A supplements, unless told to do so by a physician, as too much vitamin A can cause birth defects. The maximum safe intake for women who could become pregnant is currently being reevaluated; however, doses of less than 10,000 IU (3,000 mcg) per day is generally accepted as safe.

Results of a clinical trial by Cartmel, et al. (*Am J Clin Nutr* 1999;69: 937–943) revealed that people taking 25,000 IU of vitamin A each day for approximately four years experienced an 11 percent increase in triglycerides, a 3 percent increase in total cholesterol and a 1 percent decrease in "good" HDL cholesterol, suggesting that people at high risk of developing heart disease should be cautious when thinking about taking supplementary vitamin A.

Melhus, et al. (*Ann Int Med* 1998;129:770–778) found that a daily intake of just 5,000 IU of vitamin A (the U.S. RDA) was associated with a significant reduction in bone mineral density. The decrease in bone mineral density was so great that it approximately doubled the risk of hip fracture. More recently, in 2003, Michaelsson, et al. (*N Engl J Med* 2003;348:287–294) found that men in their forties and fifties who have the highest blood levels of vitamin A are 2.5 times more likely than men with lower levels to break their hip when they are older. Based on these findings, people at high risk of developing osteoporosis—in particular menopausal and postmenopausal women—may benefit from taking beta-carotene supplements instead of vitamin A.

Vitamin A should not be taken by people using the acne medications isotretinoin, resorcinol, topical sulfur, and tazarotene.

SOLUBILITY

Fat soluble.

Beta-Carotene (Pro-vitamin A)

GENERAL DESCRIPTION

Beta-carotene is a **natural source of vitamin A**. The majority of people in Western countries obtain sufficient vitamin A from their diet; however, beta-carotene may be prescribed for people with certain conditions that increase the need for the vitamin—for example, cystic fibrosis, chronic illness, and intestinal malabsorption. Beta-carotene is found in yellow fruit; dark-green, yellow, and leafy vegetables; carrots; yams; cantaloupe; yellow squash; spinach; apricots; spirulina; wheat grass; alfalfa; and barley grass. More than 400 carotenoids have been isolated from natural sources.

ROLE IN ANTI-AGING

Beta-carotene is an important **free-radical fighter** for various forms of cancer as it protects against ultraviolet damage and enhances the immune system. It carries many of the same functions as vitamin A. The liver and the intestinal wall obtain useable vitamin A by converting beta-carotene.

Research published in 2001 (Liu S, Lee IM, Ajani U, et al. *Int J Epidemiol.* 2001;30:130–135) revealed that people who ate two-and-a-half servings of beta-carotene-rich vegetables a day were significantly less likely to develop coronary heart disease than those who consumed less than one serving of beta-carotene-rich vegetables.

DEFICIENCY SYMPTOMS

Beta-carotene is not an essential nutrient; therefore, it is not possible to develop a true deficiency. However, alcohol consumption decreases beta-carotene in the liver, and people with hypothyroidism and diabetes may have trouble converting beta-carotene into vitamin A. Research has also found that elderly people with type II diabetes have significantly lower blood levels of carotenoids. Thus, such people may benefit from supplementary beta-carotene.

THERAPEUTIC DAILY AMOUNT

20,000 to 50,000 IU. No RDA has been established. Nontoxic. Many experts suggest that people should avoid synthetic beta-carotene and only supplement with natural beta-carotene. Some research has linked synthetic beta-carotene with an increased risk of lung cancer among smokers, while other research has found that the natural form has antioxidant properties that the synthetic version lacks.

MAXIMUM SAFE LEVEL

Not established.

SIDE EFFECTS/CONTRAINDICATIONS

The effect of beta-carotene on pregnant women has not been studied. However, no problems with fertility or pregnancy have been reported in women taking up to 30 mg of beta-carotene a day. Beta-carotene may cause complications in patients with liver disease or kidney disease, and those taking cholestyramine or colestipol mineral oil, neomycin, and vitamin E. Therefore, such patients should consult a doctor before taking any supplements. Smokers are currently advised to avoid taking both natural and synthetic beta-carotene as two separate studies have shown that taking synthetic beta-carotene may increase the risk of lung cancer in smokers.

SOLUBILITY
Fat soluble.

Vitamin B$_1$ (Thiamine)

GENERAL DESCRIPTION
Found in yellow fruit, green and leafy vegetables, carrots, yams, cantaloupe, organ meats (especially liver), pork, dried beans, peas, soybeans, wheat germ, brewer's or nutritional yeast, egg yolks, poultry, fish and seafood, dried yeast, brown rice, rice husks or rice bran, whole grain products, oatmeal, nuts, most vegetables, milk, raisins, and prunes.

ROLE IN ANTI-AGING
Known as the "morale" vitamin, vitamin B$_1$ **converts carbohydrates (sugar) into energy, promotes growth, aids digestion**, and is **essential for nerve, muscle, and heart tissues**. It also plays a vital role in the functioning of some important enzymes and is essential for the **transmission of certain nerve signals between the brain and the spinal cord**. Vitamin B$_1$ helps **repel insects and mosquitoes and is used in the treatment of alcoholics and drug addicts**.

DEFICIENCY SYMPTOMS
Vitamin B$_1$ deficiency causes the condition beri-beri, which includes mental illness, paralysis of some eye muscles, foot drop, and decreased sensation in the feet and legs. Other symptoms of deficiency include loss of appetite; fatigue; weakness; neuritis; muscle atrophy; head pressures; poor sleep; feeling tense and irritable; aches and pains; subjectively poor memory, difficulty concentrating; constipation; impaired growth; and "pins and needles" sensation in the toes and "burning" sensation in the feet. Alcohol consumption interferes with absorption of vitamin B$_1$.

THERAPEUTIC DAILY AMOUNT
1.4–100 mg. RDA is 1.4 mg; pregnant or lactating women should increase the RDA by 0.4 mg.

MAXIMUM SAFE LEVEL
100 mg (long and short term; no adverse effects have been reported).

SIDE EFFECTS/CONTRAINDICATIONS
No side effects are associated with the normal use of supplementary vitamin B_1. Pregnant women should consult their physician before taking vitamin B_1.

SOLUBILITY
Water soluble.

Vitamin B_{12} (Cobalamin or Cyanocobalamin)

GENERAL DESCRIPTION
Vitamin B_{12} is vital for normal nerve cell activity, DNA replication, the production of red and white blood cells and blood platelets (thrombocytes), the manufacture of substances needed for correct cell functioning, the metabolism of nutrients necessary for cell growth, and production of the mood-affecting substance SAMe (S-adenosyl-L-methionine). It is essential for the recycling of certain enzymes that maintain the health of blood, nerve, and other cells. It also aids the metabolism of proteins, fats, and carbohydrates. Vitamin B_{12} acts together with folic acid and vitamin B_6 to control homocysteine levels. Elevated homocysteine levels are associated with an increased risk of heart disease, stroke, and possibly Alzheimer's disease and osteoporosis.

Cyanocobalamin is a synthetic form of vitamin B_{12}, which is prescribed to correct vitamin B_{12} deficiency.

Vitamin B_{12} is found in organ meats, liver, beef, pork, eggs, whole milk, cheese, whole wheat bread, and fish. As vitamin B_{12} is not found in plant foods unless they are fortified (for example, breakfast cereal), vegans are likely to benefit from vitamin B_{12} supplementation.

ROLE IN ANTI-AGING
High plasma levels of the amino acid homocysteine have been implicated in the development of vascular diseases, including stroke. Hankey and Eikelboom (*CNS Drugs* 2001;15:437–443) found that elevated plasma levels of total homocysteine are present in less than 5 percent of the general population, but in as many as 50 percent of patients with stroke and athlersclerotic diseases. It is now well accepted that plasma levels of **total homocysteine can be lowered** effectively by folic acid, vitamin B_6, and vitamin B_{12} supplementation. Many studies concerned with lowering homocysteine levels used doses of 400–1,000 mcg of folic acid per day, 10–50 mg of vitamin B_6 per day, and 50–300 mcg of vitamin B_{12} per day. Elevated homocysteine levels have been implicated in

numerous diseases, including stroke, thromboembolism (blood clots that can dislodge and cause stroke, heart attack, and other complications), osteoporosis, inflammatory bowel disease (Crohn's disease and ulcerative colitis), Alzheimer's disease, diabetes, complications of pregnancy, and hypothyroidism. Thus vitamin B_{12} can help to protect against these diseases.

Ronco et al. (*Lipids.* 2005;40:259–264.) it was found that vitamin B_{12} reduces the oxidation of LDL-cholesterol or "bad" cholesterol, which is implicated in atherosclerosis. In a double blind, randomized trial by Till et al. (*Atherosclerosis.* 2005;181:131–135.) 50 patients at risk of cerebral ischemia received daily 2.5mg folic acid, 25mg Vitamin B_6, and 0.5mg Vitamin B_{12} or placebo for 1 year. Results showed that the vitamins significantly reduced carotid intima-media thickness (IMT), an accepted marker of atherosclerotic changes. The fact that vitamin B_{12} lowers homocysteine levels, and reduces carotid IMT and oxidation of LDL-cholesterol suggests that it may help to prevent cardiovascular disease.

Supplementation with vitamin B_{12} **may improve cognitive function** in elderly people diagnosed with a vitamin B_{12} deficiency. In a preliminary trial by Martin, et al. (*J Am Geriatr Soc* 1992;40:168–172), patients were given intramuscular injections of 1,000 mcg of vitamin B_{12} daily for one week, then weekly for a month, and finally monthly for between six and twelve months. The researchers noted significant improvements in cognitive function among participants with vitamin B_{12} deficiency and cognitive decline. It should be noted that cognitive disorders due to vitamin B_{12} deficiency may also occur in people who do not exhibit the anemia that often signifies vitamin B_{12} deficiency. This is demonstrated by a study by Lindenbaum, et al. (*N Engl J Med* 1988; 318:1720–1728). Of the elderly people with cognitive abnormalities due to vitamin B_{12} deficiency studied, 28 percent were not anemic. All deficient participants were given intramuscular injections of vitamin B_{12}, and cognitive function improved significantly in 100 percent, suggesting that B_{12} may exert some protective activity against homocysteine, an emerging marker for both heart disease and cognitive decline.

Vitamin B_{12} deficiency causes fatigue. Back in the 1970s, a small, double-blind trial by Ellis, et al. (*Br J Nutr* 1973;30:277–283) revealed that even some people who did not have a vitamin B_{12} deficiency had increased energy after being given vitamin B_{12} injections. More recently, the vitamin has been studied as a **treatment for chronic fatigue syndrome** (CFS). In one preliminary trial by Lapp and Cheney (*CFIDS Chronicle Physicians' Forum,* 1993;Fall: 19–20), 50 percent to 80 percent of CFS patients given 2,500–5,000 mcg of vitamin B_{12} via injection every two to three day saw a significant improvement in their condition.

DEFICIENCY SYMPTOMS

Deficiency of vitamin B_{12} is associated with pernicious anemia including weakness, a sore and inflamed tongue that appears smooth and shiny, numbness and tingling in extremities, pallor, weak pulse, stiffness, drowsiness, irritability, depression, mental deterioration, senile dementia, paranoid psychosis, chronic fatigue syndrome, diarrhea, poor appetite, and growth failure in children. Health experts estimate that as many as one in five adults have a vitamin B_{12} deficiency. The elderly, people whose gastrointestinal status is compromised (by gastritis or gastrectomy), those with autoimmune disorders (including type I, or insulin-dependent, diabetes mellitus and thyroid disease), and individuals receiving long-term therapy with gastric acid inhibitors or biguanide drugs may all benefit from vitamin B_{12} supplementation. As vitamin B_{12} is not found in plant foods unless they are fortified (for example, breakfast cereal), vegans are vulnerable to vitamin B_{12} deficiency and are likely to benefit from supplementation.

THERAPEUTIC DAILY AMOUNT

500–1,000 mcg (micrograms) with a complete B-complex vitamin. Sublingual form is best absorbed with tablets placed under the tongue. RDA is 2.4 mcg. For pregnant women, the RDA is 2.6 mcg, while for lactating women, it is 2.8 mcg. The European RDA is 1 mcg. The National Academy of Science of the U.S. recommends that adults over age fifty meet most of their recommended intake with synthetic B_{12} from fortified foods or vitamin supplements.

MAXIMUM SAFE LEVEL

3,000 mcg (long and short term; no adverse effect established) is a generally accepted upper safe limit, although no official tolerable upper intake level has been established.

SIDE EFFECTS/CONTRAINDICATIONS

Oral vitamin B_{12} is not associated with any side effects. However, serious allergic reactions to injections of vitamin B_{12} have been reported, although such side effects are rare. Patients with the rare eye disease Leber's disease should consult their doctor before taking vitamin B_{12}. Vitamin B_{12} should not be taken at the same time as the antibiotic tetracycline.

SOLUBILITY

Water soluble.

Vitamin B₂ (Riboflavin)

GENERAL DESCRIPTION

Vitamin B_2 is manufactured in the body by the intestinal flora, although very small quantities are stored in the body. Vitamin B_2 plays an important role in the metabolism of amino acids, fatty acids, and carbohydrates. There is evidence to suggest that it may play a role in red blood cell formation and antibody production. Natural sources of riboflavin include brewer's yeast, almonds, peanuts, organ meats, poultry, whole grains, wheat germ, wild rice, mushrooms, lentils, soybeans, milk, cheese, yogurt, eggs, broccoli, Brussels sprouts, and spinach. Flour and breakfast cereals are often fortified with vitamin B_2. Vitamin B_2 decomposes upon exposure to heat and light. Thus, milk, which is a major source of vitamin B_2, will have reduced levels of the vitamin if it is left in bright light or sunlight for long periods. Supplementary vitamin B_2 may be useful in people with **severe burns, chronic diarrhea, cirrhosis of the liver, alcoholism, and cancer.**

ROLE IN ANTI-AGING

Vitamin B_2 is vital for the formation of FAD (flavin adenine dinucleotide) and FMN (flavin mononucleotide), both of which are essential for metabolizing carbohydrates, proteins, and fats and make energy available in the body. The vitamin is also important to maintain metabolism and for the health and proper functioning of the cardiovascular and nervous systems. It also protects against free-radical damage and is necessary for good vision, skin, hair, and nails. Physical exercise increases the body's need for vitamin B_2.

Vitamin B_2 is believed to benefit the immune system by stimulating the multiplication of neutrophils and monocytes, and by activating macrophages.

Research also suggests that vitamin B_2 may help to prevent or slow the development of cataracts, and reduce the frequency of migraines.

DEFICIENCY SYMPTOMS

Symptoms include cheilosis or cracks and sores in the corners of the mouth; frayed or scaling lips; inflamed tongue with purplish or magenta color; eczema or seborrhea; flaking skin around the nose, eyebrows, chin, cheeks, earlobes, or hairline; oily appearance of nose, chin, and forehead with fatty deposits accumulating under the skin; bloodshot, watering, itching, burning, fatigued eyes with a keen sensitivity to light; increase in cataract formation; nervous symptoms such as "pins and needles" sensation, difficulty walking, muscular weakness, trembling and a lack of stamina or vigor; behavioral changes such as depression, moodiness, nervousness, and irritability.

Results of a study published in 2000 (Wacker J, Fruhauf J, et al. *Obstet Gynecol.* 2000;96:38–44) revealed that pregnant women with a vitamin B_2 deficiency may be at higher risk of developing the dangerous condition preeclampsia.

THERAPEUTIC DAILY AMOUNT

25–100 mg. The RDA is 1.3 mg for men, 1.1 mg for women, 1.4 mg for pregnant women, and 1.6 mg for women who are breastfeeding. The European RDA is 1.6 mg.

MAXIMUM SAFE LEVEL

200 mg (long and short term).

SIDE EFFECTS/CONTRAINDICATIONS

Vitamin B_2 is not associated with any serious side effects. However, prolonged use of very high doses may cause itching, numbness, burning or prickling sensations, and sensitivity to light. Riboflavin should not be taken at the same time as the antibiotic tetracycline, anti-malarial medications such as chloroquine and mefloquine, the anti-cancer drug doxorubicin, the Parkinson's drug selegiline, and sulfa-containing medications, for example, trimethoprim-sulfamethoxazole.

Patients taking propantheline, phenothiazines, tricyclic antidepressants, or probenecid should seek medical advice before supplementing their diet with vitamin B_2.

SOLUBILITY

Water soluble.

Vitamin B_3 (Niacin, Niacinamide, Nicotinic Acid, Nicotinamide)

GENERAL DESCRIPTION

Found in lean meats, organ meats, fish, brewer's yeast, whole grains, nuts, dried peas and beans, white meat of turkey or chicken, milk and milk products. Vitamin B_3 can also be synthesized by the body from the essential amino acid tryptophan.

ROLE IN ANTI-AGING

Vitamin B_3 is vital for **energy release in tissues and cells**, as it helps form the coenzymes NAD (nicotinamide adenine dinucleotide) and NADP (nicotinamide adenine dinucleotide phosphate), which are involved in the release of energy from food. The vitamin also helps to maintain a healthy **nervous and digestive**

system and is essential for **normal growth** and for **healthy skin**. It can also help to **lower "bad" cholesterol and triglyceride levels, while raising "good" HDL cholesterol levels**. Vitamin B$_3$ also plays a role in the production of bile salts and the synthesis of sex hormones. Some studies have also suggested that the vitamin may help to alleviate the symptoms of arthritis. Note: claims that vitamin B$_3$ prevents heart attack have not been clinically proven.

DEFICIENCY SYMPTOMS

Vitamin B$_3$ deficiency can cause the condition pellagra (symptoms include dermatitis, diarrhea, and dementia). Other symptoms of deficiency are bright red tongue; sore tongue and gums; inflamed mouth, throat, and esophagus; canker sores; mental illness; perceptual changes in the five senses; schizophrenic symptoms; rheumatoid arthritis; muscle weakness; general fatigue; irritability; recurring headaches; indigestion; nausea; vomiting; bad breath; insomnia; and small ulcers.

THERAPEUTIC DAILY AMOUNT

50–100 mg of niacinamide included in daily B-complex supplement. To lower cholesterol, researchers use the niacin form, 250–1,500 mg spread throughout the day. RDA is 16 mg for men and 14 mg for women. The European RDA is 18 mg.

MAXIMUM SAFE LEVEL

Nicotinamide—450 mg (long-term usage); 1,500 mg (short-term usage); Nicotinic acid—150 mg (long-term usage); 500 mg (short-term usage). Note: Dose of nicotinic acid in excess of these levels may cause temporary flushing of the skin in some individuals.

SIDE EFFECTS/CONTRAINDICATIONS

People with bleeding problems, diabetes mellitus, glaucoma, gout, liver disease, low blood pressure, or stomach ulcers should consult their doctor before taking vitamin B$_3$ supplements, as the vitamin may worsen their condition.

SOLUBILITY

Water soluble.

Vitamin B$_5$ (Pantothenic Acid, Calcium Pantothenate, Panthenol)

GENERAL DESCRIPTION

Vitamin B$_5$ is needed to make the neurotransmitter acetylcholine, as well as coenzyme A and the acyl carrier protein—both of which play important roles in the release of energy from fats, protein, and carbohydrates. It also helps to synthesize cholesterol, steroids, and fatty acids, and is required for healthy growth and the production of antibodies to help fight infection. Vitamin B_5 is important for the normal functioning of the adrenal glands and the production of cortisone.

Vitamin B_5 is sometimes referred to as the "anti-stress" vitamin because it is believed to enhance the activity of the immune system and increase the body's ability to withstand stressful conditions.

The best food sources of vitamin B_5 are brewer's yeast, corn, cauliflower, kale, broccoli, tomatoes, avocado, legumes, lentils, egg yolks, beef, turkey, duck, chicken, milk, split peas, peanuts, soybeans, sweet potatoes, sunflower seeds, whole-grain breads and cereals, lobster, wheat germ, and salmon. Vitamin B_5 is quite stable and little is lost during cooking.

ROLE IN ANTI-AGING

It has been suggested that vitamin B_5 may serve as an **effective weight-reducing agent**. Typically, ketogenesis and ketosis follow fasting or aggressive dieting. Leung (*Med Hypotheses* 1995;44:403–405) believes that ketone bodies are formed as a direct consequence of a deficiency in dietary pantothenic acid, and that supplementation of pantothenic acid would facilitate complete catabolism of fatty acids and thus circumvent the formation of ketone bodies. Leung suggests that a sufficient amount of energy would be released from storage fat to relieve dieters of the sensation of hunger and weakness.

Vaxman, et al. (*Eur Surg Res* 1996;28:306–14) found that (0.2 or 0.9 g/day) of vitamin B_5 may **aid wound healing**. Research by Kapp and colleagues from the University of Freiburg in Germany suggests calcium panthothenate, the stable salt form of vitamin B_5, may aid wound healing by inhibiting an inflammatory response triggered by granulocytes that impairs the skin's healing abilities.

Slyshenkov, et al. (*Acta Biochim Pol.* 1999;46:239–248) found that vitamin B_5 helps to **protect cells against low-dose gamma radiation**, thus suggesting that vitamin B_5 may have radioprotective properties.

Some people believe that vitamin B_5 may be beneficial to people with **rheumatoid arthritis**, although there is little evidence to support this claim.

Several studies suggest that pantethine, a byproduct of vitamin B_5, may help reduce the amount of cholesterol made by the body. Several preliminary and at least two controlled trials have found that pantethine significantly **lowers serum cholesterol levels and may also increase HDL or "good" cholesterol levels**. It has also been shown to **lower triglyceride levels**. However, none of these effects have been seen with vitamin B_5.

DEFICIENCY SYMPTOMS

Deficiency symptoms include a burning sensation in the feet; enlarged beefy, furrowed tongue; skin disorders such as eczema; duodenal ulcers, inflammation of the intestines and stomach; decreased antibody formation; upper respiratory infections; vomiting; restlessness; muscle cramps; constipation; sensitivity to insulin; adrenal exhaustion; physical and mental depression; overwhelming fatigue; reduced production of hydrochloric acid in the stomach; allergies; arthritis; nerve degeneration; spinal curvature; disturbed pulse rate; gout; and graying hair.

Vitamin B_5 deficiencies are rare. Alcoholics are at the highest risk of developing a deficiency.

THERAPEUTIC DAILY AMOUNT

Pantothenic acid comes in two forms: calcium pantothenate, which is typically used for treating conditions such as stress and heartburn, and pantethine—a byproduct of pantothenic acid—which is used to lower cholesterol levels.

A typical dose is 10–25 mg in a B-complex supplement or up to 50 mg in divided doses. No RDA for vitamin B_5 has been established in the United States as the Food and Nutrition Board of the Institute of Medicine felt the existing scientific evidence was insufficient to calculate an RDA. Therefore they set an adequate intake level (AI) of 5 mg for men and women. The European RDA is 6 mg.

Studies using pantethine to lower cholesterol typically used dosages of 900 mg, split into three 300-mg doses.

MAXIMUM SAFE LEVEL

1,000 mg—doses of around 10,000 mg cause diarrhea and gastrointestinal disturbances.

SIDE EFFECTS/CONTRAINDICATIONS

Vitamin B_5 is not known to cause side effects, except in excessively large doses. Vitamin B_5 should not be taken at the same time as the antibiotic drug tetracycline.

SOLUBILITY

Water soluble.

Vitamin B₆ (Pyridoxine)

GENERAL DESCRIPTION

Found in brewer's yeast, sunflower seeds, wheat germ, liver and other organ meats, blackstrap molasses, bananas, walnuts, roasted peanuts, canned tuna, and salmon. Breakfast cereals are often fortified with vitamin B_6. Vegetarians and vegans, women taking the combined contraceptive pill, people aged fifty-five and above, and heavy drinkers may all benefit from taking supplementary vitamin B_6.

ROLE IN ANTI-AGING

Vitamin B_6 **metabolizes proteins, fats, and carbohydrates**; it **forms hormones for adrenaline and insulin,** and is essential for maintaining a **healthy nervous system**. It is also required for the formation of **hemoglobin** in red blood cells and **antibodies** that help fight infection. Vitamin B_6 is used in the synthesis of RNA and DNA, and is needed for the production of hydrochloric acid. It also helps to regulate body fluids. Several studies have shown that vitamin B_6 helps to lower blood levels of the amino acid homocysteine. Elevated homocysteine levels are associated with an increased risk of heart disease and stroke, Alzheimer's disease, Parkinson's disease, and osteoporosis.

In a double blind, randomized trial by Till et al. (*Atherosclerosis.* 2005; 181:131–135.) 50 patients at risk of cerebral ischemia received daily 2.5 mg folic acid, 25 mg Vitamin B_6, and 0.5 mg Vitamin B_{12} or placebo for 1 year. Results showed that the vitamins significantly reduced carotid intima-media thickness (IMT), an accepted marker of atherosclerotic changes, thus suggesting that vitamin B_6 may help to prevent cardiovascular disease. Results of a study by Larsson et al. (*Gastroenterology.* 2005;128:1830–1837.) suggest that vitamin B_6 may help to prevent colorectal cancer, particularly among women who drink alcohol.

Vitamin B_6 can help to relieve carpal tunnel syndrome and symptoms of PMS; when used alongside magnesium, it can help to prevent kidney stones. Some research has suggested that vitamin B_6 may be useful in alleviating the symptoms of asthma; however, this remains inconclusive.

DEFICIENCY SYMPTOMS

Symptoms of vitamin B_6 deficiency include greasy, scaly dermatitis between the eyebrows and on body parts that rub together; low blood sugar; numbness and tingling in the hands and feet; neuritis; arthritis; trembling hands in the aged; water retention and swelling during pregnancy; nausea; motion sickness;

mental retardation; epilepsy; kidney stones; anemia; excessive fatigue; nervous breakdown; mental illness; acne; and convulsions. Babies and newborn infants may develop crusty yellow scabs on the scalp called "cradle cap." Government surveys suggest that as many as one-third of U.S. adults suffer from vitamin B_6 deficiency.

THERAPEUTIC DAILY AMOUNT

50–100 mg combined with a B-complex supplement. RDA is 2 mg. The RDA for men and women aged 19 to 50 years is 1.3 mg. For men aged 51 years and older the RDA is 1.7 mg, and for women aged 51 years and older it is 1.5 mg. The European RDA is 2 mg.

MAXIMUM SAFE LEVEL

Doses of up to 100 mg per day on a long-term basis are safe, although no adverse effects have been seen with doses of up to 200 mg. Doses in excess of 200 mg may cause nerve damage in the long term.

SIDE EFFECTS/CONTRAINDICATIONS

No side effects are associated with recommended dosages of vitamin B_6. Vitamin B_6 can cause neurological disorders, such as loss of sensation in legs and imbalance, when taken in doses of 200 mg or more per day over a long period of time. However, discontinuing the use of such high doses usually leads to a complete recovery within 6 months. There have also been reports of allergic skin reactions to high doses of vitamin B_6 supplements, however such reactions are extremely rare. People taking the antibiotic tetracycline, levodopa (a medication used to treat Parkinson's disease), phenytoin (a medication used to treat seizures), and hydralazine (a medication used to treat high blood pressure) should consult their doctor before taking supplementary vitamin B_6.

SOLUBILITY

Water soluble.

Folic Acid (Folacin, Folate)

GENERAL DESCRIPTION

Folic acid is needed for RNA and DNA synthesis, red blood cell production, and the metabolism of protein. It also increases the activity and production of antibodies and may reduce susceptibility to infection. Supplementary folic acid may help to strengthen the immune system of older people. Results of a study published in January 2006 (Field CJ, et al. *J Nutr Biochem.* 2006;17:37–44.) revealed that folic acid improves age-related decreases in lymphocyte (white blood cell) function. As folic acid is vital for the correct development of the neural tube, it is particularly important that women who are trying to conceive and those who are in the first trimester (three months) of pregnancy consume enough folic acid. Some research has shown that folic acid supplementation can reduce the risk of neural tube defects, such as spina bifida, by as much as 72 percent. Folic acid can also protect against other birth defects, including heart defects, defects of the upper lip and mouth, urinary tract defects, and limb-reduction defects. Research published in 2003 suggests that folic acid may also reduce the risk of Down's syndrome, and almost halve the risk of the unborn child's developing leukemia in childhood.

Folic acid is found in dark-green leafy vegetables, liver, brewer's yeast, whole grains, bran, asparagus, lima beans, lentils, and orange juice.

ROLE IN ANTI-AGING

Research published in 2002 found that people with the highest intakes of dietary folic acid were 21 percent **less likely to have a stroke** (*Stroke*. 2002; 33:1183–1188). This is likely to be due to folic acid's ability to **lower levels of the amino acid homocysteine**. High plasma levels of homocysteine have been implicated in the development of vascular diseases, including stroke, thromboembolism (blood clots that can dislodge and cause stroke, heart attack, and other complications), and other diseases, such as osteoporosis, inflammatory bowel disease (Crohn's disease and ulcerative colitis), Alzheimer's disease, diabetes, complications of pregnancy, and hypothyroidism. It is now well accepted that plasma levels of total homocysteine can be lowered effectively by supplementation with folic acid, vitamin B_6, and vitamin B_{12}. Many studies concerned with lowering homocysteine levels used doses of 400–1,000 mcg of folic acid per day, 10–50 mg of vitamin B_6 per day, and 50–300 mcg of vitamin B_{12} per day. It is estimated that 50,000 deaths from cardiovascular disease could be prevented each year in the United States if people consumed enough folic acid. Research by Thambyrajah, et al. (*Journal of the American College of Cardiology* 2001;37:1858–1863) suggests that folic acid may **lower the risk of heart disease by preventing damage to the endothelium**, the inner lining of arteries. Research by Seshadri, et al. (*N Engl J Med*. 2002;346:476–483) published in 2002 showed that people with the highest blood level of homocysteine were nearly twice as likely to develop dementia or Alzheimer's disease as those with the lowest levels; thus, folic acid may help to **ward off cognitive decline** by keeping homocysteine levels under control. Results of a study by Bazzano et al. (*Stroke*. 2002;33:1183–1188.) found that people with the highest intakes of dietary folic acid were 21% less likely to have a stroke. In a double blind, randomized trial by Till et al. (*Atherosclerosis.* 2005;181:131–135.) 50 patients at risk of cerebral ischemia received daily 2.5 mg folic acid, 25 mg Vitamin B_6, and 0.5 mg Vitamin B_{12} or placebo for 1 year. Results showed that the vitamins significantly reduced carotid intima-media thickness (IMT), an accepted marker of atherosclerotic changes.

Folic acid also appears to protect against cancer of the colon and rectum. Research by Terry, et al. (*International Journal of Cancer* 2002;97:864–867) found that women with the highest intakes of folic acid were 40 percent **less likely to develop colorectal cancer**. Folic acid may play a role in depression and depressive illness. Research has shown that people with major depressive illnesses commonly have low levels of plasma, serum, or red blood cell folate, and that supplementing antidepressant medication with folic acid enhances the therapeutic effect of these drugs. Abou-Saleh et al. (*J Psychosom Res.* 2006; 61:285–287.) recommend that 2 mg of folic acid should be given during treatment of depression, whilst Coppen et al. (*J Psychopharmacol.* 2005;19: 59–65.) recommend that oral doses of both folic acid (800 mcg daily) and vitamin B_{12} (1 mg daily) should be tried to improve treatment outcome in depression.

DEFICIENCY SYMPTOMS

Folic acid deficiency symptoms include anemia; poor growth; weakness; an inflamed and sore tongue that may appear smooth and shiny; numbness or tingling in the hands and feet; indigestion; diarrhea; depression; irritability; pallor; drowsiness; a slow, weakened pulse; graying hair; mental illness; impaired wound healing; reduced resistance to infection; birth defects resulting in spina bifida and other neural tube defects; toxemia; insomnia; leg numbness and cramps in pregnant women; premature birth and after birth hemorrhaging; cervical cancer; and dysplasia.

THERAPEUTIC DAILY AMOUNT

400–800 mcg (micrograms) combined with B-complex vitamin. RDA for men and women is 400 mcg; women who are planning to or who may become pregnant, and those in the first trimester of pregnancy are advised to take 600 mcg of folic acid every day. The RDA for nursing women is 500 mcg. The European RDA is 200 mcg.

MAXIMUM SAFE LEVEL

The maximum safe levels are 400 mcg (long-term usage), 700 mcg (short-term usage). The National Academy of Sciences recommends that the daily intake of folic acid in adults should not exceed 1,000 mcg. Very high doses of folic acid may trigger seizures in people with epilepsy.

SIDE EFFECTS/CONTRAINDICATIONS
Individuals taking antiepileptic drugs should seek doctor's advice before taking supplements.

SOLUBILITY
Water soluble.

Inositol Hexanicotinate

GENERAL DESCRIPTION
Inositol hexaphosphate, or IP6, is a naturally occurring component of plant fiber that is thought to possess antioxidant, anticancer, and other beneficial properties. It can be found in the germ of bran portion of whole grains (especially whole kernel corn) and legumes. Inositol hexanicotinate consists of six molecules of niacin (also known as vitamin B_3, niacinamide, nicotinic acid, or nicotinamide) surrounding a molecule of inositol. It is an unofficial B vitamin, and is occasionally referred to as vitamin B_8.

ROLE IN ANTI-AGING
As inositol hexanicotinate is slowly metabolized by the body and releases niacin over a period of time, it generally has the same anti-aging benefits as niacin; however, some research suggests that inositol hexanicotinate is safer and better tolerated.

Niacin is vital for energy release in tissues and cells, as it helps form the coenzymes NAD (nicotinamide adenine dinucleotide) and NADP (nicotinamide adenine dinucleotide phosphate), which are involved in the release of energy from food. The vitamin also helps to maintain a healthy nervous and digestive system and is essential for normal growth and for healthy skin. Niacin can also help to **lower cholesterol and triglyceride levels**—some research suggests that inositol hexanicotinate is slightly more effective than niacin in this regard. Niacin also plays a role in the production of bile salts and the synthesis of sex hormones. Some studies have suggested that the vitamin may help to **alleviate the symptoms of arthritis**.

IP6 is also thought to prevent tumor development by controlling cell development, and may assist in the treatment of existing cancer by helping natural killer cells to enter cancer cells and by triggering cancer cells to undergo apoptosis (cellular suicide). El-Sherbiny et al. (*Anticancer Res.* 2001;21:2393–2403.) found that IP6 prevents cancer cells from proliferating by halting cells in the G0/G1-stage of the cell cycle and inhibiting cells in the S-stage where DNA is normally synthesized. Animal studies have shown that supplementation with IP-6 can protect against colon cancer and possibly breast cancer. An *in vivo* study on pancreatic cancer cell lines by Somasundar et al. (*J Surg Res.* 2005;126:199–203.) revealed that IP6 lead to significant reductions (37%–95%) in cell proliferation and increased early and late apoptotic activity. These findings led the researchers to conclude that IP6 may be an effective adjunct for pancreatic cancer treatment.

DEFICIENCY SYMPTOMS

Inositol hexanicotinate is not essential for health, thus no deficiency symptoms are recognized. However, people displaying symptoms of niacin (vitamin B_3) deficiency may benefit from inositol hexanicotinate. Niacin deficiency can cause the condition pellagra (symptoms include dermatitis, diarrhea, and dementia). Other symptoms of deficiency are bright red tongue; sore tongue and gums; inflamed mouth, throat, and esophagus; canker sores; mental illness; perceptual changes in the five senses; schizophrenic symptoms; rheumatoid arthritis; muscle weakness; general fatigue; irritability; recurring headaches; indigestion; nausea; vomiting; bad breath; insomnia; and small ulcers.

THERAPEUTIC DAILY AMOUNT

500–1,500 mg. A typical dose of IP6 as a preventive supplement is 1–2 g/day. Higher doses are used for the treatment of cancer, however if used for this reason, IP6 should only be taken under the direction of a qualified health professional.

MAXIMUM SAFE LEVEL

Not established.

SIDE EFFECTS/CONTRAINDICATIONS

Inositol hexanicotinate has not been linked with the side effects associated with niacin supplementation.

IP6 can interfere with iron absorption, thus it should only be taken under medical supervision. People with cancer or immune-related illnesses should talk to their specialist before taking IP6.

Pyrroloquinoline Quinone (PQQ)

GENERAL DESCRIPTION

Pyrroloquinoline quinone (PQQ) was discovered in 1979; however, in 2003, scientists Takaoki Kasahara and Tadafumi Kato (*Nature.* 2003;422:832) found that PQQ is needed to produce an enzyme that is needed for the body to degrade the amino acid lysine in mice. As a result, PQQ has, somewhat controversially, been newly classed as a B vitamin. Tests show that **PQQ appears to play an important role in immune response and fertility** in mice, and the scientists suspect that PQQ may have a similar function in humans.

PQQ can be found in vegetables such as parsley, green peppers, and kiwi fruit, and some meats.

ROLE IN ANTI-AGING

Not yet known; however, it may help to keep the immune system healthy, and aid in reproduction. No clinical human trials on PQQ have been published to date.

DEFICIENCY SYMPTOMS

Mice fed a PQQ-deficient diet grew slowly, had fragile skin, and a reduced immune response.

THERAPEUTIC DAILY AMOUNT

Not established.

MAXIMUM SAFE LEVEL

Not established.

SIDE EFFECTS/CONTRAINDICATIONS

Not established.

PABA (Para-Amino-Benzoic Acid)

GENERAL DESCRIPTION

PABA is found in liver, brewer's yeast, wheat germ, molasses, eggs, organ meats, yogurt, and green leafy vegetables.

ROLE IN ANTI-AGING

PABA stimulates intestinal bacteria, which aids in **production of pantothenic acid** (vitamin B_5). PABA is a coenzyme and is involved in the **production of blood cells, metabolism of protein**, and is important for **healthy skin, hair pigmentation, and intestinal health**. It may also help with **vitiligo** (a disease characterized by abnormal white blotches of skin due to loss of pigmentation). PABA is used to treat many skin conditions.

DEFICIENCY SYMPTOMS

Similar to symptoms caused by folic acid or pantothenic acid deficiency; but including vitiligo, fatigue, irritability, depression, nervousness, headache, constipation, and other digestive disorders.

THERAPEUTIC DAILY AMOUNT
50–100 mg included in a B-complex vitamin. No RDA has been established.

MAXIMUM SAFE LEVEL
Not established.

SIDE EFFECTS/CONTRAINDICATIONS
No serious side effects have been reported at doses of 300–400 mg per day. However, excessive doses of PABA (upward of 8 grams per day) have been linked to hypoglycemia, rash, fever, and liver damage.

PABA should not be used by people taking dapsone, methotrexate, sulfamethoxazole, sulfasalazine, or trimethoprim.

SOLUBILITY
Water soluble.

Vitamin C (Ascorbic Acid)

GENERAL DESCRIPTION
Vitamin C is a potent antioxidant and protects against free radical cellular damage. It is vital for the formation and maintenance of collagen (the skin's "cement"), for healthy skin, and for the formation of other structural materials in bones, teeth, and capillaries. Vitamin C also protects against industrial pollutants, certain eye disorders, and bleeding gums, and is the best known of the immune system-boosting nutrients. Vitamin C is found in rose hips, citrus fruit and juices, strawberries, blueberries, cantaloupes, tomatoes, and raw vegetables such as red bell peppers. Vitamin C is easily destroyed by cooking and levels are reduced during storage.

ROLE IN ANTI-AGING
Vitamin C is a potent antioxidant and studies suggest that it may help to prevent cancer in a number of ways—it reduces lipid peroxidation, which has been linked to degeneration and the aging process, and it protects DNA from free radical-induced damage.

Research has shown that vitamin C raises HDL, or "good," cholesterol, and prevents "bad" LDL cholesterol from oxidation, which subsequently prevents the build-up of atherosclerotic plaques on the blood vessel wall. It has also been shown to improve nitric oxide activity and reverse endothelial dysfunction (abnormal functioning of the cells that line blood vessels), which is linked to the development of atherosclerosis. Thus, vitamin C may be useful in preventing cardiovascular disease.

Results of a study by Kurl, et al. (*Stroke* 2002;33:1568–1573) suggest that vitamin C may help to **lower the risk of stroke**. Men who had relatively low blood levels of vitamin C were 2.4 times more likely to have a stroke than men with the highest blood levels of the nutrient. The results also revealed that men who consumed little vitamin C and were overweight or had high blood pressure were nearly three times as likely to suffer a stroke compared with non-hypertensive men of normal weight who had a high vitamin C intake. Vitamin C may protect against Alzheimer's disease. Results of a study by Zandi et al. (*Arch Neurol.* 2004;61:82–88.) suggest that it may be possible to reduce the risk of Alzheimer's disease by taking vitamins E and C in combination. Participants taking both vitamins were 78% less likely to show signs of Alzheimer's disease than those not taking the combination. They found no benefit from taking either of the vitamins in isolation, or from taking multivitamins alone. The researchers concluded "Antioxidant supplements merit further study as agents for the primary prevention of Alzheimer's disease."

It is also vital for the **formation and maintenance of collagen** (the skin's "cement"), for healthy skin, and for the formation of other structural materials in bones, teeth, and capillaries. Vitamin C assists with **wound healing and burns**, especially for those recovering from surgery, and helps to keep the **nervous system** functioning properly. It also increases the **absorption of iron and calcium** from plant sources, and heightens **resistance to infection**. Large doses of the vitamin may help to relieve **cold and flu** symptoms. Some research has found that vitamin C may help to prevent male infertility. Some research suggests that vitamin C may help to prevent cataracts. Results of a study by Jacques et al. (*Am J Clin Nutr.* 1997;66:911–916) showed that women who took vitamin C supplements for at least ten years were 77 percent less likely to develop "lens opacities"—the beginning stage of cataracts—than women who didn't take supplementary vitamin C.

Research published in 2003 suggests that some post-surgery complications could be avoided in some critically ill patients by giving them the antioxidant vitamins C and E while they are in the hospital. Nathens, et al. (*Annals of Surgery* 2003;236:814–822) found that trauma patients who received the vitamins from the time of admission until the time of release from the hospital spent less time in intensive care following surgery, were significantly less likely to have multiple organ failure, and also spent less time on a mechanical ventilator.

DEFICIENCY SYMPTOMS

Vitamin C deficiency can cause the disease scurvy; however, this is uncommon in developed countries. Symptoms of vitamin C deficiency include bruising easily, bleeding gums, tooth decay, nosebleeds, swollen or painful joints, anemia, poor wound healing, lowered resistance to infection, general weakening of connective tissue, easily fractured bones, weakened arteries that rupture or hemorrhage, extreme muscle weakness, painful joints, and wounds and sores that will not heal.

THERAPEUTIC DAILY AMOUNT

1,000–2,000 mg, depending on need. RDA is 90 mg for men and 75 mg for women. The European RDA is 60 mg.

Research suggests that vitamin C may enhance the effects of some chemotherapy drugs; however, cancer patients should always consult their oncologist before taking dietary supplements.

MAXIMUM SAFE LEVEL

2,000 mg (long-term usage); 3,000 mg (short-term usage).

Note: Research has found that blood levels of the vitamin do not increase further when vitamin C doses exceed 250–500 mg per day. High doses of vitamin C can cause kidney stones in people with a history of the condition and those who regularly undergo hemodialysis.

SIDE EFFECTS/CONTRAINDICATIONS

No side effects are associated with vitamin C; however, large doses of the vitamin can deplete the body's supplies of the essential nutrient copper.

People with a glucose-6-phosphate dehydrogenase deficiency, iron overload (hemosiderosis or hemochromatosis), history of kidney stones, or kidney failure should consult their doctor before taking supplementary vitamin C.

Women taking the contraceptive pill should not take excessively large doses of vitamin C as it may reduce the effectiveness of the pill. People taking ampicillin, indomethacin, salsalate, or tetracycline should not take supplementary vitamin C without consulting their doctor.

SOLUBILITY

Water soluble.

Ascorbyl Palmitate

GENERAL DESCRIPTION

Ascorbyl palmitate is a fat-soluble form of vitamin C.

ROLE IN ANTI-AGING

Ascorbyl palmitate is a **potent antioxidant** that has been shown to help **prevent infections, bruising, colds and flu, sinusitis, sore throats, blood clots, atherosclerosis, and high blood pressure**. There is some evidence to suggest that it may help to strengthen the immune system, **improve blood cholesterol profile, protect the liver from toxic chemicals, and enhance collagen formation**.

DEFICIENCY SYMPTOMS

Not applicable.

THERAPEUTIC DAILY AMOUNT

500 mg of ascorbyl palmitate is typically taken with each meal.

MAXIMUM SAFE LEVEL

Not established.

SIDE EFFECTS/CONTRAINDICATIONS

None known.

SOLUBILITY

Fat soluble.

Vitamin D (Ergocalciferol)

GENERAL DESCRIPTION

Vitamin D is derived from sunshine (manufactured through the skin), fish liver oils such as cod liver oil, liver, and egg yolks. Margarine and cereals are often fortified with vitamin D. It is unlikely that food alone will provide sufficient vitamin D; therefore, several sources recommend trying to obtain five to fifteen minutes of exposure to sunshine each day.

ROLE IN ANTI-AGING

Vitamin D enhances the **absorption of calcium** from the intestine and the **utilization of calcium and phosphorus** in the body, thus ensuring that calcium and phosphorus levels are high enough to support the constant breakdown and rebuilding of bone tissue. It is therefore essential for strong and healthy bones. There is mounting evidence to suggest that vitamin D not only makes bone stronger, but also has a positive affect on the muscles. Bischoff-Ferrari et al. (*JAMA.* 2004;291:1999–2006.) found that vitamin D supplementation appears to make seniors more stable on their legs and reduce their risk of falling by more than 20 percent. Vitamin D is also necessary for the proper **functioning of the thyroid and pituitary glands**. It is used to improve **psoriasis** and maintenance of **cell membrane fluidity**. Vitamin D is a potent immune system modulator. Research has shown that the vitamin D receptor is expressed by most cells of the immune system, including T-cells (white blood cells that are crucial to the immune system) and antigen-presenting cells (cells that present foreign substances capable of eliciting an immune response, such as bacteria, to the immune system), such as dendritic cells (specialized cells that present antigens (foreign substances) to specific cells of the immune system) and macrophages (a type of white blood cell that protects the body against infection.) There is also evidence to suggest that vitamin D exerts a variety of effects on immune system function that may enhance innate immunity and help to prevent the development of autoimmunity. Both animal and human studies suggest that vitamin D may protect people from multiple sclerosis, autoimmune arthritis, and type I diabetes.

A study of nearly 190,000 women by Munger et al. (*Neurology.* 2004;62: 60–65.) found that those who took vitamin D supplements were 40 percent less likely to develop multiple sclerosis. Other research has shown that vitamin D supplements can prevent or favorably affect the course of a disease similar to multiple sclerosis in mice. Recent studies suggest that vitamin D may also protect against breast, colon, and prostate cancers. John et al. (*Cancer Res.* 2005;65:5470–5479.) found that men exposed to a high amount of sun had half the risk of prostate cancer than those exposed to a low amount. The researchers believe that this protective effect is a result of the fact that the body manufactures vitamin D when exposed to sunlight. Previous research has shown that the prostate uses vitamin D to promote the normal growth of prostate cells and to inhibit the invasiveness and spread of cancer cells to other parts of the body. Other research suggests that vitamin D may benefit people with lung cancer. Zhou et al. (*Cancer Epidemiol Biomarkers Prev.* 2005;14:2303–2309.) found that lung cancer patients who have surgery in the winter are 40 percent more likely to die of the disease than those operated on in the summer. Vitamin D may also protect against breast and colon cancers. Research also suggests that vitamin D may help to protect against cardiovascular disease. Some intervention studies have shown that vitamin D can lower blood pressure in hypertensive patients, and results of a study by researchers at the University of California San Francisco published in 2002 revealed that women over the age of sixty-five who regularly took vitamin D were nearly one-third less likely to die from heart disease, compared with women who did not take the vitamin.

DEFICIENCY SYMPTOMS

Osteomalacia (softening of the bones) in adults, rickets in children, irritability, restlessness, fitful sleeping, frequent crying, heavy perspiration behind the neck in babies, delayed eruption of teeth, soft and yielding skull, bowed legs, knock knees, depressions in the chest, pigeon-chest deformity of the rib cage, swayback, overly prominent forehead causing the appearance of sunken eyes, and delayed walking.

Results of a study by Tangpricha, et al. (*American Journal of Medicine* 2002;112:659–662) revealed that many young adults suffer from vitamin D deficiency. Thirty percent of young adults were found to be deficient in vitamin D at the end of winter, and 11 percent in the summer. The most-affected age group was the eighteen to twenty-nine year olds, 36 percent of whom were suffering from vitamin D deficiency by the time spring arrived.

THERAPEUTIC DAILY AMOUNT

400–800 IU from fish liver oil. The RDA for vitamin D is 200 IU a day for men and women aged nineteen to fifty, 400 IU for those aged fifty-one to seventy, and 600 IU for people aged seventy-one and over. The European RDA is 5 mcg. Hollis (*J Nutr.* 2005;135:317–322.) believes that the current RDA's for vitamin D are very inadequate when one considers that a 10–15 min whole-body exposure to peak summer sun will generate and release up to 20,000 IU vitamin D into the circulation. Hollis argues that humans did not evolve to live in a "sunshy" culture, and therefore "normal" with respect to circulating vitamin D levels should not be defined by the current average or median population level. Hollis suggests that the requirements for vitamin D should be re-examined, and that re-examination may likely reveal the need for vitamin D intakes exceeding 2000 IU/d for adults.

MAXIMUM SAFE LEVEL

10 mcg (long-term usage); 50 mcg (short-term usage). A daily intake (both from fortified food and supplements) of more than 1,000 IU of vitamin D is not advisable. Regular consumption of vitamin D at doses greater than 1,000 IU day may cause high blood pressure, premature hardening of the arteries, deterioration of bone, calcium buildup in muscles and soft tissues, and kidney damage.

SIDE EFFECTS/CONTRAINDICATIONS

Pregnant or breast-feeding women should limit their vitamin D intake to no more than 800 IU a day as higher doses have been linked to birth abnormalities.

Vitamin D supplements should not be used by people taking antacids containing magnesium and thiazide diuretics, such as hydrochlorothiazide. People with high blood calcium or phosphorus levels, heart problems, and kidney disease, such consult their physician before taking supplementary vitamin D.

SOLUBILITY

Fat soluble.

Vitamin E (Tocopherol)

GENERAL DESCRIPTION

Vitamin E is found in wheat germ oil, soybean oil, safflower oil, peanuts, whole grains (wheat, rice, oats), leafy green vegetables, cabbage, spinach, asparagus, broccoli, and egg yolks.

ROLE IN ANTI-AGING

Vitamin E is a potent **antioxidant** that helps to neutralize potentially damaging free radicals, and prevents polyunsaturated oils from breaking down. It may also be useful in **gangrene, diabetes mellitus, congenital heart disease, phlebitis, and other leg problems due to poor circulation**. It also helps with varicose veins. Some research has suggested that vitamin E can help to prevent stroke and other cardiovascular problems. A handful of studies have found that 400–800 IU of natural vitamin E per day lowers the risk of heart attack; however, other trials have obtained conflicting results.

Results of the Alpha Tocopherol-Beta Carotene Study, which involved more than 29,000 men, revealed that men who took vitamin E supplements were 32 percent less likely to develop prostate cancer and 41 percent less likely to die from the disease. Results of the largest ever trial on vitamin E supplementation by Lee et al. (*JAMA*. 2005;294:56–65) suggest that supplementary vitamin E is unlikely to prevent heart disease or cancer. However, results of the study of nearly 40,000 women did find that women taking the high-dose natural alpha-tocopherol supplements had a significantly lower risk of death and also a much lower risk of heart attack and stroke if they were over the age of 65. Thus, the value of vitamin E for these purposes remains inconclusive.

Vitamin E may help to normalize the **activity of ovaries** in women, hence improving periods and preventing excessive bleeding and vaginal dryness.

Morris, et al. (*Archives of Neurology* 2002;59:1125–1132) found that consuming high levels of vitamin E can **slow the rate of mental decline** by more than one-third. Results showed that the rate of decline among those with the highest intake was 36 percent slower than that of those who consumed the least. The same researchers have also published research suggesting that a high intake of vitamin E could **lower the risk of developing Alzheimer's disease** by as much as 70 percent.

Research suggests that vitamin E may boost the immune system, and if applied externally, it **eliminates radiation burns** and **reduces scarring**. It may also benefit patients with osteoarthritis and may help relieve **menopausal symptoms**. Finally, vitamin E may **increase stamina** in athletes and **improve the action of insulin**.

Research published in 2003 suggests that some **post-surgery complications could be avoided** in some critically ill patients by giving them the antioxidant vitamins C and E while they are in the hospital. Nathens, et al. (*Annals of Surgery* 2003;236:814–822) found that trauma patients who received the vitamins from the time of admission until the time of release from the hospital spent less time in intensive care following surgery, were significantly less likely to have multiple organ failure, and also spent less time on a mechanical ventilator.

DEFICIENCY SYMPTOMS

Vitamin E deficiencies are extremely rare. Symptoms include decreased survival time of red blood cells, faulty fat absorption, anemia in premature infants, degeneration of the brain and spinal cord, premature births and higher risk of miscarriage, decrease in sex hormones, and a higher risk of skin cancer.

THERAPEUTIC DAILY AMOUNT

400–1,200 IU. To obtain these potencies, one should use natural vitamin E supplements, as d-alpha tocopherol or the dry form, d-alpha tocopherol succinate. The US RDA for vitamin E has recently been updated and is now 15 mg (22.5 IU) for both men and women, which is the same as the European RDA.

MAXIMUM SAFE LEVEL

800 IU (long and short term). The daily tolerable upper intake level for adults established by the National Academy of Sciences is 1,000 mg of vitamin E, which is equivalent to 1,500 IU of natural vitamin E or 1,100 IU of synthetic vitamin E.

SIDE EFFECTS/CONTRAINDICATIONS

Vitamin E should not be taken in combination with anticoagulant drugs such as warfarin and aspirin. People taking tricyclic antidepressants, the antipsychotic medication chlorpromazine, beta-blockers, and anti-malarial medication should consult their physician before taking supplementary vitamin E. Due to vitamin E's blood-thinning properties people scheduled for elective surgery (including dental surgery) are advised to avoid supplementary vitamin E for two days before and after surgery. Much controversy concerning the safety of vitamin E supplementation arose following the publication of a study by Miller et al. in 2005 (*Ann Intern Med.* 2005;142:37–46), in which supplementary vitamin E was linked to an increased risk of death in elderly people. It should be noted that the study population in Miller's study was elderly and many of the participants had pre-existing serious illnesses, such as heart disease. Following the publication of the study by Miller et al., Hathcock et al. (*Am J Clin Nutr.* 2005;81:736–745) published a review of the safety of both vitamin C and Vitamin E, in which the authors concluded: "The fact that adverse effects are rarely reported for vitamins E at amounts higher than the RDA is testimony to the safety of such dietary supplementation up to the upper limit. Several literature reviews have concluded, on the basis of a survey of published evidence, that such intake does not cause adverse side effects or create other safety issues.The recommendations are entirely based on the available scientific evidence; the main caveat is that healthy persons should not "routinely" take vitamin E in amounts higher than the upper limit. Beyond that, the recommendations support the consensus of published studies that vitamin E doses up to 1000 mg/day are safe for use by the general population."

SOLUBILITY

Fat soluble.

Vitamin K (Phylloquinone)

GENERAL DESCRIPTION

Vitamin K can be found in yogurt, kefir, acidophilus milk, alfalfa, spinach, cabbage, cauliflower, tomatoes, pork liver, lean meat, peas, carrots, soybeans, potatoes, and egg yolk.

ROLE IN ANTI-AGING

Vitamin K is essential for the **formation of several proteins, called "clotting factors,"** that regulate blood clotting within the body. Vitamin K is also required for the formation of some proteins that are important for **proper bone mineralization** and **healthy teeth**. Vitamin K has been beneficial to people with Crohn's disease and gastrointestinal disorders.

DEFICIENCY SYMPTOMS

Dietary deficiencies of vitamin K are rare, because vitamin K is normally manufactured by bacteria present in the intestine. However, symptoms may include hypoprothrombinemia (a condition in which the time it takes for the blood to clot is prolonged), hemorrhages, bloody urine and stools, nosebleeds, and miscarriages. Deficiency in newborn babies results in bloody stools or vomiting (fairly common since newborns have no intestinal bacteria). Recent studies suggest that many men and women aged eighteen to forty-four regularly consume less than the RDA of vitamin K.

THERAPEUTIC DAILY AMOUNT
Most vitamin and mineral supplements do not contain vitamin K as it is readily available in the diet and synthesized in the body. Consult your physician for further information on this vitamin. RDA for women is 65 mcg; 80 mcg for men. There is no European RDA for vitamin K.

MAXIMUM SAFE LEVEL
Not known.

SIDE EFFECTS/CONTRAINDICATIONS
People taking any over-the-counter or prescribed medicines, especially salicylates and anticoagulants, and pregnant or breast-feeding women should consult their doctor before taking supplementary vitamin K.

SOLUBILITY
Fat soluble.

CO-VITAMINS AND COFACTORS

Alpha Lipoic Acid

GENERAL DESCRIPTION
Alpha lipoic acid is a sulfur-containing fatty acid found inside each and every body cell. Lipoic acid has a key role in the metabolism as it helps to convert glucose into cellular energy.

ROLE IN ANTI-AGING
Alpha lipoic acid is a potent antioxidant. Unlike other antioxidants, which work only in water or fatty tissues, lipoic acid can function in both water and fat. It is also thought to help recycle other antioxidants such as vitamin C and vitamin E. Because lipoic acid is fat soluble, it can help prevent free-radical damage from occurring inside nerve cells. Alpha lipoic acid's antioxidant properties mean that it can help to protect against diseases caused by oxidative damage—for example, cancer and cardiovascular disease.

Alpha lipoic acid may be of benefit to diabetics as it has been shown to enhance glucose uptake in non-insulin dependent diabetes and inhibit glycosylation. It may also help to protect against some of the complications associated with diabetes and has been shown to improve diabetic peripheral and autonomic neuropathy and improve renal function by lowering glycemia.

Alpha lipoic acid may have anti-obesity properties. Dogrell (*Expert Opin Investig Drugs*. 2004;13:1641–1643.) found that when added to the standard chow of rats, alpha lipoic acid was found to reduce body weight and food intake. Alpha lipoic acid also increased whole-body energy expenditure. Alpha lipoic acid is thought to exert its effects by suppressing hypothalamic AMP-activated protein kinase. However, the author stresses that long-term studies to determine whether these anti-obesity effects are maintained in animals are required before alpha lipoic acid is considered for clinical trial in human obesity.

Some research has also indicated that it can improve vision in patients with glaucoma. *In vitro* studies have shown that alpha lipoic acid can inhibit replication of the HIV virus; however, this has not been replicated in *in vivo* research.

DEFICIENCY SYMPTOMS

Humans are not known to develop deficiencies of alpha lipoic acid as the body manufactures it on demand.

THERAPEUTIC DAILY AMOUNT

The usual dose for antioxidant purposes is 20–50 mg per day; however, doses between 300 and 600 mg can be given to treat diabetic neuropathies.

MAXIMUM SAFE LEVEL

Alpha lipoic acid appears to have no significant side effects at daily dosages up to 1,800 mg.

SIDE EFFECTS/CONTRAINDICATIONS

None known. Pregnant women and people suffering from any type of medical condition should consult their doctor before taking alpha lipoic acid.

Bioflavonoids (Flavonoids, Rutin, Hesperidin, OPCs, Vitamin P)

GENERAL DESCRIPTION

Bioflavonoids are a group of anti-inflammatory and antioxidant plant compounds found in the pith (white part) and pulp of oranges (including the center part), lemon and grapefruit, apricots, rose hips, cherries, grapes, green peppers, tomatoes, papayas, broccoli, cantaloupe, and dark-pigmented fruit and vegetables. OPCs (oligomeric proanthocyanidin complexes) are also a type of bioflavonoid, see page 332 for a discussion about this nutrient.

ROLE IN ANTI-AGING

Bioflavonoids protect **vitamin C from oxidation and increase absorption of vitamin A.** Their antioxidant properties mean that they help to protect the body from aging and disease-causing free radicals.

Flavonoids are known to possess cardioprotective properties. Maccha and Mustafa (*J Cardiovasc Pharmacol.* 2005;46:36–40) found that bioflavonoids protect against endothelial dysfunction in rats. Other studies suggest that they can prevent the oxidation of LDL or "bad" cholesterol, lower blood pressure, and inhibit platelet aggregration. There is the possibility of the ability to ease pain of varicose veins and help certain types of hemorrhoids.

DEFICIENCY SYMPTOMS

Edema or accumulation of fluid in the tissue, bleeding into the tissue (noticeable as red spots and splotches when it occurs close under the skin) resulting from fragile, faulty capillaries.

THERAPEUTIC DAILY AMOUNT

500–2,000 mg, depending on need. No RDA has been established. People who eat a healthy, balanced diet should obtain adequate supplies of bioflavonoids from their food.

MAXIMUM SAFE LEVEL

Not established.

SIDE EFFECTS/CONTRAINDICATIONS

None known.

Biotin

GENERAL DESCRIPTION

Biotin is a water-soluble vitamin that **works synergistically with the B vitamins.** It can be found in yeast, liver, organ meats, egg yolk, grains, nuts, cauliflower, peas, beans, and fish. The majority of people obtain adequate amounts of biotin from their diet; however, individuals with a genetic deficiency of the enzyme biotinidase (needed by the body to utilize biotin), intestinal malabsorption, and an inability to absorb biotin as a result of surgical removal of the stomach require supplementary biotin. People taking antibiotics or sulphonamide antibacterial drugs may also derive benefit from taking biotin supplements. Biotin deficiency may lead to hair loss, dermatitis, high blood cholesterol levels, and heart problems.

ROLE IN ANTI-AGING

Biotin is one of the B vitamins required for the formation of glucose and fatty acids, and for the metabolism of amino acids and carbohydrates. Biotin is needed to maintain healthy hair, nails, skin, sweat glands, nerves, bone marrow, and normal bone growth. It may help prevent sudden infant death syndrome (SIDS; or crib death).

DEFICIENCY SYMPTOMS

Scaly dermatitis, inflamed sore tongue, loss of appetite, nausea, depression, muscle pain, sitophobia (morbid dread of food), pallor, anemia, abnormalities of heart function, burning or prickling sensations, sensitive skin, insomnia, extreme lassitude, increased cholesterol, and depression of immune system.

THERAPEUTIC DAILY AMOUNT

50–200 mcg (micrograms) combined with B-complex vitamin. No RDA has been established in the United States; therefore, daily dosages of 30–100 mcg are recommended. In the European Union (EU), the RDA for biotin is 150 mcg.

MAXIMUM SAFE LEVEL

2.5 mg (long and short term).

SIDE EFFECTS/CONTRAINDICATIONS

Diabetics should consult their doctor before taking very high doses of biotin (upward of 8 mg daily). Unless advised to do so by a doctor, biotin should not be taken in combination with the anticonvulsant drugs gabapentin, phenobarbital, and valproic acid.

SOLUBILITY

Water soluble.

Carotenoids

GENERAL DESCRIPTION

Carotenoids are a class of natural fat-soluble pigments found in plants, algae, and photosynthetic bacteria. Humans, and all other animals, appear to be incapable of synthesizing carotenoids; however, many obtain carotenoids from the diet—for example, beta-carotene, lycopene, and lutein. Carotenoids are potent antioxidants.

ROLE IN ANTI-AGING

Carotenoids have several important functions in humans. The most widely studied and well-understood nutritional role for carotenoids is their **provita-**

min A activity. Deficiency of vitamin A is a major cause of morbidity and mortality in developing nations. However, the body can synthesize vitamin A from some carotenoids, namely beta-carotene. Other provitamin A carotenoids include alpha-carotene (found in carrots, pumpkin, and red and yellow peppers) and cryptoxanthin (from oranges, tangerines, peaches, nectarines, and papayas). Carotenoids also act as potent **antioxidants**, protecting cells and tissues from the damaging effects of free radicals, thus protecting the body from cancer and other diseases whose pathogenesis is concerned with oxidative damage. Carotenoids have been linked to a decreased risk of premenopausal breast cancer, lung cancer, and cervical study. Lycopene, a carotenoid found in tomatoes, is of particular benefit to humans because it is an important free-radical scavenger. Results of a recent study of more than 47,000 men by researchers at Harvard School of Public Health revealed that men who consumed the greatest amounts of lycopene were 23 percent less likely to develop prostate cancer, compared with men who consumed the least lycopene. Carotenoids may also help to **prevent macular degeneration**, as both lutein and zeaxanthin, xanthophylls found in corn and in leafy greens such as kale and spinach, are thought to protect the macular region of the human retina from damaging free radicals.

DEFICIENCY SYMPTOMS
Not applicable.

THERAPEUTIC DAILY AMOUNT
People who eat at least five servings of fruit and vegetables each day should obtain plentiful supplies of carotenoids from their diet. However, some experts recommend that most people would benefit from a daily supplement of up to 15 mg (25,000 IU) of beta-carotene, and 6 mg each of alpha-carotene, lutein, and lycopene.

Note: only take natural beta-carotene. Smokers are currently advised not to take any supplementary beta-carotene as it has been linked to an increased risk of lung cancer in smokers.

MAXIMUM SAFE LEVEL
Not established.

SIDE EFFECTS/CONTRAINDICATIONS
None known.

Choline

GENERAL DESCRIPTION

The body uses choline to manufacture other valuable biochemicals, for example the neurotransmitter acetylcholine, the cell membrane constituents phosphatidylcholine and sphingomyelin, and the methyl donor betaine. Thus choline is necessary for the structural integrity of cell membranes, methyl metabolism, cholinergic neurotransmission, transmembrane signaling, and lipid and cholesterol transport and metabolism. Choline is found in green leafy vegetables, fish, peanuts, organ meat, soybeans, yeast, wheat germ, and lecithin.

ROLE IN ANTI-AGING

Choline is an essential dietary component. *In vitro* tests on human cells grown in culture have shown that choline is needed for them to survive. Numerous studies have shown that cells deprived of choline die by apoptosis. Animal studies suggest that choline may protect cell membranes by accelerating the resynthesis of phospholipids, and attenuate the progression of ischemic cell damage. There is some evidence indicating that choline may help improve cognitive functions such as memory and behavior in at least the short to medium-term, however, this remains unproven. Choline is frequently prescribed for the treatment of cognitive impairment in several European countries, principally when cognitive impairment is predominantly a result of cerebrovascular disease. Choline was originally thought to **lower cholesterol levels**; however, extensive clinical trials have failed to find any evidence that choline does have a beneficial effect upon cholesterol levels. Although recent findings suggest that when used with other methyl donors like folate, methionine, and vitamins B_{12} and B6, choline may help to **lower levels of homocysteine**. Choline may also have anticancer properties.

DEFICIENCY SYMPTOMS

Choline deficiency symptoms include fatty liver and liver damage.

THERAPEUTIC DAILY AMOUNT

RDA is 550 mg for men, 400 mg for women. Refer to packaging, as different supplements contain varying amounts of choline itself.

MAXIMUM SAFE LEVEL

3.5 g.

SIDE EFFECTS/CONTRAINDICATIONS

When taken as recommended, choline should not cause any side effects; however, if the recommended dosage is exceeded, it may cause abdominal pain and discomfort, nausea, and diarrhea. Large doses of choline (upward of 9 g daily) may cause depression.

Coenzyme Q_{10}

GENERAL DESCRIPTION

Coenzyme Q_{10} (CoQ_{10}) was discovered by scientists at the University of Wisconsin in 1957. It is also known as ubiquinone, from the word "ubiquitous" meaning "everywhere." CoQ_{10} is a powerful antioxidant found in every cell of the body, where it has important functions within the mitochondria—the "powerhouses" of cells.

ROLE IN ANTI-AGING

CoQ_{10} is a potent antioxidant. Antioxidants slow the aging process by promoting cellular repair, inhibiting inflammation, and preventing production of the inflammatory substances that accelerate aging.

CoQ_{10} is popular as a supplementary treatment for several heart conditions in Europe, Israel, and Japan. CoQ_{10} is a potent antioxidant and is known to prevent the oxidation of LDL cholesterol, a known risk factor for atherosclerosis. CoQ_{10} is a crucial component in the electron transport chain in mitochondria, as it acts as an electron and proton carrier. Researchers believe that CoQ_{10} aids the heart during times of stress, possibly by helping it to use energy in a more efficient manner. As such it is most commonly used for the treatment of congestive heart failure (CHF). However, it is also of potential therapeutic use for the treatment of myocardial ischemia, hypertension, mitral valve prolapse, infiltrative cardiomyopathy, stable and unstable angina, ventricular arrhythmia, and toxin-induced cardiotoxicity. Several clinical trials suggest that CoQ_{10} offers myocardial protection during cardiac surgery. Results of a recent study by Rosenfeldt et al. (*J Thorac Cardiovasc Surg.* 2005;129:25–32) found that giving oral CoQ_{10} therapy to patients for two weeks before undergoing cardiac surgery, increases myocardial and cardiac mitochondrial coenzyme Q(10) levels, improves mitochondrial efficiency, and increases myocardial tolerance to in vitro hypoxia-reoxygenation stress. Together these results suggest that CoQ_{10} given in the weeks before surgery and during surgery may be of benefit to the patient.

Research by Shults, et al. (*Archives of Neurology* 2002;59:1541–1550) suggests that coenzyme Q_{10} could **slow down the progression of Parkinson's disease** in people in the early stage of the disease. Results after eight months of treatment with 1,200 mg a day of coenzyme Q_{10} revealed that patients treated with the supplement were fairing significantly better than those given a placebo. So much so that they exhibited a 44 percent reduction in disease progression, compared with the placebo group. Even patients treated with the lowest dose of the supplement (300 mg a day) were more able to carry out simple daily activities (for example, dressing and washing), and demonstrated better mental functioning and mood. McCarthy et al. (*Toxicol Appl Pharmacol.* 2004;201:21–31.) found that CoQ_{10} can prevent oxidative stress and neuronal damage induced by the pesticide paraquat, thus suggesting that CoQ_{10} may be of use for the prevention and treatment of neurodegenerative diseases, such as Parkinson's disease, that are thought to be caused by environmental toxins.

CoQ_{10} is also known to help **prevent aging of the skin**, and is a common ingredient in many moisturizers. Research has suggested that CoQ_{10} may be of benefit in the treatment of other illnesses, including AIDS, angina, cancer, diabetes, male infertility, muscular dystrophy, and obesity. However, there is no clinical proof of its effectiveness in treating these conditions.

DEFICIENCY SYMPTOMS
None known.

THERAPEUTIC DAILY AMOUNT
The recommended dosage of CoQ_{10} ranges from 30–300 mg daily, usually taken in two to three doses. The majority of research on CoQ_{10} for the treatment of heart conditions has used doses ranging between 90 and 150 mg. No RDA has been established.

MAXIMUM SAFE LEVEL
Not established.

SIDE EFFECTS/CONTRAINDICATIONS
CoQ_{10} can interact with many different types of drugs; therefore, anyone taking any form of medication, especially cholesterol-lowering drugs, should consult their doctor before taking CoQ_{10}.

Pregnant and breast-feeding women should check with their physician before taking CoQ_{10}.

CHAPTER 11

Minerals

Boron

GENERAL DESCRIPTION

Boron is a little-studied mineral found naturally in fresh fruits and vegetables.

ROLE IN ANTI-AGING

Boron helps **retain calcium in bones** and **prevents calcium and magnesium loss** through the urine. It also helps **bone mineralization** and **prevents osteoporosis**. Epidemiological data implies that boron may help to **prevent arthritis**. There is evidence to suggest that boron is involved in estrogen and testosterone metabolism. In postmenopausal women, it increases estrogen naturally. Results of a study by Nielsen et al. (*FASEB J.* 1987;1:394–397.) led the researchers to conclude: "supplementation of a low-boron diet with an amount of boron commonly found in diets high in fruits and vegetables induces changes in postmenopausal women consistent with the prevention of calcium loss and bone demineralization." Several studies carried out over recent years have led the U.S. Department of Agriculture (USDA) to conclude that boron is an important nutrient for brain and psychological function in humans.

DEFICIENCY SYMPTOMS

None are officially recognized, yet some studies have linked boron deficiency to hyperthyroidism.

THERAPEUTIC DAILY AMOUNT

1–3 mg daily combined with calcium, magnesium, and all other minerals. No RDA has been established; however, data obtained in animal studies suggests that humans probably require roughly 1 mg of boron a day. Thus, people who eat plenty of fruits, vegetables, nuts, and legumes are unlikely to require supplementary boron.

MAXIMUM SAFE LEVEL

Not established.

SIDE EFFECTS/CONTRAINDICATIONS

One study found that 2.5 mg of boron per day for two months worsened hot flashes, and night sweats worsened in 50 percent of participants. Thus, women who suffer from such menopausal symptoms and take supplementary boron may wish to stop taking the supplements to see if their symptoms improve. Results of another study found that taking 3 mg of boron a day elevated estrogen and testosterone levels. Increased estrogen has also been reported in women taking daily doses of just 2.5 mg. In theory, such an increase in estrogen levels may increase the risk of several cancers. Because of this, some experts recommend that supplementary boron intake should be limited to 1 mg a day.

SOLUBILITY

Water soluble.

Calcium

GENERAL DESCRIPTION

Calcium is essential for the maintenance of many body functions, including the **transmission of nerve impulses**, the **regulation of muscle contraction and relaxation, blood clotting**, and various **metabolic activities**. It can be found in milk, egg yolk, fish or sardines (eaten with bones), yogurt, soybeans, green leafy vegetables (such as turnip greens, mustard greens, broccoli and kale), roots, tubers, seeds, soups and stews made from bones, blackstrap molasses, almonds, figs, and beans.

ROLE IN ANTI-AGING

Calcium maintains acid-alkaline balance in the body and normalizes contraction and relaxation of the heart muscles. Taken for strong bones and teeth, the mineral helps to protect against osteoporosis, rickets, and osteomalacia. It also helps to lower high blood pressure, lowers cholesterol, and aids in preventing cardiovascular disease. Used with vitamin C, it can help to relieve backaches and menstrual cramps and to induce a more sound sleep (due to its natural tranquilizing effects). Calcium can also help to prevent cancer, especially colorectal cancer.

DEFICIENCY SYMPTOMS

Nervous spasms, facial twitching, weak feeling muscles, cramps, rickets, slow growth in children, osteoporosis (porous and brittle bones), osteomalacia (a bone-softening disease), heart palpitations and slow pulse rate, height reduction, and colon cancer.

THERAPEUTIC DAILY AMOUNT

1,000–1,500 mg with half to equal parts of magnesium. Some researchers say menopausal women need 1,500 mg, with added boron and magnesium. RDA is 1,000 mg daily for adults aged nineteen to fifty, 1,200 mg for adults aged fifty-one and over, and 1,200 mg during pregnancy and lactation. The European Union (EU) RDA is 800 mg daily.

MAXIMUM SAFE LEVEL

The maximum safe level for calcium supplementation is 1,500 mg (long-term usage), 1,900 mg (short-term usage). Taking more than 1,500 mg on a long-term basis is not recommended.

SIDE EFFECTS/CONTRAINDICATIONS

Side effects are only associated with excessively high dosages. They include constipation, diarrhea, dry mouth, increased thirst and frequency of urination, persistent headache, loss of appetite, metallic taste, nausea and vomiting, and unusual fatigue. Advanced symptoms of calcium overdose are bone and muscle pain, irregular heartbeat, persistent itching, extreme drowsiness, and mental changes. People taking thiazide diuretics or supplementary vitamin D, and those suffering from kidney or thyroid disease should consult their doctor before taking calcium supplements.

Note: severe calcium toxicity may be fatal.

SOLUBILITY

Soluble in solvents such as alcohol and other dilute acids.

Chloride

GENERAL DESCRIPTION

Chloride is obtained from table salt (sodium chloride) and salt substitute (potassium chloride).

ROLE IN ANTI-AGING

Chloride stimulates production of hydrochloric acid for digestion and maintains **fluid and electrolyte balance**. Chloride has also been shown to assist **liver function**.

DEFICIENCY SYMPTOMS

Impaired digestion and loss of hair and teeth. However, chloride deficiencies are rare as the body usually produces enough.

THERAPEUTIC DAILY AMOUNT

No RDA has been established. The daily adequate intake (AI) is 2.3 g.

MAXIMUM SAFE LEVEL

The upper limit is 3.6 g.

SIDE EFFECTS/CONTRAINDICATIONS

Not established.

SOLUBILITY

Water soluble.

Chromium

GENERAL DESCRIPTION

Chromium is an essential trace mineral that helps the body to make glucose available for energy and to maintain normal blood sugar levels. It is also important for the metabolism of amino acids and fats.

It is obtained from brewer's yeast, blackstrap molasses, black pepper, meat (especially liver), whole wheat bread and cereals, broccoli, cheese, nuts, legumes, beets, and mushrooms.

ROLE IN ANTI-AGING

Chromium has been shown to **improve glucose sensitivity** in people with type I diabetes, type II diabetes, gestational diabetes, steroid-induced diabetes, and glucose intolerance, which is often seen as a precursor to type II diabetes.

Preuss (*J Am Coll Nutr* 1997;16:397–403) reports that the efficacy of chromium in the general population relates to its prevention of deficiency, or a reduction in the risk of chronic diseases. He suggests that doses above the estimated safe and adequate daily dietary intake are necessary for the treatment of certain chronic disease states—for example, in a study performed in China, the use of 1,000 mcg of chromium per day (five times above the upper limit of the estimated safe and adequate daily dietary intake) was highly effective in relieving many of the symptomatic manifestations of type II diabetes, including a return of the HbA1C (glycosylated hemoglobin) levels into the normal range. In addition to type II diabetes mellitus, Preuss reports that chromium supplementation may be useful to direct overall weight decrements specifically toward **fat loss with the retention of lean body mass** and to ameliorate many manifestations of aging.

Chromium helps stabilize blood sugar levels, and is therefore effective against diabetes and hypoglycemia. Many studies have shown that it can improve glucose sensitivity in people with type I, type II, gestational diabetes, steroid-induced diabetes, and glucose intolerance, which is often seen as a precursor to type II diabetes.

Chromium may **lower total cholesterol, LDL or "bad" cholesterol, and triglyceride levels**—all of which are risk factors for heart disease—while also **raising levels of "good" HDL cholesterol.** Results of a double-blind study by Boyd, et al. (*J Nutr Biochem* 1998;9:471–475) revealed that taking 500 mcg of chromium each day in combination with regular exercise lowered total cholesterol levels by nearly 20 percent within just thirteen weeks. In support of chromium's apparent cardiovascular benefits, results of a study by Newman, et al. (*Clin Chem* 1978;24:541–544) suggest that **people with higher blood levels of chromium are at lower risk of developing heart disease.**

Results of a study by Guallar et al. *Am J Epidemiol.* 2005;162:157–164.) further support the theory that chromium is important for cardiovascular health. To determine whether low toenail chromium concentrations were associated with risk of nonfatal myocardial infarction, the authors conducted an incident, population-based, case-control study of men with a first diagnosis of myocardial infarction. Toenail chromium concentration of the men was assessed by neutron activation analysis, and results showed that toenail chromium concentration was inversely associated with the risk of a first myocardial infarction in men.

DEFICIENCY SYMPTOMS

Chromium deficiency can cause a diabetic-like state, impaired growth, elevated blood lipids, increased aortic plaque formation, and decreased fertility and longevity.

People aged fifty-five and over and those who exercise regularly are at risk of deficiency and therefore may benefit from taking supplementary chromium.

THERAPEUTIC DAILY AMOUNT

200–400 mcg of GTF (glucose tolerance factor) taken with other minerals. Chromium polynicotinate (bound to niacin) and chromium picolinate (bound to picolinic acid) are natural forms. An RDA has not been established for chromium, although the National Academy of Sciences recommends a daily intake of 50–200 mcg. The EU recommends 25 mcg per day as a safe and effective dose. Urinary chromium losses have been reported in elderly people. Offenbacher (*Biol Trace Elem Res.* 1992;32:123–31.) reports that data indicates that chromium retention decreases with aging, and that aging alters chromium metabolism. He expresses concern that the diets of healthy older people typically contain less than 30 micrograms of chromium, which may not be sufficient to protect against the stresses and illnesses associated with aging.

MAXIMUM SAFE LEVEL

Not established. There have been reports of toxicity at doses of 1,000 mcg and above; however, the majority of research suggests that there is little risk of toxicity at this dose.

SIDE EFFECTS/CONTRAINDICATIONS

Some chromium supplements contain yeast, which can interfere with certain prescription medicines. Supplementation with chromium (or brewer's yeast) may enhance the effects of drugs used to treat diabetes—for example, insulin; therefore, people with diabetes should only take such supplements under the advice and supervision of a doctor. Chromium supplements are not suitable for pregnant or nursing women, or for people with epilepsy.

SOLUBILITY

Insoluble in water.

Copper

GENERAL DESCRIPTION

Copper can be found in nuts, organ meats, seafood, mushrooms, chocolate, and legumes. It is required for the formation of proteins involved in growth, nerve function, and energy release. It is stored in the liver.

ROLE IN ANTI-AGING

Accompanied by iron and protein, copper is able to **form hemoglobin**, which is necessary for transporting oxygen around the body. It **forms melanin** (pigment in skin and hair) and helps form connective tissues such as collagen and elastin. Copper also has the ability to assist in **lowering cholesterol**, help **prevent rancidity of fatty acids**, and **maintain cellular structure**. It may help as an anti-inflammatory against arthritis, and at least one study has shown that copper supplementation increases levels of the antioxidant enzyme superoxide dismutase (SOD).

DEFICIENCY SYMPTOMS

Anemia, loss of hair, loss of taste, general weakness, impaired respiration such as emphysema, brittle bones, chronic or recurrent diarrhea, hair depigmentation, low white blood cell count (which leads to reduced resistance to infection), retarded growth, water retention, nervous irritability; high cholesterol, abnormal ECG patterns, development of ischemic heart disease, birth defects, miscarriage, and neural tube defects. Antacid use creates copper deficiency. Recent research has linked copper deficiency to an increased risk of colon cancer.

THERAPEUTIC DAILY AMOUNT

2–3 mg taken with zinc at a 10 to 1 or 15 to 1 ratio (zinc: copper). The RDA is 900 mcg. The European RDA is 1.2 mg.

MAXIMUM SAFE LEVEL

5 mg (long-term usage); 8 mg (short-term usage). Doses of 10 mg and above may cause stomach ache, nausea, muscle pain, and other side effects. Copper is toxic and extremely high doses may be lethal.

SIDE EFFECTS/CONTRAINDICATIONS

None known except in overdose.

SOLUBILITY

Insoluble in water.

Fluoride

GENERAL DESCRIPTION

Fluoride is added to drinking water, toothpastes, and mouthwashes to prevent dental caries.

ROLE IN ANTI-AGING

Fluoride is necessary for **formation of strong bones and teeth** and may protect against osteoporosis.

DEFICIENCY SYMPTOMS

None.

THERAPEUTIC DAILY AMOUNT

No RDA has been established.

MAXIMUM SAFE LEVEL

Do not take additional fluoride.

SIDE EFFECTS/CONTRAINDICATIONS

Side effects are only evident in fluoride overdose.

SOLUBILITY

Fluoride salts are water soluble.

Iodine

GENERAL DESCRIPTION

Iodine stimulates the thyroid gland to produce the thyroid hormones thyroxin and tri-iodothyronine, which regulate metabolic rate. The trace element is also present in more than a hundred enzyme systems involved in energy production, nerve function, and hair and skin growth.

Iodine is found in seaweed (especially kelp), seafood, iodized salt and sea salt, eggs, garlic, turnip greens, and watercress. Vegans and others who don't eat dairy products or fish may benefit from taking iodine.

ROLE IN ANTI-AGING

Iodine promotes the conversion of body fat to energy, thereby **regulating basal metabolic rate**. It also **protects against toxic effects from radioactive material**.

Research shows that iodine can help to **relieve pain and soreness associated with fibrocystic breast disease**, and can loosen clogged mucus in breathing tubes. New research suggests that iodine solution may **prevent dental caries** in infants and young children.

DEFICIENCY SYMPTOMS

A deficiency of iodine can cause goiter (characterized by enlarged thyroid gland, which may thicken the neck, restrict breathing, and cause bulging of the eyes), hypothyroidism (low thyroid), physical and mental sluggishness, poor circulation and low vitality, dry hair and skin, cold hands and feet, obesity, cretinism (characterized by physical and mental retardation in children born to mothers deficient in iodine), and hearing loss.

THERAPEUTIC DAILY AMOUNT

Since the introduction of iodized salt, iodine supplements are generally unnecessary and not recommended for most people. Very strict vegetarians who exclude salt from their diet and do not eat sea vegetables, such as kelp, may benefit from 150 mcg a day. Therapeutic daily amount (if advised by a physician that iodine supplementation is necessary) is 150–300 mcg (micrograms). The RDA is 150 mcg. Liquid iodine for medicinal uses (as a topical antiseptic for wounds) should NOT be used orally.

MAXIMUM SAFE LEVEL

Iodine supplementation is usually only necessary upon medical advice. The upper safe level is 500 mcg (long-term usage); 700 mcg (short-term usage).

SIDE EFFECTS/CONTRAINDICATIONS

None if taken as recommended. Only take supplementary iodine when advised to do so by a physician; high amounts (several milligrams per day) of iodine can interfere with normal thyroid function. People taking lithium and antithyroid drugs such as methimazole and propylthiouracil should not take supplementary iodine without consulting their doctor.

SOLUBILITY

Slightly soluble in water; soluble in many other solvents such as alcohol.

Iron

GENERAL DESCRIPTION

Found in liver, heart, kidney, lean meats, shellfish, dried beans, fruit, nuts, leafy green vegetables, whole grains, and blackstrap molasses.

ROLE IN ANTI-AGING

Iron is essential for the **formation of hemoglobin**, which is present in red blood cells, and myoglobin, a molecule that transports oxygen in muscles. By taking an iron supplement, it is possible to cure and prevent **iron-deficiency anemia**, as well as stimulate the **immune system**. Iron can be used to **improve muscular and athletic performance**, and **prevent fatigue**. People who may benefit from iron supplements include vegetarians and vegans, athletes, those who have recently undergone surgery, and women of childbearing age.

Results of a study by Ames, et al. (*PNAS* 2002; 10.1073/pnas.192585799) suggests that iron deficiency may play a role in the degeneration of brain cells that occurs in Alzheimer's disease. Experiments on both human and animal brain cells revealed that reducing the production of heme (a form of iron present in cells) caused cells to degenerate in a way similar to that seen in aging and Alzheimer's disease. Furthermore, interfering with heme levels also caused cells to make abnormal versions of proteins called APP—the proteins that accumulate to form the amyloid plaques characteristic of Alzheimer's disease. Senior study author Dr. Ames said that although it was too soon to say whether iron helps protect against Alzheimer's, he recommends taking a multivitamin containing iron as "an insurance pill."

DEFICIENCY SYMPTOMS

Anemia (pallor, weakness, persistent fatigue, labored breathing on exertion, headaches, and palpitation). Young children suffer diminished coordination, and unbalanced attention span and memory; older children have poor learning, reading and problem-solving skills; depressed immune system with decreased ability to produce white blood cells to fight off infection; and concave or spoonlike fingernails and toenails.

THERAPEUTIC DAILY AMOUNT

The RDA for men and postmenopausal women is 8 mg. The European RDA is 14 mg. This should be adequate. Experts recommend consuming vitamin C-rich food or drinks, such as orange juice, at the same time as taking supplementary iron since vitamin C improves iron absorption. Do not use inorganic iron (ferrous sulfate) as a supplement as it destroys vitamin E; use organic iron (ferrous fumarate, ferrous citrate, or ferrous gluconate) instead.

MAXIMUM SAFE LEVEL

The maximum safe level for iron is 15 mg for long-term usage and 80 mg for short-term usage.

SIDE EFFECTS/CONTRAINDICATIONS

Iron can cause side effects such as abdominal pain and diarrhea, nausea, and vomiting. All side effects of iron supplementation should be reported to a doctor. Do not supplement iron without first having a laboratory diagnosis of anemia. Elevated iron or ferritin blood levels is thought to increase free-radical damage, and has also been linked to an increased risk of cancer, diabetes, heart attack, infection, systemic lupus erythematosus (SLE), and Huntington's disease. Excess iron may also worsen the symptoms of rheumatoid arthritis. Overdose of iron is dangerous.

SOLUBILITY

Insoluble in water.

Magnesium

GENERAL DESCRIPTION

Magnesium is essential for life, as it plays a major role in the metabolism of glucose. It is also used in the production of cellular energy and to create protein. Magnesium is vital for the nervous system, muscle contraction, and the formation of healthy bones and teeth. Because magnesium is involved in hundreds of enzyme reactions, a deficiency can adversely affect the immune system. The ability of immune cells to adhere to other substances requires magnesium.

Magnesium is present in the chlorophyll of all green plants. The main food sources are unrefined cereals, figs, lemons, grapefruit, apples, leafy green vegetables, peanuts, and whole-meal bread.

ROLE IN ANTI-AGING

Magnesium may help to protect against cardiovascular disease, as some research suggests that it may help to lower high blood pressure. Magnesium appears to be particularly effective in people who are taking potassium-depleting diuretics, which deplete the body's supply of magnesium.

Results of a review by Paolisso, et al. (*Diabetologia* 1990;33:511–514) showed that people with diabetes tend to have low magnesium levels. Supporting this research, a study by Kao, et al. (*Arch Intern Med* 1999;159: 2151–2159) found that middle-aged people with the lowest serum magnesium levels were twice as likely as those with the highest to develop type II diabetes. Other research by Paolisso, et al. (*Diabetes Care* 1989;12:265–269) showed that magnesium supplementation **improves insulin production** in elderly people with type II diabetes. However, other studies have not been able to replicate this effect.

People who regularly suffer from migraines have been found to have lower blood and brain levels of magnesium. A number of studies suggest that magnesium may help to **reduce the frequency of migraines**. For example, preliminary research by Weaver (*Headache* 1990;30:168) found that supplementing with 200 mg of magnesium a day reduced the frequency of migraines in 80 percent of participants. Mauskop, et al. (*Clin Sci* 1995;89:633–636) found that giving intravenous magnesium to people with low serum magnesium levels at the onset of an attack can significantly reduce, and sometimes completely relieve, symptoms, typically within fifteen minutes or less.

Magnesium was found to benefit restless legs syndrome and periodic limb movement disorder by Hornyak, et al. (*Sleep* 1998;21:501–505). When the researchers supplemented people experiencing insomnia due to these conditions, Hornyak found **significant improvement in sleep efficiency**. Magnesium is also a good general muscle relaxant, and so it may help to alleviate muscle-related aches and pains that may cause some people to experience sleep difficulties.

Other research suggests that magnesium may help to **minimize the severity of asthma attacks, and alleviate the symptoms of PMS**.

DEFICIENCY SYMPTOMS

Deficiency of magnesium can result in depression, apprehensiveness, confusion, disorientation, vertigo (a condition in which the room seems to spin), muscular weakness and twitching, over-excitability of the nervous system (which may lead to muscle spasms or cramps), insomnia, jumpiness, sensitivity to noise, irritability, poor memory, and tremors or convulsions.

THERAPEUTIC DAILY AMOUNT

Magnesium supplementation is important for people taking diuretics and digitalis. Heavy drinkers and those concerned about osteoporosis may also benefit from taking supplements of the mineral. Many doctors recommend taking a supplement containing 250–350 mg each day. The RDA of magnesium is 400 mg a day for men aged nineteen to thirty, 420 mg a day for men aged thirty-one to seventy. For women, the RDA is 310 mg a day for those aged nineteen to thirty, and 320 mg for those aged thirty-one to seventy. The European RDA is 300 mg.

MAXIMUM SAFE LEVEL

The tolerable upper limit (UL) is 350 mg for magnesium obtained from supplementation only and not through the diet.

SIDE EFFECTS/CONTRAINDICATIONS

The most common problem caused by magnesium is diarrhea; however, the amounts of magnesium found in nutritional supplements are unlikely to cause such problems.

People with kidney disease or heart disease should consult their doctor before taking supplementary magnesium.

SOLUBILITY

Insoluble in water.

Manganese

GENERAL DESCRIPTION

Manganese is found in whole grains, wheat germ, bran, peas, nuts, leafy green vegetables, beets, egg yolks, bananas, liver, organ meats, and milk.

ROLE IN ANTI-AGING

Manganese is required for the initiation of **vital enzyme reactions** and **proper bone development** as well as **synthesis of mucopolysaccharides**. It is also essential for the formation of certain enzymes, one of which is superoxide dismutase, a powerful antioxidant that neutralizes potentially damaging free radicals. It is also helpful with osteoarthritis. The pancreas needs manganese in order to function normally, and it is also a requirement for normal carbohydrate metabolism. It plays an important part in the formation of thyroxin, a hormone secreted by the thyroid gland. Some research has suggested that manganese may also improve memory and reduce nervous irritability.

DEFICIENCY SYMPTOMS
Weight loss, dermatitis, nausea, slow growth and color changes of hair, low cholesterol, disturbances in fat metabolism and glucose tolerance, and myasthenia gravis (severe loss of muscle strength). A deficiency is suspected in diabetes. Deficiency during pregnancy may be a factor in epilepsy in the offspring.

THERAPEUTIC DAILY AMOUNT
5–10 mg in combination with other minerals. No RDA has been established; however, recent recommendations of an adequate intake level are 1.8 mg for women and 2.3 mg for men.

MAXIMUM SAFE LEVEL
The maximum safe level is 11 mg per day (note: this is the total intake from food, water, and dietary supplements, not dietary supplements alone). This dose is based on a recent study, where no adverse effects were seen when 11 mg was consumed over an extended period. A dose of 15 mg per day was found to cause Parkinson's-like symptoms. Note that the National Research Council's "estimated safe and adequate daily dietary intake" is 2.5 mg.

SIDE EFFECTS/CONTRAINDICATIONS
Too much manganese is known to cause nervous system disorders. The element is neurotoxic and can cause Parkinson's-like symptoms when taken in excess. People with cirrhosis of the liver, cholestasis, and diabetes should consult their doctor before taking supplementary manganese.

SOLUBILITY
Manganese salts are water soluble.

Molybdenum

GENERAL DESCRIPTION
Molybdenum is obtained from organ meats (liver, kidney), milk, dairy products, legumes, whole grains, and leafy green vegetables.

ROLE IN ANTI-AGING
This mineral is required for the activity of several enzymes in the body, and is

a **vital component of the enzyme responsible for iron utilization**. Molybdenum can help to prevent anemia, and is able to **detoxify potentially hazardous substances**. It can be an antioxidant and protects teeth from cavities. It aids in **carbohydrate and fat metabolism**.

DEFICIENCY SYMPTOMS

Molybdenum deficiency may be linked to esophageal cancer. Epidemiological studies have shown that the incidence of esophageal cancer is significantly higher than normal in people who live in areas with molybdenum deficient soil.

THERAPEUTIC DAILY AMOUNT

The RDA for men and women is 45 mcg. The European Union has not set an RDA for molybdenum.

MAXIMUM SAFE LEVEL

The maximum safe level for long-term use is 2,000 mcg. No adverse effects were observed with supplementation of 10,000 mcg for short periods.

SIDE EFFECTS/CONTRAINDICATIONS

Molybdenum usually causes side effects only when taken in excess; these include gout-like symptoms and, in one case, psychosis. Excess molybdenum can also inhibit certain enzymes.

SOLUBILITY

Insoluble in water.

Phosphorus

GENERAL DESCRIPTION

Phosphorus is found in virtually all types of food, especially high-protein foods such as meat, fish, poultry, eggs, milk, cheese, nuts, legumes, and cereals. Many processed foods and soft drinks preserved with phosphates adversely affect the body's calcium-phosphorous balance.

ROLE IN ANTI-AGING

Phosphorus is essential for **bone mineralization**, for normal bone and tooth structure. It may help with **muscular fatigue** and is involved in cellular activity. Studies have shown that phosphorus is important for **heart regularity** and the mineral is also needed for the **transference of nerve impulses**. Phosphorus aids normal growth and body repair mechanisms.

DEFICIENCY SYMPTOMS

Phosphorus deficiencies can cause muscle weakness (to the point of respiratory arrest), anemia, and increased susceptibility to infection. The typical diet usually makes a phosphorus deficiency rare in the United States. Those with kidney failure or gastrointestinal diseases can have severe deficiencies; alcoholics and those taking antacids may be deficient.

THERAPEUTIC DAILY AMOUNT

No supplementation needed as the diet should supply sufficient amounts. The RDA is 700 mg for adults. The European RDA is 800 mg.

MAXIMUM SAFE LEVEL

The maximum safe level is 4,000 mg per day for adults.

SIDE EFFECTS/CONTRAINDICATIONS

None known; however, excess phosphorus can lower blood calcium levels.

SOLUBILITY

Insoluble in water.

Potassium

GENERAL DESCRIPTION

Found in bananas, apricots, lettuce, broccoli, potatoes, fresh fruits and fruit juices, sunflower seeds, unsalted peanuts, nuts, squash, wheat germ, brewer's yeast, desiccated liver, fish, bone meal, watercress, blackstrap molasses, and unsulfured figs.

ROLE IN ANTI-AGING

Potassium is important for intracellular chemical reactions, and regulates the transfer of nutrients to the cells. It also helps to **regulate water balance** in the body, balance fluid with sodium inside the cells, and distribute fluids on both sides of the cell membrane. As potassium is an **electrolyte**, it has important roles in **maintaining heart and muscle contraction**, and **nerve transmission**. The mineral also assists red blood cells in carrying oxygen and helps to **eliminate water waste** through the kidneys. Potassium is required for **proper carbohydrate metabolism** and to store energy in the muscles and liver. Research has shown that potassium can reduce high blood pressure, allergies, and colic in babies and help to prevent heart attacks.

Potassium may also lower the risk of stroke and fatal stroke. One study of people with high blood pressure revealed that those who ate at least one serving of potassium-rich foods each day were 40 percent less likely to suffer a fatal stroke. Meanwhile, results of a study by Green et al. (*Neurology* 2002;59:314–320) suggest that eating bananas and other potassium-rich foods could lower the risk of stroke. The study of more than 5,600 seniors by researchers from The Queen's Medical Center in Honolulu, Hawaii, revealed that those with the lowest dietary intake of potassium were 1.5 times more likely to have a stroke within the next eight years. Furthermore, this risk was increased by 2.5 times in individuals taking diuretics, and a staggering 10 times higher in people suffering from atrial fibrillation who took diuretics and had a low dietary intake of the mineral.

DEFICIENCY SYMPTOMS

General weakness of muscles, mental confusion, muscle cramping, poor reflexes, nervous system disruption, soft and flabby muscles, constipation, acne in young people, and dry skin in adults. Severe deficiency leads to heart attack.

Potassium supplementation is important for those using diuretics.

THERAPEUTIC DAILY AMOUNT

2,000–4,000 mg. Generally, potassium supplementation is unnecessary as adequate amounts of the mineral are obtained in the diet. Athletes generally require more (3,000–6,000 mg) because of heavy perspiration. The maximum potency allowed by the government in supplement form is 99 mg. Discuss higher potencies with a physician.

MAXIMUM SAFE LEVEL

See above.

SIDE EFFECTS/CONTRAINDICATIONS

Side effects are unusual, unless one takes too much of the mineral. Possible side effects include black stool, bloody stool, diarrhea, fatigue, and upset stomach. Many drugs can cause potentially dangerous increases in potassium levels; therefore, those taking any form of medication should seek medical advice before taking potassium supplements.

SOLUBILITY

Potassium salts are water soluble.

Selenium

GENERAL DESCRIPTION

Selenium is an essential trace element found in organ meats, tuna, seafood, brewer's yeast, fresh garlic, mushrooms, wheat germ, and some whole grains.

ROLE IN ANTI-AGING

Selenium is necessary for the body's growth and **protein synthesis**. It helps to increase effectiveness of vitamin E, and acts as an **antioxidant** to protect cells from the free-radical damage that causes aging and is linked to many age-related diseases. Ryan-Harshman and AldooriIt (*Can J Diet Pract Res.* 2005; 66:98–102.) write that selenium may be of benefit to people whose oxidative stress loads are high, such as those with inflammatory or infectious diseases like rheumatoid arthritis or HIV/AIDS, or those who are at high risk for cancers, particularly prostate cancer. Selenium appears to offer protection against a number of different types of cancer. Results of two five-year-long studies at Cornell University and the University of Arizona revealed that taking just 200 mcg of supplementary selenium each day cut the incidence of prostate cancer by 63 percent, colorectal tumors by 58 percent, and lung cancer by 46 percent. Altogether, the death rate from cancer of people who took 200 mcg of selenium was found to be 39 percent lower than that of the general population. Selenium may help to prevent heart disease by increasing levels of "good" HDL cholesterol and lowering levels of "bad" LDL cholesterol, and reduce heart attack and stroke risk by decreasing the "stickiness" of the blood, and therefore reducing the risk of blood clots. Results of research published in 2001 revealed that people with the highest intake of selenium were 50 percent less likely to have asthma, compared with those who consumed the least. Low selenium levels have also been linked to an increased risk of prostate cancer. Selenium also protects against toxic pollutants for sexual reproduction, helps to eliminate arsenic, and protect against the effects of cadmium and mercury. The mineral is also a **component of glutathione peroxidase**, which protects tissues from the effects of polyunsaturated fatty acid oxidation. Studies suggest that selenium and glutathione may play a key role in slowing the spread of HIV infection in the body. Research suggests that selenium is vital for the proper functioning of the immune system, and that it can increase levels of white blood cells, therefore enhancing the body's ability to fight illness and infection. Selenium may also inhibit viral replication. A number of studies have found that selenium deficiency is linked to increased occurrence or progression of viral infections, thus supporting the theory that the mineral inhibits viral replication. Broome et al. (*Am J Clin Nutr.* 2004;80:154–162) found that selenium supplementation improved immune function and increased the rate of clearance of poliovirus vaccine in humans. A study of elderly men and women by Girodon (*Arch Intern Med.* 1999;159:748–754) revealed that those who received zinc and selenium supplements demonstrated a better immune response to the influenza vaccine than those who received placebo, thus suggesting that supplementary selenium and zinc may help to boost immunity in older people and improve their resistance to infections, such as influenza.

Results of a study by Smorgan et al. (*Arch Gerontol Geriatr Suppl.* 2004; 9:393–402) suggest that selenium may offer some protection against cognitive impairment. Research has shown that selenium can help to **alleviate hot flashes and other symptoms of menopause**.

DEFICIENCY SYMPTOMS

Dandruff, decreased growth, premature aging, infertility, and increased risk of cancer and heart disease. Infant deaths have also been associated with selenium and/or vitamin B deficiency.

THERAPEUTIC DAILY AMOUNT

The RDA of selenium is 55mcg, however many experts recommend a daily intake of 100–200 mcg. The European Union has not set an RDA for selenium.

MAXIMUM SAFE LEVEL

The maximum safe level is 400 mcg for long-term usage and 700 mcg for short-term usage. Supplementation at levels greater than 800 mcg a day may be toxic. The Food and Nutrition Board states that overt selenium toxicity may occur in humans ingesting 2,400–3,000 mcg.

SIDE EFFECTS/CONTRAINDICATIONS

Side effects are rare, but can include dizziness, nausea, brittle fingernails, and hair loss. People taking cholesterol-lowering medications, such as statins, should consult their physician before taking supplementary selenium as it may reduce their effectiveness.

Selenium has recently been reported to adversely effect blood glucose metabolism in older individuals with metabolic or diabetic syndrome. If taking selenium at high doses, have your physician check your fasting blood sugar and glycosylated hemoglobin (HbA1c) levels, to ensure neither is elevated due to supplemental selenium.

SOLUBILITY

Insoluble in water.

Silicon

GENERAL DESCRIPTION

Silicon is a trace element found in flaxseed, steel cut oats, almonds, peanuts, sunflower seeds, onions, alfalfa, fresh fruit, brewer's yeast, and dietary fiber.

ROLE IN ANTI-AGING

Silicon is needed for a healthy bone structure, normal growth, and the production of the connective tissue collagen. Thus, the mineral is also important for **healthy nails, skin, hair, and bone.** Most people take silica as a form of silicon, to help with hair, skin, and nails. Silicon also helps to **maintain healthy arteries via its anti-atherosclerotic actions**, and prevents cardiovascular disease, as well as counteracting the effects of aluminum toxicity and improving calcium intake.

DEFICIENCY SYMPTOMS

Aging of skin (wrinkles), thinning or loss of hair, poor bone development, and soft or brittle nails.

THERAPEUTIC DAILY AMOUNT

Adequate amounts are found in the diet. No RDA has been established. Supplements typically contain 1–2 mg.

MAXIMUM SAFE LEVEL

Not established.

SIDE EFFECTS/CONTRAINDICATIONS

None known.

SOLUBILITY

Insoluble in water.

Sodium (Sodium Chloride, Salt)

GENERAL DESCRIPTION

Sodium is most commonly obtained from table salt and sea salt. However, it is also found in many types of food, especially foods from animal sources, including, shellfish, meat, poultry, milk, and cheese. Other sources of sodium are kelp, powdered seaweed, and most processed foods.

ROLE IN ANTI-AGING

Sodium works with potassium to **maintain proper fluid balance** between cells. It is an electrolyte, and is a vital **component of nerves** as it stimulates muscle contraction. Sodium also helps to keep calcium and other minerals soluble in the blood, as well as **stimulating the adrenal glands**. High sodium levels can cause high blood pressure. Finally, sodium aids in **preventing heat prostration** or sunstroke.

DEFICIENCY SYMPTOMS

Sodium deficiencies are rare since most foods contain sodium; however, symptoms include headaches, excessive sweating, heat exhaustion, respiratory failure, muscular cramps, weakness, collapsed blood vessels, stomach and intestinal gas, chronic diarrhea, weight loss, kidney failure, tuberculosis of kidneys, and streptococci infections.

THERAPEUTIC DAILY AMOUNT

Supplementary sodium is rarely needed, as an ordinary diet provides enough sodium. A gram of sodium chloride has been suggested for each kilogram of water ingested. The adequate intake (AI) for sodium is 1.5 g for people aged 9 to 50, 1.3 g for people aged 51 to 70, and 1.2 g for those aged 70 and above. The US Food and Nutrition Board states that the AI is based on being able to obtain a nutritionally adequate diet for other nutrients and to meet the needs for sweat losses for individuals engaged in recommended levels of physical activity.

MAXIMUM SAFE LEVEL

The upper limit (UL) for sodium is 2.3 g per day. The US Food and Nutrition Board states that the UL applies to apparently healthy individuals without hypertension, and that the UL is too high for individuals who already have hypertension or who are under the care of a health care professional. It is important not to exceed the UL. Sodium toxicity can be serious.

SIDE EFFECTS/CONTRAINDICATIONS

Sodium only causes side effects when taken in excess. Excess sodium intake is associated with hypertension and increased risk of cardiovascular disease and stroke.

SOLUBILITY

Water soluble.

Sulfur

GENERAL DESCRIPTION

The trace element sulfur is found in protein foods, especially eggs, lean beef, fish, onions, kale, soybeans, and dried beans.

ROLE IN ANTI-AGING

Sulfur is found in cells; the amino acids cysteine, cystine, and methionine; hemoglobin; collagen; keratin; insulin; beparin; hair, skin, and nails; and many other biological structures. Sulfur is required for the **metabolism of several vitamins**, including thiamine, biotin, and pantothenic acid, in addition to normal **carbohydrate metabolism**. The element is also essential for **cellular respiration** and the **formation of the connective tissue collagen**. Sulfur aids in **bile secretion** in the liver and helps to convert toxins to less-hazardous substances. Sulfur is also needed to maintain normal functioning of the nerves and muscles, and to control glandular secretions. It is necessary for **healthy hair, skin, and nails**. It also helps maintain oxygen balance necessary for **brain function**.

DEFICIENCY SYMPTOMS

Deficiency symptoms are rare, but may include excessive sweating, chronic diarrhea, nausea, respiratory failure, heat exhaustion, muscular weakness, and mental apathy.

THERAPEUTIC DAILY AMOUNT

A diet sufficient in protein should be adequate in sulfur. No RDA has been established.

MAXIMUM SAFE LEVEL

Supplementary sulfur is not required.

SIDE EFFECTS/CONTRAINDICATIONS

Side effects are not associated with normal sulfur levels.

SOLUBILITY

Insoluble in water.

Vanadium

GENERAL DESCRIPTION

The richest sources of vanadium are fish, black pepper, and dill seed; however, the mineral can also be found in whole grains, meats, and dairy products.

ROLE IN ANTI-AGING

Vanadium is needed for **cellular metabolism** and in the **formation of bones, cartilage, and teeth**. It is required for normal growth and development, and mimics the action of insulin on glucose uptake and metabolism in fat cells, increases glucose metabolism and conversion into lipids, activates glycogen synthesis, and improves glucose tolerance and the efficiency of insulin in the muscle cells. Thus, vanadium may be **beneficial to diabetics**. Vanadium may have cardioprotective properties. Research has shown that vanadium compounds have the ability to improve cardiac performance and smooth muscle contractility, and lower blood pressure in various models of hypertension and insulin resistance.

DEFICIENCY SYMPTOMS

Little is known at present, but high blood pressure and hardening of the arteries have been implicated.

THERAPEUTIC DAILY AMOUNT

More needs to be known before recommendations can be made. No RDA has been established. The average diet is estimated to provide 15–30 mcg of vanadium a day.

MAXIMUM SAFE LEVEL

Not established.

SIDE EFFECTS/CONTRAINDICATIONS

Vanadium can cause mild gastrointestinal intolerance. High blood levels of vanadium have been associated with manic-depressive disorders.

SOLUBILITY

Insoluble in water.

Zinc

GENERAL DESCRIPTION

Zinc is one of the most important trace elements in the body for many biological functions. It is a vital ingredient of more than 300 enzymes needed for a healthy immune system, to repair wounds, maintain fertility in adults and growth in children, synthesize protein, help cells reproduce, preserve vision, boost immunity, and protect against free radicals. It is also an important structural component of many proteins, hormones, neuropeptides, and hormone receptors. Due to its role in cell division and differentiation, programmed cell death, gene transcription, biomembrane functioning, and many enzymatic activities, zinc is considered a major element in assuring the correct functioning of an organism, from the very first embryonic stages to the last periods of life.

Fresh oysters, herring, wheat germ, pumpkin seeds, milk, steamed crab, lobster, chicken, pork chops, turkey, lean ground beef, liver, and eggs are all good natural sources of zinc.

ROLE IN ANTI-AGING

Many scientists subscribe to the theory that many of the degenerative diseases have their origin in deleterious free-radical reactions. These diseases include atherosclerosis, cancer, inflammatory joint disease, asthma, diabetes, senile dementia, and degenerative eye disease. There is also a lot of evidence to suggest that the process of biological aging might also have a free-radical basis.

Most free-radical damage to cells involves oxygen free radicals or, more generally, activated oxygen species (AOS), which include non-radical species as well as free radicals. The AOS can damage genetic material, cause lipid peroxidation in cell membranes, and inactivate membrane-bound enzymes. As an antioxidant, zinc serves as an **important free-radical scavenger** to protect cells from increased AOS activity. Dr. Florence from the Centre for Environmental and Health Science in Australia believes that antioxidant supplementation including zinc is important to ensuring the health of the older population.

Zinc **promotes resistance to infections**, particularly in aging, a time when the immune system slows down. According to Fabris, et al. (*Exp Gerontol 1997;32:*415–429), data obtained both in animal and human studies suggests that zinc supplementation may help to **restore thymic activity and even regrow the thymus** by normalizing the altered zinc pool seen in aging. Low zinc ion bioavailability and impaired cell-mediated immunity combine during aging to result in increased susceptibility to infection. Mocchegiani, et al. (*Biogerontology* 2000;1:133–143) report that dietary supplementation with the recommended daily allowance of zinc significantly **decreases the incidence of infection, prolongs survival, and reduces the risk of death from infections and tumors**. It has also been shown to **increase the activity of natural killer cells and to boost the production of antibodies** in response to infections.

Zinc **may have antiviral properties**. It has been shown to interfere with viral replication *in vitro,* and it is thought that it may also impair the ability of viruses to enter cells. Research suggests that it can help immune cells to fight a cold, and may relieve cold symptoms when taken as a supplement. New research by Mossad (*QJM* 2003;96:35–43) published in 2003 revealed that a zinc-based nasal spray was able to **cut the duration of a cold in half** if treatment is started within two days of the onset of symptoms.

Zinc plays an important role in **wound healing**. Research shows that even a mild zinc deficiency can impair recovery from everyday tissue damage. A controlled trial conducted by Pores, et al. (*Ann Surg* 1967;165:432–436) found that the healing time of a surgical wound was reduced by 43 percent when patients were supplemented with oral zinc in the form of zinc sulfate at a dose of 50 mg of zinc three times a day. However, it remains uncertain as to whether oral supplementation is useful if the patient is not deficient. Topical zinc-containing treatments have been shown to aid wound healing even when the patient has no zinc deficiency.

DEFICIENCY SYMPTOMS

Symptoms of zinc deficiency include fingernails with white spots or bands or an opaquely white appearance; loss of taste, smell, and appetite; delayed sexual development in adolescence; underdeveloped penis and less full beard and underarm hair in boys; irregular menstrual cycle in girls; infertility and impaired sexual function in adults; poor wound healing; loss of hair; increased susceptibility to infection; reduced salivation; skin lesions; stretch marks; reduced absorption of nutrients; impaired development of bones, muscles, and nervous system; deformed offspring; and dwarfism.

THERAPEUTIC DAILY AMOUNT

15–50 mg (take with copper to yield a zinc to copper ratio of 10:1). The RDA is 15 mg for men and 12 mg for women. Coffee drinkers should take zinc supplements at least one hour before or two hours after drinking coffee, as it reduces the body's ability to absorb zinc by 50 percent.

MAXIMUM SAFE LEVEL

The maximum safe level for long-term use is 15 mg; for short-term use, 50 mg can be taken safely, although doses of 50 mg and more should be taken only under medical advice and supervision. Supplementation at levels greater than 150 mg per day may suppress immunity and cause other side effects.

SIDE EFFECTS/CONTRAINDICATIONS

High doses of zinc affect the absorption of iron and copper, suppress the immune system, raise LDL cholesterol (the "bad" form of cholesterol), and lower HDL cholesterol (the "good" form of cholesterol) levels. Zinc should be taken with food to avoid irritating the stomach. People with liver damage or an intestinal disorder should consult their doctor before taking supplementary zinc. Zinc should not be taken with corticosteroids, cyclosporine, or other medications intended to suppress the immune system. Zinc may reduce the effectiveness of NSAIDs (nonsteroidal anti-inflammatory drugs, for example aspirin and ibuprofen) therefore people taking such drugs should consult their physician before taking supplementary zinc.Results of several studies conducted over the last few years have linked zinc to Alzheimer's disease. However, one study found that the zinc appeared to improve mental performance in Alzheimer's patients. Until the effect of zinc on Alzheimer's disease is understood more clearly, people diagnosed with Alzheimer's and those deemed at high risk of developing the disease may wish to avoid taking supplementary zinc.

SOLUBILITY

Insoluble in water.

CHAPTER 12

Amino Acids

Acetyl L-Carnitine

GENERAL DESCRIPTION

Acetyl L-carnitine (ALC) is a "conditionally essential" nutrient for humans, which is made in the body from the amino acids lysine and methionine. One of the functions of ALC is to transport fats into the mitochondria. Carnitine from dietary sources or supplementation is required to maintain normal plasma or serum carnitine concentrations in humans of all ages. In fact, researchers observe that nutritional or pharmacological intervention with carnitine may be beneficial for very premature infants, infants and children with various clinical conditions associated with low circulating carnitine concentrations, and for people with some chronic diseases associated with the aging process. It is important to note that Vitamin B_{12} is necessary for carnitine metabolism. ALC occurs in many common foods, including milk.

ROLE IN ANTI-AGING

Numerous clinical trials suggest that ALC can **delay the onset of age-related cognitive decline and improves overall cognitive function** in the elderly. In a controlled clinical trial conducted by Cipolli and Chiari (*Clin Ter* 1990;132(6 Suppl):479–510), 1,500 mg of ALC a day was given to elderly people suffering from mild cognitive impairment. Results showed that participants exhibited significant improvements in cognitive function after just forty-five days of treatment. Meanwhile, research by Salvioli and Neri (*Drugs Exp Clin Res* 1994;20:169–176) found that ninety days of treatment with 1,500 mg of ALC per day significantly improved memory, mood, and responses to stress. Furthermore, these benefits persisted for at least thirty days after supplementation was discontinued.

Several clinical trials have suggested that ALC supplementation may **delay**

the progression of Alzheimer's disease. Abdul et al. (*J Neurosci Res.* 2006; 84:398–408.) found that ALC protects cortical neuronal cells against Abeta(1-42)-mediated oxidative stress and neurotoxicity. Amyloid-beta peptide, particularly the 42-amino-acid peptide Abeta(1-42), is a principal component of senile plaques and is thought to be central to the pathogenesis of Alzheimer's disease. ALC also increased cellular levels of the amino acid glutathione, a potent antioxidant. The results led the researchers to conclude: "Our results suggests that ALC exerts protective effects against Abeta(1-42) toxicity and oxidative stress in part by up-regulating the levels of glutathione. This evidence supports the pharmacological potential of ALC in the management of Abeta(1-42)-induced oxidative stress and neurotoxicity. Therefore, ALC may be useful as a possible therapeutic strategy for patients with Alzheimer's disease." There is also some evidence that the amino acid may help to improve the memory and overall cognitive performance in some Alzheimer's patients.

In 2001, Rani and Panneerselvam (*J Gerontol A Biol Sci Med Sci* 2001; 56:B140–141) studied the activity of acetylcholinesterase, which is responsible for utilization of acetylcholine and is important in neurotransmission, in various regions of young and aged rat brain before and after L-carnitine supplementation. Results showed that ALC treatment is able to **restore the level of acetylcholinesterase** in the cerebral cortex, hippocampus, hypothalamus, striatum, and cerebellum. Research by Lohninger, et al. (*Arch Gerontol Geriatr* 2001;32:245–253) tested the effect of ALC supplementation on the ability of elderly rats to learn the outlay of a maze. Results showed that compared with untreated rats, those treated with ALC made significantly fewer errors and significantly more animals reached the goal of the mazes. Thus suggesting that carnitine treatment **improves the learning ability** of old rats, and seems to be able to reduce the loss of cognitive functions that occur with aging.

Recent studies have confirmed that ALC can **reduce both lipid peroxidation and lipofuscin concentration in brain cells**. Carnitine is an important free-radical scavenger. Carnitine plays an important role in biochemical processes that occur between the mitochondria of cells that synthesize acetylcholine in the brain. Dr. Juliet and colleagues from University of Madras in India have shown that L-carnitine suppresses oxidative damage during aging. The team followed up this finding with a study to evaluate the effect of L-carnitine on the status of non-enzymatic antioxidants and accumulation of lipofuscin (age pigments that result with brown spots) in various regions of the aged rat brain. Dr. Juliet's group observed a decrease in the status of ascorbic acid, glutathione, and vitamin E—all important antioxidants that combat free radicals—in aged rats. Lipofuscin increased as a function of age. In administering L-carnitine supplementation, Dr. Juliet's team was able to improve the antioxidant status in a duration dependent manner. The accumulation of lipofuscin was also found to be decreased after L-carnitine administration. This research suggests that decrement of lipofuscin accumulation by L-carnitine may be partially due to its antioxidant promoting action.

ALC has been demonstrated to **reduce necrotic damage and infarct size**, and **decrease the incidence of arrhythmias** in animal studies. In fact, ALC pre-treatment has been shown to preserve myocardial levels of ATP and partially normalizing metabolic functioning of the heart following ischemia. Animal studies also indicate that L-carnitine increases the contractility of the heart, decreases heart rate, and dilates the coronary artery to promote coronary blood flow. Human studies with L-carnitine supplementation have yielded similarly encouraging results. Both human (*Tumori.* 2005;91:135–138.) and animal studies (*Neurosci Lett.* 2006;397:219–223.) suggest that ALC may help to reduce chemotherapy-induced peripheral neuropathy.

Carnitine is utilized in exercise, and numerous studies have established that L-carnitine supplementation is effective for **increasing maximal aerobic power** and promoting glycogen sparing in the course of prolonged heavy exercise.

DEFICIENCY SYMPTOMS

None known

THERAPEUTIC DAILY AMOUNT

ALC is distributed in 250 mg and 500 mg tablets, and sometimes in oral liquid form. Pharmaceutical trade name preparations include Branigen, Ceredor, Nicetile, Normobren and Zibren. Follow instructions on packaging.

Specific segments of the population that have a requirement for supplementary carnitine include: infants (premature and full-term), patients on long-term parenteral nutrition, and possibly children.

MAXIMUM SAFE LEVEL

1,500 mg per day.

SIDE EFFECTS/CONTRAINDICATIONS

Side effects are uncommon. They may include skin rash, increased appetite, nausea, vomiting, dizziness, headache, agitation, and body odor. People with kidney or liver disease should consult their doctor before taking supplementary ALC.

Arginine

GENERAL DESCRIPTION

Arginine is a non-essential amino acid that the body can synthesize in the liver; however, in times of stress or trauma arginine becomes an essential amino acid. The end-products of arginine metabolism produced by the enzymes arginase, arginine decarboxylase (ADC), and nitric oxide synthase (NOS) have been shown to play roles in wound healing, immune response, tumor biology, and the regulation of inflammation. In men, low arginine has been associated with decreased sperm count.

Arginine is found in beans, brewer's yeast, chocolate, dairy products, eggs, fish, legumes, meat, nuts, oatmeal, popcorn, raisins, seafood, seeds, sesame seeds, soy, sunflower seeds, whey, whole grains.

ROLE IN ANTI-AGING

Arginine **stimulates the pituitary to release growth hormone**. Arginine appears to enhance growth hormone releasing hormone-induced growth hormone secretion by blocking the hormone, somatostatin, which acts as a brake within the pituitary gland lowering the production and release of HGH. Furthermore, the responsiveness of growth hormone-secreting somatotrope cells to growth hormone releasing hormone is reduced in older people; however, research suggests that arginine is able to restore this decreased responsiveness. In a controlled trial by Elam (*J Sports Med Phys Fitness* 1988;28:35–39), when arginine and ornithine (500 mg of each, twice per day, five times per week) were combined with weight training, a greater decrease in body fat was obtained after only five weeks, than in participants taking a placebo but doing the same amount of exercise.

Arginine supplementation may help to **reduce the risk of cardiovascular disease**. Arginine boosts nitric oxide (NO) production, making it potentially useful in the treatment of congestive heart failure, intermittent claudication, angina, impotence, and sexual dysfunction in women. Arginine relaxes blood vessels and keeps arteries flexible. L-arginine supplementation has been proposed to reverse endothelial dysfunction in such diverse pathophysiological conditions as hypercholesterolemia, coronary heart disease, and some forms of animal hypertension. Additionally, chronic oral administration of L-arginine has prevented the blood pressure rise induced by sodium chloride loading in salt-sensitive rats. L-arginine has also been shown to lower blood pressure in humans. Siani et al. (*Am J Hypertens.* 2000;13:547–551.) found that a moderate increase in L-arginine administered to healthy adults was able to significantly lower blood pressure and beneficially affect renal function and carbohydrate metabolism.

Arginine helps to **give the immune system a boost** and, therefore, is useful for people recovering from illness or surgery. It is a known **T-lymphocyte stimulator**. Daly, et al. (*Ann Surg.* 1988;208:512–523) found that arginine has immunomodulatory effects in surgical patients. Results of their study showed that supplemental arginine significantly enhanced the mean T-lymphocyte response and increased the mean CD4 phenotype postoperatively. Li, et al. (*J Tongji Med Univ.* 1993;13:111–115) observed that there is a significant reduction in interleukin 2 (IL-2) production, interleukin 2 receptor (IL-2R) expression, and lymphocyte response in patients with obstructive jaundice as a result of surgery. However, supplementation of such patients with arginine around the time of surgery was able to enhance immune function by **increasing IL-2 production** and IL-2R expression. In animal tests, Barbul, et al. (*J Parentel Enteral Nutr* 1980;4:446–449) found that arginine supplementation caused a significant **increase in thymic weight** (average increase 22 percent), thymic lymphocyte content (average increase 45 percent), and the *in vitro* reactivity of thymic lymphocytes.

Arginine is also important in **promoting healthy permeability and adaptive responses of the gut**. Research suggests that supplementation with arginine may positively promote gut mucosal barrier function, which is particularly important for patients recovering from surgery. Arginine promotes wound healing. Shi et al. (*Wound Repair Regen.* 2003;11:198–203.) found that L-arginine supplementation partially corrected the impaired healing of diabetic wounds. Whilst Farreras et al. (*Clin Nutr.* 2005;24:55–65.) found that postoperative enteral nutrition with a formula supplemented with arginine, omega 3 fatty acids and ribonucleic acid increased improved surgical wound healing and significantly lowered the incidence of surgical wound healing complications in patients undergoing gastrectomy for gastric cancer.

Arginine can also help to protect sperm from oxidative damage, and increase sperm vitality.

DEFICIENCY SYMPTOMS

Decreased sperm count.

THERAPEUTIC DAILY AMOUNT

A typical therapeutic dosage of arginine is 2–3 g per day. Most people do not need to take supplementary arginine. People suffering from serious burns, infections, or other trauma may need extra arginine; however, a doctor should decide the dosage. Doses used in studies to improve immune function ranged between 25 and 43 grams per day.

MAXIMUM SAFE LEVEL

Not established. However, oral supplementation with L-arginine at daily doses of up to 15 grams is generally well tolerated.

SIDE EFFECTS/CONTRAINDICATIONS

The most common adverse reactions of higher doses—from 15 to 30 grams daily—are nausea, abdominal cramps and diarrhea. Individuals with renal or hepatic insufficiency and those with insulin-dependent diabetes should avoid large doses of arginine, as should people who are allergic to eggs, milk, or wheat. Some doctors suggest that people with herpes should not take arginine supplements, because it aids herpes virus replication. Arginine can interfere with the metabolism of lysine, which can reactivate the herpes simplex virus. People taking non-steroidal anti-inflammatory drugs (NSAIDs) such as aspirin, and drugs that alter potassium levels, for example ACE inhibitors, should be cautious if taking supplementary arginine. People with kidney or liver disease should consult their doctor before taking supplementary arginine.

Note: Arginine and lysine are antagonistic amino acids, meaning that concomitant intake could compromise the absorption of one over the other. When taking a product containing both arginine and lysine, ask the manufacturer about how to best take the product so that absorption of these two amino acids is optimized.

Branched-Chain Amino Acids (BCAAs)— Leucine, Isoleucine, and Valine

GENERAL DESCRIPTION

The branched-chain amino acids (BCAAs) leucine, isoleucine, and valine are used by the body to manufacture proteins. Muscles have a high content of BCAAs. Adequate amounts of BCAAs are usually obtained from the diet; however, injury can increase the body's need for BCAAs in order to repair damage. BCAAs are found in all protein-containing foods, but the best sources are red meat and dairy products.

ROLE IN ANTI-AGING

BCAAs are often used for their **muscle-building properties**; however, the majority of evidence obtained from clinical studies suggests that they do not improve performance, reduce fatigue, or increase the body's muscle/fat ratio.

Results of a 1999 study suggest that BCAAs might improve the symptoms of **tardive dyskinesia**, a movement disorder caused by long-term use of antipsychotic drugs. Other studies have found that supplementary BCAAs may reduce the symptoms of **Lou Gehrig's disease** (amyotrophic lateral sclerosis; ALS), and may be of benefit to people with liver disease to preserve or to restore muscle mass and to improve hepatic encephalopathy.

BCAAs may be of benefit to restore appetite in people with cancer and other chronic diseases. According to Laviano et al. (*Curr Opin Clin Nutr Metab Care*. 2005;8:408–414.) BCAAs "appear to exert significant antianorectic and anticachectic effects, and their supplementation may represent a viable intervention not only for patients suffering from chronic diseases, but also for those individuals at risk of sarcopenia due to age, immobility or prolonged bed rest, including trauma, orthopedic or neurologic patients."

DEFICIENCY SYMPTOMS

There are no known deficiency symptoms for leucine and valine; however, a severe deficiency of isoleucine may cause hypoglycemia (this is extremely unlikely).

THERAPEUTIC DAILY AMOUNT

The therapeutic dose is 1–5 g per day, depending upon requirements.

MAXIMUM SAFE LEVEL

The maximum safe level has not been established. When taken in excess, BCAAs are simply converted into other amino acids; therefore, they are generally regarded as safe, even in large doses.

SIDE EFFECTS/CONTRAINDICATIONS

People with kidney or liver disease should consult their doctor before taking supplementary leucine, isoleucine, or valine. BCAAs can reduce the effectiveness of anti-Parkinson's drugs, for example levodopa.

Cysteine, N-Acetyl Cysteine (NAC)

GENERAL DESCRIPTION

Cysteine is a nonessential amino acid that can be manufactured in the liver. It is obtained in the diet from beans, brewer's yeast, broccoli, Brussels sprouts, dairy products, eggs, fish, garlic, legumes, meat, nuts, onions, red peppers, seafood, seeds, soy, whey, and whole grains. N-acetyl cysteine (NAC) is a modified form of cysteine. NAC helps the body make the antioxidant enzyme glutathione.

ROLE IN ANTI-AGING

Cysteine may help to diminish the effects of aging, **protect against heart disease** and **cancer, boost the immune system, promote metabolism of fats and production of muscle tissue, aid healing after surgery, promote hair growth, and prevent hair loss.** It is also known to work synergistically with vitamin E and selenium as an antioxidant, **protecting against the damaging effects of radiation, acetaldehyde, acrolein in tobacco smoke, alcohol, and environmental pollutants.**

Several studies have found that NAC is beneficial to patients with **chronic bronchitis** and **angina.** NAC's power as an immune system booster stems from its ability to enhance the production of the enzyme glutathione, a potent antioxidant vital for the correct functioning of the immune system. NAC may also reduce the severity and duration of influenza by thinning mucus and weakening the flu virus. De Flora et al. (*Eur Respir J.* 1997;10:1535–1541.) gave 262 people 600 mg NAC or placebo twice daily for six months. Results showed that treatment with NAC resulted in a significant decrease in the frequency of influenza-like episodes, severity, and length of time confined to bed. The results led the authors to conclude: "Administration of N-acetylcysteine during the winter, thus, appears to provide a significant attenuation of influenza and influenza-like episodes, especially in elderly high-risk individuals." Some experts believe that NAC increases the efficacy of chemotherapy drugs and helps to alleviate their side effects; however, there is little clinical evidence to support this. Very high doses of NAC are given to patients in hospitals to treat acetaminophen poisoning.

DEFICIENCY SYMPTOMS

Symptoms of cysteine deficiency include apathy, loss of pigmentation in hair, edema, lethargy, liver damage, muscle loss, skin lesions, weakness, fat loss, and slowed growth in children.

THERAPEUTIC DAILY AMOUNT

Optimal levels of NAC and cysteine have not been determined. 250–1,500 mg of NAC per day has been used in clinical studies with no adverse effects.

MAXIMUM SAFE LEVEL

Not established—there are no known signs of toxicity from cysteine.

NAC appears to be a very safe supplement even in high doses; however, an animal study found that 60 to 100 times the normal dose could cause liver injury. Note: NAC is known to have antioxidant activity; however, one study found that daily doses of 1.2 g or more increased oxidative stress.

SIDE EFFECTS/CONTRAINDICATIONS

People with diabetes mellitus and allergies to eggs, milk, or wheat should not take supplementary cysteine. People taking the drug may experience severe headaches when taking NAC. Cysteine supplements must be taken with vitamin C to prevent cysteine's being converted to cystine, which may form kidney or bladder stones. People with kidney or liver disease should consult their doctor before taking supplementary cysteine.

Gamma Aminobutyric Acid (GABA)

GENERAL DESCRIPTION

GABA is a nonessential amino acid and is the most prevalent inhibitory neurotransmitter in the central nervous system. GABA is found in large amounts in the hypothalamus, thus implying that it has a fundamental role in hypothalamic-pituitary function, and thus neuroendocrine metabolism.

GABA can be found naturally in beans, brewer's yeast, dairy products, eggs, fish, legumes, meat, nuts, seafood, seeds, soy, whey, and whole grains.

ROLE IN ANTI-AGING

GABA is an excellent substitute for growth hormone and several clinical studies have found that ingestion of GABA, especially after exercise, **stimulates the pituitary to secrete growth hormone**. Thus, it may help to **increase lean body mass**.

Because of its inhibitory effects upon the central nervous system, supplemental GABA can be useful for aiding relaxation, preventing anxiety, and promoting sleep. GABA exerts its anti-anxiety effects by acting on the membrane of the cell receiving the neurotransmitter, and exerting a strong calming (inhibitory) effect on brain neurons. This creates a biochemical environment conducive to sleep. In research by Murck et al. (*Neurobiol Aging*. 1999;20: 665–668.) GABA was found to exert a protective action on brainwave patterns in sleep and hormone secretion under conditions of sleep deprivation.

GABA can help to decrease epileptic seizures and muscle spasms by inhibiting message transmission in neurons. This helps control nerve cells from firing too fast, which would overload the system. GABA also lowers blood pressure and helps control hypoglycemia.

DEFICIENCY SYMPTOMS
There are no known signs of GABA deficiency.

THERAPEUTIC DAILY AMOUNT
Refer to packaging. Some sources recommend 200 mg up to four times daily.

MAXIMUM SAFE LEVEL
Not established.

SIDE EFFECTS/CONTRAINDICATIONS
Side effects can include a tingling sensation in the face and a slight shortness of breath shortly after taking the supplement. Both effects only last for a few minutes. GABA may cause drowsiness; therefore, it is best to take it shortly before going to bed. People with kidney or liver disease should consult their doctor before taking supplementary GABA.

Glutamic Acid (Glutamate)

GENERAL DESCRIPTION
Glutamic acid is a nonessential amino acid that the body uses to build proteins. It can be obtained from eating meat, poultry, fish, eggs, and dairy products.

ROLE IN ANTI-AGING
The fluid produced by the prostate gland contains significant amounts of glutamic acid. This has led scientists to believe that glutamic acid may play a role in the normal **functioning of the prostate**. One clinical study found that supplementary glutamic acid significantly improved the symptoms of benign prostatic hyperplasia (BPH). There is some evidence to suggest that glutamic acid may have protective effects on heart muscle. Results of one study revealed that intravenous injections of glutamic acid (as monosodium glutamate) increased exercise tolerance and heart function in people with stable angina pectoris. However, whether a similar effect would be seen with oral glutamic acid is uncertain.

DEFICIENCY SYMPTOMS
There are no known glutamic acid deficiency symptoms.

THERAPEUTIC DAILY AMOUNT
As glutamic acid is abundant in common foods, supplementation is not necessary unless directed by a physician or nutritionist, who will prescribe a relevant dose.

MAXIMUM SAFE LEVEL

Not established.

SIDE EFFECTS/CONTRAINDICATIONS

Glutamic acid is generally free of side effects. People with renal or liver disease should consult their doctor before taking supplementary glutamic acid. People who are hypersensitive to monosodium glutamate (MSG), that is, those who suffer from "Chinese meal syndrome" should not take supplementary glutamic acid as it can exacerbate their symptoms. People with kidney or liver disease should consult their doctor before taking supplementary glutamic acid.

Glutamine

GENERAL DESCRIPTION

The most abundant amino acid in muscles and blood, glutamine provides fuel for various cells of the immune system and is a critical component in wound repair. The body can make glutamine, but may not make enough when the body is under stress. Glutamine is found naturally in beans, brewer's yeast, brown rice, dairy products, eggs, fish, legumes, meat, nuts, seafood, seeds, soy, whey, and whole grains.

ROLE IN ANTI-AGING

Preliminary evidence suggests that glutamine might help **prevent infections** in people who are overstressed and athletes who are overtrained—and thus immunosuppressed. Scientists have proposed that the decrease in plasma glutamine concentration in catabolic conditions—including strenuous exercise—results in a lack of glutamine for cells of the immune system. This mechanism is suspected to be responsible for the phenomena of transient postexercise immunosuppression. Antonio and colleagues from the University of Nebraska examined the potential utility of glutamine for athletes engaged in heavy exercise training. They found positive effects of glutamine supplementation on **muscle protein mass, immune system function, and glucose regulation** in athletes. Based on their studies, the team suggests that glutamine is potentially useful as a dietary supplement for athletes engaged in heavy exercise training.

Griffiths et al. (*Nutrition.* 1997;13:295–302.) found that intravenous glutamine supplementation increased the survival rate of critically ill people. Furthermore the total cost of intensive care per survivor was reduced by 50 percent in those treated with glutamine. There is also evidence that supplemental glutamine can help to maintain muscle protein mass and immune system function in critically ill patients. Thus, glutamine may be useful as a nutritional supplement for people undergoing recovery from illness.

Some scientists have also suggested that glutamine could be useful as a **treatment for food allergies**. This speculation is based on a theory called "leaky gut syndrome," where proteins leak through the wall of the digestive tract and enter the blood, causing allergic reactions. There is some evidence to support this theory as several studies have suggested that glutamine supplements might reduce leakage through the intestinal walls. Because of this, glutamine supplements have been suggested for people with other digestive problems, such as irritable bowel syndrome, Crohn's disease, and ulcerative colitis. However, there have also been trials that have found that glutamine supplements were of no benefit to these people. Glutamine may be of benefit to patients with HIV as it has been shown to **increase levels of glutathione**, which interferes with viral activation, as well as significantly increases lean body mass.

Glutamine may be of benefit to people with cancer. Yoshida et al. (*Ann Surg.* 1998;227:485–491.) found that lab animals with tumors utilize more glutamine, as was shown by measurements of plasma and skeletal muscle concentrations. In concurrent studies of people with esophageal cancer the team found that oral supplementation of glutamine enhanced lymphocyte function and reduced permeability of the gut during radiochemotherapy treatment. Meanwhile Chen et al. (*Asian J Surg.* 2005;28:121–124.) gave patients with gastric carcinoma who had undergone major surgery an enteral immunonutrition formula enriched with glutamine, arginine and omega-3 fatty acids for seven days. Those given the immunonutrition group had higher levels of immunoglobulin, CD4 cell counts, CD4/CD8 ratio and IL-2 than those in the control group, whereas IL-6 and TNF-alpha levels were significantly lower in the immunonutrition group. The authors conclude: "enteral immunonutrition can improve defence mechanisms and modulate inflammatory action after major elective surgery for gastric carcinoma." There is also evidence that supplemental glutamine can help to maintain immune system function in critically ill patients. Thus, glutamine may be useful as a nutritional supplement for people undergoing recovery from illness.

Glutamine is particularly important in **promoting growth hormone levels**. Dr. Tomas Welbourne (*Am J Clin Nutr* 1995;61:1058–1061) showed that a surprising small oral dose (about 2 g of glutamine) raised HGH levels more than four times than when the subjects were given a placebo. Even more exciting, age did not diminish the response, at least in this small study of volunteers, who ranged from thirty-two to sixty-four years old. Indeed, it appears that there exists a direct relationship between glutamine and growth hormone. Biolo, et al. (*Am J Physiol Endocrinol Metab.* 2000;279:E323–332) studied the effects of human growth hormone administration on glutamine metabolism in hypercatabolic trauma patients (experiencing excessive catabolic breakdown). They found that net glutamine release from muscle into circulation significantly decreased after growth hormone administration. They suspect this served to compensate for reduced availability of glutamine precursors as occurs with the catabolic trauma state. Confirmation of the glutamine-growth hormone control mechanism is also offered by research by Parry-Billings, et al. (*Horm Metab Res* 1993;25:292–293). When they administered human growth hormone, they found the concentrations of glutamine in both skeletal muscle and plasma, and the rate of glutamine release, were increased. Their research confirms that growth hormone plays an important role in controlling glutamine metabolism in muscle.

DEFICIENCY SYMPTOMS

There are no known symptoms of glutamine deficiency. Glutamine deficiencies are very rare as the body manufactures its own glutamine. However, people with cirrhosis, AIDS, cancer, and critical illnesses in general may develop deficiencies.

THERAPEUTIC DAILY AMOUNT

Doses range from 1.5–6 grams daily, divided into several separate doses. The majority of healthy people do not need to take supplementary glutamine.

MAXIMUM SAFE LEVEL

Not established. Glutamine is generally regarded as safe.

SIDE EFFECTS/CONTRAINDICATIONS

People who are hypersensitive to monosodium glutamate (MSG) should use glutamine with caution, as the body metabolizes glutamine into glutamate. Individuals taking antiseizure medications—for example, carbamazepine, phenobarbital, Dilantin (phenytoin), Mysoline (primidone), and valproic acid (Depakene)—should only take supplementary glutamine under medical supervision. People with kidney or liver disease should consult their doctor before taking supplementary glutamine.

Glutathione

GENERAL DESCRIPTION

Glutathione is a tripeptide composed of the three amino acids—glycine, glutamic acid (glutamate), and cysteine. Dietary glutathione can be found in fruit and vegetables, especially asparagus, avocado, walnuts, fish, and meat.

ROLE IN ANTI-AGING

Glutathione has been called **the "master antioxidant."** In addition to its own potent antioxidant powers, glutathione helps to recycle other antioxidants such as vitamins C and E. Thus, glutathione can help to protect against aging, cancer, and other diseases caused by oxidative damage.

Glutathione plays an important role in the regulation of immune cells, and results of several studies suggest that glutathione has antiviral properties. Research has shown that glutathione inhibits activation and replication of the influenza virus. Scientists from Emory University reported at the Experimental Biology 2000 meeting in San Diego that glutathione, could help prevent infection by the influenza virus if administered directly to the tissues lining the mouth and upper airway. The scientists suggested that glutathione concentrated in a lozenge or spray might be the most effective way to use the compound as a flu preventive. Research has shown that glutathione inhibits activation of the HIV virus, therefore it may be beneficial to people with HIV and AIDS. Vogel et al. (*Med Microbiol Immunol* (Berl). 2005;194:55–59.) found that glutathione acts as an antiviral agent against herpes simplex virus-1 (HSV-1) both *in vitro* and *in vivo,* thus suggesting that it may be of benefit in the adjunctive therapy of HSV-1 infection.

Glutathione is a potent detoxifying agent.

Low levels of glutathione have been associated with hepatic dysfunction, immune dysfunction, cardiac disease, and premature aging. It is also important in DNA synthesis and repair, protein and prostaglandin synthesis, and amino acid transport.

DEFICIENCY SYMPTOMS

There are no known symptoms of glutathione deficiency; however, some medical conditions, such as diabetes, low sperm count, and liver disease, are associated with glutathione deficiency. Heavy smokers may have low levels as certain chemicals in tobacco smoke increase the rate at which the body utilizes glutathione.

THERAPEUTIC DAILY AMOUNT

Refer to dosage instructions on packaging. People with a proven glutathione deficiency should be treated by a doctor, and may require intravenous or intramuscular injections.

Some research suggests that taking oral glutathione may not be the best way of raising blood glutathione levels. One study showed that healthy people could raise their blood glutathione levels by nearly 50 percent by taking 500 mg of vitamin C each day for two weeks. Other nutritional compounds that may help to boost glutathione levels include alpha lipoic acid, glutamine, methionine, S-adenosyl methionine (SAMe), and whey protein.

MAXIMUM SAFE LEVEL
Not established.

SIDE EFFECTS/CONTRAINDICATIONS
People with kidney or liver disease should consult their doctor before taking supplementary glutathione.

Glycine

GENERAL DESCRIPTION
Glycine is a nonessential amino acid found naturally in beans, brewer's yeast, dairy products, eggs, fish, gelatin, legumes, meat, nuts, seafood, seeds, soy, sugar cane, whey, and whole grains.

Glycine is important in the control of gluconeogenesis—the manufacture of glucose from glycogen in the liver. Glycine is also one of the few amino acids that can spare glucose for energy by improving glycogen storage. Therefore, **inappropriate blood glucose control** may be managed by increased glycine intake. Glycine is also known to serve as a **source of nitrogen** for the manufacture of many other amino acids and is useful in the synthesis of hemoglobin, glutathione, DNA, and RNA. Glycine is required by the body for the maintenance of the central nervous system, and the synthesis of the porphyrin core of hemoglobin. It also enhances the activity of neurotransmitters (chemical messengers) in the brain that are important for memory and cognition. The amino acid is also required for the prostate gland to function correctly.

ROLE IN ANTI-AGING
Glycine may be useful in treating stroke victims. One study found that relatively small doses of the amino acid were able to significantly reduce the damage to brain cells that occurs after a stroke. However, some studies have found evidence to suggest that high doses of glycine could actually increase stroke damage. Thus, the benefits of glycine in limiting stroke damage remain inconclusive. Results of a study by Amin et al. (*Cancer Biol Ther.* 2003;2:173–178.) suggest that dietary glycine is a potent anti-angiogenic agent

that can reduce tumor growth through reduction of inducible nitric oxide synthase (iNOS) expression.

Animal studies have found that dietary glycine may protect against chemical damage to the liver and kidneys; however, there is no human data to back up these findings.

Results of at least two studies have shown that supplementary glycine taken in combination with equal amounts of the amino acids alanine and glutamic acid significantly improves the symptoms of benign prostatic hyperplasia (BPH). Several studies have found that high doses of glycine, in combination with standard therapy, may be useful in the treatment of schizophrenia. Finally, there is some evidence to suggest that topically applied glycine may aid in wound healing.

DEFICIENCY SYMPTOMS

There are no known symptoms of glycine deficiency.

THERAPEUTIC DAILY AMOUNT

Dosage depends on a number of factors; doses ranging from 2–60 g daily have been used for therapeutic purposes in clinical trials.

MAXIMUM SAFE LEVEL

Not established; however, no serious adverse effects from using glycine have been seen even with doses as high as 60 g per day.

SIDE EFFECTS/CONTRAINDICATIONS

Some studies have shown that glycine may be harmful when taken in combination with newer antipsychotic drugs, such as clozapine. Therefore, people taking such medications should not take glycine. People with kidney disease or liver disease should consult their doctor before taking glycine.

Histidine

GENERAL DESCRIPTION

Histidine is occasionally referred to as a semi-essential amino acid. This means that the body can usually produce adequate amounts of histidine; however, in certain circumstances, such as periods of rapid growth, the body cannot supply enough to meet demand. Histidine is found in beans, brewer's yeast, dairy products, eggs, fish, legumes, meat, nuts, seafood, seeds, soy, whey, and whole grains.

ROLE IN ANTI-AGING

The body uses histidine to **produce histamine**, a substance that plays a central role in allergic reactions and other functions of the immune system. Histidine also helps to **chelate trace minerals and copper**, thus aiding their removal from the body.

People with rheumatoid arthritis may have low blood levels of histidine. This discovery led to speculation that histidine supplements may be of benefit to patients with rheumatoid arthritis. However, as of yet no clinical studies have been able to find any evidence to support these theories.

DEFICIENCY SYMPTOMS

There are no known symptoms of histidine deficiency.

THERAPEUTIC DAILY AMOUNT

A typical therapeutic dosage of histidine is 4–5 g per day.

MAXIMUM SAFE LEVEL

Not established. However, large doses of histidine can cause premature ejaculation, reduce zinc levels, and possibly trigger an allergic or asthmatic reaction.

SIDE EFFECTS/CONTRAINDICATIONS

People with kidney or liver disease should consult their doctor before taking supplementary histidine.

Homocysteine

GENERAL DESCRIPTION

Homocysteine (Hcy), a sulfur-containing amino acid involved in methionine metabolism, is now recognized as a **major independent risk factor for cardiovascular disease**—joining the ranks of dyslipidemia, hypertension, and smoking. An elevated level of Hcy in the blood increases the risk of atherosclerosis, and consequently heart attacks and strokes. Hcy causes direct damage to the lining of blood vessels, weakening them and opening them to the accumulation of plaque. There is also some evidence to suggest that Hcy may be a thrombogenic agent that triggers the formation of blood clots. Interestingly, it was recognized more than thirty years ago that individuals with an inborn error of metabolism, cystathionine betasynthase deficiency, had a 50 to 100–fold elevation in circulating Hcy and excreted large amounts of Hcy in the urine. Premature vascular disease and implicated subclinical deficiencies of B vitamins are contributing factors. It was estimated that a 5 umol/L increase in serum Hcy is associated with a 60 to 80 percent increased risk of coronary artery disease (CAD).

Homocysteine has also been linked to Alzheimer's disease, Parkinson's disease, and osteoporosis.

ROLE IN ANTI-AGING
Not applicable.

DEFICIENCY SYMPTOMS
Not applicable.

THERAPEUTIC DAILY AMOUNT
Not applicable.

MAXIMUM SAFE LEVEL
Not applicable.

SIDE EFFECTS/CONTRAINDICATIONS
Not applicable.

Lysine

GENERAL DESCRIPTION
Lysine is an essential amino acid that helps to regulate the pineal gland, mammary glands, and ovaries. It is important for growth and bone development; promotes calcium absorption; maintains nitrogen balances; aids in the production of antibodies, hormones, and collagen; and helps to build muscle tissue.

Beans, brewer's yeast, cheese, dairy products, eggs, fish, legumes, lima beans, meat, milk, nuts, potatoes, seafood, seeds, soy, whey, whole grains, and yeast are natural sources of lysine.

ROLE IN ANTI-AGING
Lysine is needed for the production of antibodies, and studies have shown that lysine-deficiency in animals is associated with a reduced antibody response and cell-mediated immune response to infection. Lysine is a natural protease inhibitor (a compound that interferes with the ability of certain enzymes to break down proteins), and therefore it can help to prevent bacteria and viruses from replicating, and therefore limit infection.

Several studies have found that regular use of lysine supplements may **reduce the frequency and intensity of herpes virus** flare-ups. Both cold sores and genital herpes are caused by the herpes simplex virus. After the initial infection with herpes, the virus hides in nerves cells and causes flare-ups of the disease at times of stress—for example, when the body is immunocompromised. *In vitro* studies suggest that lysine combats the herpes virus by blocking the amino acid arginine, which the herpes virus requires in order to replicate. Walsh, et al. (*J Antimicrob Chemother.* 1983;12:489–496) studied 1,543 men and women after six months of lysine supplementation following diagnosis of cold sores, canker sores, and genital herpes. Eighty-four percent said that lysine supplementation prevented recurrence or decreased the frequency of herpes infection. While 79 percent described their symptoms as severe or intolerable without lysine, only 8 percent used these terms when taking lysine. Furthermore, lysine also appears to speed healing of sores; 90 percent indicated that healing took six to fifteen days, but with lysine 83 percent stated that lesions healed in five days or less. Overall, 88 percent considered supplemental lysine an effective form of treatment for herpes infection.

Studies in animals have shown that dietary supplements with certain amino acids—particularly lysine—can increase calcium absorption. Civitelli, et al. (*Nutrition* 1992;8:400–405) found that lysine can both enhance intestinal calcium absorption and improve the renal conservation of absorbed calcium. Together, these effects may contribute to a positive calcium balance; Civitelli suggests that lysine supplements may help to prevent and treat osteoporosis.

DEFICIENCY SYMPTOMS

Symptoms and signs of lysine deficiency include anemia, apathy, bloodshot eyes, depression, edema, fatigue, fever blisters, hair loss, inability to concentrate, infertility, irritability, lethargy, liver damage, loss of energy, muscle loss, retarded growth, stomach ulcers, and weakness.

THERAPEUTIC DAILY AMOUNT

Most people do not require lysine supplementation. 1,000–3,000 mg of lysine per day is recommended for the treatment of herpes. For the treatment or prevention of influenza sources recommend a dose of 6,000 mg each day, to be taken in three doses of 2,000 mg at mealtimes.

MAXIMUM SAFE LEVEL

Not established. However, lysine supplements should not be taken for any longer than six months, as prolonged use may cause an imbalance of the amino acid arginine.

SIDE EFFECTS/CONTRAINDICATIONS

People who are allergic to eggs, milk, or wheat, and diabetics should not take supplementary lysine. People with kidney disease or liver disease should consult their doctor before taking lysine.

Methionine

GENERAL DESCRIPTION

Methionine is an essential amino acid that is required for the **absorption, transportation, and bioavailability of zinc and selenium in the body**. Methionine also facilitates the **breakdown of fats** and prevents accumulation of fat in the liver and arteries. Methionine is obtained in the diet from brewer's yeast, dairy products, eggs, fish, meat, seafood, and whey.

ROLE IN ANTI-AGING

Methionine appears to prevent bacteria from adhering to the wall of the bladder; this property of methionine has led to its being suggested as a treatment for recurrent urinary tract infections (UTIs). One trial has found evidence to support this claim, yet the use of methionine in preventing UTIs has not been confirmed.

Methionine has been shown to be effective in the prevention of acetaminophen toxicity, and some experts have suggested selling acetaminophen in combination with the amino acid to prevent acetaminophen poisoning. However, there has been some speculation that chronic use of methionine can increase homocysteine levels.

DEFICIENCY SYMPTOMS

Methionine deficiency can cause apathy, loss of pigmentation in hair, edema, lethargy, liver damage, muscle loss, fat loss, skin lesions, weakness, and slowed growth in children.

THERAPEUTIC DAILY AMOUNT

Not established. However, one study that used methionine supplements to treat urinary tract infections found that 500 mg taken three times a day had a therapeutic effect.

MAXIMUM SAFE LEVEL

Not established.

SIDE EFFECTS/CONTRAINDICATIONS

Some research suggests that methionine may help to relieve some symptoms of Parkinson's disease. However, several studies have found that S-adenosylmethionine (SAMe)—another form of methionine—worsens symptoms of the disease. Therefore, some experts suggest that Parkinson's disease patients should avoid taking methionine and SAMe at present. Furthermore, methionine may interfere with the absorption or action of the anti-Parkinson's drug levodopa.

Animal studies suggest that a high intake of methionine, in the presence of B-vitamin deficiencies, may increase the risk of developing atherosclerosis by increasing blood cholesterol and homocysteine levels.

People taking supplementary methionine should ensure that they obtain recommended amounts of folate, vitamin B_6, and vitamin B_{12}. People with kidney disease or liver disease should consult their doctor before taking methionine.

Ornithine Alpha-Ketoglutarate

GENERAL DESCRIPTION

Ornithine alpha-ketoglutarate (OKG) is a combination of the amino acids ornithine and glutamine. OKG enhances the body's release of muscle-building hormones, such as growth hormone and insulin, and increases arginine and glutamine levels in muscle. OKG also encourages synthesis of polyamine, helps prevent the breakdown of muscle, increases muscle growth, and improves immune function.

The amino acids that comprise OKG are present in protein foods such as meat, poultry, and fish; however, the OKG compound itself can only be obtained from supplements.

ROLE IN ANTI-AGING

The concentration of free glutamine in skeletal muscle decreases characteristically after surgical trauma. Wernerman, et al. (*Metabolism* 1989;38:63–66) found that administration of glutamine and OKG after surgery **reduced the loss of muscle glutamine** from 40 percent to 25 percent. Coudray-Lucas, et al. (*Crit Care Med.* 2000;28:1772–1176) administered OKG in enteral nutrition to a group of severe burn patients. Results showed that the average wound healing time for patients receiving OKG was sixty days, whereas that of the control group was ninety days. In separate research conducted on burn victims by De Bandt, et al. (*J Nutr.* 1998;128:563–569), OKG administration **significantly improved wound healing** and nitrogen balance, and reduced urinary elimination of proteins necessary for wound healing. In addition, patients receiving OKG tended to need enteral nutrition for less time than control patients.

OKG may also have other benefits in people recovering from surgery or illness. Results of a study by Brocker, et al. (*Age Aging* 1994;23:303–306) revealed that elderly patients given 10 grams per day of OKG as they recovered from various illnesses or surgery showed **improved appetite, weight gain, muscle growth, reduced need for medical care, and improved quality of life**.

Animal studies suggest that OKG may help to **prevent the spread of bacterial infection**. Research published in 2000 by Schlegel, et al. (*J Nutr.* 2000; 130:2897–2902) found that OKG supplementation limits bacterial spread and adverse metabolic changes that occur after infection. The authors of this study suggest that OKG supplementation may help to prevent gut-derived sepsis in critically ill patients.

DEFICIENCY SYMPTOMS

A deficiency of OKG has not been reported.

THERAPEUTIC DAILY AMOUNT

The optimum dosage of OKG has not been established. Several clinical trials of OKG have used doses of approximately 10 g per day.

MAXIMUM SAFE LEVEL

Not yet established.

SIDE EFFECTS/CONTRAINDICATIONS

None known.

Phenylalanine

GENERAL DESCRIPTION

Phenylalanine is an essential amino acid that can be obtained from eating almonds, avocado, bananas, beans, brewer's yeast, cheese, corn, cottage cheese, dairy products, eggs, fish, legumes, lima beans, meat, nuts, peanuts, pickled herring, pumpkin seeds, seafood, seeds, sesame seeds, soy, whey, and whole grains. Once inside the body, phenylalanine is converted into the amino acid tyrosine, which is then converted into the neurotransmitters L-dopa, norepinephrine, and epinephrine. Phenylalanine governs the release of the hormone cholecystokinin (CCK) that signals the brain to feel satisfied after eating.

ROLE IN ANTI-AGING

Phenylalanine is used to treat a variety of medical problems. Because some antidepressants work by raising norepinephrine levels, **phenylalanine has been used to treat depression**, with varying degrees of success. D-phenylalanine has been suggested as a treatment for chronic pain caused by **rheumatoid arthritis, muscle pain, and osteoarthritis**, as it blocks enkephalinase, an enzyme that may act to increase pain levels in the body. There is some evidence to support the use of phenylalanine to alleviate chronic pain, although it has not been clinically proven. Some studies have suggested that the various forms of phenylalanine may be useful as a treatment for vitiligo (a disease characterized by abnormal white blotches of skin due to loss of pigmentation), when used in combination with UV light therapy.

DEFICIENCY SYMPTOMS

Symptoms and signs of phenylalanine deficiency include low serum levels of essential blood proteins, apathy, loss of pigmentation in hair, edema, lethargy, liver damage, muscle loss, fat loss, skin lesions, weakness, and slowed growth in children.

THERAPEUTIC DAILY AMOUNT

When used as a treatment for depression, the initial dose of L-phenylalanine is typically 500 mg per day; the dose is then gradually increased to 3–4 g daily. However, some people may suffer side effects at doses of 1.5 mg and above.

D- or DL-phenylalanine can also be used as a treatment for depression; however, the typical dosage is much lower at 100–400 mg per day.

For the treatment of chronic pain, doses of D-phenylalanine can be as high as 2.5 g.

MAXIMUM SAFE LEVEL

Not established. However, doses of 1.5 g and above can cause side effects.

SIDE EFFECTS/CONTRAINDICATIONS

Phenylalanine does not generally cause side effects. However, daily doses of approximately 1.5 g and above have been reported to cause anxiety, headaches, and mildly elevated blood pressure.

People who suffer from the metabolic disease phenylketonuria (PKU) should avoid all forms of phenylalanine (L-phenylalanine, D-phenylalanine, and DL-phenylalanine). Phenylalanine can cause potentially dangerous hypertension when taken with monoamine oxidase inhibitors (MAOIs). It should also not be taken alongside the amino acid tyrosine.

There is some evidence to suggest that using phenylalanine in combination with antipsychotic drugs may increase the risk of developing the movement disorder tardive dyskinesia.

As with other amino acids, phenylalanine may interfere with the absorption and action of the anti-Parkinson's drug levodopa.

People with kidney disease or liver disease should consult their doctor before taking phenylalanine.

SAMe (S-adenosyl-L-methionine, S-adenosylmethionine)

GENERAL DESCRIPTION

SAMe is a compound made from methionine, a sulfur-containing amino acid, and adenosine triphosphate (ATP)—the body's "energy" molecule. SAMe was discovered by an Italian biochemist in 1952, and was first studied as a treatment for depression; during these studies, it was found that SAMe also helped to relieve the symptoms of arthritis. At present, SAMe is classed, along with glucosamine and chondroitin, as a potential "chondroprotective" agent—that is, a substance that not only relieves the symptoms of arthritis but also helps to slow its progression. However, this use of SAMe is yet to be clinically proven.

The body usually produces adequate amounts of SAMe, thus there is no dietary requirement. However, methionine, folate, or vitamin B_{12} deficiencies can reduce SAMe levels and as it is not found in significant quantities in foods, it must be obtained from a supplement.

ROLE IN ANTI-AGING

Numerous clinical studies have found that SAMe is an effective treatment for **osteoarthritis**. Results of a study by Najm et al. (*BMC Musculoskelet Disord.* 2004;5:6.)revealed that SAMe was as effective at managing the symptoms of knee osteoarthritis as the COX-2 inhibitor celecoxib (Celebrex).

SAMe may be useful in the treatment of depression. Mischoulon and Fava (*Am J Clin Nutr.* 2002;76:1158S–61S.) wrote: "trials with oral SAMe have shown that, at doses of 200–1,600 mg/d, SAMe is superior to placebo and is as effective as tricyclic antidepressants in alleviating depression . . . SAMe may have a faster onset of action than do conventional antidepressants and may potentiate the effect of tricyclic antidepressants."

SAMe may be of benefit to people with certain liver conditions, for example cirrhosis, pregnancy-related jaundice, and Gilbert's syndrome. Three out of four clinical trials found that SAMe significantly improved the symptoms of **fibromyalgia**. However, all but one of these trials involved the intravenous or intramuscular injection of SAMe. Thus, it is unclear if the results would be replicated with oral doses.

DEFICIENCY SYMPTOMS

None known.

THERAPEUTIC DAILY AMOUNT

A typical therapeutic dose of SAMe is 400 mg taken three to four times a day.

MAXIMUM SAFE LEVEL

Not established.

SIDE EFFECTS/CONTRAINDICATIONS

The most common side effect is mild gastrointestinal upset. People with bipolar disease should avoid SAMe as it can trigger manic episodes. Furthermore, people taking antidepressants or the anti-Parkinson's drug levodopa should avoid SAMe unless under medical supervision. People with kidney disease or liver disease should consult their doctor before taking SAMe.

Serine

GENERAL DESCRIPTION

Serine is a nonessential amino acid needed for the metabolism of fats and fatty acids, muscle growth, and to maintain a healthy immune system—as it aids the production of immunoglobulins and antibodies. It also plays an important role in the manufacture of cell membranes, and the synthesis of both muscle tissue and the sheath that surrounds nerve cells. Serine can be obtained from beans, brewer's yeast, dairy products, eggs, fish, lactalbumin, legumes, meat, nuts, seafood, seeds, soy, whey, and whole grains. When necessary, the body can synthesize serine from the amino acid glycine.

Phosphatidylserine (PS) is a serine compound made by the body. Supplemental PS is widely used in Italy, Scandinavia, and other parts of Europe to treat various forms of age-related dementia as well as normal age-related memory loss.

ROLE IN ANTI-AGING

PS supplements increase the cerebral cortex's output of the neurotransmitter acetylcholine, which is associated with **thought, reasoning, and concentration**. PS also stimulates the synthesis and release of dopamine. PS also appears to be associated with the brain's **response to stress**. One clinical study found that the stress response of healthy men who had been exposed to exercise-induced stress was lower in those who had taken PS. Stress response was determined by measuring blood ACTH levels. ACTH is a hormone secreted by the pituitary gland, which in turn promotes the adrenal glands to secrete the stress hormone cortisol.

PS is primarily used to treat dementia (both Alzheimer's disease and non-Alzheimer's dementia) as well as normal age-related memory loss.

DEFICIENCY SYMPTOMS
There are no known symptoms of serine deficiency.

THERAPEUTIC DAILY AMOUNT
Refer to packaging.

MAXIMUM SAFE LEVEL
Not established. However, excessively high doses of serine may cause immune suppression and psychological symptoms.

SIDE EFFECTS/CONTRAINDICATIONS
People with kidney disease or liver disease should consult their doctor before taking PS.

Taurine

GENERAL DESCRIPTION
Taurine is a conditionally essential nutrient. As such, taurine is derived directly from the breakdown of food, but the body can produce its own stores from other pre-proteins (the amino acids methionine and cysteine) as well. Taurine is found abundantly in tissues that are excitable, rich in membranes, and that generate oxidants. Thus, it is the most prevalent of all the amino acids in the tissues comprising the skeletal and cardiac muscles and the brain. As such, it is critical to the proper function of the brain, heart, lungs, and blood.

Brewer's yeast, dairy products, eggs, fish, meat, ox bile, and seafood are natural sources of taurine.

ROLE IN ANTI-AGING
Taurine **protects cell membranes from damage**, and enhances the immune system by **stimulating the release of interleukin-1 in macrophages**, and **increasing the phagocytic and bactericidal activity of neutrophils**. It also helps to **detoxify toxic substances** such as retinoids and environmental toxins. Several studies have found that taurine might be useful in the treatment of **congestive heart failure** (CHF), and at least one study has found that it may also be useful for **acute viral hepatitis**. Taurine also increases levels of the neurotransmitter acetylcholine and helps to regulate the nervous system.

Taurine is found at consistently high concentrations in the brain, with levels declining with age. Dawson et al. (*Brain Res Bull.* 1999;48:319–324) showed that the spatial learning ability of older rats was impaired, with the impairment correlated to the reduction in taurine in the striatum of the brain. Aged rats without this learning difficulty showed only modest reductions in taurine. Additionally, striatal dopamine was markedly lower in aged learning-impaired rats, demonstrating a potential interaction between taurine and dopamine that may have implications for Parkinson's disease.

Taurine **promotes the activity of superoxide dismutase**, a copper-containing protein enzyme that breaks down superoxide, a reactive free radical, into harmless oxygen and hydrogen peroxide. Researchers have shown that the activity of glutathione peroxidase, an antioxidant also involved in free-radical binding, is notably higher in fetal brain cells exposed to taurine-rich media. Taurine also serves to stabilize the fluidity of the membrane lipids, and as such, participates in **postponing the aging process of brain neural cells**.

Taurine has numerous beneficial effects upon the cardiovascular system. It makes up nearly 50 percent of the free amino acids in the heart cells, and has a dramatic effect on the success of recovery from life-threatening cardiac conditions. Taurine may help to **prevent the formation of clots** (thrombi) in the cardiovascular system in the hours following myocardial infarction, by lowering levels of serum endothelin levels. Taurine **lowers arterial pressure** by promoting diuresis and vasodilation, and research in mice suggests that taurine may **prevent the progression of arteriosclerosis** by regulating calcium flux in aortic and myocardial tissue. Azuma, et al. (*Jpn Circ J* 1992;56:95–99) conducted a six-week comparative study of oral supplementation of taurine versus coenzyme Q_{10} in patients with congestive heart failure attributed to cardiomyopathy (including ischemia) and exhibiting a grossly compromised ejection fraction (the ability of the heart to pump blood). A **significant improvement in systolic left ventricular function** was seen in the taurine-treated group; however, there was no change in the CoQ_{10} group. Taurine is valuable in its role to **protect the heart from oxidative stress and post-ischemic injury**. It reduces lipoperoxidation (free-radical damage). In a study by Milei et al. (*Am Heart J.* 1992;123:339–345.) of patients undergoing coronary artery bypasses who were pre-treated with taurine, results showed that heart cell mitochondria were subjected to far less extensive damage. Taurine's ability to scavenge free radicals means that is plays a potent cardioprotective role. When taurine is administered to people recovering from ischemia, the rate of the heart's action is notably different than non-treated counterparts. Both the quantity of lactate (a marker of ischemic challenge) and quantity of glutathione (a marker of oxidative stress) are attenuated with taurine. ATP levels (denoting cellular energy production) are also suppressed in ischemia. Through the modulation of lactate, glutathione, and ATP, taurine influences the ability and extent of recovery.

Taurine may **reduce the risk of Alzheimer's disease** by promoting vascular nitric oxide production, which protects nerve cells from taking in the excessive amounts of calcium characterized by the activity of beta-amyloid— the main constituent of the amyloid plaques characteristic of the disease.

People with type I diabetes have been found to have lower blood levels of taurine than nondiabetics. Trachtman, et al. (*Am J Physiol* 1995;269: F429– 438) demonstrated the therapeutic and preventative effects of taurine in diabetic rats. Taurine administration reduced the total proteinuria and albuminuria by approximately 50 percent, prevented glomerular hypertrophy, and diminished glomerulosclerosis and tubulointerstitial fibrosis, overall **ameliorating diabetic nephropathy by reducing renal oxidant injury**. Taurine is also able to affect changes in the adverse blood lipid profile that are associated with the diabetic condition. Researchers found that elevated plasma triglycerides and LDL cholesterol in diabetics were countered through administration of taurine. Some research suggests that taurine may help to correct the metabolic anomalies in vascular smooth muscle produced by type II diabetes.

Taurine is essential to the proper function of the kidney. Without it, renal capacity is adversely changed such that the process of excretion of unwanted substances from the blood is grossly impaired. People with chronic renal failure have elevated levels of urea in the blood, a condition called uremia. They also exhibit markedly low levels of taurine despite an adequate or elevated concentration of precursor amino acids such as cysteine and methionine. An impaired ability to metabolize the precursors to taurine may exacerbate taurine depletion. Left uncorrected, low taurine levels, combined with elevated homocysteine (an undesirable byproduct of cysteine metabolism), causes an increased incidence of cardiovascular disease in patients with uremia.

DEFICIENCY SYMPTOMS

Symptoms of taurine deficiency include anxiety, epilepsy, hyperactivity, and impaired brain function. Low levels of the amino acid cysteine and vitamin B_6 can cause taurine deficiency.

THERAPEUTIC DAILY AMOUNT

1.5–6 g a day.

MAXIMUM SAFE LEVEL

Not established.

SIDE EFFECTS/CONTRAINDICATIONS

Although rare, taurine can cause memory loss and depression of the central nervous system (CNS). People with kidney disease or liver disease should consult their doctor before taking taurine.

Threonine

GENERAL DESCRIPTION

Threonine is an essential amino acid. It is obtained in the diet from beans, brewer's yeast, dairy products, eggs, fish, legumes, meat, nuts, seafood, seeds, soy, whey, and whole grains.

As of all amino acids, threonine is important for the formation of proteins; however, it is especially required for the production of tooth enamel, collagen, and elastin. Threonine helps to metabolize fat and prevents the development of a buildup of fat in the liver; it is also useful for intestinal disorders and indigestion.

ROLE IN ANTI-AGING

Threonine can help to **stabilize the blood sugar** as it can be converted into glucose in the liver by gluconeogenesis. People who have been burned, wounded, or undergone surgery have higher than normal levels of threonine in their urine. This indicates that the amino acid is released from the tissues following **trauma**. Recent research indicates that increasing threonine intake during these periods may aid the recovery process.

Several study findings have suggested that threonine might be able to decrease the **muscle spasticity** that often occurs with MS; however, this use of threonine has not been clinically proven.

DEFICIENCY SYMPTOMS

There are no known signs or symptoms of threonine deficiency.

THERAPEUTIC DAILY AMOUNT

There is no official RDA for threonine; however, suggested doses for therapeutic purposes range from 300–1,200 mg per day.

MAXIMUM SAFE LEVEL

Not established.

SIDE EFFECTS/CONTRAINDICATIONS

None known. People with kidney disease or liver disease should consult their doctor before taking threonine.

Tryptophan

GENERAL DESCRIPTION

Tryptophan is an essential amino acid. It is obtained in the diet from bananas, beans, brewer's yeast, cottage cheese, dairy products, dates, eggs, fish, legumes, meat, milk, nuts, peanuts, protein (hydrolysis), seafood, seeds, soy, turkey, whey, and whole grains.

ROLE IN ANTI-AGING

Tryptophan is required for the production of vitamin B_3 (niacin), which is vital for the brain to manufacture serotonin. Tryptophan is a precursor of the transmitter serotonin, and its ability to boost serotonin levels suggests that it may help to improve mood in people who are low or depressed. Tryptophan may also be of use to people suffering from insomnia, as serotonin is regarded as an effective sleep-inducing agent. Hartman and Spinweber (*J Nerv Ment Dis.* 1979;167:497–499.) found that tryptophan is an effective hypnotic that can significantly reduce the time of onset of sleep (sleep latency) without affecting the various stages. Tryptophan also **boosts the release of growth hormones** and helps to **suppress the appetite.**

DEFICIENCY SYMPTOMS

Signs and symptoms of tryptophan deficiency include apathy, loss of pigmentation in hair, edema, lethargy, liver damage, muscle loss, fat loss, skin lesions, weakness, and slowed growth in children.

THERAPEUTIC DAILY AMOUNT

Therapeutic doses range from 1.5–6 g per day, depending upon need. Tryptophan is best taken between meals with a low-protein food, for example, bread.

MAXIMUM SAFE LEVEL

Not established.

SIDE EFFECTS/CONTRAINDICATIONS

People taking monoamine oxidase inhibitors (MAOIs) should be cautious when taking tryptophan as it can increase the risk of central nervous system (CNS) excitation. People with kidney disease or liver disease should consult their doctor before taking tryptophan.

5 Hydroxytryptophan (5-HTP)

GENERAL DESCRIPTION

The body uses 5 hydroxytryptophan (5-HTP) to manufacture the neurotransmitter serotonin. Due to its effects upon serotonin levels, 5-HTP is often used as an antidepressant.

ROLE IN ANTI-AGING

5-HTP is well absorbed from an oral dose. It easily crosses the blood-brain barrier and effectively increases central nervous system (CNS) synthesis of serotonin. In the CNS, serotonin levels have been implicated in the regulation of sleep, depression, anxiety, aggression, appetite, temperature, sexual behavior, and pain sensation. Therapeutic administration of 5-HTP has been shown to be effective in treating a wide variety of conditions, including depression, fibromyalgia, binge eating associated with obesity, chronic headaches, and insomnia.

5-HTP may also aid weight loss as it promotes earlier feelings of satiety. Ceci, et al. (*J Neural Transm* 1989;76:109–117) studied obese female subjects with body mass index ranging between thirty and forty. The participants were administered oral 5-HTP or a placebo for five weeks—no restrictions were placed on their diet during the study period. Results showed that participants treated with 5-HTP ate less food and lost weight. Meanwhile, research by Cangiano, et al. (*Int J Obes Relat Metab Disord.* 1998;22:648–654) who studied obese people with type II diabetes revealed that supplementation with 5-HTP decreased their daily energy intake, by reducing carbohydrate and fat intake, and reduced their body weight. These findings suggest that 5-HTP may be safely utilized to improve the compliance to dietary prescriptions in type II diabetes.

Serotonin precursors are used in the treatment of depression based on the mechanism that a cerebral serotonin deficiency plays a role in the cause of depression. As the immediate precursor to serotonin, 5-HTP has been evaluated in double-blind studies of depression sufferers to be as effective as many of the popular SSRIs (selective serotonin reuptake inhibitors), such as Prozac and Zoloft, while demonstrating a much milder side effect profile. Serotonin deficit also plays a role in Parkinson's patients with depression. *Griffonia simplicifolia* (see page 315) is a botanical source of moderate levels of 5-HTP so this herb may be helpful to Parkinson's patients.

5-HTP also has a value in pain management. 5-HTP can induce a significant decrease of the cropping out of migraine, the commonest primary pain. The latest medical research on migraine headaches indicates that migraine sufferers experience periods of unusually high MAO activity during their headaches. MAO (monoamine oxidase) is an enzyme that breaks down serotonin. Thus, boosting serotonin levels should help to counter the elevated MAO activity.

5-HTP is an effective, clinically proven way to treat symptoms of fibromyalgia. Fibromyalgia sufferers will notice that the beneficial effects of the 5-HTP will increase over time. Nicolodi and Sicuteri (*Adv Exp Med Biol.* 1996;398:373–379) studied the effect of 5-HTP and monoamine oxidase inhibitors for treating fibromyalgia. They found that the combination of MAOIs with 5-HTP significantly improved fibromyalgia syndrome.

5-HTP has been shown to decrease the time required to get to sleep and to decrease the number of awakenings. It works well in conjunction with herbs such as valerian and hops to promote quality sleep.

Finally, 5-HTP has been studied as an antihypertensive agent. Fregly, et al. (*J Hypertens.* 1987;5:621–628) administered 5-HTP to rats with salt-induced hypertension. 5-HTP was able to prevent the elevation of blood pressure and cardiac hypertrophy, and provided modest protection against reduction of urinary concentrating ability. These results suggest that chronic administration of L-5-HTP provides significant protection against the development of deoxycorticosterone acetate-salt-treated-induced hypertension, polydipsia, polyuria, and cardiac hypertrophia.

DEFICIENCY SYMPTOMS
Not applicable.

THERAPEUTIC DAILY AMOUNT
100–200 mg of 5-HTP three times daily is the recommended initial dose; however, once 5-HTP starts to work, the dosages can usually be reduced.

MAXIMUM SAFE LEVEL
Not established.

SIDE EFFECTS/CONTRAINDICATIONS
5-HTP should not be used alongside the Parkinson's drug carbidopa as it can cause skin changes similar to those that are seen with the disease scleroderma. 5-HTP should not be combined with drugs that raise serotonin levels—for example, SSRIs (such as Prozac) and other antidepressants. People with kidney disease or liver disease should consult their doctor before taking 5-HTP.

Trimethylglycine (TMG, Betaine)

GENERAL DESCRIPTION

TMG is a natural compound found in small quantities in some plant foods. However, humans do not need to obtain it from their diet because the body can manufacture it from other nutrients.

ROLE IN ANTI-AGING

Trimethylglycine is a methyl donor supplement that **assists in methylation** and may help **protect cellular DNA from mutation**. Trimethylglycine helps to keep the liver healthy by assisting the detoxification process, and animal studies suggest that the compound's methyl group-donating properties may help to protect the liver from chemical damage. Trimethylglycine aids in the conversion of homocysteine to methionine, and thus helps to **lower levels of the amino acid homocysteine**, high levels of which have been linked to an increased risk of heart disease, heart attack, stroke, Alzheimer's disease, Parkinson's disease, and osteoporosis. However, results of a study by Olthof et al. (*PLoS Med.* 2005 May;2(5):e135.) revealed that TMG supplementation increased blood LDL cholesterol and triacylglycerol concentrations in healthy humans, a side effect that has been observed in other studies. This finding led the researchers to conclude: "The adverse effects on blood lipids may undo the potential benefits for cardiovascular health of betaine [TMG] supplementation through homocysteine lowering. Folic acid supplementation does not seem to affect blood lipids and therefore remains the preferred treatment for lowering of blood homocysteine concentrations."

DEFICIENCY SYMPTOMS

None known.

THERAPEUTIC DAILY AMOUNT

No optimal therapeutic dosage of TMG has been established as of yet; however, one manufacturer recommends dosages between 375 and 1,000 mg daily. Refer to packaging.

MAXIMUM SAFE LEVEL

Not established.

SIDE EFFECTS/CONTRAINDICATIONS

TMG has been shown to increase blood LDL cholesterol and triacylglycerol levels. People with kidney disease or liver disease should consult their doctor before taking TMG.

Tyrosine

GENERAL DESCRIPTION

Tyrosine is a nonessential amino acid found naturally in almonds, avocados, bananas, beans, brewer's yeast, cheese, cottage cheese, dairy products, eggs, fish, lactalbumin, legumes, lima beans, meat, milk, nuts, peanuts, pickled herring, pumpkin seeds, seafood, seeds, sesame seeds, soy, whey, and whole grains.

ROLE IN ANTI-AGING

Tyrosine is a precursor for the neurotransmitters L-dopa, dopamine, norepinephrine, and epinephrine. Due to its effect on neurotransmitters, it is thought that tyrosine may benefit people with **Parkinson's disease, dementia, depression, and other mood disorders**. Tyrosine may counter some of the deletorius effects of sleep deprivation. Magil et al. (*Nutr Neurosci.* 2003;6: 237–246.) found that tyrosine improved scores of cognitive and motor performance in healthy men suffering from sleep deprivation. While results of a study by Neri et al. *Aviat Space Environ Med.* (1995;66:313–319.) led the authors to conclude: "tyrosine may prove useful in counteracting performance decrements during episodes of sustained work coupled with sleep loss." Skin cells use tyrosine to **form melanin**, the pigment that protects the skin against the damaging effects of ultraviolet light. Thyroid hormones, which play many important roles throughout the body, also contain tyrosine as part of their structure. In fact, tyrosine is used to **produce the hormone thyroxin**, which is important in the regulation of growth and metabolism, and is required for healthy skin and the maintenance of mental health. Finally, tyrosine may be of benefit to people who suffer from phenylketonuria (PKU).

DEFICIENCY SYMPTOMS

Signs and symptoms of tyrosine deficiency include apathy, blood sugar imbalances, depression, edema, fat loss, fatigue, lethargy, liver damage, loss of pigmentation in hair, low serum levels of essential blood proteins, mood disorders, muscle loss, skin lesions, slowed growth in children, and weakness.

THERAPEUTIC DAILY AMOUNT

The therapeutic dosage of tyrosine is 7–30 g daily, depending upon requirements.

MAXIMUM SAFE LEVEL

A maximum safe level for tyrosine has not been established. Furthermore, it is not known whether long-term, high-dosage (that is, doses in excess of 1,000 mg a day) use of L-tyrosine is safe. For this reason, long-term use of tyrosine at any dosage should be monitored by a doctor.

SIDE EFFECTS/CONTRAINDICATIONS

Supplementary tyrosine can cause hypertension, hypotension, and migraine headaches in susceptible individuals.

People who are allergic to eggs, milk, and wheat, and those who suffer from migraine headaches, phenylketonuria (PKU), melanoma, and hypertension should not take tyrosine.

If taken in combination with monoamine oxidase inhibitor (MAOI) antidepressants (for example, isocarboxazid, phenelzine, and procarbazine), tyrosine can cause potentially dangerous hypertension.

People with kidney disease or liver disease should consult their doctor before taking tyrosine.

CHAPTER 13

Additional Cutting-Edge Anti-Aging Nutrients

FATTY ACIDS, LIPIDS, AND OILS

Alkylglycerols

GENERAL DESCRIPTION

Alkylglycerols (AKGs) are lipids (fats) with a glycerol backbone that stimulate the production of white blood cells (leukocytes) to normal levels and encourage the growth of antibodies. AKGs are found in human breast milk, cow's milk, and the livers of most animals and fish. Shark liver contains an exceptionally high level of AKGs. Alkylglycerols are considered critical to the development of a healthy immune system in children.

ROLE IN ANTI-AGING

Animal studies suggest that AKGs may **inhibit cancer** growth by selectively destroying cancer cells via their ability to induce apoptosis. Some studies have also found that AKGs help the body to **eliminate toxic heavy** metals such as mercury and that they may help protect healthy tissue from the effects of radiation therapy. Because of the immune system enhancing effects of alkylglycerols, they also help the body to **fight bacterial, viral, and parasitic infections.**

DEFICIENCY SYMPTOMS

People deficient in alkylglycerols may be prone to infections.

THERAPEUTIC DAILY AMOUNT

500–1,500 mg per day.

MAXIMUM SAFE LEVEL

No side effects have been seen with doses as high as 6,000 mg per day.

SIDE EFFECTS/CONTRAINDICATIONS

None known.

Borage Oil

GENERAL DESCRIPTION

The borage plant (*Borago officinalis*) has been exploited for its medicinal properties for more than 400 years. Although research has found little evidence to suggest that the herb itself has any health benefits, borage oil, which is derived from the seeds, may be useful in treating a number of conditions. Borage oil is a **rich source of gamma linoleic acid (GLA),** an omega-6 essential fatty acid that the body converts to the anti-inflammatory prostaglandin E1 (PGE1).

ROLE IN ANTI-AGING

Borage oil may be of benefit to people suffering from **rheumatoid arthritis.** Results of one study by Leventhal et al. (*Ann Intern Med.* 1993;119:867–873) revealed that high doses of borage oil (1.4 grams a day) significantly **reduced pain and swelling in arthritic joints.** Other studies suggest that borage oil **combats inflammation and reduces joint damage;** however, it should be noted that participants in these studies were given very high doses of the oil.

There is some evidence to suggest that borage oil may help people with **multiple sclerosis.** Some researchers believe that high levels of essential fatty acids present in borage oil could help to combat the inflammation associated with the disease; furthermore, these acids may also help to prevent nerve damage.

In addition to its anti-inflammatory properties, GLA also **enhances the transmission of nerve impulses.** Together, these facts suggest that borage oil may be useful in treating Alzheimer's-memory disorders. Animal research also suggests that the oil may help to combat stress and high blood pressure (hypertension).

Borage oil is also cited as a treatment for **acne, eczema, endometriosis, female infertility, gout, impotence, lupus (SLE), PMS, psoriasis, respiratory infections, and rosacea.**

DEFICIENCY SYMPTOMS

Not applicable.

THERAPEUTIC DAILY AMOUNT

1,000–1,300 mg of borage oil a day will provide roughly 240–300 mg of GLA. Taking borage oil with food may improve GLA absorption.

MAXIMUM SAFE LEVEL

Many studies using borage oil employ relatively high dosages of borage oil.

However, study participants are always under close medical supervision. Borage seeds contain small amounts of liver toxins called pyrrolizidine alkaloids (PAs). Some research suggests that high-levels of amabiline, a PA present in borage oil, could be carcinogenic and may cause liver damage. There is as yet no established maximum safe level for borage oil; furthermore, no studies have been conducted to prove that long-term use or high-dose use of the product poses no threat to health. For these reasons it is important to take borage oil as directed on packaging.

SIDE EFFECTS/CONTRAINDICATIONS

Borage oil may cause bloating, nausea, headache, and indigestion. Taking borage oil with food may reduce the risk of side effects.

Epileptics and people taking anticoagulant drugs such as warfarin should consult their doctor before taking borage oil. Because of the potential health hazards of the supplement, pregnant women, nursing women, and children should not take borage oil.

People with liver disease should not take borage oil because of the potential risk of liver damage.

Several countries discourage the use of borage oil because of the unestablished long-term supplementation effects.

Evening Primrose Oil

GENERAL DESCRIPTION

Evening primrose oil (EPO) is derived from the seeds of the evening primrose plant (*Oenothera biennis*), native to North America, Europe, and parts of Asia. Native Americans used EPO to treat bruises, hemorrhoids, sore throats, and stomach aches. The active ingredient in EPO is **gamma linolenic acid (GLA),** an omega-6 essential fatty acid that the body converts to the anti-inflammatory prostaglandin E1 (PGE1).

ROLE IN ANTI-AGING

EPO may be considered as an important botanical in combating the general effects of aging. The body loses its ability to convert dietary fats into GLA with age, thus EPO may be helpful in age-related conditions resulting from GLA deficiency. As such, EPO is often used to relieve the symptoms of **rheumatoid arthritis.**

Some research suggests that EPO may be of benefit to **diabetics,** as the GLA in EPO has been shown to prevent, and in some cases, **reverse nerve damage (neuropathy),** which is a common complication of the disease. As GLA helps to keep nerves healthy and combat inflammation, EPO may be helpful in **multiple sclerosis.** The supplement is also recommended for people suffering from **Alzheimer's-related memory problems,** as GLA boosts the transmission of nerve impulses.

Some studies have produced evidence to suggest that EPO may lower cholesterol levels; however, other studies have produced conflicting results. EPO is often marketed as a treatment for PMS; however, research to support these claims is inconclusive.

DEFICIENCY SYMPTOMS
Not applicable.

THERAPEUTIC DAILY AMOUNT
The optimal daily intake of EPO is yet to be established. A typical daily dose is 3,000–6,000 mg, which contains roughly 270–540 mg of GLA. Taking EPO with foods boosts GLA absorption. Some experts recommend taking a supplement containing magnesium, zinc, vitamin C, niacin, and vitamin B_6 at the same time as EPO, as the body needs all of these nutrients in order to produce PGE1.

MAXIMUM SAFE LEVEL
A maximum safe level of EPO has not been established. Nor is there any evidence to confirm the safety of long-term use of EPO; however, there have been no reports of any significant toxic side effects associated with EPO.

SIDE EFFECTS/CONTRAINDICATIONS
EPO may worsen symptoms of temporal lobe epilepsy. It should also be avoided by schizophrenics who are prescribed phenothiazine epileptogenic drugs.

Flax Oil

GENERAL DESCRIPTION
The brown seeds of the flax plant (*Linum usitatissimum*) were used many centuries ago in Europe to promote healing and combat constipation. Flax oil, which is produced by pressing the seeds, is a rich source of **essential fatty acids,** including linoleic acid and alpha linoleic acid (ALA).

ROLE IN ANTI-AGING
As well as being a rich source of essential fatty acids, flax oil also contains **high concentrations of lignans**—antioxidant compounds that may **benefit hormone-related conditions.** They are also thought to guard against aging, and aid the body in its **fight against certain bacteria and viruses.** There is some

evidence to suggest that lignans may also help to **prevent breast, colon, prostate, and skin cancers.** However, other research has suggested that the ALA contained in flax oil may increase the risk of breast and prostate cancer. On the whole, the effect of flax oil on cancer risk is inconclusive.

Research suggests that flax oil may have several **heart-friendly** benefits. Several studies have found that the oil can help to **lower cholesterol,** while others have revealed that it may **protect against high blood pressure and angina.** The antioxidant properties of lignans present in flax oil may also help to **guard against the oxidation of "bad" LDL cholesterol.** Research by Joshi et al. (*Prostaglandins Leukot Essent Fatty Acids.* 2006;74:17–21.) suggests that flax oil may help to treat Attention Deficit Hyperactivity Disorder (ADHD). Results showed that giving flax oil to children with ADHD led to a significant improvement in the symptoms of the disorder.

DEFICIENCY SYMPTOMS
Not applicable.

THERAPEUTIC DAILY AMOUNT
The most commonly recommended daily dose is 1 tablespoon (15 ml) of flax oil. Note: the majority of flax oil capsules contain 1,000 mg of oil per capsule, thus to obtain a similar dose to that obtained from 1 tablespoon of oil you would have to take roughly 14 capsules. Always refer to dosage instructions on packaging.

MAXIMUM SAFE LEVEL
Not established.

SIDE EFFECTS/CONTRAINDICATIONS
There are no known side effects for flax oil if taken as directed; however, some people may suffer an allergic reaction.

People with bowel obstructions should not take flax oil or ground flax seeds.

Some studies suggest that the ALA present in flax oil may increase breast and prostate cancer risk, although other research does not support these claims.

Omega-3 Fatty Acid, Fish Oil, DHA (Docosahexaenoic Acid), and EPA (Eicosapentaenoic Acid)

GENERAL DESCRIPTION
Omega-3 fatty acids, which are found primarily in fish oils but are also present in vegetable oils, are essential fatty acids—in that they are not made by the

body and must be supplied by the diet or supplements. Scientists first became interested in omega-3 fatty acids when it was reported that the Eskimo population, who eat a diet rich in fish oil, had a low rate of heart disease. Mackerel, salmon, sea bass, trout, herring, sardines, sablefish (black cod), anchovies, and tuna, as well as cod liver oil supplements, are rich sources of both DHA and EPA. Fish oil contains two types of omega-3 fatty acids: DHA (docosahexaenoic acid) and EPA (eicosapentaenoic acid). The majority of fish oil supplements contain 18 percent EPA and 12 percent DHA.

ROLE IN ANTI-AGING

Omega-3 fatty acids have profound anti-inflammatory effects when taken at a therapeutic dosage. In recent years it has become clear that chronic, low-level, or "silent" inflammation (SI) plays an important role in a number of age-related diseases, including heart disease, Alzheimer's disease, arthritis, Parkinson's disease, and cancer. Omega-3 fatty acids may help to reduce the risk of these diseases by combating SI. Recent research has found that omega-3 acids taken in supplement form can significantly **lower the risks associated with heart disease.** Some studies have found that while omega-3s appear to have little effect on total cholesterol levels, they can significantly **decrease serum triglyceride levels, lower blood pressure,** and **reduce blood levels of homocysteine,** high levels of which are associated with an increased risk of heart disease and stroke. Elevated homocysteine levels have also been linked to Alzheimer's disease, Parkinson's disease, and osteoporosis. Omega-3s also help to **thin the blood** by discouraging platelets in the blood from clumping together, thus reducing the risk that blood will clot and cause a heart attack. Preliminary research also suggests that omega-3 fatty acids from fish oil may help regulate the rhythm of the heart, as both EPA and DHA have been reported to help prevent **cardiac arrhythmias.** Results of a study by Maresta et al. (*Am Heart J.* 2002;143:E5.) showed that taking a supplement of fish oils for a month before and after surgery led to a significant decrease in the rate of restenosis (reclogging of the arteries) after percutaneous transluminal coronary angioplasty (PTCA). However, other studies have produced conflicting results.

Potent anti-inflammatory agents, omega-3s help curb an overactive immune system and thus are helpful in the **treatment of autoimmune diseases** such as rheumatoid arthritis, chronic inflammatory bowel disease, Crohn's disease, and psoriasis. Omega-3s are also **effective in curbing the inflammatory response to severe burns, sepsis, systemic inflammatory response syndrome (SIRS) and asthma.** Nordvik et al. (*Acta Neurol Scand.* 2000;102:

143–149.) found that omega-3s can improve the clinical outcome for newly diagnosed multiple sclerosis patients.

A daily dose of the omega-3 fatty acid **eicosapentaenoic** acid (EPA) may help to **shift depression in patients who do not respond to conventional antidepressant drugs.** Peet and Horrobin (*Archives of General Psychiatry* 2002;59:913–919) found that twelve weeks of treatment with a daily dose of 1 gram of EPA led to a significant improvement in symptoms, such as anxiety, sleeping problems, feelings of sadness, and suicidal thoughts. In fact, the treatment was so successful that 69 percent of patients experienced a 50 percent reduction in their symptoms, compared with just 25 percent of patients given a placebo.

In a review of the use of Omega-3 fatty acids in the treatment of psychiatric disorders Peet and Stokes (*Drugs.* 2005;65:1051–1059.) write: "Epidemiological studies indicate an association between depression and low dietary intake of omega-3 fatty acids, and biochemical studies have shown reduced levels of omega-3 fatty acids in red blood cell membranes in both depressive and schizophrenic patients. Five of six double-blind, placebo-controlled trials in schizophrenia, and four of six such trials in depression, have reported therapeutic benefit from omega-3 fatty acids.particularly when EPA is added on to existing psychotropic medication. Individual clinical trials have suggested benefits of EPA treatment in borderline personality disorder and of combined omega-3 and omega-6 fatty acid treatment for attention-deficit hyperactivity disorder. The evidence to date supports the adjunctive use of omega-3 fatty acids in the management of treatment unresponsive depression and schizophrenia."

DEFICIENCY SYMPTOMS

Omega-3 fats are required for normal brain development during pregnancy and during the first two years of life. If mother and infant are deficient in Omega-3 fatty acids, the infant's immune and nervous systems may not develop correctly.

THERAPEUTIC DAILY AMOUNT

Eat fish several times a week for naturally occurring omega-3s and the nutrients that accompany them. Use canola oil in cooking and salad dressings. Fish oil capsules should be taken only with guidance from a qualified nutritionist.

The majority of research into the effects of DHA and EPA in humans have used doses of at least 3 grams of DHA plus EPA supplements. To obtain a similar amount of DHA and EPA from fish oil, it may be necessary to consume as much as 10 grams, as most fish oils contains only 18 percent EPA and 12 percent DHA. It is important to buy a good quality, mercury-free, fish oil supplement.

MAXIMUM SAFE LEVEL

Not established. Burns et al. (Clin Cancer Res. 1999;5:3942–3947.) found that the maximum amount of fish oil tolerated by people being treated for cancer-related weight loss was roughly 21g per day. However, the maximum tolerated amount in people without cancer may well be different. High doses of fish oil (3 g and above) should only be taken if directed to do so by an expert.

SIDE EFFECTS/CONTRAINDICATIONS

People with heart disease or diabetes should consult their doctor before taking more than 3 grams of fish oil a day as there is some evidence to suggest that the supplement may raise cholesterol levels and blood sugar levels. Omega-3 fatty acids should be used cautiously by people who have a bleeding disorder or take blood-thinning medications, as excessive amounts of omega-3 fatty acids may lead to bleeding. People who consume more than three grams of omega-3 fatty acids per day (equivalent to 3 servings of fish per day) may be at an increased risk for hemorrhagic stroke.

BOTANICAL AGENTS

Aloe

GENERAL DESCRIPTION

The Aloe Vera plant is native to North Africa. Aloes have been used all over the world throughout the ages for their various medicinal properties. Manufacturers sell the transparent gel from the plant's leaf as a topical remedy; they also process it into "juice" and pills, which are taken internally for **gastrointestinal benefits** or as a tonic (a substance that works to balance the body's systems instead of addressing a specific ailment). For topical use, aloe gels work well on **sunburn, rashes, and other minor irritations** (look for products containing 95 to 100 percent pure aloe). Aloe-based ointments and sprays are also available for other skin traumas. Aloe for internal use comes in liquids, tablets, and capsules.

ROLE IN ANTI-AGING

The gel of the aloe leaf contains several chemicals, a polysaccharide, enzymes, nutrients, and other compounds that seem to fight bacteria and fungi, reduce inflammation and encourage wound healing. Furthermore, aloeride and acemannan, two isolated compounds in the gel of the aloe leaf, have been shown to stimulate the immune system and improve skin-healing time. A number of studies suggest that Aloe vera may be of use in the treatment of diabetes. Rajasekaran et al. (*Pharmacol Rep.* 2005;57:90–96.) found that oral administration of Aloe vera gel extract at a concentration of 300 mg/kg to diabetic rats significantly decreased levels of blood glucose, glycosylated hemoglobin and increased hemoglobin. Furthermore, the increased levels of lipid peroxidation and hydroperoxides in tissues of diabetic rats were reverted back to near normal levels after the treatment with gel extract. Bolkent et al. (*Indian J Exp Biol.* 2004;42:48–52.) found evidence to suggest that Aloe leaf gel and pulp extracts has a protective effect on kidney damage caused by type-II diabetes, thus suggesting that it may be useful in preventing, or ameliorating, some of the complications of diabetes. While Okyar et al. (*Phytother Res.* 2001;15:157–161.) found that Aloe leaf gel extract has hypoclglycemic properties. The results led the researchers to conclude that Aloe may be useful in the treatment of non-insulin dependent diabetes mellitus.

THERAPEUTIC DAILY AMOUNT
Check product labels for dosage recommendations.

MAXIMUM SAFE LEVEL
Aloe juice products for oral consumption are generally considered safe, although drinking more than a pint a day may lead to diarrhea.

SIDE EFFECTS/CONTRAINDICATIONS
Gel preparations used topically have not been associated with side effects. Products made from the plant's latex can cause side effects such as intestinal cramping due to their laxative effect. Because of these side effects, the latex form of aloe should not be used by elderly people, children, pregnant or breastfeeding women, and anyone with inflammatory intestinal diseases, such as Crohn's disease, ulcerative colitis, or appendicitis.

Arabinogalactan

GENERAL DESCRIPTION
Arabinogalactan (AG) is a phytochemical extracted from the timber of the larch tree. The immune-enhancing herb echinacea also contains AG, as do leeks, carrots, radishes, pears, wheat, red wine, and tomatoes.

ROLE IN ANTI-AGING
AG is an important source of dietary fiber. Research has shown that AG increases the production of short-chain fatty acids (SCFAs), principally

butyrate and proprionate, which are essential for the **health of the colon.** AG also acts as a food supply for "friendly" bacteria, in that it helps to **increase levels of "good" bacteria** such as bifidobacteria and lactobacillus, while eliminating "bad" bacteria. AG has a beneficial effect upon the immune system as it **increases the activity of natural killer cells** and other immune-system components, thus helping the body to fight infection.

THERAPEUTIC DAILY AMOUNT
1,000–3,000 mg per day.

MAXIMUM SAFE LEVEL
Not established.

SIDE EFFECTS/CONTRAINDICATIONS
May cause bloating. Doses of up to 10 grams per day are seemingly well tolerated. However, very high doses (30 grams or more per day) may cause gastrointestinal side effects. Larch arabinogalactan contains galactose, therefore people with who require a low galactose diet and those with lactose intolerance should avoid taking this supplement. Pregnant women and nursing mothers should avoid larch arabinogalactan supplements.

Ashwagandha Root (*Withania somniferum*)

GENERAL DESCRIPTION
Ashwagandha root has extensive historical use in traditional Indian and Ayurvedic medicine. It is most commonly used to treat inflammatory conditions, such as arthritis, fever, tumors, and a wide range of infectious diseases. Recent scientific analysis of ashwagandha has discovered compounds known as withanolides that are steroidal in molecular construction and are similar, both in their action and appearance, to the active constituents of Panax ginseng's ginsenosides. As such, ashwagandha has been called "Indian ginseng" by some.

ROLE IN ANTI-AGING
Wagner, et al. (*Phytomed* 1994;1:63–76) showed that **ashwagandha stimulates the activation of immune system cells,** such as lymphocytes, thus helping the immune system to ward off infectious disease agents such as bacteria and viruses. Research by Iuvuno (*Life Sci* 2003;72:1617–1625) suggests that ashwagandha's immune-stimulating properties may be due in part to its ability to induce the synthesis of inducible nitric oxide synthase (NOS) in macrophages. Ashwagandha is particularly effective against Staphylococcus aureus, a strain of bacteria that has become increasingly resistant to antibiotic drugs; there-

fore, ashwagandha may prove to be an important natural combatant against this infectious agent.

Anabalgan and Sadique (*Indian J Exp Biol* 1981;19:245–259) found that ashwagandha **inhibits inflammation,** and thus is a natural anti-inflammatory. Numerous animal studies point to its potential therapeutic use for rheumatologic conditions.

Ashwagandha is an important **antioxidant nutrient.** It has been demonstrated to reduce free-radical damage, specifically within cells of the brain. Studies of ashwagandha supplementation in lab animals by Bhattacharya, et al. (*Phytother Res* 1995;9:110–113) found that it can improve cognitive performance in both healthy subjects and animal models of Alzheimer's disease.

When given to lab animals, ashwagandha has **conveyed improved physical stress** tolerance. It has been demonstrated to improve the animals' anabolic activity and reduce their nervous exhaustion.

Ashwagandha has also been shown to **increase hemoglobin, serum iron, and other blood markers** in children. Similarly, a study of healthy men in their fifties demonstrated that ashwagandha supplementation for a one-year period could increase hemoglobin and red blood cell count. In this study, additional benefits were reported: more than 70 percent of the subjects remarked that their sexual performance improved, and for many of the men, their graying hair regained color (hair melanin levels increased).

THERAPEUTIC DAILY AMOUNT
3–6 grams of the dried root, taken each day in capsule or tea form.

MAXIMUM SAFE LEVEL
Not established.

SIDE EFFECTS/CONTRAINDICATIONS
No significant side effects have been reported. Ashwagandha has been used in children in India for many years, with no reports of any ill effects. Its safety during pregnancy and lactation is unknown; thus, it is best avoided at this time.

Astragalus (*Astragalus membranaceous*)

GENERAL DESCRIPTION
The astragalus or Huang Qi plant hails from China. It has been used in traditional Chinese medicine for more than two thousand years. The part of the plant used medicinally is the root, which is collected in the spring and dried

for four to seven years. Astragalus stimulates the adrenal glands, and it is thought that it may help to promote a healthy response to physical and emotional stressors that otherwise could suppress the adrenal glands and lead to sleep difficulties.

ROLE IN ANTI-AGING

Astragalus may help to **combat anxiety and promote sleep** as it contains a number of chemical constituents that are important for sleep. Several dozen flavonoids have been found in the root and flower of this plant. Flavonoids are potent antioxidants, and antioxidants have been shown to have anti-anxiety effects. Astragalus also contains GABA, an amino acid that is important in modulating stress and anxiety.

Astragalus has also gained interest for potential cardiovascular and circulatory benefits. It has a vasodilation effect upon blood vessels, which lends credence to its use to **lower elevated blood pressure, to promote renal function, and to treat seizures.** Zhang, et al. (*J Vasc Res.* 1997;34:273–280) discovered that lipids unique to astragalus affect the pathway through which blood clots occur, thus suggesting that it may help to reduce the risk of heart attack, coronary heart disease, and stroke. Chang found that astragalus **restored regular heart rhythm** to lab animals experiencing tachycardia, while Hong, et al. (*Am J Chin Med* 1994;22:63–70) showed that it **improved congestive heart failure** in animal models. Work by Zhang, et al. (*Zhongguo Zhong Xi Yi Jie He Za Zhi* 2002;22:346–348 [in Chinese]) revealed that astragalus injections are effective at **reversing left ventricular remodeling and improving left ventricular function** in heart attack patients.

Astragalus is considered to be a **potent immune-system booster** in traditional Chinese medicine. Practitioners report that astragalus **reduces the production of T-suppressor cells** (responsible for terminating the immune response) and **increases the activity of T cells** (white blood cells that seek and destroy infectious agents). In turn, astragalus is thought to **increase the production of white blood cells** in the bone marrow and lymph tissue. Jaio, et al. (*Chin J Integrated Trad West Med* 2001;7:117–120) found that the flavonoids in astragalus restored proper immune responses in lab animals whose immune systems were suppressed by steroids. Studies performed by the National Cancer Institute and five other leading cancer research institutions over the past ten years have reported that astragalus **strengthens the immune system in cancer patients,** quite possibly by increasing the number of white blood cells. Additionally, cancer patients given astragalus during chemotherapy and radiation recovered significantly faster and lived longer than those not given the supplement.

Finally, the saponins and betaine present in astragalus have been reported to improve liver function and heal liver injury.

THERAPEUTIC DAILY AMOUNT

One drop of tincture is taken two to three times per day. The dried root is taken in dosages of 1–4 grams three times per day. Some Chinese medicine texts recommend taking 9–15 grams of the crude herb per day in decoction form. The most potent astragalus supplements contain a standardized extract of the root, with 0.5 percent glucosides and 70 percent polysaccharides. Research suggests that the body can develop a tolerance to immune-stimulating herbs such as astragalus if it is taken for long periods. Therefore, some experts recommend alternating astragalus with other immune system-enhancing herbs such as echinacea.

MAXIMUM SAFE LEVEL

Not established.

SIDE EFFECTS/CONTRAINDICATIONS

No side effects have been reported. Pregnant women should not take astragalus without consulting their physician first. Astragalus has been found to have a synergistic effect with interferon; therefore, those on interferon therapy should discuss whether supplementation with this herb is appropriate. Because some reports have suggested that fresh astragalus contains chemicals known as exudate gums that cause allergic reactions in some people, those with gum allergies should consult a physician before taking this herb.

Bilberry (*Vaccinium myrtillus*)

GENERAL DESCRIPTION

The bilberry plant is closely related to blueberries and currants, all of which belong to the genus *Vaccinium*. The specific activity of bilberry comes from concentrated fruit pigments called "anthocyanins," which have beneficial effects on the cardiovascular system. The bilberry fruit contains important tannins, which act as antibacterial and antiviral agents, as well as vitamins A and C. The most popular products are extracts standardized to contain 15 to 25 percent of a chemical called anthocyanosides. Bilberry is also available as tinctures and concentrated drops. An average dose of an encapsulated extract standardized for 20 to 25 percent anthocyanosides is 60–120 mg.

ROLE IN ANTI-AGING

The anthocyanosides in bilberries can **improve circulation, protect fragile capillaries, and cause biochemical reactions in the eye;** they have a **positive effect on enzymes crucial to vision and the eye's ability to adapt to the dark.** Anthocyanosides have also been shown to alleviate symptoms of diabetes and heart disease. The herb's short-term effect on vision is most noticeable within the first four hours of taking it; thus, it can be useful if taken before a visually demanding task like driving all night or reading the entire Sunday paper. Research suggests that bilberry supplements may also help to **slow the progression of cataracts** and **reduce the effects of diabetic retinopathy** (a common complication of diabetes and the leading cause of blindness in the United States and many other Western countries). In lab tests, bilberry has been shown to prevent the oxidation of "bad" LDL cholesterol, which may help to reduce the risk of heart disease. However, whether bilberry has the same effect *in vivo* remains to be seen. Although scientists don't know what components of the bilberry leaf are responsible for these effects, recent research has shown that taking a dried leaf extract will cause a drop in glucose levels. The same research also showed that bilberry leaf can lower blood triglyceride levels, a heart disease risk factor. In vitro screening tests have suggested that components of the hexane/chloroform fraction of bilberry may also have potent anticarcinogenic properties.

THERAPEUTIC DAILY AMOUNT

20–60 grams dried fruit. 240–280 mg of extract standardized to 25 percent anthocyanosides.

MAXIMUM SAFE LEVEL

Not established.

SIDE EFFECTS/CONTRAINDICATIONS

Tests have shown bilberry to be completely nontoxic, even when taken in large doses for an extended period of time. Bilberry is safe for use during pregnancy and may even be beneficial for the prevention and treatment of varicose veins and hemorrhoids.

Black Currant Seed Oil (*Ribes nigrum*)

GENERAL DESCRIPTION

This thornless shrub belongs to the red currant family. The leaves and berries are used medicinally. In European folk medicine, black currant once had a considerable reputation for controlling diarrhea, promoting urine output (as a diuretic) and reducing arthritic and rheumatic pains. Black currant oil is a **source of gamma-linoleic acid (GLA)** to treat a wide range of ailments.

ROLE IN ANTI-AGING

Factors such as high cholesterol, aging, stress, alcohol, diabetes, premenstrual syndrome (PMS), aging, viral infections, and other conditions may interfere with the normal conversion of linoleic acid into GLA. Thus, people who obtain little GLA from their diet and those whose systems are unable to metabolize linoleic acid into GLA may benefit from taking GLA-rich supplements like black currant seed oil. Dayong et al. (*American Journal of Clinical Nutrition.* 1999;70:536–543.) found that 4.5 g daily of black currant seed oil was able to promote cell-mediated immune function in healthy elderly subjects. The researchers believe that black currant seed oils immune-enhancing effect is attributable to its ability to reduce prostaglandin E (2) (a compound that modifies inflammatory responses) production. Other studies have found that the extract has anti-inflammatory properties due to its capability of stimulating the production of prostaglandin-1, an anti-inflammatory hormone.

THERAPEUTIC DAILY AMOUNT

A daily dosage of 600–6,000 mg is typical. Capsules containing black currant oil are available in 200–400 mg doses—the capsules typically have a fixed oil component, and usually contain 14 to 19 percent GLA.

MAXIMUM SAFE LEVEL

Not established.

SIDE EFFECTS/CONTRAINDICATIONS

No side effects have been reported; however, German health authorities warn that people with fluid accumulation, because of heart or kidney problems, should not take the leaf preparations. It should be noted that no studies appear to have been done to determine the safety of black currant seed extract over the long term, although preliminary findings for other GLA-rich oils suggest that the supplements are relatively safe.

Calendula (*Calendula officinalis*)

GENERAL DESCRIPTION

Calendula was enormously popular in medieval Europe for treating blemishes, bedsores, and skin infections. Present day herbalists continue to use the plant extract in topical form for inflamed or damaged skin: poorly healing wounds and ulcers, bites, stings, burns (including sunburn), infectious sores such as herpes zoster (shingles), and varicose veins. Gargles and rinses are used for mouth and throat inflammation. Calendula tea promotes sweating and lowers fever. The plant contains several beneficial chemicals, including flavonoid, a gelatinous substance called mucilage, an essential oil, and alcohols. Calendula is sold in liquid forms (such as juice, concentrated drops and tinctures) and as an ingredient in herbal combination ointments, salves, lotions, and creams. It is also used to make homeopathic calendula remedies and an essential oil, both of which are used topically to treat skin irritations, burns, and scrapes. (An easy way to use the herb is to soak a gauze pad in calendula tincture and apply directly to the skin.)

ROLE IN ANTI-AGING

Research suggests that calendula may have anti-inflammatory, anti-viral, and anti-genotoxic properties. Results of a study by Jimenez-Medina et al. (*BMC Cancer.* 2006;6:119.) revealed that an aqueous calendula extract inhibited in vitro and in vivo tumor growth and prolonged the survival of mice. The extract was found to inhibit tumor growth by triggering cell cycle arrest in the G0/G1 phase and Caspase-3-induced apoptosis. *In vitro* studies have demonstrated that calendula can **stimulate lymphocyte proliferation.** Animal studies have indicated that calendula extracts may counter high lipid levels, produce sedation, help treat hepatitis, and reduce signs of systemic inflammation when taken internally. Results of a study published in 2002 suggest that low-concentrations of calendula may have chemoprotective properties.

THERAPEUTIC DAILY AMOUNT

Ointments typically contain 2–5 percent calendula.

MAXIMUM SAFE LEVEL

Not established.

SIDE EFFECTS/CONTRAINDICATIONS

Calendula has not been associated with toxicity or side effects.

Cayenne (*Capsicum annuum*)

GENERAL DESCRIPTION

The hot fruit of the cayenne plant has been used as medicine for centuries. Cayenne was frequently used to treat diseases of the circulatory system and is still traditionally used in herbal medicine as a circulatory tonic. The active ingredient in cayenne is a pungent substance known as capsaicin. Capsaicin appears to alter the action of the bodily compound (called "substance P") that transfers pain messages to the brain, **reducing pain and inflammation by short-circuiting the pain message.**

ROLE IN ANTI-AGING

Capsaicin is used in many over-the-counter and prescription creams for the treatment of arthritis, shingles (herpes zoster), post-operative pain, cluster headaches, and psoriasis and other skin conditions. Some studies have also suggested that capsaicin may protect against the damage aspirin can cause to the stomach. Beyond this, a recent study found that cayenne has antimicrobial effects, meaning it could be used to fight infection. When taken orally, cayenne stimulates circulation, aids digestion, and promotes sweating. Because perspiration works to cool the body, cayenne is sometimes used to break a fever. There is also evidence to suggest that cayenne may be useful in the treatment of **obesity.** Yoshioka et al. (*Br J Nutr.* 1999;82:115–123.) found that consumption of 10g of cayenne pepper with meals helped to reduce appetite and energy intake. Results of a study by Lee et al. (*J Nutr Sci Vitaminol* [Tokyo]. 2004; 50:144–148.) suggest that capsaicin exerts its anti-obesity effects by altering the levels of the orexigenic or anorexigenic peptides, neuropeptide Y (NPY) and cholecystokinin (CCK) and thereby promoting satiety. Results of several studies suggest that capsaicin increases the metabolism of dietary fats.

THERAPEUTIC DAILY AMOUNT

Cayenne is also sold in capsules, concentrated drops and tinctures, which are taken orally. Popular products are standardized for 5 to 10 percent capsaicin. An average dose of an oral extract standardized for eight percent capsaicin is 100 mg.

MAXIMUM SAFE LEVEL

Not established.

SIDE EFFECTS/CONTRAINDICATIONS

Cayenne is potent and can cause serious tissue irritation if used improperly. Be sure to wash your hands thoroughly after using capsaicin-containing creams; avoid any contact with eyes, mucous membranes, or open wounds. Excessive ingestion may cause gastroenteritis, liver, or kidney damage. Cayenne is reported to possibly interfere with MAO inhibitors and antihypertensive therapy, and may increase hepatic metabolism of drugs. Follow label directions carefully and do not exceed the recommended doses.

Chamomile (*Matricaria chamomilla* and *Matricaria recutita*)

GENERAL DESCRIPTION

Chamomile is a member of the daisy family native to Europe and western Asia. Most of us are familiar with chamomile by way of chamomile tea. Chamomile can promote relaxation and it is a reliable remedy for skin irritation.

ROLE IN ANTI-AGING

Chamomile contains active chemical constituents that **reduce inflammation,** which are responsible for the herb's association as a tea in soothing a sore throat, but also points to its potential usefulness in improving inflammatory conditions such as arthritis and joint problems that may keep some people awake at night. Safayhi, et al. (*Planta Med.* 1994;60:410–413) found that two chemical constituents of chamomile inhibited the accumulation of prostaglandins and leukotrienes—molecules that circulate in blood and are released in great quantities when the body mounts an inflammatory response.

Chamomile also contains flavonoids, most notably apigenin, which exerts both **antioxidant and anti-anxiety effects.** Viola, et al. (*Planta Med.* 1995;61:213–216) found that the apigenin in chamomile produced a **sedating effect** along with a reduction in excess movement, both of which help to explain its apparent sleep promoting properties.

The concentration of apigenin present in chamomile has important potential anti-aging implications, particularly relating to **cancer prevention.** Wei, et al. (*Cancer Res.* 1990;50:499–502) found that cancer-prone skin cells grown in culture but concurrently treated with apigenin from chamomile became cancerous three weeks later than untreated cells. In related research, Chaumontet, et al. (*Carcinogenesis.* 1994;15:2325–2330) reported that the apigenin in chamomile retarded the ability of skin cells in culture to become cancerous. More recently, Lin, et al. (*J Cell Biochem Suppl.* 1997;28–29:39–48) reported that apigenin in chamomile inhibited TPA-induced tumor promotion. Meanwhile, Liang, et al. (*Carcinogenesis.* 1999;20:1945–1952) published a separate study that found that apigenin in chamomile suppresses the activation of two blood components (cyclooxygenase-2 and inducible nitric oxide synthase) that, when found in excess in the blood, have been associated with cancer.

Chamomile may also **benefit the cardiovascular system.** Jannssen, et al. (*Am J Clin Nutr.* 1998;67:255–262) found that the apigenin present in chamomile significantly **inhibits the aggregation of collagen and platelets.** Yamamoto, et al. (*Chem Pharm Bull* [Tokyo]. 2002;50:47–52) discovered a new substance in chamomile that modulates blood pressure. The substance discovered by these researchers was effective in countering tachykinin, an excess of which can lead to hypotension (low blood pressure).

Chamomile's immune system-protecting properties are due to its heteropolysaccharides. Laskova, et al. (*Antibiot Khimioter.* 1992;37:15–18 [in Russian]) found that lab animals exposed to this constituent in chamomile were **more able to resist immune compromise when subjected to physical stress.** In follow-up research, Laskova found that the chamomile heteropolysaccharides stimulated key immune cells and **increased the sensitivity of immune cells to signals that prompt their activation.**

Chamomile also has **antibacterial and fungicidal activity.** It is very effective against Candida albicans and against *Staphylococcus* and *Streptococcus*—infection-causing bacteria that are becoming antibiotic resistant. The herb also has been shown to be of benefit in healing a variety of skin disorders. In Germany, where chamomile has been sold to the public under a leading brand-name for over 80 years, company case reports have shown beneficial results in the treatment of skin ulcers, dermatitis, and eczema. Topical applications of chamomile have been shown to be moderately **effective in the treatment of eczema,** while a double-blind trial by Albring, et al. (*Meth Find Exp Clin Pharmacol* 1983;5:75–77) found it to be approximately 60 percent as effective as 0.25 percent hydrocortisone cream.

Chamomile also has **antispasmodic properties;** therefore, it may help to reduce epileptic convulsions, and may be useful in the treatment of diverticular disorders and inflammatory bowel conditions such as Crohn's disease. As it relaxes smooth muscle, chamomile may also help to reduce menstrual cramps.

THERAPEUTIC DAILY AMOUNT
Chamomile is available as a dried whole herb (to be used as a tea or bath infusion) and in packaged teas, tablets, capsules, concentrated drops, tinctures, and extracts. It is often taken three to four times daily between meals as a tea. Standardized extracts containing 1 percent apigenin and 0.5 percent volatile oils may also be used. One to two capsules containing 300–400 mg of extract may be taken three times daily. Follow dosage directions on labels.

MAXIMUM SAFE LEVEL
Not established.

SIDE EFFECTS/CONTRAINDICATIONS
Both oral and topical chamomile products are considered very nontoxic and

are gentle enough for use in children, or during pregnancy and lactation. Medicinal chamomile has a low risk of allergic reactions, however Hausen et al. (*L. Planta Med.* 1984;50:229–234.) reported that so-called "chamomile allergy" may actually be the result of the substitution of dog chamomile (which contains the allergenic compound anthecotulide) for the medicinal-grade varieties. An extremely remote concern is that people with an allergy to some other herb in the daisy family would also be allergic to chamomile. The herb has been reported as being a potential trigger of severe anaphylaxis, for this reason people with allergies to plants of the Asteraceae family (ragweed, aster and chrysanthemums) should avoid using chamomile. The herb may also increase the risk of bleeding or potentiate the effects of warfarin therapy. Chamomile-based skin creams should not come into contact with the eyes.

Chrysin

GENERAL DESCRIPTION

Chrysin is a naturally occurring isoflavone chemically extracted from the plant Passiflora coerulea. Chrysin has many actions on the body, including **anti-anxiety, anti-inflammatory, anticancer** properties. In addition, studies carried out in Europe found that chrysin can increase testosterone levels by 30 percent or more.

ROLE IN ANTI-AGING

Chrysin, like some other flavonoids, has been found to be a potent inhibitor of P-form phenolsulfotransferase-mediated sulfation, a reaction affecting drug interactions and metabolism. This implies that chrysin is a potential **chemo-preventive agent** in sulfation-induced carcinogenesis. In addition, Lautraite, et al. (*Mutagenesis* 2002;17:45–53) revealed that cells exposed to toxic concentrations of cancer-causing substances along with chrysin *in vitro* were less likely to develop DNA damage. Chrysin can, therefore, be seen as an effective antioxidant phytonutrient, and may be useful in **treating conditions related to oxidative stress.**

Wolfman, et al. (*Pharmacol Biochem Behav.* 1994;47:1–4) discovered that chrysin has **strong anti-anxiety properties.** Zanoli, et al. (*Fitoterapia.* 2000;71 Suppl 1:S117–S123) concluded from their studies that chrysin exerts its anti-anxiety activity by activating receptors of the neurotransmitter GABA, which is responsible for calming brain activity. Wolfman, et al. (*Pharmacol Biochem Behav.* 1994;47:1–4) found that chrysin obtained from passionflower was as effective in countering anxiety as benzodiazepene-type prescription sleeping medications.

Chrysin **relaxes smooth muscle** and thus has been used to relieve pain. Because chrysin relaxes smooth muscle, it has been studied for the treatment of cardiovascular diseases. Villar, et al. (*Planta Med. 2002;*68:847–850) found that a six-week long supplementation of chrysin in the diet of rats **reduced hypertension** and improved the performance of veins and arteries. Furthermore, Duarte, et al. (*Planta Med.* 2001;67:567–569) found that chrysin relaxed the aorta after it was stimulated by the stress hormone noradrenaline.

A discovery by Shin, et al. (*Bioorg Med Chem Lett.* 1999;9:869–874) suggests that chrysin may be **useful in the treatment of diabetes.** Results of their study showed that compounds derived from chrysin were found to have a hypoglycemic effect on the diabetic state.

Some studies have also found that chrysin inhibits HIV-1 activation by interfering with factors responsible for viral transcription. Such findings indicate that chrysin could be of use as an anti-AIDS drug.

THERAPEUTIC DAILY AMOUNT
1–3 grams of chrysin daily is a safe and effective dosage.

MAXIMUM SAFE LEVEL
Not established.

SIDE EFFECTS/CONTRAINDICATIONS
Chrysin should be not be taken by pregnant or lactating women, or by those with prostate or reproductive abnormalities.

Coleus forskohlii (Makandi)

GENERAL DESCRIPTION
Coleus forskohlii is a member of the mint (Lamiaceae) family native to India. The root is used medicinally. Ancient Sanskrit texts show that coleus was commonly used to treat heart and lung diseases, intestinal spasms, insomnia, and convulsions. Today, it is employed in the treatment of glaucoma.

ROLE IN ANTI-AGING
Forskolin is a diterpene found in coleus that **inhibits the enzyme adenylate cyclase.** Adenylate cyclase regulates the formation of cAMP, a compound that controls many cellular activities. Forskolin-induced elevation of cAMP levels has been shown to cause **blood vessel dilation, inhibition of mast cells** (hence the herb is a powerful agent for reducing inflammation caused by allergies),

an **increase in thyroid hormone secretion,** and the **stimulation of fat release from fat cells.** As an extension of its cAMP regulation activities, forskolin also has been shown to **stimulate growth hormone release** within twenty minutes of exposure to the herbal extract. Additionally, forskolin produces a gradual and **sustained increase in LH** (luteinizing hormone), a hormone important in women's reproductive health.

Forskolin has been shown to be of benefit for disorders in which the lung tissue becomes inflamed. Tsukawaki, et al. (*Lung* 1987;165:225–237) investigated the relaxant effects of forskolin by measuring the isometric tension of tracheal smooth muscle during histamine provocation. Forskolin caused dose-dependent relaxant effects on resting tone and on leukotriene-induced contraction of tracheal smooth muscle. The team observed that forskolin raised tissue cyclic AMP levels, and submits that as the mechanism by which forskolin **relaxes airway smooth muscle.**

Forskolin's beneficial impact on smooth muscle extends to heart function. One study on humans has shown that forskolin can **reduce blood pressure and improve heart function** in people with cardiomyopathy. Metzger and Lindher (*Arzneimittelforschung* 1981;31:1248–1250) found that in heart tissue, forskolin was able to activate membrane-bound cAMP-dependent protein kinase. The researchers observed that the adenylatecyclase activation enhanced calcium uptake by the heart muscle cell. They suggest that forskolin is a positive inotropic-acting and effective blood pressure-lowering agent.

Forskolin is also a potent platelet aggregation inhibitor. Researchers have examined it for its effects on tumor-induced human platelet aggregation and pulmonary tumor colonization. Research carried out in 1983 by Agarwal and Parks (*Int J Cancer* 1983;32:801–804) suggests that forskolin is able to **inhibit the spread of cancer cells.** In addition, Li and Wang (Cell Biol Int. 2006 Jul 5; [Epub ahead of print]) found that FSK88, a forskolin derivative, was able to induce apoptotic death of human gastric cancer cells in a dose and time-dependent manner. Thus suggesting that the derivative may prove useful. In lab animals, forskolin strongly inhibits melanoma cell-induced human platelet aggregation. Moreover, a single dose of forskolin was able to reduce tumor colonization in the lungs by more than 70 percent. These findings raise the possibility that forskolin could be valuable in the **prevention of cancer metastasis.**

Direct application of forskolin to the eyes has consistently been shown to lower the pressure inside the eye; therefore, the herb can be useful **for treat-**

ing glaucoma. In research conducted by Caprioli, et al. (*Invest Ophthalmol Vis Sci.* 1984;25:268–277), it was determined that the ability for forskolin to stimulate adenylate cyclase is critical in the ability of the nutrient to reduce aqueous inflow, which is characteristic of intraocular disease. As such, forskolin represents a potentially useful class of antiglaucoma agents.

A human study by Kramer, et al. (*Arzneim Forsch* 1987;37:364–367) showed that forskolin can **reduce blood pressure and improve heart function in people with cardiomyopathy.**

Colenol, a diterpenoid isolated from the roots of *Coleus forskohlii* **stimulates the release of insulin and glucagon** from the islets both *in vitro* and *in vivo*. In a study by Ahmad, et al. (*Acta Diabetol Lat.* 1991;28:71–77), colenol stimulated release of glucagon from islets in a much more pronounced manner compared to that of insulin. Feeding of coleonol to diabetic rats caused a 36.5 percent increase in blood glucose level, compared to control. Oral feeding of coleonol for seven days to normal rats caused increase in blood glucose, serum insulin, glucagon, and free fatty acid levels with corresponding increase in glucose-6–phosphatase activity and depletion of liver glycogen. Ahmad suggests that coleonol's ability to stimulate A-cells is responsible for these effects. Taken collectively, the studies of coleus and insulin suggest a role for Forskolin in the **management of weight.**

THERAPEUTIC DAILY AMOUNT

Coleus extracts standardized to 10 to 18 percent forskolin are available. Some doctors recommend 50–100 mg two to three times per day of standardized extract. Fluid extract can be taken in the amount of 2–4 ml three times per day. The majority of clinical studies have used injected forskolin, so it is unclear if oral ingestion of coleus extracts will provide similar benefits in the amounts recommended above.

MAXIMUM SAFE LEVEL

Not established.

SIDE EFFECTS/CONTRAINDICATIONS

Coleus is thought to be free from side effects; however, it should be avoided in people with stomach ulcers as it may increase stomach acid levels. There are reasons to suggest that coleus could potentiate antiplatelet drugs such as aspirin; however, such an effect has never been documented. The safety of coleus in pregnancy and lactation is unknown.

Cranberry (*Vaccinium macrocarpon*)

GENERAL DESCRIPTION

Cranberry is a member of the same family as bilberry and is native to North America. The medicinal part of cranberry is the juice obtained from ripe berries. Cranberry has been used to **prevent kidney stones** as well as to remove toxins from the blood. The plant has long been recommended for people with **recurrent urinary tract infections** (UTIs).

ROLE IN ANTI-AGING

The proanthocyanidins present in cranberry prevent *E. coli,* the most common cause of UTIs and recurrent UTIs, from adhering to the cells lining the wall of the bladder and urinary tract. The berries have also been shown to reduce bacteria levels in the urinary bladder, an action that may help to prevent future infections.

Preliminary results of a study by researchers from the University of Michigan suggest that cranberry juice could help **lower the risk of developing lung and ear infections** by inhibiting strains of a bacteria called *Haemophilus influenzae.* Dr. Kirk McCrea and colleagues discovered that chemicals present in cranberry juice called proanthocyanidins bind to block the action of strains of *Haemophilus influenzae,* a bacterium present in the throat and nose of three-quarters of the population. *Haemophilus influenzae* is a common cause of ear and lung infections in children, and is thought to be responsible for as many as 40 percent of bacterial middle ear infections.

A study carried out in 2000 by Wang and Jiao revealed that cranberry is an **effective scavenger of free radicals;** therefore, the plant has antioxidant properties. Cranberry is also rich in flavonoids, citric and other acids, and vitamin C; exactly which compounds are most active in promoting good urinary tract health (and delivering cranberry's other health benefits) is still being determined. Patients taking the protein pump inhibitors Lansoprazole and Omeprazole may benefit from cranberry extracts as the plant has been shown to increase the absorption of vitamin B_{12}.

THERAPEUTIC DAILY AMOUNT

Most tablets and capsules contain dried, unsweetened juice powder or concentrated extract. An average dose is 500–1,000 mg per day. Unsweetened cranberry juice (available in some health foods stores) is the most potent cranberry drink, but many people find it difficult to get down; sweetened drinks are more palatable. "Cranberry juice drinks" typically contain 10 to 20 percent juice;

"cranberry juice cocktails" typically have 25 to 35 percent real juice. Some observers have wondered whether these products were too diluted or sugar-laden to have any therapeutic effects but a number of recent studies have found that they can be quite beneficial. For instance, a 1994 study found that 10 ounces per day of commercially available cranberry juice cocktail was almost twice as effective as a placebo in reducing bacteria in urine. When buying the "juice drinks," one will have to drink roughly twice the amount, 20 ounces a day. Results of a study by Stothers (*Can J Urol.* 2002;9:1558–1562.) revealed that cranberry tablets were twice as cost effective as organic juice for prevention of UTIs.

MAXIMUM SAFE LEVEL

Not established.

SIDE EFFECTS/CONTRAINDICATIONS

Ingestion of large amounts (more than 3–4 liters per day) often results in diarrhea and other gastrointestinal symptoms. Therefore, large doses of cranberry should be avoided if one is taking drugs for urinary or kidney problems, or is pregnant or breast-feeding.

People taking drugs that affect the kidneys or the urinary tract should consult their doctor before taking supplementary cranberry. In summer 2006 the United Kingdom's Committee on Safety of Medicines alerted clinicians to a potential interaction between warfarin and cranberry juice and has advised that patients avoid their concurrent use. Analysis of data by Aston et al. (*Pharmacotherapy.* 2006 Sep;26(9):1314–9.) revealed that ingestion of large volumes of cranberry juice destabilizes warfarin therapy.

Dong Quai (*Angelica sinensis*)

GENERAL DESCRIPTION

Dong quai is a member of the celery family. It has been used for many years in traditional Chinese medicine; however, it is rarely used alone and is typically used in combination with herbs such as peony and ligusticum. The root is used in herbal medicine.

ROLE IN ANTI-AGING

In traditional Chinese medicine, dong quai is often referred to as "the female ginseng," and is thought to have **a balancing effect on the female hormonal system.** For this reason, it is often included in preparations to **treat abnormal menstruation, suppressed menstrual flow, dysmenorrhea (painful menstruation), and uterine bleeding.** However, it does not qualify as a phytoestrogen and does not appear to have any hormonelike actions in the body.

Dong quai is also used, in both men and women, for **the treatment of high blood pressure and peripheral circulatory disorders.** It also has a traditional use as a way to **promote formation of red blood cells.** A widely cited case study by Bradley, et al. (*Am J Kidney Dis* 1999;34:349–354) profiles a man with kidney failure who exhibited a significant improvement in anemia due to dialysis while drinking a tea made from dong quai and peony. However, there is currently no evidence obtained from clinical trials to substantiate the use of dong quai alone for this purpose, or for the treatment of other forms of anemia.

Results of a study by Yang et al. (*Int J Biol Macromol.* 2006 Mar 6; [Epub ahead of print]) indicate that Dong quai may possess immunomodulatory properties. Study results showed that a polysaccharide purified from the fresh root of the plant was able to regulate the expression of Th1 and Th2 related cytokines and activate macrophages and natural killer T cells.

THERAPEUTIC DAILY AMOUNT

The powdered root of dong quai is available in capsule and tablet form. The recommended dose for women is 3–4 grams daily in three divided doses. A tincture is also available, 3–5 ml of which can be taken three times a day.

MAXIMUM SAFE LEVEL

Not established.

SIDE EFFECTS/CONTRAINDICATIONS

Dong quai may cause some fair-skinned people to become more sensitive to sunlight; it is therefore recommended that people using it on a regular basis avoid prolonged exposure to the sun or other sources of ultraviolet radiation. Dong quai is not recommended for pregnant or breast-feeding women.

Echinacea (*Echinacea purpurea*)

GENERAL DESCRIPTION

An herb native to North America, echinacea (purple coneflower) is an important component of Native American medicine, traditionally used as both an anti-inflammatory and an antiseptic, especially for skin problems. Echinacea was introduced into medical practice in the United States in 1887 and touted for use in conditions ranging from colds to syphilis. Modern research into the plants properties began in Germany in the 1930s. The active ingredients of echinacea are found in both the root and the aboveground parts of the plant.

Echinacea is one of the most popular herbal supplements on the market. More than $300 million a year is spent on Echinacea supplements in the United States. In recent years, echinacea has been studied for its antiviral, immune-boosting, and antibody-producing properties. Echinacea increases the production of white blood cells and helps them move into the circulatory system more quickly. Currently, one of the most popular uses for echinacea is to relieve the symptoms and shorten the duration of the common cold. Whether or not echinacea can prevent colds is a matter of some debate.

ROLE IN ANTI-AGING

Echinacea has been shown to **boost the immune system, short-circuit colds and flu, fight bacterial and viral infections, lower fever,** and **calm allergic reactions** when taken internally. Many studies have found that echinacea (when taken at the first sign of a cold for 8 to 10 days) reduces cold symptoms and/or shortens their duration. For example, Lindenmuth et al. (*J Altern Complement Med.* 2000;6:327–334.) studied 95 people with early symptoms of cold and flu (such as runny nose, scratchy throat, and fever), those who drank five to six cups of echinacea tea every day for five days felt better sooner than those who drank tea without echinacea. Other studies have found that echinacea reduces cold symptoms by roughly 34 percent. Many people taken echinacea to try prevent a cold or flu by taking the herb throughout cold and flu season or just after exposure to an infection. Despite the popularity of this approach, several studies suggest that it does not work. The consensus seems to be that echinacea may help treat but not prevent the common cold.

Echinacea has also been found to have anti-inflammatory properties, and some research suggests that this may be due to the plant's ability to modulate COX-2 expression. Several constituents of echinacea have been shown to work together to increase the proliferation and activity of white blood cells. These include alkylamides/polyacetylenes, caffeic acid derivatives, and polysaccharides. Researchers have also determined that echinacea increases levels of the antiviral substance interferon as well as an immune-related blood protein known as properdin. In addition, a recent study found that echinacea contains a number of antioxidant compounds, which suggests that echinacea extracts would protect the skin from sunlight-induced free-radical damage. Results of a study by Melchart et al. (*Phytother Res.* 2002;16:138–142) suggest that echinacea may help to alleviate some of the **side effects associated with chemotherapy.**

THERAPEUTIC DAILY AMOUNT

Echinacea products vary widely and often include other ingredients such as zinc and goldenseal. There are three different types of echinacea (*E. purpurea,* *E. pallida,* and *E. angustifolia*), and various formulations contain different parts of the plant (leaves, flowers, roots). Studies indicate that the best results occur in people who use a liquid or tincture form, rather than a pill or capsule. To treat colds, flu, or upper respiratory tract infections, one of the following should be taken three times a day: 1–2 grams dried root or herb, drunk as tea; 2 to 3 ml of standardized tincture extract; 200 mg of powdered extract containing 4 percent phenolics; Tincture (1:5): 1–3 ml; Stabilized fresh extract: 0.75 ml.

MAXIMUM SAFE LEVEL
Not established.

SIDE EFFECTS/CONTRAINDICATIONS
Echinacea is one of the least toxic herbs around; it is not known to cause any side effects. Allergic reactions are rare, but one should take only a small dose at first if one is allergic to any other plants in the Compositae family (which includes sunflowers, daisies, and dandelions). Echinacea should only be taken on an as-needed basis. German health authorities recommend that people should not take echinacea if they have an autoimmune illness, such as lupus (SLE), are HIV-positive, or have progressive systemic diseases, such as tuberculosis and multiple sclerosis. People with liver disease are also advised to avoid echinacea. They also recommend that no one should take echinacea either internally or externally for more than eight weeks in a row. Efficacy may decline if used for an extended period, so holidays (where you do not take it daily) are recommended. Echinacea may also interfere with immunosuppressive drugs, and its use is not recommended during pregnancy.

Elderberry (*Sambucus nigra*)

GENERAL DESCRIPTION
Every part of the elder tree has a food or medicinal purpose. For centuries, the elderberry has been used to treat colds and flu. Scientists believe that antioxidant flavonoids found in the elderberry fight viral infection. Elderberry is most commonly used to treat the runny nose and sore throat of the common cold and to help reduce the fever, muscle pain, and other symptoms of the flu. Elderberry **induces sweating** and **stimulates circulation;** it also has **slight laxative and cough-suppressant effects.** The berries are rich in vitamin C, flavonoids such as anthocyanins, substances called tannins, and other phyto- (or "plant") nutrients. The flowers contain flavonoids, an essen-

tial oil, mucilage, tannins, and other compounds, whose main effects appear to be reducing fever and promoting sweating.

ROLE IN ANTI-AGING

An animal study carried out in 1987 reported that elder flowers had moderately strong anti-inflammatory properties; however, no further research to back this claim has been carried out. Recent research carried out at Tufts University has revealed that elderberry contains four anthocyanins that work to protect endothelial cells, which line artery walls, from oxidative damage caused by free radicals. It is thought that certain compounds in elderberry may help counter the effects of some strains of influenza by binding to the virus and preventing it from attacking cells. An extract from elderberry called Sambucol has proven effective at treating—not preventing—influenza (type A and B). In a study by Zakay-Rones et al (*J Int Med Res*. 2004;32:132–140.) of 60 patients who had been suffering with flu symptoms for 48 hours or less, half the group took 15 ml of Sambucol four times a day for five days, whilst the other half took a placebo. Patients in the Sambucol group had "pronounced improvements" in flu symptoms after just three days, and nearly 90 percent of patients were completely cured within two to three days. In comparison, the placebo group took at least six days to recover.

THERAPEUTIC DAILY AMOUNT

Elderberry comes in tinctures, liquid extracts, lozenges, syrups, standardized extract capsules, and throat sprays. Follow dosage directions on labels. For the treatment of flu 15 ml of Sambucol four times a day should be taken at the onset of symptoms.

MAXIMUM SAFE LEVEL

Not established.

SIDE EFFECTS/CONTRAINDICATIONS

No adverse reactions to elderberry are known to exist. Raw berries are edible but may cause nausea and vomiting. Herbal products made from the leaves, stems or bark of the elderberry tree should NOT be taken internally as they contain the potentially fatal poison cyanide.

Feverfew (*Tanacetum parthenium*)

GENERAL DESCRIPTION

Feverfew was commonly used by the early Europeans and Greeks to treat fevers, headaches, arthritis, menstrual problems, and other generalized aches and pains. Today, the plant is most commonly used to **reduce the frequency and severity of migraines**—several placebo-controlled human trials have confirmed feverfew's effectiveness in this area. The active ingredient in feverfew is a compound called parthenolide, which belongs to a group of compounds known as sesquiterpene lactones. Parthenolide prevents the excessive clumping of platelets in addition to inhibiting the release of certain chemicals, including serotonin and some inflammatory mediators. Feverfew's antimigraine action was originally attributed to its parthenolide content; however, this has been a subject of recent debate.

ROLE IN ANTI-AGING

Research carried out by Mazor et al. (*Cytokine.* 2000;12:239–245.) suggests that sesquiterpene lactones inhibit the expression of the immunoreactive molecule Interleukin (IL) 8, a discovery that could account for feverfew's anti-inflammatory actions.

Feverfew may have anti-cancer properties. Parthenolide has been shown to exhibit *in vitro* and *in vivo* anti-tumor and anti-angiogenic activity. Won et al. (*Carcinogenesis.* 2004;25:1449–1458.) found that parthenolide had chemopreventive effects on UVB-induced skin cancer in mice. While several recent studies have found that parthenolide appears to induce apoptosis in cancer cells.

THERAPEUTIC DAILY AMOUNT

Feverfew is sold dried and in capsules, concentrated drops, tinctures and extracts. The newest products are standardized for 0.1 to 0.2 percent of the chemical parthenolide; however, standardized leaf extracts may contain as much as 0.7 percent. An average daily dose is 125 mg of feverfew (standardized for 0.2 percent parthenolide) or 250 mcg parthenolide. A number of studies done in the last ten years indicate that several commercial feverfew products contained none of the active compound parthenolide (in addition, parthenolide levels of the dried herb were found to fall during storage). These studies emphasize the importance of using high-quality standardized extracts of this herb in order to obtain proper dosage and reliable effects.

MAXIMUM SAFE LEVEL

Not established.

SIDE EFFECTS/CONTRAINDICATIONS

Few side effects have been associated with feverfew products, although eating the fresh leaves can cause swelling of the lips and tongue and mouth ulcers. A withdrawal syndrome called "post-feverfew syndrome" has been described, with symptoms including nervousness, tension headaches, joint stiffness, and tiredness. People who are allergic to other plants in the daisy family, such as chamomile or ragweed should not take feverfew. The herb is not recommended during pregnancy or lactation and should not be used by children under the age of two. It has also been reported that the drug may interact with anticoagulant medicines.

Fo-Ti Root Extract (*Polygonum multiflorum*) (He-Shou-Wu)

GENERAL DESCRIPTION

Fo-ti root extract has a long history in traditional Chinese medicine. The unprocessed root is sometimes used medicinally. However, if the root has been boiled in a special liquid made from black beans, it is considered as a different medicine. The unprocessed root is often called white fo-ti, and the processed root red fo-ti. The unprocessed root is used to relax the bowels and detoxify the blood, while the processed root is used to strengthen the blood, invigorate the kidneys and liver, and serve as a tonic to increase overall vitality.

ROLE IN ANTI-AGING

The major active constituents of fo-ti are anthraquinones, phospholipids, tannins, and tetrahydroxystilbene glucoside. In traditional Chinese medicine the processed root has been used to **lower cholesterol levels.** Animal research supports this use as it has been shown to **decrease fat deposits in the blood,** and possibly **prevent atherosclerosis.** However, human clinical trials to support this use are lacking. Research by Yim, et al. (*Planta Medica* 1998;64: 607–611) suggests that the extract can exert a **protective effect on heart cells.** Their research showed that lab animals pretreated with fo-ti extract before being subjected to heart injury were better able to recover than their untreated counterparts. Fo-ti's ability to protect the heart appears to be due to its **ability to reduce the depletion of glutathione,** an important cellular antioxidant.

In vitro studies suggest that fo-ti's ability can **boost the immune system** and **increase red blood cell formation.** It may also help to **combat bacterial infection.**

The unprocessed roots have a mild laxative action.

THERAPEUTIC DAILY AMOUNT

The typical intake of processed root powder is 4–8 grams per day. A tea can be made from processed roots by boiling 3–5 grams in 250 ml of water for ten to fifteen minutes. Three or more cups are suggested each day. Fo-ti is also available in tablet form; the recommended dose is 500 mg three times a day, but follow instructions on packaging.

MAXIMUM SAFE LEVEL

Not established.

SIDE EFFECTS/CONTRAINDICATIONS

The unprocessed roots may cause mild diarrhea, and some cases of skin rash have been reported. Taking 15 grams or more of processed root powder may cause numbness in the arms or legs.

Garlic (*Allium sativum*)

GENERAL DESCRIPTION

Garlic has been renowned for its medicinal properties throughout history. It is referred to in both the Bible and the Talmud, and Hippocrates, Galen, and Dioscorides all mention the use of garlic for many conditions, including parasites, respiratory problems, poor digestion, and low energy. By 1500 B.C., the Egyptians had identified twenty-two different uses for garlic ranging from headaches to general physical weakness. Today, the herb figures in a seemingly endless array of remedies for everything from insect bites and fever to intestinal ailments. The main active ingredient of garlic is the sulfur compound allicin, produced by crushing or chewing fresh garlic, which in turn produces other sulfur compounds, including ajoene, allyl sulfides, and vinyldithiins.

ROLE IN ANTI-AGING

Garlic contains amino acids, various vitamins and trace minerals, flavonoids, enzymes, and at least 200 additional compounds. Researchers have documented garlic's potential to reduce heart attacks by **lowering the levels of blood fats,** including triglycerides and LDL ("bad") cholesterol, and raising "good" HDL cholesterol levels. In one recent study, Russian researchers determined that garlic's beneficial effects on cardiovascular health could be attributed to both direct actions on the walls of heart arteries and to indirect preventive actions at the cellular level. In other words, garlic is a double-barreled weapon against heart disease. Garlic extracts have also been shown to inhibit smooth muscle cell proliferation, normalize vascular reactivity, and improve exercise tolerance (*Indian J Physiol Pharmacol.* 2005;49:115–118).

Among the most active medicinal compounds are dozens of sulfur compounds found in few other plants; these are thought to be responsible for garlic's documented antibacterial (Louis Pasteur confirmed the antibacterial

action of the bulb in 1858), antiviral, antifungal, and other healthful properties. Research published in 2001 suggests that allicin, the main active ingredient of garlic, could be useful in the fight against potentially fatal hospital
acquired infections. Researchers found that that topical creams containing
just 32 parts per million (ppm) of allicin inhibited the growth of thirty different samples of the antibiotic-resistant bacterium methicillin-resistant **Staphylococcus aureus** (MRSA), and that concentrations of 256 ppm were enough to
kill the bacteria. Meanwhile, results of another study by Josling (*Adv Ther.*
2001;18:189–193) revealed that people who took a daily allicin-containing garlic supplement were more than 50 percent less likely to catch a cold. Furthermore, those taking the supplement and were unlucky enough to catch a cold
tended to recover much more quickly and were significantly less likely to
become re-infected with the disease.

Epidemiological studies have shown that eating garlic regularly can **reduce the risk of developing esophageal, stomach, and colon cancers.** Research
by Hsing, et al. (*Journal of the National Cancer Institute* 2002;94:1648–1651)
suggests that eating plenty of **garlic and onions could help men to lower their
risk of developing prostate cancer.** The study of 238 men diagnosed with
prostate cancer and 471 healthy men revealed that those who ate more than a
third of an ounce (10 grams) of onions, garlic, chives or scallions each day
were significantly less likely to be in the group with cancer. What's more, men
who ate the most vegetables were 50 percent less likely to develop prostate
cancer than those who are the least. Garlic's apparent anticancer abilities are
thought to be attributable, at least in part, to its ability to prevent the formation of carcinogenic compounds. Animal and *in vitro* studies have also demonstrated that the sulfur compounds found in garlic can inhibit the growth of
different types of cancer, in particular breast and skin tumors. Numerous studies also indicate that garlic can boost immunity, balance blood sugar, and prevent digestive ailments (it may also help the liver to neutralize toxins).

THERAPEUTIC DAILY AMOUNT

Garlic is available fresh or juiced, as well as in tablets, capsules, and tinctures.
Odor-controlled powders, concentrates, and capsules are popular forms, as are
enteric-coated tablets (which have a coating that prevents the destruction of
active compounds by stomach acids). Supplement manufacturers are increasingly standardizing their products for desirable garlic compounds (principally
one called allicin, but also total sulfur, allin, and S-allyl cysteine), but debate
rages on as to which of these compounds are most important and which for-

mulations are most effective. The potency of garlic products may be described in terms of fresh or whole garlic equivalent; an average dose is 1,500–1,800 mg of fresh garlic equivalent, approximately equal to eating one-half clove of fresh garlic. To fight infection, 3 or 4 chopped, crushed or chewed cloves should be consumed per day or, in supplement form (1.3 percent allicin), 600–900 mg divided into two to three doses per day. Garlic can help to treat colds and flu, however it is best seen as a preventative. The use of garlic against colds and flu seems to be most effective when applied before the infection is caught, or immediately the symptoms begin to show. In Josling's study, which showed that garlic offers protection against the common cold, participants took one capsule of Allimax, an allicin-containing garlic supplement, each day.

MAXIMUM SAFE LEVEL
Not established.

SIDE EFFECTS/CONTRAINDICATIONS
Garlic is extremely safe but taking very large daily doses (more than 10 g) of some products may cause flatulence, stomach irritation, or indigestion. Because of garlic's anticlotting properties, persons taking anticoagulant drugs, such as warfarin and Ticlopidine, should check with their doctor before taking garlic. In addition, people scheduled for surgery should inform their surgeon if they are taking garlic supplements. People taking drugs for the treatment of HIV infection and AIDS should consult their specialist before taking supplementary garlic.

Women should avoid taking garlic supplements during pregnancy as laboratory studies suggest that they may cause irregular uterine contractions.

Ginger (*Zingiber officinale*)

GENERAL DESCRIPTION
Ginger grows in India, China, Mexico, and several other countries. The medical part of the plant is the underground stem, which is called the rhizome. Zesty flavor notwithstanding, ginger is often taken for its **calming effects on a churning stomach.** It is also taken to treat morning sickness, seasickness, and motion sickness. In some people, it also can help reduce a fever or lessen the symptoms of a cold. Ginger contains an essential oil and other compounds (including gingerol and shogaol) that apparently **prevent nausea** through effects on the stomach and gastrointestinal system rather than through the nervous system. Doctors recently have tested ginger's ability to prevent nausea and vomiting after surgery and during chemotherapy treatment. One study

found that ginger was better than a placebo and as effective as the conventional anti-emetic drug metoclopramide for preventing nausea after gynecological surgery.

ROLE IN ANTI-AGING

A study carried out in Israel in 2000 found that ginger extract significantly reduced the development of atherosclerotic lesions and lowered LDL-cholesterol levels in mice. Components of ginger, called flavonoids, also have antioxidant potential. Results of a study by Altmann and Marcussen (*Arthritis Rheum.* 2001;44:2531–2538) suggest that highly purified ginger extracts may be useful for **alleviating the pain caused by osteoarthritis** (OA) of the knee. The study of 247 patients with OA of the knee revealed that the extract lessened the pain experienced by sufferers when walking or standing.

THERAPEUTIC DAILY AMOUNT

Ginger comes in a variety of forms including fresh, dried, tablets, capsules, tinctures, extracts, syrups, and teas; follow dosage directions on labels. You can also buy ginger essential oil, which can be diffused into the air for inhalation, or diluted in a vegetable oil for inhalation or topical application (or massage).

MAXIMUM SAFE LEVEL

Not established.

SIDE EFFECTS/CONTRAINDICATIONS

Ginger has a long history of being taken in relatively large doses (up to several grams) without causing any toxicity or side effects. Many pregnant women use it to help control morning sickness; however, there have been no studies in which women have taken large doses of ginger during pregnancy. Studies carried out in Europe found that ginger may enhance absorption of sulphaguanidine. In addition, excessive consumption of ginger (dosage not stated) may interfere with cardiac, antidiabetic, or anticoagulant therapy. Do not ingest the essential oil and be sure to dilute it before applying to your skin.

Ginkgo (*Ginkgo biloba*, Maidenhair tree)

GENERAL DESCRIPTION

The ginkgo tree grows most prominently in the southern and eastern United States, southern France, China, and Korea. The leaves of the tree are used medicinally for treating various conditions, including **asthma, allergies, and coughs.** Ginkgo **stimulates circulation in the brain, ears, and other parts of the body;** it is also an **antioxidant.** Plant scientists believe that the most active constituents of ginkgo are the flavonoid compounds flavoglycosides and ginkgoheterosides.

ROLE IN ANTI-AGING

Bioflavonoids are primarily responsible for ginkgo's antioxidant activity and these may inhibit platelet aggregation. These actions may help ginkgo protect against cardiovascular diseases such as atherosclerosis and support the brain and central nervous system. Unique terpene lactone components found in ginkgo leaves, called ginkgolides and bilobalide, are associated with increased circulation to the brain and other parts of the body; they also help to protect nerve cells from oxidative damage. Recent animal studies indicate that bilobalide protects neurons from apoptosis (programmed cell death) and excitotoxic damage. Research suggests that Gingko extracts may be of use in the treatment and management of Alzheimer's disease and other neurodegenerative diseases. Results of a study by Bate et al. (*J Neuroinflammation.* 2004;1:4.) suggest that ginkgolides inhibit platelet-activating factor, and that platelet-activating factor antagonists block the toxicity of the amyloid-beta protein, which is implicated in Alzheimer's disease. Gingko is often touted as being able to boost memory, however clinical research to support these claims is somewhat contradictory. A study of patients with Alzheimer's type senile dementia revealed that those who took ginkgo extract three times per day experienced significant improvements in memory and attention. The changes were evident after one month and continued to accumulate over the three-month period of the study. However, results of a study of healthy seniors published in 2002 suggest that it does not help to boost memory. Solomon, et al. (*JAMA* 2002; 288:835) studied the effects of ginkgo on 230 men and women aged sixty and results showed that the herb had no measurable benefit on the memory, attention, or concentration of healthy adults.

Results of a study by Chen et al. (*World J Gastroenterol.* 2005;11:3746–3750.) suggest that Gingko may help to protect against gastric ulcers. For the study researchers induced gastric ulcers in rats with ethanol. Results showed that Gingko extract provided a dose-dependent protection against the ethanol-induced gastric ulcers in rats. The researchers suggest that the preventive effect of Gingko extract may be due to inhibition of lipid peroxidation, preservation of gastric mucus, and blockade of cell apoptosis.

THERAPEUTIC DAILY AMOUNT

The most popular ginkgo products are encapsulated extracts standardized to 24 percent of chemicals called flavoglycosides; you can also find liquid herbal concentrates and the powdered whole herb. An average dose of the standardized extract is 40–60 mg. IMPORTANT: Ginkgo leaves contain a group of potentially toxic chemicals known as alkylphenols. The German health commission, Commission E, states that ginkgo supplements must not contain more than 5 parts per million of these toxic compounds. The ginkgo extracts EGb 761 and LI 1370 both conform to these strict safety limits.

MAXIMUM SAFE LEVEL
Not established.

SIDE EFFECTS/CONTRAINDICATIONS
Ginkgo has been associated with no long-term toxicity and few side effects. However, newcomers to the herb who take single doses in excess of 300 mg or so may experience headaches or dizziness. Some ginkgo users may also experience a mild upset stomach. Until recently, ginkgo was not contraindicated for pregnant and lactating women; however, in August 2001 Petty et al. (*Chem Res Toxicol.* 2001;14:1254–1258) found that women taking one type of the supplement had high levels of the toxin colchicine, which can cause birth defects. For this reason alone, pregnant women, breast-feeding women, and women planning to conceive should not take ginkgo supplements.

Ginseng, Panax (*Panax quinquefolius*)

GENERAL DESCRIPTION
Panax ginseng has been a staple in traditional Chinese medicine for more than 2,000 years. The first reference to the use of Panax ginseng dates to the first century A.D. Ginseng is commonly used by elderly people in the East to improve mental and physical vitality. Ginseng is not so much a cure-all as a **prevent-all,** a strengthening "tonic" herb taken to rejuvenate and revitalize the body. Ginseng has been shown to act on both the cardiovascular and central nervous systems. Among ginseng's key ingredients are chemicals called saponins or glycosides, particularly a group called ginsenosides. Thirteen ginsenosides have been identified in Panax ginseng. Two of them, ginsenosides Rg1 and Rb1, have been closely studied. These chemicals appear to affect the nervous system, blood flow to the brain, and certain neurotransmitters.

ROLE IN ANTI-AGING
Long-term intake of Panax ginseng may be linked to a **reduced risk of some forms of cancer.** Yun et al. (*J Korean Med Sci.* 2001;16 Suppl:S19–27) found that people who regularly used ginseng had a dramatically reduced risk of

developing cancer of the ovaries, pancreas, and stomach. Individuals who had been taking ginseng the longest had the lowest overall risk of cancer. Ginseng may also be of benefit to cancer patients undergoing radiotherapy. In a recent review concerning the radioprotective properties of ginseng, Lee et al. (*Mutagenesis.* 2005;20:237–243.) wrote: "In addition to its anti-tumor properties, ginseng appears to be a promising radioprotector for therapeutic or preventive protocols capable of attenuating the deleterious effects of radiation on human normal tissue, especially for cancer patients undergoing radiotherapy."

A double-blind study determined that Panax ginseng supplementation could **improve blood sugar levels in people with type II diabetes.** Results of the study on mice bred to develop diabetes showed that the extract normalized blood sugar levels, **improved insulin secretion and insulin sensitivity, and lowered cholesterol levels** by 30 percent. Furthermore, the treated animals lost more than 10 percent of their body weight, ate 15 percent less, and were 35 percent more active than untreated mice. In addition, Liu et al. (*Horm Metab Res.* 2005;37:146–151.) found that oral administration of Panax ginseng improves insulin sensitivity and could delay the development of insulin resistance in rats. Yun et al. (*Arch Pharm Res.* 2004;27:790–796.) investigated the preventative anti-diabetic and anti-obese effects of wild ginseng ethanol extract (WGEE). Results showed that WGEE co-administered with a high fat diet significantly inhibited body weight gain, fasting blood glucose, triglyceride, and free fatty acid levels in a dose-dependent manner. WGEE also significantly increased the insulin resistance index. The authors conclude: "WGEE has potential as a preventive agent for type 2 diabetes mellitus (and possibly obesity) and deserves clinical trial in the near future."

Several studies have shown that ginseng **supports the thymus and spleen, and therefore boosts the immune system.**

Panax ginseng may **enhance athletic performance.** One study suggests that it may help those in poor physical condition to tolerate exercise better. In another study, when combined with some vitamins and minerals, ginseng reduced fatigue. A separate study found Panax ginseng to be helpful for **relieving fatigue and stress.**

Other constituents of Panax ginseng, include the panaxans, which may help lower blood sugar, and the polysaccharides (complex sugar molecules), which are thought to support immune function.

Panax ginseng may also support the normal function of the hypothalamic-pituitary-adrenal axis—seat of the hormonal stress system of the body. With these characteristics, Panax ginseng has been suggested to be useful for people with chronic fatigue syndrome (CFS).

Panax ginseng may be important in male sexual health. A double-blind trial of a large group of infertile men by Chen et al. (*Am J Chin Med.* 1999;27: 123–128) found that Panax ginseng **improved sperm count and sperm motility.** Panax ginseng has been found in clinical studies to improve libido and the ability to maintain an erection in men with erectile dysfunction.

THERAPEUTIC DAILY AMOUNT

Ginseng comes in a variety of forms, from the whole root to teas to standardized extracts. Potency varies considerably, depending on the type, place of origin, and how it was cultivated, stored, and prepared. The most predictable results come from using products standardized for one or more ginsenosides (chemicals isolated from the whole plant); an average dose is 100 mg of an extract standardized for 7 percent ginsenosides.

MAXIMUM SAFE LEVEL

Not established.

SIDE EFFECTS/CONTRAINDICATIONS

Ginseng may occasionally cause insomnia, but no long-term adverse effects from taking average doses have been identified. However, a few contraindications exist: Ginseng is best used with caution by anyone with high blood pressure or cardiovascular disease and should not be used by pregnant or nursing women. Children should not take ginseng, as the structure of some of the ginsenosides is chemically similar to certain steroid hormones that have unknown effects on children's growth and development.

Ginseng, Siberian (*Eleutherococcus senticosus, Eleuthero*)

GENERAL DESCRIPTION

Siberian ginseng is native to the southeastern part of Russia, northern China, Korea, and Japan. The root and the rhizomes (underground stem) of the plant are used medicinally. It supports the working of the adrenal glands and prevents the worst effects of nervous tension. It tends to increase energy, extend endurance, and fight fatigue. Chemists have isolated more than three-dozen compounds in Siberian ginseng that may affect the mind and body; foremost among these are the eleutherosides, which occur in the plant's roots and, to a lesser degree, in the leaves. Studies have determined that the eleutherosides differ from the ginsenosides isolated from the Panax ginsengs, although some of their effects on the body are similar; exactly how these compounds affect the body is still being determined. (The effects, in fact, may be available only from the whole herb. The isolated components of Siberian ginseng do not have the same tonic action as the whole plant.) The effects of Siberian ginseng also vary from person to person.

ROLE IN ANTI-AGING

Studies on Siberian ginseng have shown that it has considerable promise for increasing longevity and improving overall health. The plant may also play a role in the treatment of hypertension, blood sugar irregularities, and depression. Siberian ginseng is known to **boost overall immune function** and preliminary findings also suggests that it may prove valuable in the long-term management of various diseases of the immune system, including HIV infection and chronic fatigue syndrome. Healthy people who were given a daily supplement of Siberian ginseng were found to have increased numbers of T lymphocytes. Siberian ginseng also supports the body by helping the liver detoxify harmful toxins. Studies carried out in Russia have confirmed that ginseng can also exert a **protective effect on the body during radiation exposure.** Therefore, it may be of benefit to patients undergoing radiotherapy to treat cancer. The plant also helps the liver to detoxify harmful toxins. Animal studies have shown that Siberian ginseng helps to protect against ethanol, sodium barbital, and the tetanus toxoid, and chemotherapeutic agents, among others. Siberian ginseng has also been shown to **enhance mental acuity and physical endurance** without the side effects associated with caffeine. Research suggests that Siberian ginseng improves oxygen utilization by exercising muscle; thus, it would be logical to assume that it may help to increase endurance and speed recovery from exercise. However, research in this area has produced somewhat contradictory results. In research conducted on people of average athletic abilities, for instance, people given Siberian ginseng have shown marked improvements in endurance. However, the validity of some of these studies is questionable. In a recent review on the use of Siberian ginseng on endurance performance by Goulet and Dionne (*Int J Sport Nutr Exerc Metab.* 2005;15:75–83), the authors concluded: "Eleutherococcus senticosus supplementation (up to 1,000 to 1,200 mg/d for one to six weeks) offers no advantage during exercise ranging in duration from 6 to 120 minutes."

THERAPEUTIC DAILY AMOUNT

Siberian ginseng is sold in capsules, tinctures, and extracts. Standardized Siberian ginseng products often specify the content of one or more of a series of chemicals known as eleutherosides. An average dose is 100 mg of an extract standardized for 1 percent eleutherosides. Siberian ginseng should not be used continuously for more than six to eight weeks, with a break of one to two weeks between use.

MAXIMUM SAFE LEVEL
Not established.

SIDE EFFECTS/CONTRAINDICATIONS
Siberian ginseng is considered to be safe for daily consumption even in doses many times larger than average, though some people may experience insomnia and other side effects from taking high amounts. Siberian ginseng should be avoided, or taken with caution, by individuals with uncontrolled high blood pressure and those who are hysteric, manic, or schizophrenic. It should not be taken with stimulants, including coffee, with antipsychotic drugs, or during treatment with hormones. People taking digoxin should consult their doctor before taking Siberian ginseng.

Goldenseal (*Hydrastis Canadensis*)

GENERAL DESCRIPTION
Goldenseal is native to eastern North America. The dried root and rhizome are used medicinally. With **anti-inflammatory and antibiotic properties,** the herb goldenseal is effective against bacteria and fungi. Goldenseal can also be made into a paste and applied directly to the skin to **treat impetigo, ringworm, and other skin infections.**

ROLE IN ANTI-AGING
The primary active ingredients in goldenseal are the alkaloids hydrastine and berberine, along with smaller amounts of canadine. Berberine, which has been extensively researched, appears to have a wide spectrum of antimicrobial activity against pathogens, including *Chlamydia, E. coli,* and *Salmonella typhi,* as well as viruses and protozoans. Goldenseal is often combined with echinacea in preparations designed to strengthen the immune system. Many herbalists recommend goldenseal in herbal remedies for hay fever, colds, and flu. The herb also appears to stimulate the activity of macrophages, the immune cells that attack harmful bacteria, and increase immunoglobulin production.

THERAPEUTIC DAILY AMOUNT
Standardized extracts supplying 8 to 12 percent alkaloids are available; the recommended dose is 250–500 mg three times per day. Goldenseal should not be

used continuously for more than three weeks, with a break of at least two weeks between use.

MAXIMUM SAFE LEVEL

Not established.

SIDE EFFECTS/CONTRAINDICATIONS

Taken as recommended, goldenseal is generally regarded as safe; however, the herb should be avoided during pregnancy and lactation and by those with heart disease, high blood pressure, and diabetes. Some studies have suggested that goldenseal may reduce the efficacy of doxycycline and tetracycline. Goldenseal may be contraindicated if allergic to ragweed.

Grapefruit Seed Extract

GENERAL DESCRIPTION

Grapefruit seed extract (GSE) has a proven track record as a powerful and non-toxic **antimicrobial agent** with a broad spectrum of activity. Research has demonstrated that grapefruit seed extract can be effective in treating **candidiasis,** including *Candida albicans* vaginitis. Researchers have also had positive results using GSE as an antimicrobial on food and as a **deep cleanser for skin.** Added to toothpaste and mouthwash, GSE may **protect against both viral and bacterial infection in the mouth.**

ROLE IN ANTI-AGING

Grapefruit seed extract can be used in a variety of ways to boost protection against pathogens. Some asthmatics have used the extract in nebulizers, with great success, in order to prevent against lung and bronchial infections. Zayachkivska et al. (*J Physiol Pharmacol.* 2005;56:219–231.) found that pre-treatment with GSE protected the gastric mucosa of rats from ethanol-induced lesions. Thus suggesting that GSE may help to protect against gastric ulcers.

THERAPEUTIC DAILY AMOUNT

Refer to dosage information on labels. Be careful not to confuse GSE with "grape seed extract."

MAXIMUM SAFE LEVEL

Not established.

SIDE EFFECTS/CONTRAINDICATIONS

Grapefruit seed extract is not associated with any side effects, drug interactions, or contraindications. However, a number of medications should not be taken with grapefruit juice itself. These include certain immunosuppressants, cholesterol-lowering drugs, and antihistamines—if in doubt, consult a physician. Furthermore, when taken as recommended, it does not destroy the "healthy" bacteria that reside in the gastrointestinal tract.

Green Tea (*Camellia sinensis*)

GENERAL DESCRIPTION

Green tea, unlike black and oolong tea, is not fermented; therefore, the active ingredients remain unaltered in the herb.

ROLE IN ANTI-AGING

Drinking green tea may substantially cut the risk of dying from a range of illnesses, a Japanese study has found. The Ohsaki National Health Insurance Cohort Study, by Kuriyama et al. (*JAMA*. 2006;296:1255–1265) followed 40 530 Japanese adults aged 40 to 79 years (without history of stroke, coronary heart disease, or cancer at the start of the study) for 11 years (1995–2005) for all-cause mortality and for up to 7 years (1995–2001) for cause-specific mortality. Results showed that green tea consumption was inversely associated with mortality due to all causes and due to cardiovascular disease, particularly stroke mortality. Compared with people who drank less than one cup per day of green tea, those who consumed five or more were found to have a 16 percent lower risk of dying from any cause during the 11-year study. They also had a 26 percent lower risk of dying from CVD in the seven years of follow-up. For some reason the benefits of green tea appear to be greater in women. Women who drank five cups or more of green tea each day had a 31 percent lower risk of dying from cardiovascular disease compared with those who had less than one. However, no significant association between green tea consumption and death from cancer was found in men or women.

Green tea contains numerous cancer-fighting polyphenol compounds, including antioxidant flavonoid catechins. The primary catechin in green tea is epigallocatechin gallate (EGCG). Studies indicate that green tea may help protect against cancers of the lungs, skin, liver, pancreas, and stomach. Numerous studies have shown that green tea catechin inhibit the growth of many cancer cell types by inducing apoptosis, or programmed cell death.

Green tea may be useful as a weight-loss agent as it known to increase fat metabolism, and help to regulate blood sugar and insulin levels. Lin et al. (*Obes Res*. 2005;13:982–990) found that EGCG increased apoptosis in mature adipocytes, and inhibited lipid accumulation in maturing preadipocytes in a dose-dependent manner. The authors conclude: "These results demonstrate that EGCG can act directly to inhibit differentiation of preadipocytes and to induce apoptosis of mature adipocytes and, thus, could be an important adjunct in the treatment of obesity."

Green tea is also thought to prevent cardiovascular disease by lowering cholesterol levels, inhibiting LDL oxidation, reducing the tendency of blood platelets to stick together, promoting the loss of body weight, and lowering systolic and diastolic blood pressure. According to Hernandez Figueroa et al. (*Arch Latinoam Nutr.* 2004;54:380–394): "The positive effects found suggest that a daily intake of 7 cups of green tea (3.5 g catechins) is a good choose for coronary heart disease prevention."

The evidence for green tea's potent antioxidant effects continues to accumulate. In a recent study, researchers found that green tea compounds not only directly scavenge free radicals but also enhance the effectiveness of the body's natural antioxidant systems. Research conducted at the University of California, San Francisco (UCSF), revealed that two chemicals found in green tea called gallotannin and nobotanin B may help to prevent the brain damage that occurs after strokes and other brain injuries. Results of their study showed that the two chemicals prevent brain cell death by inhibiting the action of the enzyme PARG (poly-ADP-ribose glycohydrolase), which is thought to play a key role in the destruction of brain cells that occurs after a stroke. More recent research suggests that antioxidants present in green tea may slow down the muscle wasting seen that occurs in muscular dystrophy. The study of mice with a Duchenne muscular dystrophy-like disease revealed that daily doses of green tea extract appeared to slow down deterioration of some muscle tissue, possibly by combating oxidative stress in the muscle.

Green tea polyphenols are also known to stimulate the production of several immune system cells, as well as possess antibacterial properties. Drinking green tea may also be a key flu-fighting strategy. Research has shown that drinking green tea stimulates gamma-delta T-cells that boost immunity against viruses. Furthermore, a substance in green tea called L-theanine causes T cells to secrete 10 times their normal output of the virus-fighting interferon. Results of a study by Yamamoto et al. (*Biofactors.* 2004;21:119–121) suggest that EGCG may be a potential immunotherapeutic agent against respiratory infections in immunocompromised patients, such as heavy smokers.

THERAPEUTIC DAILY AMOUNT

It is possible to buy encapsulated extracts standardized for chemicals called polyphenols. An average dose is 200mg of an extract standardized for 25 percent polyphenols. An alternative is to buy the dried herb and make tea; which is available in various grades, from twiggy, inexpensive Kikich to choice Sencha. For maximum benefit, drink up to four or five cups of green tea per day.

MAXIMUM SAFE LEVEL
Not established.

SIDE EFFECTS/CONTRAINDICATIONS
The most worrisome chemical in green tea is caffeine, which occurs in small amounts (an average of 20–30 mg per cup, if brewed for two to three minutes). This is much less caffeine than in coffee; however, an 8-ounce cup of coffee typically contains more than 100 mg of caffeine. Unless caffeine has been added, the caffeine content in green tea capsules should be approximately 5–15 mg. Breast-feeding women are advised to avoid drinking green tea and take supplements instead, as caffeine may have unwanted effects on a breast-fed baby's sleep patterns.

Griffonia simplicifolia

GENERAL DESCRIPTION
Griffonia simplicifolia is a plant native to Africa. The seeds of *Griffonia simplicifolia* are used medicinally as they are a rich source of 5–hydroxytryptophan (5-HTP; see page 265), the precursor of the neurotransmitter serotonin.

ROLE IN ANTI-AGING
The 5-HTP content of *Griffonia simplicifolia* is well absorbed from an oral dose. It easily crosses the blood-brain barrier and effectively **increases central nervous system (CNS) synthesis of serotonin.** In the CNS, serotonin levels have been implicated in the regulation of sleep, depression, anxiety, aggression, appetite, temperature, sexual behavior, and pain sensation. Therapeutic administration of 5-HTP has been shown to be effective in treating a wide variety of conditions, including depression, fibromyalgia, binge eating associated with obesity, chronic headaches, and insomnia.

 Griffonia simplicifolia may also **aid weight loss** as 5-HTP promotes earlier feelings of satiety. Ceci, et al. (*J Neural Transm.* 1989;76:109–117) studied obese female subjects with body mass index ranging between thirty and forty. The participants were administered oral 5-HTP or a placebo for five weeks—no restrictions were placed on their diet during the study period. Results showed that participants treated with 5-HTP ate less food and lost weight.

Meanwhile, research by Cangiano, et al. (*Int J Obes Relat Metab Disord.* 1998; 22:648–654) who studied obese people with type II diabetes revealed that supplementation with 5-HTP decreased their daily energy intake, by reducing carbohydrate and fat intake, and reduced their body weight. These findings suggest that 5-HTP may be safely utilized to **improve the compliance to dietary prescriptions in type II diabetes.**

Serotonin precursors are used in the **treatment of depression** based on the mechanism that a cerebral serotonin deficiency plays a role in the cause of depression. As the immediate precursor to serotonin, 5-HTP has been evaluated in double-blind studies of depression sufferers to be as effective as many of the popular SSRIs (selective serotonin reuptake inhibitors), such as Prozac and Zoloft, while demonstrating a much milder side effect profile. Serotonin deficit also plays a role in Parkinson's patients with depression. Thus, supplementation with *Griffonia simplicifolia* may be of benefit to people suffering from depression.

Griffonia simplicifolia may help to **reduce the symptoms of migraine.** 5-HTP can induce a significant decrease of the cropping out of migraine—the commonest primary pain. The latest medical research on migraine headaches indicates that migraine sufferers experience periods of unusually high MAO activity during their headaches. MAO (monoamine oxidase) is an enzyme that breaks down serotonin. Thus, boosting serotonin levels should help to counter the elevated MAO activity.

Griffonia simplicifolia may be of **benefit to people suffering from fibromyalgia,** as 5-HTP is an effective, clinically proven way to treat symptoms of the disease. Fibromyalgia sufferers will notice that the beneficial effects of the 5-HTP will increase over time. Nicolodi and Sicuteri (*Adv Exp Med Biol.* 1996; 398:373–379) studied the effect of 5-HTP and monoamine oxidase inhibitors (MAOIs) for treating fibromyalgia. They found that the combination of MAOIs with 5-HTP significantly improved fibromyalgia syndrome.

It may also help **alleviate some sleep problems.** 5-HTP has been shown to decrease the time required to get to sleep and to decrease the number of awakenings. It works well in conjunction with herbs such as valerian and hops to promote quality sleep.

Finally, *Griffonia simplicifolia* may help to **prevent hypertension.** 5-HTP has been studied as an antihypertensive agent. Fregly, et al. (*J Hypertens.* 1987;5:621–628) administered 5-HTP to rats with salt-induced hypertension. 5-HTP was able to prevent the elevation of blood pressure and cardiac hypertrophy, and provided modest protection against reduction of urinary concentrating ability. These results suggest that chronic administration of 5-HTP provides significant protection against the development of deoxycorticosterone acetate-salt-treated-induced hypertension, polydipsia, polyuria, and cardiac hypertrophia.

THERAPEUTIC DAILY AMOUNT
Refer to packaging.

MAXIMUM SAFE LEVEL
Not established.

SIDE EFFECTS/CONTRAINDICATIONS
Griffonia simplicifolia should not be combined with drugs that raise serotonin levels, for example SSRIs (such as Prozac) and other antidepressants.

People using the Parkinson's drug carbidopa are advised not to take 5-HTP as it can cause skin changes similar to those that are seen with the disease scleroderma; thus, they should also avoid *Griffonia simplicifolia*. People with kidney disease or liver disease should consult their doctor before taking *Griffonia simplicifolia*.

Hawthorn (*Crataegus laevigata, Crataegus oxyacantha, Crataegus monogyna*)

GENERAL DESCRIPTION
Hawthorn is commonly found in Europe, western Asia, North America, and North Africa. Modern medicinal preparations make use of the leaves and flowers, whereas traditional preparations use the ripe fruit.

ROLE IN ANTI-AGING
Hawthorn helps the heart because it tends to **normalize blood pressure, prevent palpitations and arrhythmias,** and **relieve angina.** Studies have confirmed that the plant is a rich source of healthy chemical compounds, including procyanidins and the flavonoids rutin, quercetin, hyperoside, and vitexin, which have been shown to dilate blood vessels of the heart and thus improve blood flow (these cardiovascular effects result from taking the herb over a prolonged period). Walker et al. (*Br J Gen Pract.* 2006;56:437–443.) gave patients with type 2 diabetes were 1200 mg hawthorn extract or placebo for 16 weeks. Results showed that there was a significant drop in mean diastolic blood pressure among those given hawthorn extract compared with those receiving the placebo. However, there was no significant group difference in systolic blood pressure reduction. Clinical trials have confirmed that hawthorn is beneficial

for people with stage II congestive heart failure. Researchers in Germany recently gave hawthorn extract to patients suffering from congestive heart failure and found the patients experienced fewer overall symptoms and showed improvements in stamina and a reduction in blood pressure and heart rate during exercise. Hawthorn is also good for arthritis as it helps **stabilize collagen,** the protein found in joints, and thus protects the joints from damage inflicted by inflammatory diseases. The bioflavonoids present in hawthorn also have potent **antioxidant** properties.

THERAPEUTIC DAILY AMOUNT

Hawthorn is sold as dried berries, capsules, and tinctures. Extracts are often standardized for one of two different chemical compounds: total flavonoids (usually calculated as vitexin) or procyanidins. An average dose is 200 mg of an extract standardized for approximately 1.5 percent vitexin or 2.0 percent flavonoids.

MAXIMUM SAFE LEVEL

Not established.

SIDE EFFECTS/CONTRAINDICATIONS

While the herb is considered nontoxic if taken as directed, consumers should be warned against taking this or any other natural remedy to treat a self-diagnosed heart condition. People taking medication for a preexisting heart condition should consult their doctor before taking products containing hawthorn. Hawthorn is not contraindicated during pregnancy or while breast-feeding.

Hops (*Humulus lupus*)

GENERAL DESCRIPTION

The hop plant is native to Europe, Asia, and North America. Hops has a reputation of promoting a calm and mellow disposition. Its **mild sedative properties** result in it being a **common ingredient in herbal sleeping remedies.** It is also used to soothe the stomach and **aid digestion.**

ROLE IN ANTI-AGING

Hops strobiles, the female flowers of the cultivated hop plant, contains two active ingredients that combine to form hop resin, a substance that causes tiredness and sleepiness. Additionally, bitter acids in hops strobiles have been found to effect sedation. As a **sleep aid,** hops is most often combined with other herbs, such as valerian and passionflower.

Hops contain prenylflavonoids. In a study published in 2000, Miranda, et al. (*Drug Metab Dispos*. 2000;28:1297–1302) found that the prenylflavonoids present in hops are potent inhibitors of the metabolic activation of hetero-cyclic amine 2-amino-3-methylimidazo [4,5-f] quinoline, or IQ, which is a car-cinogen found in cooked food—thus suggesting that hops has the potential to serve as a **cancer fighter.**

Hops also **contains oligomeric proanthocyanidin complexes (OPCs),** which many nutritional scientists consider to be today's most potent and most promising antioxidant nutrient (see discussion on OPCs later in this chapter). Hops contains OPCs in about 5 percent dry weight concentration.

THERAPEUTIC DAILY AMOUNT

The German Commission E monograph recommends a single dose of 500 mg for the treatment of anxiety and insomnia. Hops tea can be made by pouring 150 ml of boiling water over 5–10 grams of the dried fruit. Dried hops are also available in tablet or capsule form. Follow the recommended dosages given on the labels.

MAXIMUM SAFE LEVEL

Not established.

SIDE EFFECTS/CONTRAINDICATIONS

Use of hops is generally regarded as safe. Hops may increase the activity of cer-tain medications, including antidepressants, anti-anxiety, and antipsychotics. People suffering from depression are advised to avoid hops. Beer consumption is not to be considered an equivalent to supplementation with extract of the botanical.

Jujube (*Zizyphus jujuba;* Red Date Fruit)

GENERAL DESCRIPTION

Jujube (*Zizyphus jujuba*) is a dark red plumlike fruit harvested from trees originally native to northern China. Jujube has been a mainstay of traditional Chinese medicine for more than 2,000 years, and is considered to bring the heart into energy balance with other organs and the rest of the body. By bal-ancing the heart meridian, jujube is thought to calm the nerves.

ROLE IN ANTI-AGING

Jujube seed is the most widely used herb in Chinese medicine for the **treat-ment of insomnia.** Jujube seeds that are heat-treated have been shown to help treat insomnia. This is supported by a study by Han, et al. (*Saengyak Hakhoechi* 1986;16:233–238) that determined that roasting or boiling jujube seeds modestly before use increased their sedative activity. Scientific study of jujube seed has revealed several chemical constituents that are relevant to the herb's sedative properties. Han found that jujube contains chemical constituents known as alkaloids: fourteen alkaloids specific to jujube seed, collectively known as sanjoinines, have been identified and are believed to lend this herb its sleep-inducing action. Subsequently, Hwang, et al. (*Arch Pharm Res* 2001; 24: 202–206) published a study that found the alkaloids present in jujube seed inhibit a specific cellular pathway (Ca2+-ATPase) that is associated with wakefulness. Jujube also contains a noticeable concentration of flavonoids, which are a type of antioxidant. Research has shown that antioxidants have anti-anxiety effects. Meanwhile, in 1995 Weinges and Schick (*Phytochemistry* 1995; 28:505–507) found that jujube contains a compound known as dodeca-acetylprodelphinidin B3, which is composed of **oligomeric proanthocyanidins (OPCs),** an important and emerging antioxidant nutrient (see discussion on OPCs later in this chapter). In addition to helping combat insomnia, jujube has also been shown to **improve sleep quality.**

Jujube also contains chemical constituents called jujubosides. Matsuda, et al. (*Chem Pharm Bull* (Tokyo). 1999;47:1744–1748) reported that jujubosides **demonstrate potent immune-boosting activity.** Additionally, Wu, et al. (*China J Chinese Materia Medica* 1993; 18:685–687) found that jujubosides interact with the amino acid phenlyalanine, which is involved in moderating pain perception, thereby lending evidence for its traditional use as an **analgesic.**

Jujube seed extract also can **protect cells** from various insults. Kim, et al. (*Han'guk Sikp'um Yongyang Kwahak Hoechi* 1999;28:698–704) exposed spleen cells to radiation and then applied jujube seed extract. They found that the cellular DNA of the cells was far less damaged than that of irradiated cells that did not receive the extract. The mechanism for this protection, however, is yet to be discovered. Wan, et al. (*Shengwu Huaxue Yu Wuli Jinzhan* 1995;22:540–542) discovered that jujube seed extract **protected heart cells *in vivo* from oxygen-deprivation damage,** suggesting a possible value for this botanical in heart disease.

Jujube has **muscle-relaxing effects,** and in Chinese medicine it has been used to treat convulsions and arrhythmia. Animal studies suggest that jujube seed can **lower blood pressure.**

THERAPEUTIC DAILY AMOUNT

Take as directed by your practitioner.

MAXIMUM SAFE LEVEL

Not established.

SIDE EFFECTS/CONTRAINDICATIONS

Because jujube can stimulate the uterus, pregnant women should not take this supplement.

Kava (*Piper methysticum*)

GENERAL DESCRIPTION

Kava is a member of the pepper family. The rhizome (underground stem) is used medicinally. Kava root is used to **calm body and mind** and **promote restful sleep;** it is also helpful as a solution to **low mood, muscle spasms or tightness, and anxiety.** Kava's relaxant properties are created by certain oxygen-containing lipidlike compounds known as lactones or pyrones. Researchers have identified six major kavalactones (a class of lactones) and another dozen minor ones. Exactly how the kavalactones act on the brain is still being determined. Like Valium and related synthetic drugs, they may influence GABA, the neurotransmitter that acts as a brake on the central nervous system.

ROLE IN ANTI-AGING

Kava is well-known for its ability to combat anxiety and stress, and there is plenty of research to support these claims. An epidemiological study carried out in 2000 uncovered a close inverse relationship between cancer incidence and kava consumption, thus implying that the herb may also have anticancer properties.

THERAPEUTIC DAILY AMOUNT

Look for kava in capsules, liquids, and standardized extracts; a few sources offer dried kava in root pieces, cut and sifted, and as a powder. For a mildly relaxing, anxiety-relieving effect, an average dose is 200–250 mg of an extract standardized for 25 to 25 percent kavalactones.

MAXIMUM SAFE LEVEL

Not established.

SIDE EFFECTS/CONTRAINDICATIONS

IMPORTANT: Following reports linking kava to six cases of liver failure and one death in mainland Europe, products containing kava were withdrawn from sale in Spring 2002 by a number of countries, including the United Kingdom, Germany, Switzerland, France, and Ireland. Health Canada has advised consumers not to use kava or kava-containing products until it has completed a safety review of the herb. In March 2002, the U.S. FDA warned consumers about using products containing kava. In November 2002, an article published in *Morbidity and Mortality Weekly Report* (2002;29: 1065–1067) reported that two people in the United States required liver transplants after using kava for only a short time. Despite this, the official stance of the U.S. FDA Center for Food Safety and Applied Nutrition (CFSAN) remains the same. They recommend that persons who have liver disease or liver problems, or persons who are taking drug products that can affect the liver, should consult a physician before using kava-containing supplements. They also advise that consumers who use a kava-containing dietary supplement and who experience signs of illness associated with liver disease should consult their physician immediately. The FDA also warns that kava has many commonly used names, and thus consumers should be careful when checking product ingredients. Common names for kava include ava, ava pepper, intoxicating pepper, kawa, kava kava, kew, rauschpfeffer, sakau, tonga, wurzelstock, and yangona. Sorrentino et al. (*Phytomedicine.* 2006;13:542–549) conducted a chronic toxicity study of kava extract in rats. Their results found no evidence to link kava with liver toxicity. Thus, the safety of Kava remains uncertain.

Aside from recently reported cases of liver toxicity, kava is associated with few side effects. However, occasional or moderate use of the herb may cause mild nausea and other gastrointestinal disturbances. High doses of potent kava products, however, can reduce one's motor control and lead to accidents, including fatal ones if one unwisely attempts to drive or operate heavy equipment after taking it. Persistent heavy consumption of kava may cause diarrhea, an overall lethargy and apathy, or a scaly skin condition. Eliminating or cutting back on kava consumption reverses these conditions. People suffering from depression and those using drugs that act upon the central nervous system such as alcohol, barbiturates, antidepressants, and antipsychotics should avoid kava. The herb is not recommended during pregnancy and lactation.

Lemon Balm (*Melissa officinalis*)

GENERAL DESCRIPTION

The lemon balm (*Melissa officinalis*) plant is native to southern Europe; however, it can now be found throughout the world. Lemon balm has been used as a natural calming agent as early as the Middle Ages. Terpenes and eugenol have been isolated from the leaves of lemon balm, and these chemicals are associated with sedative and muscle-relaxing properties.

ROLE IN ANTI-AGING

The active ingredients in lemon balm include terpenes, flavonoids, and polyphenolics.

Lemon balm has proven **anti-herpes properties.** Dimitrova, et al. (*Acta Microbiol Bulg.* 1993;29:65–72) reported that lemon balm extract started to kill the herpes virus both in cells in culture and in the body within three hours of administration. Within just twelve hours after exposure, the virus was rendered inactive. Koytchev, et al. (*Phytomedicine* 1999;6:225–230) found that a cream made with lemon balm reduced the severity of herpes sores as early as on the second day of treatment (when the sores are the most intense). Lemon balm also reduced the spread of the infection and reduced itching, tingling, burning, redness, and other symptoms that make the sores difficult to bear. Additionally, the herpes virus was unable to become resistant to the lemon balm extract, suggesting that the herb may be valuable in treatment of recurring flare-ups.

Lemon balm may also help to combat other viral and bacterial pathogens. Englberger, et al. (*Int J Immunopharmacol.* 1988;10:729–737) found that the rosmarinic acid present in lemon balm suppressed the ability of certain bacteria to attack once inside the host organism. Mikus, et al. (*Planta Med.* 2000; 66:366–368) found that lemon balm was **highly toxic to *Trypanosoma* bacteria,** the bacteria responsible for Chagas disease, with which the chronic form is associated with a decrease in life expectancy by nine years. Yamasaki, et al. (*Biol Pharm Bull.* 1998;21:829–833) found that lemon balm extract was **highly effective in inhibiting HIV-1 infection.** In addition to the active chemical ingredients mentioned so far, lemon balm also contains tannins, which are thought to lend **antiviral effects,** and eugenol, which **kills bacteria.** Taken collectively, this research suggests that lemon balm has **potent anti-infective properties.**

Lemon balm is also now recognized as an **important antioxidant.** Hohmann, et al. (Planta Med. 1999;65:576–578) found that lemon balm contains a very high concentration of phenols, chemicals that act as potent scavengers of free radicals. The antioxidant capacity of lemon balm is still being discovered today, in 2002 Patora and Klimek (*Acta Pol Pharm.* 2002;59: 139–143) isolated three new flavonoids previously unidentified in this herb.

Lemon balm may also help in the **treatment of gastric ulcers.** Khayyal, et al. (*Arzneimittelforschung* 2001;51:545–553) found that lemon balm extract was as effective as the ulcer medication cimetidine in reducing the acid output and mucin secretion typical of gastric ulcers. The authors suspect the apparent anti-ulcerogenic activity may be due to their flavonoid content and to their free-radical-scavenging properties.

Exciting new research indicates a potential role for lemon balm in **improving memory.** In a study by Wake, et al. (*J Ethnopharmacol.* 2000;69:105–114), lemon balm demonstrated a high capacity to **enhance the activity of nerve cell receptors involved in memory.** In an important study by Kennedy, et al. (*Pharmacol Biochem Behav.* 2002;72:953–964), researchers administered lemon balm to twenty healthy young men and women for one week. Cognitive testing revealed **significant sustained improvement in attention and memory.** Additionally, the study participants reported feeling calmer yet more alert. According to the researchers, lemon balm acts on one of the biochemical pathways that may become debilitated with Alzheimer's disease; thus, they are hopeful that future studies may prove lemon balm to be a suitable natural agent in the fight against Alzheimer's disease.

Paladini, et al. (*J Pharm Pharmacol.* 1999;51:519–526) isolated the antioxidant apigenin in lemon balm, from which they synthesized a potent sleep-promoting chemical. Wagner and Sprinkmeyer (*Dtsch Apoth Z* 1973; 113:1159 [in German]) conducted the only experimental study to date on lemon balm in which its **sleep-promoting properties** were verified. Dressing, et al. (*Therapiewoche* 1992;42:726–736 [in German], *Psychopharmakotherapie* 1996;6: 32–40) found that **lemon balm and valerian taken in combination are particularly effective at combating insomnia and improving sleep quality.** Lemon balm may also promote sleep in an indirect manner by **improving pain associated with inflammatory conditions,** such as arthritis and chronic joint problems. Work by Soulimani, et al. (*Planta Med* 1991;57:105–109) revealed an analgesic (painkilling) action of lemon balm extract when it was administered to lab animals. Related work by Peake, et al. (*Int J Immunopharmacol.* 1991; 13:853–857) identified the presence of the chemical rosmarinic acid in lemon balm. Rosmarinic acid is known to inhibit one of the pathways involved in triggering the inflammatory response.

Finally, lemon balm has been found to be useful in **treating Graves' disease,** a disorder in which the disease's antibodies bind to thyroid stimulating hormone (TSH) and cause the thyroid gland to become overactive. A hyperactive thyroid gland can cause sleeplessness, fatigue and weakness, feeling warm and sweating, rapid irregular heartbeat, and other symptoms. Auf'mkolk, et al.

(*Endocrinology.* 1985;116:1687–1693) found that extracts of lemon balm were able to inactivate the antibodies of Graves' disease and prevent them from binding to TSH.

THERAPEUTIC DAILY AMOUNT

Refer to packaging. The German Commission E recommends drinking several cups of lemon balm tea (containing 1.5–4.5 grams of the herb) each day. Some sources recommend taking 160–200 mg of concentrated lemon balm extract thirty minutes to one hour before bed for the treatment of insomnia. Highly concentrated topical extract ointments for herpes can be applied three to four times per day to lesions.

MAXIMUM SAFE LEVEL

Not established.

SIDE EFFECTS/CONTRAINDICATIONS

No adverse effects from lemon balm have been reported. People with Graves' disease or other thyroid conditions should not use lemon balm without consulting a physician. Because lemon balm can promote menstruation, women who are pregnant should not use it. Because some animal studies have found that the herb may raise pressure in the eye, people suffering from glaucoma should avoid lemon balm.

Licorice (*Glycyrrhiza glabra, Glycyrrhiza uralensis*)

GENERAL DESCRIPTION

Licorice is an extract prepared from the sweet-tasting dried roots and underground stems of a shrub that grows in subtropical climates. For more than three thousand years, licorice has been used to treat **coughs, colds, congestion, rashes, arthritis, constipation, cancer,** and **hepatitis,** and to promote **healing of stomach and mouth ulcers.**

ROLE IN ANTI-AGING

The herb's natural sweetness and flavor (it is fifty times sweeter than sugar) are due to its high content of glycyrrhizin. Glycyrrhizin is also responsible for most of licorice's medicinal properties, including its ability to reduce inflammation, soothe throat tissues, and reduce allergy symptoms.

The ulcer-healing compounds in licorice are thought to be flavonoids. They apparently work by promoting the overall health of the gastrointestinal system rather than reducing the secretion of stomach acid that triggers ulcers. One study found that licorice extract exerted a cytotoxic effect upon N-nitrosamines—carcinogenic compounds found in foods. A recent Russian study discovered that the antitumor and antimetastatic effects of cyclophosphan (cyclophosphamide) are potentiated by licorice extract. This research implies that this commonly used herb may have useful anticancer properties.

THERAPEUTIC DAILY AMOUNT
Retailers sell licorice in powders, capsules, lozenges, concentrated drops, tinctures, and extracts. Chewable tablets and other licorice products for extended anti-ulcer therapy now often contain very little (just 2 percent or less) of the active component glycyrrhizin (also known as glycyrrhizic acid). These deglycyrrhizinated licorice (DGL) products cause fewer side effects and are much safer for long-term use than glycyrrhizin-containing licorice. An average dose of DGL licorice is 200 mg.

MAXIMUM SAFE LEVEL
Not established.

SIDE EFFECTS/CONTRAINDICATIONS
Taking high or repeated doses of licorice extracts containing glycyrrhizin may cause serious adverse health effects related to salt and water retention (including elevated blood pressure). If you wish to use licorice medicinally, it is wise to discuss it with your doctor first. Some health authorities warn that you should not take licorice for more than four to six weeks without medical advice. Individuals with high blood pressure, glaucoma, diabetes, kidney, or liver disease; pregnant and nursing women; or those who are taking hormonal therapy should be extremely cautious if using the herb. People taking digitalis or who have had a stroke or who have heart disease should only take licorice under the direction of a doctor.

Lycium Berry Extract (Lycium Chinese Mill, Gou Qi Zi, Wolfberry)

GENERAL DESCRIPTION
In traditional Chinese medicine, lycium berry extract has been used as a liver and kidney tonic, to boost immune function, to improve male urinary function, to improve vision and hearing, to increase appetite, and to reduce sleeplessness.

ROLE IN ANTI-AGING
In clinical studies, lycium polysaccharide has been found to be an **important immune stimulator.** In lab animals, lycium has been shown to **improve**

macrophage and antibody activities. It has also been shown to inhibit sarcoma, a type of cancer, in lab animals. By doing so, lycium prolonged the life span of the animals by up to 35 percent. Case studies in human trials also suggest similar **immune-enhancing, cancer-fighting capacities.** Additionally, the immune function in cancer patients undergoing chemotherapy has been improved by administration of lycium.

Lycium contains zeaxanthin, a potent type of antioxidant, and as such this herb can convey important **cellular protection.** Research by Kim, et al. (*Research Communications in Molecular Pathology and Pharmacology.* Sept 1997;3:301–314) determined that zeaxanthins present in lycium were particularly able to **protect the liver against toxic insults.** Kim also found that the zeaxanthin present in lycium was able to inhibit the fibrotic activity of liver cells, offering a therapeutic potential for this botanical in the future prevention or treatment of liver fibrosis.

THERAPEUTIC DAILY AMOUNT
Take as directed by packaging or by a practitioner.

MAXIMUM SAFE LEVEL
Not established.

SIDE EFFECTS/CONTRAINDICATIONS
No severe side effects reported.

Milk Thistle (*Silybum marianum, Carduus marianus*)

GENERAL DESCRIPTION
Milk thistle has been used medicinally for more than 2,000 years. The well-known seventeenth-century pharmacist Nicholas Culpeper recommended the plant for the treatment of jaundice as well as citing its use for opening "obstructions" of the liver and spleen. The parts of the plant used in medicine are the seeds of the dried flower. These seeds contain a bioflavonoid complex known as silymarin. Three compounds make up the silymarin complex: silibinin, silidianin, and silicristin. Silibinin is the most active and is largely responsible for the medicinal powers of silymarin. The dried fruit (known as achenes) is used medicinally.

ROLE IN ANTI-AGING
Many people take milk thistle regularly to **protect their livers from the effects of alcohol,** heavy metals, and drugs, and as needed after exposure to solvents, pesticides, bacteria from food poisoning, and other toxins. Studies since the

1930s, conducted mainly in Germany, confirmed that silymarin works to stabilize liver cell membranes and act as an antioxidant to protect liver cells from free-radical damage. Sonnenbichler and Zetl (*Assessment and Management of Hepatobiliary Disease*, ed. L Okolicsanyi, G Csomos, G Crepaldi. Berlin: Springer-Verlag, 1987, 265–272) demonstrated that it helps **regenerate healthy liver cells** and **boosts the liver's ability to filter toxins from the blood.** Palsciano, et al. (*Curr Ther Res* 1994;S5:S37–45) found that the antioxidant activity of milk thistle seed extract reduced the liver damage typically seen in patients who take prescription antipsychotic drugs for extended periods. More recently, Schuppen, et al. (*Zeits Allgemeinmed* 1998;74:577–584) showed that silymarin has the ability to **block fibrosis,** a process that contributes to the eventual development of cirrhosis in people with inflammatory liver conditions caused by alcohol abuse or hepatitis. Double-blind clinical trials suggest that milk thistle **helps the liver return to a healthy state** once a person stops drinking. Results of studies by Ferenci, et al. (*J Hepatol* 1989;9:105–113) and Velussi, et al. (*J Hepatology* 1997;26:871–879) suggest that it may **improve the quality of life** and **possibly even improve life expectancy of people with liver cirrhosis.**

Naausato, et al. (*J Hepatol* 1991;12:290–295) found that milk thistle alters bile makeup and, therefore, **may reduce the risk of gallstones;** however, this use of milk thistle has yet to be verified with human clinical trials.

THERAPEUTIC DAILY AMOUNT

Milk thistle comes in capsules, liquids, and teas; silymarin (the chemical constituent thought to be responsible for milk thistle's medical benefits) does not dissolve well in water, so the teas are very weak. The most popular products are standardized extracts of silymarin. The recommended daily dose for treatment of liver disease and impaired liver function is 420–600 mg of an extract standardized for 80 percent silymarin.

MAXIMUM SAFE LEVEL

Not established.

SIDE EFFECTS/CONTRAINDICATIONS

Taking milk thistle products does not seem to cause any adverse effects either immediately or over the long term. In fact, the plant's young (non-spiny) leaves and stems were once consumed as food in Europe. In some individuals, milk thistle may have a mild, transient laxative effect.

Mushrooms, Medicinal: Maitake (*Grifola frondosa*), Reishi (*Ganoderma lucidum*), Shiitake (*Lentinus edodes*)

GENERAL DESCRIPTION

There are more than 100,000 varieties of mushroom on earth, some 700 of which are edible. In laboratory tests (mostly in Japan and China), about fifty species have been confirmed to have some medicinal properties. Mushrooms are available in a variety of forms, including whole, dried, powdered, tinctures, capsules, tablets, and tea. Most edible mushrooms are rich in vitamins, minerals, fiber, and amino acids.

Maitake: Known in Japan as the "dancing mushroom," the maitake mushroom is called the "hen of the woods" by American mushroom hunters.

Reishi: Reishi has been used in Chinese medicine as a treatment for fatigue, asthma, insomnia, and cough for more than 2,000 years.

Shiitake: The shiitake mushroom (*Lentinus edodes*) has been revered in Asia for centuries, both as a food and as a medicine. Its most studied active ingredient is the polysaccharide lentinan.

ROLE IN ANTI-AGING

Maitake: An extract from maitake mushrooms called D fraction is marketed in the United States and Japan as a dietary supplement. D fraction has been shown to **stimulate the production of immune cells** and increases their effectiveness. Results of a study of D-fraction by Kodama et al. (*J Med Food.* 2004;7:141–145.) led the researchers to conclude: ". . . its administration may enhance host defense against foreign pathogens and protect healthy individuals from infectious diseases." D-fraction may also prevent healthy cells from becoming cancerous, help prevent the spread of cancer (metastasis), and slow the growth of tumors. Results of a later study by Kodama et al. (*Nutrition.* 2005;21:624–629) suggest that D-Fraction can decrease the dosage of chemotherapy drugs needed to treat cancer by increasing the proliferation, differentiation, and activation of immunocompetent cells. However, results of a study by Devere, et al. (Urology 2002;60:640–644) suggest that supplements containing shiitake mushroom extract are no help in the fight against prostate cancer. The study of patients with various stages of prostate cancer, all of whom took capsules of shiitake mushroom extract three times a day for four to six months, revealed no benefits. Furthermore, 38 percent of the patients' conditions worsened during the study. Unlike other mushroom extracts, D fraction is effective not only by injection but orally as well. Two other fractions, X and ES, have been used to lessen the side effects of chemotherapy. As an HIV/AIDS treatment, maitake may help prevent the destruction of T cells. In animal studies, maitake extracts have lowered blood pressure and glucose levels. Maitake mushrooms, fresh or preserved, taste good and can be used in a variety of food preparations. Maitake tea, juice, powder, and granules are available. A liquid extract of maitake D fraction is available to health professionals.

Reishi: Reishi mushrooms contain several constituents, including sterols, coumarin, mannitol, polysaccharides, and triterpenoids called ganoderic acids. Ganoderic acids lower blood pressure, lower LDL ("bad") cholesterol levels, and reduce the "stickiness" of platelets—all of which help to **lower the risk of coronary artery disease.** Animal studies and some preliminary human studies have suggested that reishi extracts may be beneficial for the treatment of **diabetes** and **cancer.** Reishi mushrooms may be of use in the treatment of cancer. Jiang et al. (*Int J Oncol.* 2004;24:1093–1099) found that Reishi mushrooms were able to induce apoptosis, inhibit cell proliferation, and suppress cell migration of highly invasive human prostate cancer cells. Whilst another study by Jiang et al. (*Nutr Cancer.* 2004;49:209–216.) found that Reishi mushrooms suppressed the growth of breast cancer cells.

Shiitake: Shiitake extract can be used to **boost the immune system, protect the body from cancer (and even shrink existing tumors), lower blood cholesterol levels, reduce blood pressure,** and **combat viruses and bacteria.** Shiitake contains vitamins, minerals, amino acids, and a number of polysaccharides, which are linked to countering cancer, primarily by promoting immune function rather than attacking cancer cells directly. Following the discovery that cancer patients given lentinan have increased survival times and a more positive prognosis, the Japanese have recently begun prescribing the polysaccharide as an adjunct to chemotherapy. Other research also indicates shiitake extracts may assist in the treatment of AIDS.

THERAPEUTIC DAILY AMOUNT

Maitake: 3–7 grams per day of the supplement is recommended. Maitake mushrooms, fresh or preserved, taste good and can be used in a variety of food preparations. Maitake tea, juice, powder, and granules are available. A liquid extract of maitake D-fraction is available to health professionals.

Reishi: 1.5–9 grams per day of the crude dried mushroom; 1–1.5 grams per day in powdered form.

Shiitake: products vary in potency; follow dosage directions on labels.

MAXIMUM SAFE LEVEL

Not established.

SIDE EFFECTS/CONTRAINDICATIONS

Maitake: no reported side effects.

Reishi: continuous use of reishi over three to six months may produce dizziness, dry mouth and throat, nosebleeds, and abdominal upset; however, these side effects are quite rare. Reishi is not recommended for individuals taking anticoagulant drugs.

Shiitake: safe and nontoxic, even in very large doses.

Olive Leaf Extract (*Olea europa*)

GENERAL DESCRIPTION

A staple of folk medicine for centuries, olive leaves have been used for tea or chopped up as a salad ingredient. Olive leaf extract is now recognized for its ability to fight **viral and bacterial infections.** The plant chemical oleuropein is the source of olive leaf's infection-fighting ability. Oleuropein interferes with the production of amino acids that are essential to bacteria and viruses.

ROLE IN ANTI-AGING

Oleuropein **lowers blood pressure** and **dilates the coronary arteries** when given to animals intravenously. Furthermore, in vitro studies revealed that oleuropein **inhibits the oxidation of LDL "bad" cholesterol.** Combined, these facts may help to explain why the traditional Mediterranean diet is linked to a decreased risk of atherosclerosis.

Studies have indicated that olive leaf extract can kill the antibiotic-resistant, and potentially fatal, bacteria *Staphylococcus aureus.* Olive leaf may also be useful in fighting HIV and AIDS. In addition to its antimicrobial effects, oleuropein has antioxidant and anti-inflammatory properties.

THERAPEUTIC DAILY AMOUNT

Dried leaf extracts containing 6–15 percent oleuropein are available; however, a standard therapeutic amount has not been established.

MAXIMUM SAFE LEVEL

Not established.

SIDE EFFECTS/CONTRAINDICATIONS

Olive leaf can irritate the stomach lining; therefore, it should always be taken with meals.

Pregnant women should not take olive leaf extract as safety during pregnancy has not yet been established. Olive Leaf Extract may inactivate antibiotics and therefore should not be taken while taking antibiotics.

OPCs (Oligomeric Proanthocyanidin Complexes)

GENERAL DESCRIPTION

Oligomeric proanthocyanidin complexes (OPCs) are a specific category of flavonoids. Flavonoids are potent antioxidants that occur naturally in plants and offer them defense against invasions from fungi, toxins, and environmental stress. Animals, including humans, are not able to produce flavonoids, but we are able to absorb and use plant flavonoids. OPCs' ability to fight cell-damaging free radicals means that they could be useful for the prevention of any disease where oxidative stress is involved, for example cardiovascular disease and cancer, as well as aging itself. The richest sources of OPCs are found in red wine extract, grape seed extract, and pine bark extract.

ROLE IN ANTI-AGING

Red wine extract has been shown to have a number of benefits on the cardiovascular system. Halpern, et al. (*J Int Med Res.* 1998;26:171–180) found that red wine extract **prevents platelet aggregation by relaxing arterial tissue.** In a study by Fremont, et al. (*Life Sci* 1999;64:2511–2521), a red wine extract containing 50 percent proanthocyanidins prevented oxidation of LDL in pigs. Auger, et al. (*J Nutr.* 2002;132:1207–1213) determined that red wine extract **reduced levels of cholesterol, triglycerides, and apolipoprotein B** (the protein component of LDL), while also increasing the activity of an antioxidant enzyme produced by the liver by a remarkable 67 percent. In 2002, Sato, et al. (*Free Radic Biol Med.* 2001;15;31:729–737) found that red wine extract **improves post-ischemic heart function while reducing the signal that prompts for heart cell death.**

Red wine has also been shown to have **potent anticancer effects** in numerous clinical studies. Caderni, et al. (*Carcinogenesis.* 2000;21: 1965–1969) found that rats exposed to a cancer-inducing chemical were less likely to develop cancer if they received red wine extract as part of their diet. Meanwhile, Kamei, et al. (*Cancer Biother Radiopharm.* 1998;13:447–452) determined that OPCs from red wine extract suppressed the growth of human colon cancer cells.

De Ruvo, et al. (*Int J Dev Neurosci.* 2000;18:359–366) found that red wine extract **prevented the death of rat brain cells exposed to cell-damaging**

agents. Red wine extract did this better than vitamin E, and to the same extent of vitamin C. De Ruvo attributes this antidegenerative effect to the free-radical scavenging OPCs present in red wine extract.

Grape seed extract has been shown to have numerous anti-aging benefits. In a study involving rabbits fed a high-cholesterol atherosclerotic diet, Yamokoshi, et al. (*Atherosclerosis* 1999 142:139–149) found that the rabbits that also received grape seed extract avoided a ten-fold increase in their levels of peroxides (a marker of oxidation) that occurred in rabbits that did not receive the grape seed supplement. Yamokoshi's work suggests that the OPCs present in grape seed extract trap reactive oxygen species (ROS) before they can oxidize LDL. Additionally, Preuss, et al. (*J Med.* 2000;31:227–246) found that the activity of OPCs present in grape seed extract on **lowering LDL** can be boosted by coadministration of chromium in a niacin-bound form.

Singletary and Meline (*Nutr Cancer.* 2001;39:252–258) found that lab animals fed grape seed OPCs exhibited an 88 percent **inhibition of tumor growth** in the colon. Previously, the University of Illinois researchers found that topical application of grape seed extract inhibited skin tumor activity by as much as 73 percent in mice. Grape seed extract has also been shown to **inhibit the growth of breast cancer cells, lung cancer cells, and stomach cancer cells.** At the same time, it has also been shown to **promote the growth and viability of normal lung and stomach cells.**

Grape seed extract can help to **protect neurons from damage caused by free radicals,** and thus may help to prevent neurodegenerative diseases, such as Alzheimer's disease. Bagchi, et al. (*Gen Pharmacol.* 1998;30:771–776) found that OPCs from grape seed extract offered protection against damage to brain tissue commonly found with exposure to free radicals, including DNA breakage. In fact, Bagchi found that grape seed extract was far superior to vitamin C and beta-carotene in preventing DNA breakage (50 percent protection by grape seed extract, versus 14 percent by vitamin C and 11 percent by beta-carotene).

The OPCs present in grape seed extract may also help the immune system. Nair, et al. (*Clin Diagn Lab Immunol.* 2002;9:470–476) found that grape seed extract **promotes the production of interferon** (a substance that activates our defenses against viruses) by TH1 cells, thus suggesting that it may help to ward off viral infections.

Pine bark has been used medicinally by Native Americans for hundreds of years, and in the mid 1900s, Dr. Jack Masquelier of the University of Bordeaux in France found that pine bark contains oligomeric proanthocyanidin complexes (OPCs) that boosted the activity of vitamin C (now recognized as a primary anti-scurvy nutrient), which is also present in the bark, and offered its own independent health-promoting properties. Since Masquelier's discovery, pine bark extract has been shown to **protect cells from oxidative damage, treat venous insufficiency, and boost the immune system.**

Rong, et al. (*Biotechnol Ther* 1994–95;5:117–126) found that pine bark extract protected vascular endothelial cells (cells that line blood vessels) from oxidative damage. This suggests that pine bark extract may help to **guard against atherosclerosis, and thus cardiovascular disease,** as endothelial damage plays an important role in the pathology of atherosclerosis.

Some of pine barks purported immune-boosting and anticancer effects may be due to its effect upon macrophages. Park, et al. (*FEBS Lett.* 2000; 465:93–97) found that pine bark extract **increases secretion of tumor necrosis factor** (TNF-alpha) by activated macrophages. TNF-alpha is a protein that kills tumor cells. Pine bark has also been shown to be effective in treating cryptosporidiosis, a diarrheal disease caused by the microscopic parasite *Cryptosporidium parvum.*

THERAPEUTIC DAILY AMOUNT

The optimal intake of OPCs is yet to be established. Dose will vary depending upon the supplement; therefore, refer to packaging.

MAXIMUM SAFE LEVEL

Not established.

SIDE EFFECTS/CONTRAINDICATIONS

None known.

Passionflower (*Passiflora incarnata*)

GENERAL DESCRIPTION

Passionflower is a climbing vine native to North, Central, and South America. It has a long history as a folk remedy for anxiety. It recently has gained a body of scientific studies that support this action. The leaves, stems, and flowers are used medicinally.

ROLE IN ANTI-AGING

It was originally thought that a group of harman alkaloids were the active constituents in passionflower; however, recent research suggests that its benefits may be due to flavonoids. Wolfman, et al. (*Pharmacol Biochem Behav.*

1994;47:1–4) isolated a flavonoid called chrysin from passionflower, and subsequently found that it has **strong anti-anxiety properties.** Zanoli, et al. (*Fitoterapia.* 2000;71 Suppl 1:S117–S123) concluded from their studies that the chrysin in passionflower exerts its anti-anxiety activity by **activating receptors of the neurotransmitter GABA,** which is responsible for calming brain activity. In a comparison of passionflower extract versus the prescription drug oxazepam for the treatment of generalized anxiety disorder, Akhondzadeh, et al. (*J Clin Pharm Ther* 2001;26:369–373) found that passionflower extract was highly effective for the management of anxiety without causing adverse cognitive effects. Additionally, Wolfman, et al. (*Pharmacol Biochem Behav.* 1994;47:1–4) found that chrysin obtained from passionflower was as effective in countering anxiety as benzodiazepene-type prescription sleeping medications.

Chrysin relaxes smooth muscle and thus passionflower has been used to relieve pain. In particular, passionflower has been used to relieve sciatica. The scientific studies and folk use of passionflower collectively indicate usefulness of passionflower for **sleep difficulties, including insomnia, that are a direct result of worry, overworking, stress-related emotions, and pain.**

Because chrysin relaxes smooth muscle, it has been studied for the treatment of cardiovascular diseases. Villar, et al. (*Planta Med.* 2002;68:847–850) found that a six-week long supplementation of chrysin in the diet of rats **reduced hypertension** and improved the performance of veins and arteries. Furthermore, Duarte, et al. (*Planta Med.* 2001;67:567–569) found that chrysin relaxed the aorta after it was stimulated by the stress hormone noradrenaline.

A discovery by Shin, et al. (*Bioorg Med Chem Lett.* 1999;9:869–874) suggests that chrysin may be useful in the treatment of diabetes. Results of their study showed that compounds derived from chrysin were found to have a **hypoglycemic effect** on the diabetic state.

Chrysin may also **protect cells from carcinogens.** Lautraite, et al. (*Mutagenesis* 2002;17:45–53) found that cells exposed to toxic concentrations of cancer-causing substances along with chrysin *in vitro* were less likely to develop DNA damage.

Another active chemical in passionflower, the methanol extract, demonstrates important health-promoting potential as well. Dhawan and Sharma (*Fitoterapia* 2002;73:397–399) discovered that the methanol extract from the leaves of passionflower was as effective as codeine (a common ingredient in prescription cough medications) in **suppressing cough.** Methanol extract of passionflower has also been found to have value in treating drug and alcohol addiction. The extract contains a very high concentration of flavonoids, which not only reflects the anti-anxiety aspect of passionflower but also gives the extract its unique **anti-addiction properties.** In two separate studies of mice bred to be addicted to either tetrahydrocannabinol or alcohol, the mice treated with the passionflower methanol extract were able to break their addictions faster and with fewer withdrawal effects than untreated mice.

THERAPEUTIC DAILY AMOUNT

4–8 grams per day of the dried herb. 5–10 ml of passionflower tincture can be taken three to four times per day. European herbalists recommend passionflower products containing no less than 0.8 percent total flavonoids.

MAXIMUM SAFE LEVEL

Not established.

SIDE EFFECTS/CONTRAINDICATIONS

Passionflower is generally safe if used as directed. Because some of its constituent chemicals mimic the activity of antidepressant drugs known as MAO inhibitors, people taking this type of medication should not take passionflower. Passionflower also contains the compounds harman and harmaline that have been shown to affect the uterus; therefore, passionflower should not be taken during pregnancy. Because passionflower acts on smooth muscle including heart tissue, high doses should be avoided as they may cause heartbeat irregularities in some people.

Rye Extract (*Secale cereale*)

GENERAL DESCRIPTION

Rye extract is rich in vitamins, minerals, enzymes (including coenzyme Q_{10}), and phytochemicals such as lignans, isoflavones, and beta 1,3 glucan.

ROLE IN ANTI-AGING

Rye is commonly used to treat **colds and flu, rashes, wounds, burns, fatigue, teeth and gums, and cold sores.** Coenzyme Q_{10} is thought to treat heart disease and lower high blood pressure; thus, rye extract may be **beneficial for the cardiovascular system** in general. Beta 1,3 glucan, which is also found in the extract, is known to help the immune system fight **bacterial, viral, fungal, and parasitic infections** by activating key immune cells known as macrophages. Studies have shown that rye extract can also improve the symptoms of **benign prostatic hyperplasia** (BPH).

THERAPEUTIC DAILY AMOUNT

Rye extract is available in drops, creams, gels, and sprays. Follow product label instructions.

MAXIMUM SAFE LEVEL

Not established.

SIDE EFFECTS/CONTRAINDICATIONS

No side effects have been reported; however, those with an allergy to rye should not take rye extract.

Saw Palmetto (*Serenoa repens*)

GENERAL DESCRIPTION

Saw palmetto was traditionally used as a remedy for chronic cystitis (bladder inflammation), urinary tract infections, sex hormone disorders, impotence and frigidity, and respiratory tract diseases. Today, saw palmetto is most widely used as an herbal remedy for **benign prostatic hypertrophy** (BPH) symptoms, including discomfort and excessive nighttime urination.

ROLE IN ANTI-AGING

Saw palmetto contains a number of compounds with potential therapeutic effects. Researchers have not yet identified with certainty the BPH related compounds, although the evidence points to certain fatty acids and sterols with either enzyme or hormone-related effects. A recent study found that a saw palmetto extract significantly reduced excessive urination both at night and during the day. 85 percent of the study's participants had their condition either stabilize or improve over the study's three-year period. Results of a study by Goldmann, et al.. (*Cell Biol Int.* 2001;25:1117–1124) revealed that saw palmetto berry extract (SPBE) inhibited the growth of prostate cancer cells and decreased the expression of the enzyme Cox-2. Increased expression of Cox-2 is associated with an increased risk of prostate cancer. These findings suggest that saw palmetto may help to protect against this common disease. However, results of a recent study by Bonnar-Pizzorno et al. (*Nutr Cancer.* 2006;55:21–27) failed to find any evidence that saw palmetto reduces the risk of developing prostate cancer. Animal studies have suggested that the fruit and extracts also have anti-allergic and immune-system-stimulating properties.

THERAPEUTIC DAILY AMOUNT

Saw palmetto is sold in capsules, liquids, and standardized extract; it is frequently combined with pygeum (*Pygeum africanum*), an herb with a somewhat less-established reputation for improving prostate health. Although saw palmetto is also available as a tea, the fatty acids in the herb thought to be at least partly responsible for its effects do not dissolve well in water; thus, drinking a tea would not be effective against BPH. An average dose of saw palmetto is 160 mg of an extract standardized for 85 to 95 percent fatty acids and sterols.

MAXIMUM SAFE LEVEL

Not established.

SIDE EFFECTS/CONTRAINDICATIONS

No long-term toxicity has been reported. Large amounts of the berry are reported to cause diarrhea. Given saw palmetto's well-documented hormonal actions, the herb may interact with prostate medicines or hormonal treatments (including hormone replacement therapy), possibly canceling out their effectiveness or causing unwanted side effects. Saw palmetto should also be avoided in patients with a hormone-dependent illness such as breast cancer, and those who are pregnant or lactating.

St. John's Wort (*Hypericum perforatum*)

GENERAL DESCRIPTION

St. John's wort has long been used to treat anxiety, depression, insomnia, diarrhea, stomach irritation, fluid retention, bladder ailments, kidney and lung disorders, and even cancer. Today, the herb is used to alleviate menstrual cramps, as a potential tool in fighting viral infections, and as an antidepressant.

ROLE IN ANTI-AGING

Well-controlled studies show that St. John's wort alleviates symptoms of **depression.** Studies show that St. John's wort is much more effective than a placebo and provokes response rates that are similar to or even slightly better than conventional antidepressants such as Prozac. Research has also determined that St. John's wort is better tolerated than conventional antidepressants. In June 2000, German researchers announced results of a study demonstrating the value of St. John's wort in fighting bacteria. Researchers from the University of Freiburg found that low concentrations of hyperforin, one of the active ingredients in St. John's wort, **inhibited the growth of several types of bacteria,** including *Staphylococcus aureus* and *Corynebacterium diphtheria*. Particularly noteworthy is the ability of hyperforin to inhibit a bacterium (methicillin-resistant *S. aureus*) that is resistant to penicillin and other antibiotics. Researchers are currently investigating the use of hypericin, another active constituent of the herb, to fight retroviruses such as the AIDS virus HIV.

Newly published research by Lawvere et al. (*Complement Ther Med.* 2006; 14:175–184) suggests that St. John's wort may be of help to people who want to stop smoking. The researchers found that the herb appeared to help people who had recently stopped smoking remain smoke-free. The authors conclude: "St. John's wort demonstrates feasibility for use in smoking cessation. If St. John's wort proves to be effective in larger controlled studies, it could represent a less expensive, more readily accessible and well-tolerated agent to promote tobacco cessation."

THERAPEUTIC DAILY AMOUNT

St. John's wort is usually sold dried and in concentrated drops, tinctures, and extracts. Its antidepressant effects may not be apparent until it is taken daily for three to four weeks. An average dose of a standardized extract containing 0.3 percent hypericin is 200–300 mg.

MAXIMUM SAFE LEVEL

Not established.

SIDE EFFECTS/CONTRAINDICATIONS

The most common side effects from taking St. John's wort are mild nausea, stomachache, lack of appetite and tiredness, although these are not common. A very small percentage of people taking high daily doses of St. John's wort may experience increased sensitivity to sunlight. Avoid the herb during pregnancy. Excessive doses may potentiate existing MAO inhibitor therapy, and may cause an allergic reaction in sensitive individuals. St John's wort should not be used at the same time as prescription antidepressants. Recent reports suggest that St John's wort may increase the risk of organ transplant rejection by reducing the effectiveness of the antirejection drug cyclosporine. Therefore, people waiting for organ transplants should not take St. John's wort. Recent reports suggest that St. John's wort may interact with kava and cause liver toxicity. Therefore, until this potential interaction has been clarified, St. John's wort should not be taken at the same time as kava.

Tea Tree Oil (*Melaleuca alternifolia*)

GENERAL DESCRIPTION

Tea tree oil is distilled from the leaves of *Melaleuca alternifolia,* a small tree native to Australia. Tea tree oil earned widespread fame in the 1700s, when

Captain Cook enthused about the oil's wound- and burn-healing properties. Australian soldiers were issued tea tree oil as a disinfectant in World War II. Today, tea tree oil is sold as a **topical antiseptic** and remedy for a whole variety of ailments, including sunburn, sores, cuts, arthritis, bruises, insect bites, warts, acne, fungal infections, mouth ulcers, and dandruff.

ROLE IN ANTI-AGING

Tea tree oil's main infection fighting ingredient is terpinen-4-ol, a compound that weakens bacteria so that the immune system can fight them more effectively and kills a variety of microbes, including some that other standard antibiotics are ineffective against. In 1995 an in vitro study revealed that an 0.5 percent solution of tea tree oil (lower than that found in commercial concentrations) can both inhibit and **kill certain antibiotic-resistant bacteria** that are common in hospitals, such as the potentially deadly bacteria *Staphylococcus aureus*. In 2005 Messager et al. (*J Hosp Infect.* 2005;59:220–228) found that a Tea Tree Oil handwash was effective at reducing the activity of *Escherichia coli*. Results of a study by Farnan et al. (J *Laryngol Otol.* 2005;119:198–201.) suggest that Tea Tree Oil may be of use in the treatment of otitis externa or "Swimmer's Ear." Other studies have shown that the oil is also effective in fighting organisms responsible for **vaginal infections,** including trichomonas vaginalis and *Candida albicans*.

THERAPEUTIC DAILY AMOUNT

Tea tree oil is used externally in concentrations of 0.4 to 100 percent, depending on what part of the body it is applied to and for what purpose. It should not be taken internally.

MAXIMUM SAFE LEVEL

Not established.

SIDE EFFECTS/CONTRAINDICATIONS

Tea tree oil can irritate sensitive skin; however, it is generally regarded as safe to use when applied externally. Tea tree oil should never be swallowed as it may cause nerve damage.

Tribulus terrestris (Puncture Vine Fruit)

GENERAL DESCRIPTION

Tribulus terrestris has been used for centuries in traditional Ayurvedic medicine. The active ingredients are extracted from the fruits, which contain alkaloids, resins, tannins, saponins, sugars, sterols, essential oil, peroxidase, diastase, and glucoside.

ROLE IN ANTI-AGING

Tribulus terrestris is a proven herbal remedy for **depression,** as harmine, the main active ingredient of the plant, is a very effective monoamine oxidase inhibitor (MAOI). Many antidepressants used in conventional medicine are MAOIs, which work by gradually **increasing levels of the neurotransmitter dopamine.**

High dopamine levels in men are known to stimulate the pituitary gland to release lutenizing hormones, which leads to an **increase in testosterone levels.** As recent studies have suggested that older men may benefit from hormone replacement therapy, the herb may be of benefit in this area. High dopamine levels also lead to an **increased production of growth hormone,** in both men and women.

Research carried out by Lee, et al. (*J Neurochem* 2000;75:521–531) in 2000 found that harmine may help to **protect brain cells from oxidative damage,** thus *Tribulus* could be useful in treating a variety of brain disorders, particularly Parkinson's disease.

New research is elucidating the role of *Tribulus* in **cancer treatment.** In 2000, Bedir and Khan (*J Nat Prod.* 2000;63:1699–1701) identified new steroidal glycosides from the fruits of *Tribulus terrestris.* The new saponins include one compound that demonstrated cytotoxicity against a human malignant melanoma cell line. Meanwhile, Li, et al. (*Planta Med.* 1998;64:628–631) found that tribulusamides A (1) and B (2), newly discovered lignanamides, were able to prevent cell death induced by tumor necrosis factor alpha.

Arcasoy, et al. (*Boll Chim Farm.* 1998;137:473–475) investigated the effects of saponin mixtures derived from *Tribulus terrestris* on smooth muscle. The saponin mixture caused a significant decrease on peristaltic movements of gastrointestinal and urinary muscle tissue. As a result, the team suggests that *Tribulus terrestris* may be useful in **treating smooth muscle spasms** or pains associated with colic.

In related research on smooth muscle tissue, Wang, et al. (*hong Xi Yi Jie He Za Zhi* 1990;10:85–87) studied the effect of *Tribulus terrestris* in coronary heart disease. Results showed that the total efficacious rate of remission angina pectoris was 82.3 percent, fifteen points higher than the control group. The total effective rate of ECG improvement (52.7 percent) was nearly twenty points higher than control. The researchers submit these findings to demonstrate that the saponin of *Tribulus terrestris* **dilates coronary artery and improves coro-**

nary circulation, and thus improves ECG related to myocardial ischemia. Furthermore, chronic administration had no adverse reaction on blood system and hepatic and renal functions. Neither did it have side effects. These findings led the authors to suggest that *Tribulus terrestris* may be useful in **the treatment of angina pectoris.** The vasodilatory properties of the herb may make it useful for patients with **heart disease, high blood pressure, and atherosclerosis.**

THERAPEUTIC DAILY AMOUNT

Follow dosage instructions on packaging.

MAXIMUM SAFE LEVEL

Not established.

SIDE EFFECTS/CONTRAINDICATIONS

Tribulus terrestris should not be taken by pregnant women or children or by anyone with psychosis, schizophrenia, or phaeochromocytoma. In addition, it should not be taken in combination with psychoactive medicines, such as tranquillizers, sedatives, stimulants (including OTC decongestants like ephedrine), and antidepressants.

Uva Ursi (*Arctostaphylos uva-ursi*)

GENERAL DESCRIPTION

A small evergreen shrub found in the northern United States and Europe, uva ursi's most active component is arbutin, which is found in its leaves and was at one time marketed as a urinary antiseptic and diuretic. Historically, uva ursi has been used to treat bladder and kidney infections, kidney stones, and bronchitis. When given alone, arbutin is broken down by intestinal bacteria almost completely before it can have any effect. Other components in the uva ursi plant, however, prevent this degradation.

ROLE IN ANTI-AGING

The active ingredient in uva ursi is the glycoside arbutin, which is present in fairly high amounts (up to 10 percent). Arbutin has been shown to **kill bacteria,** such as *Escherichia coli* and *Staphylococcus aureus* in the urine; thus, it may be of use in treating urinary tract infections. Once in the body arbutin is converted into a molecule called hydroquinone—a powerful antimicrobial agent. Arbutin has also been shown to **increase the anti-inflammatory action of synthetic cortisone.** Arbutin is a known inhibitor of melanin, thus suggesting that it may be useful in the treatment of hyperpigmentation.

THERAPEUTIC DAILY AMOUNT

3 grams of uva ursi in 150 ml of water as an infusion to be taken three to four times daily. 250–500 mg three times per day of the herbal extract in capsules or tablets (containing 20 percent arbutin) can also be taken. Uva ursi should not be used for more than fourteen days.

MAXIMUM SAFE LEVEL

Not established.

SIDE EFFECTS/CONTRAINDICATIONS

Long-term (more than two to three weeks) use of uva ursi is not recommended. Acidic agents such as cranberry juice, prune juice, and vitamin C (more than 500 mg per day) should be avoided when taking uva ursi. Pregnant and lactating women should not take uva ursi. In 2005 Wang and Del Priore (*Am J Ophthalmol.* 2004;137:1135–1137.) reported a case of reported a case of bilateral bull's-eye maculopathy in a patient who took uva ursi for 3 years before the onset of symptoms. The authors conclude that uva ursi should be recognised as a potential retinal toxic drug.

Valerian (*Valeriana officinalis*)

GENERAL DESCRIPTION

Valerian is an extract from the underground stem and root of *Valeriana officinalis*. Valerian has been used as a sedative for more than a thousand years. The root of valerian contains more than 100 chemical compounds, most notably valepotriates and valerenic acids that, when isolated and concentrated, have been found to have a very potent sedative effect. It is one of the most popular herbal preparations in Europe and thus has been the subject of extensive scientific study. It also helps to alleviate **headaches** and **intestinal and menstrual cramps.**

ROLE IN ANTI-AGING

Valerian is very effective in **promoting sleep,** and has a much better safety record than prescription sleeping pills. Leathwood and Chauffard (*Planta Med* 1985;2:144–148) demonstrated that valerian **reduces the time it takes to fall asleep** (known as sleep latency), while Balderer and Borbely (*Psychopharmacology* (Berl). 1985;87:406–409) showed that valerian could also **decrease the number of nighttime awakenings.** A two-week-long trial of valerian extract in healthy men and women aged twenty-two to fifty-five by Donath, et al. (*Pharmacopsychiatry.* 2000;33:47–53) revealed that the herb hastened the time it took to reach deep sleep, extended the period of deep sleep, and increased the amount time spent in REM sleep. Together, these studies suggest that valerian has therapeutic benefit for the **treatment of insomnia.** In fact, some research suggests that valerian is as effective at treating insomnia as some prescription drugs. Dorn (*Forsch Komplementarmed Klass Naturheilkd.* 2000;7:79–84. [in German]) reported that 600 mg of valerian extract, taken thirty minutes before bedtime for twenty-eight days, was as effective for promoting sleep as the prescription sleep drug oxazepam, which is commonly prescribed for insomnia.

As well as helping people to get to sleep, valerian has also been shown to markedly **improve sleep quality**—as a bonus it also **promotes improved mood.** When administered to older men and women with sleep disturbances, Kamm-Kohl, et al. (*Med Welt* 1984;35:1450–1454 [in German]) found that after just two weeks, valerian supplementation improved mood, calmed aggressive behavior, and reduced difficulties in falling and staying asleep. Vorbach, et al. (*Psychopharmakotherapie* 1996;3:109–115 [in German]) reported that a month-long treatment with valerian supplements in men and women whose sleep problems persisted for a month or more produced a pronounced improvement in mood. Other studies have shown that valerian calms fear and restlessness and curbs aggression. Scientists suspect that valerian causes these benefits through the active component chemical valerenic acid. Valerenic acid has been shown in a number of animal studies to increase the release and activity of GABA, an amino acid that is important in modulating stress and anxiety. Thus, many scientists believe that valerian promotes sleep simply by **raising GABA levels.**

Valerian may also be of benefit to people suffering from muscle-related causes of sleep disturbances. Houghton (*J Ethnopharmacol* 1998;22:121–142) concluded that it is useful in **treating restless motor syndromes and muscle spasms.** As such, it has applicability to sleep-related restlessness. The volatile oils present in valerian, as well as valepotriates and valerenic acids, have been shown to have a strong ability to relax smooth muscle contractions. Additionally, as a smooth muscle relaxer, valerian **relieves tense, aching muscles,** so it may be useful when muscular aches and pains are the cause of the inability to fall asleep.

Dressing, et al. (*Therapiewoche* 1992;42:726–736 [in German], *Psychopharmakotherapie* 1996;6:32–40) found that valerian was **particularly effective at combating insomnia and improving sleep quality when taken in combination with lemon balm.**

As a smooth-muscle relaxer, valerian has a diverse range of possible anti-aging applications. It has been used **to reduce rheumatic pain, neuralgic pain, and migraine.** Valerian has also been used to **treat nervous stomach, abdominal cramps, and to heal ulcers.** Yang, et al. (*Sleep.* 2001;24:272–281) report that valerian may be valuable in treating heart palpitation, as they found that it **slowed the heart rate while also increasing the strength of the beats.** Valerian has been reported by various studies to **improve nervous tension in premenstrual syndrome** experienced by some women.

THERAPEUTIC DAILY AMOUNT

Valerian is sold in capsules, tinctures, and extracts; it is frequently combined with other calming herbs in natural insomnia remedies. Valerian root has an unpleasant smell; so many people prefer the odor-free capsules to liquid remedies. Refer to packaging.

MAXIMUM SAFE LEVEL

Not established. However, a woman who swallowed forty to fifty capsules of powdered valerian containing 470 mg each (approximately twenty times the recommended dose) in a suicide attempt suffered no long-term ill effects.

SIDE EFFECTS/CONTRAINDICATIONS

Valerian is much safer than prescription sedatives. However, as with any relaxant, one should not take it before doing tasks that require full alertness (for example, when driving or operating heavy machinery). Valerian is not contraindicated during pregnancy or lactation; however, it should not be given to children under age twelve. Valerian may be contraindicated in people with medical conditions and those who are taking medications that depress the central nervous system (including other sedatives, antihistamines, antidepressants, and anti-anxiety agents). Anyone using this herb should report its use to their physician so that he or she may monitor for any possible herb-drug interactions.

Velvet Bean (*Mucuna pruriens*)

GENERAL DESCRIPTION

Velvet bean is a botanical used in Ayurveda, the Indian system of traditional medicine. Velvet bean is a source of dopa, which the brain converts into the neurotransmitter dopamine.

ROLE IN ANTI-AGING

Modern Ayurvedic medicine has employed velvet bean seed to **treat Parkinson's disease.** The brains of Parkinson's patients are low in the neurotransmitter dopamine. Dopamine can be elevated by administering the drug L-dopa. Research has shown that velvet bean seed grown in culture contains a **very high concentration of naturally occurring L-dopa.** A Parkinson's Disease Study Group study (*J Altern Complement Med.* 1995;1:249–255) reported that Parkinson's tremor and rigidity were better controlled with a twelve-week supplementation of natural L-dopa from velvet bean than by synthetic L-dopa.

Tripathy and Udpadhyay (*Phytother Res.* 2002;16:534–538) found that the seeds of velvet bean have **antioxidant properties.** They also found that velvet bean can help to reduce the oxidation of lipids, which is important in maintaining healthy cholesterol levels.

Work by Rathi, et al. (*Phytother Res.* 2002;16:236–243) suggests that velvet bean may have some potential as a **treatment for diabetes.** The researchers gave rats with experimental diabetes velvet bean extract for four months. Results showed that those treated with velvet bean exhibited a 51 percent drop in plasma glucose levels. Previous research by Akhtar, et al. (*J Pak Med Assoc.* 1990;40:147–150) led them to conclude that the apparent anti-hyperglycemic effect of velvet bean is due to its ability to **stimulate the release of insulin.**

Prakash, et al. (*Int J Food Sci Nutr.* 2001;52:79–82) found that seeds of velvet bean are high in trypsin and chymotrypsin, enzymes that assist the gastrointestinal system with the processing of food. Thus, velvet bean may be an important **digestive aid.**

Historically, the use of velvet bean in Ayurveda originated from its ability to serve as an antidote to snake venom. Houghton, et al. (*Ethnopharmacol.* 1994;44:99–108) found that velvet bean's utility for this purpose is due to its ability to prolong the time for blood to clot. This use suggests a possible role for velvet bean as a blood-thinning agent.

As velvet bean is a good source of natural L-dopa it may **promote sleep.** A number of studies have found that its key chemical constituent, L-dopa, is a natural clock setter. Specifically, L-dopa has been shown to advance the circadian rhythm of sleep. Additionally, some scientists speculate that restless legs syndrome and periodic limb movement disorder—a frequent cause of insomnia in older people—is due to a deficiency of dopamine. This suggests a possible use of velvet bean in these sleep disorders. In addition, Rajyalakshmi and Geervani (*Plant Foods Hum Nutr.* 1994;46:53–61) found that velvet bean has a very high protein content. High-protein foods promote the release of serotonin, which is a critical neurotransmitter necessary for the onset of sleep.

THERAPEUTIC DAILY AMOUNT

As directed on packaging or recommended by practitioner.

MAXIMUM SAFE LEVEL

Not established.

SIDE EFFECTS/CONTRAINDICATIONS

Because velvet bean provides a supply of L-dopa, the precursor to dopamine, to the brain, people with medical conditions associated with elevated dopamine (schizophrenia and other neuropsychiatric conditions) should not take it. Those on Parkinson's medications, including synthetic L-dopa, as well as people taking antidepressant drugs known as MAO inhibitors, should consult their physician before taking velvet bean. Because velvet bean can prolong the time for blood to clot, those taking blood-thinning medications or nutrients, or those with blood-clotting disorders, should not take velvet bean.

Wild Yam (*Dioscorea villosa*)

GENERAL DESCRIPTION

Wild yam is native to North and Central America. Historically, wild yam has been used as an expectorant for people with coughs. It has also been used to alleviate gastrointestinal upset, nerve pain, and morning sickness. The root is used medicinally.

ROLE IN ANTI-AGING

One of the active components of wild yam—dioscoretine—has been shown in animal studies to **lower blood sugar levels.** Research by Araghiniknam, et al. (*Life Sci* 1996;11:147–157) found that an extract of wild yam has **antioxidant properties,** and can **raise HDL ("good cholesterol") levels and lower triglyceride levels** in elderly men and women.

Recent chemical analysis of wild yam has found that saponins in this herb could be synthesized commercially into steroids including cortisone, estrogens, and progesterone-like compounds. The Mexican wild yam, *Dioscorea barbasco,* contains a high amount of the saponin called diosgenin. Contrary to popular belief, the diosgenin present in wild yam cannot be converted into progesterone or dehydroepiandrosterone (DHEA) in the body. Pharmaceutical progesterone is produced from wild yam using a chemical conversion process.

THERAPEUTIC DAILY AMOUNT

Wild yam products come in capsules, tinctures, extracts, and topical creams and gels. The recommended dose for the dried, powdered root is 100 mg three times each day.

MAXIMUM SAFE LEVEL
Not established.

SIDE EFFECTS/CONTRAINDICATIONS
A number of experts recommend that wild yam should not be used by people with hormone-sensitive conditions (for example, certain types of breast cancer). Although the herb has been used as a treatment for morning sickness, its safety during pregnancy and breast-feeding has not been ascertained.

FUNCTIONAL FOODS AND FOOD COMPONENTS

Apple Cider Vinegar

GENERAL DESCRIPTION
Apple cider is a natural source of acetic acid. When taken orally, apple cider vinegar creates an internal pH environment that microbes cannot tolerate. Its use in oral form is an extension of its well-documented efficacy as a vaginal douche against yeast infections.

ROLE IN ANTI-AGING
Advocates of apple cider vinegar claim that the acetic acid and butyric acid contained in vinegar support gastrointestinal health by **promoting the growth of friendly bifidobacteria.** The vinegar also has both **antiseptic and antibiotic properties,** and can be helpful in treating **sore throat, cuts, wounds, digestive problems, and gum infections.** There has been some suggestion that apple cider vinegar may help to reverse atherosclerosis (hardening of the arteries), and break up gall and kidney stones, possibly by dissolving calcium deposits; however, these benefits have not been clinically proven. There is also some evidence to suggest that apple cider vinegar may have the potential to destroy both A and B strains of the human herpes virus-6 (HHV-6).

THERAPEUTIC DAILY AMOUNT
Refer to packaging.

In the event that taking liquid vinegar is cumbersome or inconvenient, vinegar tablets, 500 mg each (equivalent to one tablespoon of liquid vinegar), are available from health food stores. Hill et al. (*J Am Diet Assoc.* 2005;105:1141–1144) carried out a study of eight apple cider vinegar tablet products after an adverse event was reported to the authors. The products were tested for pH, component acid content, and microbial growth. Considerable variability was found between the brands in tablet size, pH, component acid content, and label claims. Furthermore, doubt remains as to whether apple cider vinegar was in fact an ingredient in the evaluated products. Thus, it is advisable to buy a reputable high-quality brand of apple cider vinegar.

MAXIMUM SAFE LEVEL
Not established.

SIDE EFFECTS/CONTRAINDICATIONS
None known.

Bee Products

GENERAL DESCRIPTION
Bees produce several substances that are useful to humans—namely, honey, propolis, pollen, and royal jelly.

ROLE IN ANTI-AGING
Honey: Used as a **skin treatment,** honey prevents infection and speeds healing by starving existing bacteria and protecting the skin from infection by new bacteria. Research by Natarajan et al. (*J Dermatolog Treat.* 2001;12:33–36) suggests that honey could prove useful in the fight against antibiotic-resistant "superbugs." Tests revealed that the high sugar content of honey slows bacterial growth, while its thick, syrupy texture acts as a seal over wounds forming a natural barrier against any potential bacterial invaders. Furthermore, in its undiluted form, the sweet substance **killed a number of antibiotic-resistant bacteria.** The researchers suspect that honey's bacteria-killing properties may be due to enzymes present in the bees themselves or in the pollen. Either way, the findings suggest that honey, which has been used medicinally by certain populations for thousands of years, could help doctors to win the battle against bugs such as methicillin-resistant *Staphylococcus aureus* (MRSA), which can be fatal.

Results of a study published in 2002 suggest that eating honey can **boost the levels of antioxidants in blood.** Gheldof et al. (*J Agric Food Chem.* 2002; 50:3050–3055) found that drinking honey mixed with water led to a significant increase in blood antioxidant levels within sixty to ninety minutes. Previous research by the same team revealed that the level of antioxidants in honey is dependent upon its color—with dark honey being the richest in the chemicals. In fact, on a per-weight basis, the darkest honey contains roughly the same levels of antioxidants as garlic and spinach. Van der Weyden (*Br J Communi-*

ty Nurs. 2005;Suppl:S21, S24, S26–S27) tested a honey impregnated alginate dressing on a man who had a long history of venous ulcers on his leg, in order to evaluate the effectiveness of honey as an alternative treatment to current wound management therapies. Results showed that the honey seemed to act as an effective antibacterial, anti-inflammatory and deodorizing dressing. Furthermore, the ulcer healed completely. Honey has also been used successfully in the treatment of diabetic foot ulcers.

Pollen: Bee pollen is essentially the male seed of a flower blossom that has been collected by bees and to which bees add certain digestive enzymes. Analysis of bee pollen shows it typically contains a **wealth of nutrients** utilized by the human body, including vitamins, minerals, enzymes, and amino acids. Several studies have found that bee pollen is of benefit to men suffering from **benign prostatic hyperplasia** (BPH). There is also some evidence to suggest that it may help to **protect the liver from toxins.**

Propolis: Consisting mostly of tree resins, propolis is used by honeybees to seal the cracks and openings in hives. Propolis is rich in **anti-inflammatory** and **antioxidant** flavonoids. It also contains terpenoids, which have **antibacterial, antiviral, antiprotozoan, and antifungal effects.** For acute internal infections, propolis can be taken along with regularly prescribed medications. It is also an effective salve for wounds, especially in combination with honey. Propolis is available in a dry powder form, which may be sprinkled onto **mouth sores** as a therapeutic dressing.

Royal jelly: Secreted from glands on the bee's head, royal jelly is used to feed bee larvae for three days. The queen bee, however, eats royal jelly exclusively and it is believed to account for her fertility and her relatively long life (five to seven years versus seven to eight weeks for worker bees). Royal jelly contains collagen and several vitamins. It is thought to be an **anti-inflammatory** agent.

THERAPEUTIC DAILY AMOUNT
Refer to packaging.

MAXIMUM SAFE LEVEL
Not established.

SIDE EFFECTS/CONTRAINDICATIONS
Pollen: Bee pollen should not be taken during pregnancy.
Propolis: Allergic reactions to topically applied propolis are quite common; typically, they involve pain, redness, swelling, and sores. Use should be discontinued immediately.

Propolis is also a known "sensitizing agent"; therefore, regular use can cause people to develop allergies to the product.

Royal Jelly: Contraindicated during pregnancy.

Colostrum, Bovine

GENERAL DESCRIPTION

Within hours of giving birth, human and animal mothers secrete colostrum as a prelude to breast milk. It gives newborns a "vaccination" of antibodies, immune system protection, and growth factors. Whole colostrum is preferred over defatted colostrum because fat is necessary to assist in transporting colostrum protein into the bloodstream. Colostrum is now available in capsules that contain its immune proteins in dry form.

ROLE IN ANTI-AGING

Colostrum is primarily taken for its immune system enhancing benefits. Crooks et al. (*Int J Sport Nutr Exerc Metab.* 2006;16:47–64) studied the effects of bovine (cow) colostrum on athletes. Results showed that supplementation with bovine colostrum for twelve weeks led to a 79 percent increase in levels of secretory IgA (an immunoglobulin (a protein that acts as an antibody) found in body fluids such as tears and saliva that protects the body's mucosal surfaces from infection) in saliva. Secretory IgA offers protection against upper respiratory tract infection (URTI). Thus, suggesting that bovine colostrum may be of benefit to people at risk of URTIs, such as influenza, and the common cold.

In addition to its **immune-system enhancing** benefits, there is some evidence that colostrum may help to **protect the stomach from damage caused by nonsteroidal anti-inflammatory drugs.** As bovine colostrum is an inexpensive, readily available source of growth factors, scientists are studying its value in the prevention of NSAID-induced gastrointestinal damage in humans. Playford, et al. (*Clin Sci* (Lond). 2001;100:627–633) investigated whether colostrum supplementation could reduce the rise in gut permeability (a non-invasive marker of intestinal injury) caused by NSAIDs. Results showed that colostrum kept the gut permeability ratio low in patients taking long-term NSAID treatment, thus suggesting that colostrum may help to prevent NSAID-induced damage. Furthermore, results of an earlier study in rats by the same researchers (*Gut* 1999;44:653–658) found that pretreatment with 0.5 or 1.0 ml of a colostrum preparation reduced indomethacin-induced gastric injury by 30 percent and 60 percent, respectively.

Results of a more recent study appear to confirm Playford's findings. Kim et al. (*Asia Pac J Clin Nutr.* 2005;14:103–107) conducted a study to determine whether bovine colostrum was able to prevent NSAID-induced small intestinal damage in rats. results showed that administration of bovine colostrum reduced the increase in intestinal permeability, enteric bacterial overgrowth, protein losing enteropathy and mucosal villous damage of the small intestine induced by the NSAID (diclofenac). Thus leading the authors to conclude that bovine colostrum may have a beneficial effect in prevention of NSAID induced small intestinal injuries.

Colostrum may **increase insulin-like growth factor 1 (IGF-1) levels.** Mero, et al. (*J Appl Physiol.* 1997; 83:1144–1151) studied the effect of bovine colostrum supplementation on hormonal and immune markers in athletes in active training. In sprinters and jumpers supplemented with colostrum, post-training increases were noticed for serum IGF-1, with the most marked IGF-1 increase associated with consumption of a higher dose of colostrum. Moreover, the change in IGF-I concentration correlated positively with the change in insulin concentration. Serum immunoglobulin G, hormone, and amino acid and saliva immunoglobulin A responses remained unchanged during supplementation.

Colostrum may also be of benefit to people with short bowel syndrome, chemotherapy-induced mouth ulcers, and inflammatory bowel disease. However, there is no conclusive scientific evidence to prove colostrum's effectiveness in treating these conditions.

THERAPEUTIC DAILY AMOUNT
1,000–4,000 mg per day of freeze-dried colostrum is often recommended by manufacturers.

MAXIMUM SAFE LEVEL
Not established.

SIDE EFFECTS/CONTRAINDICATIONS
No significant side effects of colostrums have been reported.

Lactoferrin

GENERAL DESCRIPTION
A protein found in breast milk, lactoferrin helps combat infection during the critical period when the infant's immune system is not yet fully functional. Lactoferrin is most abundant in colostrum.

ROLE IN ANTI-AGING
During inflammatory reactions, certain immune cells release lactoferrin into

the blood and tissues as a defense against infection. Lactoferrin **reduces swelling** and **facilitates circulation around the injury.** Thus, lactoferrin is thought to boost the immune system. Research has shown that lactoferrin modulates the migration, maturation, and function of immune cells. Artym et al. (*Stem Cells Dev.* 2005;14:548–855) found that lactoferrin helped to accelerate the restoration of immune responsiveness in bone marrow transplant recipients whose immune systems' had been impaired by chemotherapy. Lactoferrin has both antibacterial and antiviral properties. Research has shown that it may be useful for the treatment of HIV when taken in combination with standard antiretrovital therapy. Lactoferrin also has antioxidant properties. Studies have shown that it scavenges non-protein-bound iron in body fluids and inflamed areas in order to suppress free radical-mediated damage and decrease accessibility of iron to invading bacteria, fungi, and cancer cells.

THERAPEUTIC DAILY AMOUNT
Refer to packaging.

MAXIMUM SAFE LEVEL
Not established.

SIDE EFFECTS/CONTRAINDICATIONS
None known.

Psyllium

GENERAL DESCRIPTION
Psyllium is the main ingredient in the majority of bulk-producing nonirritant laxatives, which are milder and much safer treatments for constipation than stimulant laxative herbs, such as senna and cascara sagrada.

ROLE IN ANTI-AGING
Psyllium is mostly soluble dietary fiber but it is also rich in water-absorbing mucilage, which is not broken down in the digestive tract. Psyllium **adds bulk to stools, absorbs excess liquids in the intestines, and speeds bowel transit time.** Psyllium's **regulation of blood cholesterol and blood sugar levels** may be due to effects on cholesterol-containing bile and digestion of carbohydrates. In a recent triple-blind study (subjects, researchers, and statisticians all were unaware of who was getting what), seventeen "non-restrained eaters" tested psyllium for its effects on appetite. Taking 20 grams of seed granules with seven ounces of water, three hours prior to and again immediately before a meal, caused a significant increase in the feeling of fullness and a reduction in

the consumption of fat and calories. Psyllium may also help to prevent fluctuations in blood sugar and could therefore be of benefit to diabetics.

THERAPEUTIC DAILY AMOUNT

Psyllium is sold as dried whole seeds, powders, wafers, and liquids. An average dose is one rounded teaspoon (5–6 grams) of powdered psyllium mixed with at least eight ounces of water or other liquid, taken at meal times. Effects on the bowels are usually noticeable within one to two days.

MAXIMUM SAFE LEVEL

Not established.

SIDE EFFECTS/CONTRAINDICATIONS

Always drink plenty of water with psyllium to promote its therapeutic effect and to prevent it from causing choking or intestinal blockage. Some people may experience flatulence or upset stomach; allergic reactions are rare but possible. Pregnant women, people with bowel obstructions, and diabetics or people who have difficulty keeping their blood sugar levels under control should not use psyllium.

Schisandra Berry Extract (*Schisandra chinensis*)

GENERAL DESCRIPTION

Schisandra, or Wu-Wei-Zi, is known in traditional Chinese medicine for its usefulness as a kidney tonic and lung astringent, to treat coughs, night sweats, insomnia, thirst, and physical exhaustion. Schisandra is also used to improve the body's ability to respond to stress. The fully ripe, sun-dried fruit is used medicinally.

ROLE IN ANTI-AGING

The major constituents in schisandra are lignans (schizandrin, deoxyschizandrin, gomisins, and pregomisin) found in the berries of the fruit. Modern Chinese research suggests these lignans have a **protective effect on the liver** and an **immunomodulating** effect. Human trials conducted in China have shown that schisandra may help people with **chronic viral hepatitis.** Work by Ip, et al. (*Planta Med* 1995;61:398–401) found that the lignans present in schisandra appear to protect the liver by activating enzymes in liver cells that produce glutathione, which is an important cellular antioxidant.

Laboratory studies suggest that schisandra may also improve physical performance, build strength, and help to reduce fatigue.

THERAPEUTIC DAILY AMOUNT

Suggested intakes of schisandra range from 1.5–15 grams per day. A tincture is also available; the recommended dosage is 2–4 ml three times per day.

MAXIMUM SAFE LEVEL

Not established.

SIDE EFFECTS/CONTRAINDICATIONS

Side effects are uncommon; however, abdominal upset, decreased appetite, and skin rash have been reported.

Soy Isoflavones

GENERAL DESCRIPTION

Soy-based foods such as soymilk, tempeh, and tofu, contain potent compounds called isoflavones that are chemically similar to the female hormone estrogen. Many scientists believe that the widespread use of soy in Eastern diets may help to explain why the incidence of hormone-related cancers is much lower among Asian women.

ROLE IN ANTI-AGING

Research suggests that two **isoflavones** present in soy—genistein and daidzein—appear to **lower the risk of developing hormone-related diseases** such as breast cancer, prostate cancer, and endometriosis. Results of one study revealed that women who ate the most soy and other phytoestrogen-rich foods were 54 percent less likely to develop endometrial cancer. Researchers believe that genestein, which has been shown to inhibit angiogenesis, may also block a protein called tyrosine kinase, which promotes the growth and proliferation of tumor cells. Meanwhile, results of research published in 2002 revealed that women who eat soybeans and soy-based foods such as tofu have significantly less "high-risk" dense breast tissue, which is linked to breast cancer. In fact, women who consumed the most soy were 60 percent less likely to have dense breast tissue than women who ate the least.

In 1999 the U.S. Food and Drug Administration (FDA) decided that soy foods could be marketed as foodstuffs that can **reduce the risk of heart disease by lowering "bad" LDL cholesterol levels.** In one study, people who drank a milkshake containing 25 grams of soy protein for nine weeks experienced an average 5 percent reduction in LDL cholesterol levels, while those with the highest LDL levels experienced a drop of 11 percent—both of which could have a significant effect upon heart disease risk. As well as lowering LDL cholesterol levels, soy has been shown to inhibit the oxidation of LDL cholesterol and raise "good" HDL cholesterol levels.

Soy isoflavones may also protect against **osteoporosis.** In a study of post-menopausal women by Potter, et al., published in the *American Journal of Clinical Nutrition* in 1998, findings demonstrated that the consumption of 40 grams of soy protein each day led to a significant **increase in bone mineral density** of the spine. Although these results are encouraging, no long-term human study to date has examined the effects of soy or soy isoflavone supplements on bone density or fracture risk.

Soy isoflavones are also recommended to help lessen the symptoms of premenstrual syndrome (PMS) and menopause. Bryant et al. (*Br J Nutr.* 2005;93: 731–739.) found that soy isoflavones helped to lessen headache, breast tenderness, swelling, and cramps. Several studies have showed that soy isoflavones can reduce the frequency of hot flashes by 40 percent or more.

DEFICIENCY SYMPTOMS

Not applicable.

THERAPEUTIC DAILY AMOUNT

While it is now possible to buy soy isoflavone supplements, it is not yet proven whether such supplements have the same health benefits as soy isoflavones consumed in food. In Asian countries, where the incidence of hormone-related cancers such as breast cancer and prostate cancer is significantly lower than in the West, people obtain roughly 20–200 mg of soy isoflavones a day from their food.

MAXIMUM SAFE LEVEL

Not established. However, due to recent study findings, some experts recommend that soy intake should be limited to no more than 100 mg a day.

SIDE EFFECTS/CONTRAINDICATIONS

In laboratory studies, soy has been shown to stimulate the growth of breast cells, whether or not this increases the risk of breast cancer remains unclear, and research is ongoing. However, women with a medical history or family history of breast cancer are advised to consult their doctor before taking soy isoflavone supplements.

Numerous studies suggest that the soy isoflavone genistein may actually suppress the immune system. Results of a study in mice by Yellayi et al. (*Proceedings of the National Academy of Sciences.* 2002;99:7616–7621) showed that when mice were injected with genistein levels of several immune system cells dropped, and the thymus, a gland where T-cells mature (white blood cells that are crucial to the immune system), shrank. However, more alarmingly, the thymus also shrank when mice were fed genistein in their diet. The authors of this study recommend that soy intake should be limited to no more than roughly 100mg a day. Studies have also found evidence to suggest that feeding babies soy-based infant formulas increases their risk of autoimmune disease later in life (*J Nutr.* 2006;136:704–708.) However, there is also animal research to suggest that genistein stimulates various aspects of immune function. In conclusion, more work is needed to definitively establish the effects that genistein has on the immune system.

Several groups of people should avoid taking soy isoflavone supplements, these include: pregnant women, nursing women, women trying to conceive, and people taking estrogens, ipratropium bromide, thyroid hormones, or warfarin.

Whey Protein

GENERAL DESCRIPTION

As a derivative of milk production, the types of amino acids in whey proteins are closely related to the amino acids required by the human body. Whey proteins also have proportionately more sulfur-containing amino acids and contain a relative surplus of a variety of essential amino acids. In particular, whey protein contains about 2.5 percent cysteine, a sulfur amino acid known to increase the cellular level of glutathione, a potent antioxidant. Glutathione plays an important role in the regulation of immune cells and may possess antiviral properties. Whey also contains the protein lactoferrin, which is known to boost the immune system and modulate the migration, maturation, and function of immune cells.

ROLE IN ANTI-AGING

The proteins found in whey are widely recognized for their high biological value. A high biological value indicates the amount of protein absorbed and retained by the muscles in relation to the amount consumed. Inasmuch as protein is intimately involved in anabolism (protein synthesis and muscle growth), whey protein may be the best candidate for **maximizing muscle growth.** Whey also features one of the highest profiles of branched-chain amino acids (BCAAs) compared with other protein sources. Diets high in BCAAs demonstrate greater signs of muscle preservation when the body is in a catabolic state (breakdown of muscle tissue). Severe metabolic stresses such as sepsis, major operations, burns, strenuous exercise, and certainly fending off infection, are associated with accelerated muscle catabolism.

Of the various forms available (concentrate, peptides, hydrolysate, etc.), **whey protein isolate** is considered superior by many because of its purity, **high glutathione content,** and **increased bioavailability.** Results of an animal study by Xiao et al. (*Mol Cancer.* 2005 Jan;4:1) suggest that whey protein may have anti-cancer properties. The researchers found that rats fed a whey protein diet appeared to have some protection against chemically-induced colon cancer. Xiao et al. believe that whey protein induces the production of somatostatin, a hormone that is a known anti-proliferative agent for colon cancer cells.

Van Dissel et al. (*J Med Microbiol.* 2005;54:197–205) treated 16 patients with a history of relapsing *Clostridium difficile* diarrhea. Results showed that just two weeks of treatment with whey proteins removed all traces of the bacteria from the feces of all but one participant. When participants were followed-up one year later, none had suffered another bout of *Clostridium difficile*—associated diarrhea.

THERAPEUTIC DAILY AMOUNT

Most people should not need to take supplementary whey protein, as they should obtain enough protein from their diet. However, people who have undergone recent trauma, surgery, and those who participate in strenuous exercise may benefit from taking up to 25 grams of whey protein per day.

MAXIMUM SAFE LEVEL

Not established.

SIDE EFFECTS/CONTRAINDICATIONS

Whey may be contraindicated if you have milk allergies. Long-term, excessive intake of whey protein, as with other proteins, is not recommended as it may be associated with deteriorating kidney function and possibly osteoporosis.

OTHER NOTEWORTHY NUTRIENTS

Alpha-GPC (Alpha-Glycerylphosphorylcholine; Choline Alphoscerate)

GENERAL DESCRIPTION

Alpha-GPC is a nutrient capable of providing high levels of choline to nourish the nervous cells of the brain by protecting their cell walls. Alpha-GPC increases levels of the neurotransmitter acetylcholine, which results in an increase in human growth hormone (HGH) secretion.

ROLE IN ANTI-AGING

Studies in lab animals demonstrate the value of Alpha-GPC in **correcting age-related brain decline.** Muccioli, et al. (*Prog Neuropsychopharmacol Biol Psychiatry* 1996;20:323–339), observed that old rats showed a significant decrease in the number of muscarinic M(1) receptors—important in nerve signals involving acetylcholine—and a significant increase in membrane microviscosity in the striatum and hippocampus as compared with young animals. When Mucciolo treated the aged rats with Alpha-GPC, it restored the number of M(1) receptors to levels found in the striatum and hippocampus from young animals. It also partially restored membrane microviscosity in both regions studied and hence increased membrane fluidity. Amenta, et al. (*Mech Ageing Dev.* 1994;76:49–64) studied the anatomical changes in the aging brain, and the application of Alpha-GPC as an intervention. The researchers found that the density of nerve cells in the hippocampus and cerebral cortex in adult rat brains decreases with aging. When supplemented with Alpha-GPC, the age-dependent reduction of nerve cells in both these brain regions was counteracted. The researchers submit that **Alpha-GPC treatment is effective in slowing down the expression of structural changes occurring in aging brain.** Taken together, Alpha-GPC's ability to restore M(1) receptors in the brain and slow the reduction of nerve cells in the hippocampus and cerebral cortex suggest that the nutrient may be particularly important in **protecting cognition and learning as we age.** Schettini, et al. (*Pharmacol Biochem Behav.* 1992;43: 139–151) found that Alpha-GPC improves the performance of animals in both active and passive conditioning tasks. Furthermore, extended treatment with Alpha-GPC enhanced the transduction of the nerve signal required for learning and cognition in young animals and restored it in older ones. Taken together, Alpha GPC's ability to restore M(1) receptors in the brain and slow the reduction of nerve cells in the hippocampus and cerebral cortex, suggest that the nutrient may be particularly important in protecting cognition and learning as we age.

Alpha-GPC has a therapeutic effect on the cognitive recovery of stroke victims. In their study of men and women experiencing cognitive decline after stroke, Barbagallo, et al. (*Ann NY Acad Sci.* 1994;717:253–269) found that nearly three-quarters of the study's participants experienced no cognitive decline or forgetfulness. Their findings led them to **recommend Alpha-GPC in the cognitive recovery of stroke patients.** Similarly, patients with vascular dementia are able to gain benefit from Alpha-GPC supplementation. Di Perri, et al. (*J Int Med Res.* 1991;19:330–341) administered Alpha-GPC to 120 patients with mild to moderate vascular dementia. Throughout the ninety days of treatment, Di Perri's team observed **improvements in cognitive, memory, and depression** scales.

Ceda, et al. (*Horm Metab Res.* 1992;24:119–121) studied the effect of Alpha-GPC on growth hormone secretion, which decreases significantly with age. This decrease may be due to increased hypothalamic somatostatin release, which is inhibited by cholinergic agonists, or to decreased secretion of GHRH (growth hormone releasing hormone). Ceda's team administered Alpha-GPC to young and old men and women, and results showed that it **potentiated growth hormone secretion in elderly subjects.** As a result of increasing the cholinergic tone, Alpha-GPC serves as an important growth hormone releaser.

THERAPEUTIC DAILY AMOUNT

Refer to packaging.

MAXIMUM SAFE LEVEL

Not established.

SIDE EFFECTS/CONTRAINDICATIONS

Minor, transient side effects have been reported with the use of orally administered Alpha-GPC, although these are quite rare. Reported side effects include diarrhea, dizziness, gastralgis, heartburn, insomnia, restlessness, and skin rashes.

Beta-Glucan (Beta-1,3, and Beta-1,6 glucan)

GENERAL DESCRIPTION

Beta-glucan is derived from baker's yeast, young rye plants, and some medicinal mushrooms.

ROLE IN ANTI-AGING

Beta-glucan is known to help the immune system **fight bacterial, viral, fungal, and parasitic pathogens** by activating key immune cells known as macrophages. Taken before and after surgery, beta-glucan has been shown to help reduce infection. It also appears to **enhance the activity of conventional antibiotic therapy.** Beta-glucan also acts as a **free-radical scavenger,** removing debris and cells damaged by exposure to radiation, chemotherapy, and environmental pollutants. Results of a study by Sener et al. (*Int Immunopharmacol.* 2005;5:1387–1396) showed that beta-glucan reversed oxidant responses to induced sepsis in rats. The researchers concluded that these results suggest that beta-glucan's antioxidant properties may offer protection against sepsis-induced oxidative organ injury. Beta-glucan is thought to be responsible for the cholesterol-lowering properties of oat bran. Results of several clinical trials using beta-glucan derived from either oats or yeast, suggest that regular, long-term consumption of beta-glucan can **lower total cholesterol levels and "bad" LDL cholesterol levels** by roughly 10 percent and 8 percent, respectively, while **raising "good" HDL cholesterol** by as much 16 percent.

DEFICIENCY SYMPTOMS
Not applicable.

THERAPEUTIC DAILY AMOUNT
Not established. Most manufacturers recommend doses ranging between 50 and 1,000 mg. However, doses as high as 15,000 mg per day have been used to lower cholesterol in clinical trials.

SIDE EFFECTS/CONTRAINDICATIONS
None known.

Betaine (HCl)

GENERAL DESCRIPTION
Betaine HCl (hydrochloric acid) is used to increase the level of hydrochloric acid in the stomach. IMPORTANT: Do not confuse betaine HCl with the amino acid betaine (trimethylglycine).

ROLE IN ANTI-AGING
The stomach needs a ready supply of hydrochloric acid (HCl) to convert the inactive precursor pepsinogen into the active digestive enzyme pepsin, which is needed for the **digestion of protein.** HCl also **protects the body from orally ingested pathogens,** prevents bacterial and fungal overgrowth **in the small intestine,** and encourages the flow of both bile and pancreatic enzymes. **It also helps the body to absorb** folic acid, vitamin C, **beta-carotene, iron, calcium, magnesium, and zinc.**

DEFICIENCY SYMPTOMS
Gastric acid deficiency increases the severity and risk of contracting certain bacterial and parasitic intestinal infections. There is some evidence suggesting that people with inadequate levels of gastric acid are more susceptible to allergies, asthma, indigestion, *Candida* (thrush), arthritis, and autoimmune disorders. People with chronic disorders, such as allergies, asthma, and gallstones, are most at risk from stomach acid deficiency. The elderly are also at risk, as gastric acid levels tend to decline with age.

THERAPEUTIC DAILY AMOUNT

Betaine HCl should only be taken by people who have been diagnosed with hypochlorhydria—low levels of stomach acid. Betaine HCl is usually taken with a meal containing protein; the typical dose is 325–650 mg.

MAXIMUM SAFE LEVEL

It is not recommended to take more than 650 mg of betaine HCl unless advised to do so by a doctor.

SIDE EFFECTS/CONTRAINDICATIONS

Large quantities of betaine HCl can burn the lining of the stomach. Thus, betaine HCl use should be stopped immediately if a burning sensation in the stomach is experienced while taking the supplement.

Anyone suffering from, or with a history of, peptic ulcers, gastritis, and heartburn should consult their doctor before taking betaine HCl. Furthermore, people taking drugs that can cause peptic ulcers, such as nonsteroidal anti-inflammatory drugs (NSAIDs), and cortisone-like drugs, should avoid betaine HCl.

Bromelain (Pineapple Enzyme)

GENERAL DESCRIPTION

Bromelain is a proteolytic enzyme (an enzyme that digests proteins) found in fresh pineapple. It is often used to treat muscle injuries and as a digestive aid.

ROLE IN ANTI-AGING

Bromelain is a natural **anticoagulant** that works by breaking down the blood-clotting protein fibrin. This may help to explain why results of at least two clinical trials suggest that the enzyme can help to improve the symptoms of angina and thrombophlebitis. As well as thinning the blood, bromelain also **thins mucus,** and thus may be of benefit to asthmatics and people suffering from chronic bronchitis.

There is also evidence that bromelain can trigger beneficial changes in white blood cells, and thus may **improve immune function.** Barth et al. (*Eur J Med Res.* 2005;10:325–331) found that bromelain activates macrophages and has positive effects on other factors. The results of the study led the authors to conclude: ". . . [bromelain] may stimulate, therefore, the innate as well as the adaptive immune system." Other research has shown that bromelain also activates natural killer cells. However, whether or not the enzyme would be beneficial to immunocompromised people has not been established clinically.

Bromelain has potent **anti-inflammatory** properties and therefore may be useful in promoting the healing of minor muscle injuries such as sprains and strains. Results of one study also found evidence to suggest that it can help to improve the symptoms of **rheumatoid arthritis.** When applied topically it may help to speed **wound healing.** There has also been some suggestion that bromelain has anticancer properties, although this has not been proven. Several recent studies have linked chronic inflammation to cancer; thus, any anticancer action of bromelain could be due to its anti-inflammatory properties. Tynes et al. (*Neoplasia.* 2001;3:469–479) found that bromelain was able to significantly and reversibly reduce glioma cell adhesion, migration, and invasion. Thus suggesting that it may be of use in the treatment of glioma.

The enzyme may also **enhance the effect of the antibiotics** amoxicillin, erythromycin, penicillamine, and penicillin. In a study of people with urinary tract infections, 100 percent of participants given antibiotics in combination with bromelain and another enzyme called trypsin were cured of their infection, compared with just 46 percent who received antibiotics alone.

Bromelain aids **digestion** by enhancing the effects of the digestive enzymes trypsin and pepsin. It can also help to prevent heartburn and ease diarrhea, if either are caused by a deficiency of digestive enzymes. Hale et al. revealed that treating mice with oral bromelain each day beginning at five weeks old decreased the incidence and severity of spontaneous colitis. Bromelain also significantly decreased the clinical and histologic severity of colonic inflammation when administered to mice with established colitis. Thus suggesting that bromelain may be of benefit to people with inflammatory bowel disease.

DEFICIENCY SYMPTOMS
Not applicable.

THERAPEUTIC DAILY AMOUNT
Bromelain is measured in MCUs (milk clotting units) or GDUs (gelatin dissolving units), where one GDU equals roughly 1.5 MCU. Potent bromelain products contain approximately 2,000 MCU per gram. Some doctors recommend taking up to 3,000 MCU three times daily for several days, and then decreasing the dosage to three daily 2,000 MCU doses.

Bromelain supplements often contain a plant pigment called quercetin. The two substances are found in combination simply because they enhance each other's anti-inflammatory actions, and that bromelain appears to improve quercetin absorption.

MAXIMUM SAFE LEVEL
Not established.

SIDE EFFECTS/CONTRAINDICATIONS
Bromelain is generally regarded as being safe and free of side effects when taken as directed. However, some people may be allergic to bromelain as it is derived from pineapple. Bromelain is not recommended for people with active gastric or duodenal ulcers. People taking anticoagulant drugs such as warfarin should not take supplementary bromelain without consulting their physician.

Cetylmyristoleate (Cis-9-Cetyl Myristoleate; CMO)

GENERAL DESCRIPTION
Cetylmyristoleate (CMO) is the common name for cis-9-cetyl myristoleate, an anti-inflammatory compound discovered in 1972 by Harry W Diehl, Ph.D., a researcher at the National Institutes of Health. It is a naturally occurring compound in a number of animals, including cows, whales, beavers, and mice.

ROLE IN ANTI-AGING
Diehl's research suggests that CMO **lubricates joints** and acts as an **anti-inflammatory** agent. In one study of people with various types of arthritis who did not respond to treatment with nonsteroidal anti-inflammatory drugs, Diehl gave some 540 mg of CMO each day for thirty days, while the remainder received a placebo. Both groups were told to apply topical CMO or placebo when needed. Results showed that 63.5 percent of those receiving CMO improved significantly, compared with just 14.5 percent of the placebo group. U.S. patents were subsequently granted to Diehl for the use of CMO in the treatment of osteoarthritis and rheumatoid arthritis.

DEFICIENCY SYMPTOMS
Not applicable.

THERAPEUTIC DAILY AMOUNT
CMO is available in both capsule and tablet form for oral use, and in creams and lotions for topical application. The general recommendation for oral CMO is 400–500 mg daily for thirty days. Topically, it can be used if and when needed.

MAXIMUM SAFE LEVEL
Not established.

SIDE EFFECTS/CONTRAINDICATIONS
None known.

Lactobacillus acidophilus

GENERAL DESCRIPTION

Lactobacillus acidophilus is a "friendly" strain of bacteria, which colonizes the intestines where it helps **prevent intestinal infections.** *Lactobacillus* also flourishes in the vagina, where it **protects women against yeast infections.** Along with other "friendly" microbes, *Lactobacillus* is known as a "probiotic."

ROLE IN ANTI-AGING

Lactobacillus and other probiotics may help to prevent traveler's diarrhea and diarrhea caused by antibiotics. Approximately 30 percent of people taking an antibiotic will develop diarrhea (due to the drug's creating an imbalance in natural intestinal flora). Among people who develop antibiotic-associated diarrhea, about a third will go on to develop colitis (inflammation of the colon) Lactobacillus acidophilus in two 8-oz servings of yogurt per day can reduce the risk of antibiotic-induced diarrhea by half. There have been suggestions that Lactobacillus acidophilus may also help irritable bowel syndrome.

There is also some evidence that the bacteria may help to strengthen the immune system and protect against colorectal cancer. Le Leu et al. (*J Nutr.* 2005;135:996–1001) fed rats a combination of resistant starch (RS) and probiotic bacteria (Lactobacillus acidophilus and Bifidobacterium lactis). The results showed that the synbiotic combination of RS and the probiotic bacteria facilitated the apoptotic deletion of carcinogen-damaged cells in the rat colon. The authors suspect that ingested RS acts as a metabolic substrate, thus creating the right conditions for probiotic bacteria to exert its proapoptotic action. Results of a study by Sheih et al. (*J Am Coll Nutr.* 2001;20:149–156) led the authors to conclude:" [*Lactobacillus acidophilus*] appears to enhance systemic cellular immune responses and may be useful as a dietary supplement to boost natural immunity."

DEFICIENCY SYMPTOMS

Not applicable.

THERAPEUTIC DAILY AMOUNT

A typical daily dose of *Lactobacillus* should supply about 3 to 5 billion live organisms.

MAXIMUM SAFE LEVEL

Not known

SIDE EFFECTS/CONTRAINDICATIONS

Immunocompromised people should consult their doctor before taking probiotics.

Methyl-Sulfonyl-Methane (MSM)

GENERAL DESCRIPTION

MSM is organic sulfur, which occurs naturally in the body. Sulfur is found in every cell of the body and is structurally and functionally important to a number of hormones, enzymes, antibodies, and antioxidants. In the body, the highest concentrations of MSM are found in breast milk, which helps infants to build a strong immune system. Over time, MSM deficiencies occur as a part of the aging process. MSM is present in meat, fish, eggs, poultry, milk, grains, legumes, fruits, and vegetables (especially asparagus and cruciferous vegetables). Because MSM is lost in food processing and storage, dietary sources may not offer enough MSM for therapeutic impact.

ROLE IN ANTI-AGING

Some studies have found that MSM may be beneficial to people with **osteoarthritis** and **rheumatoid arthritis;** however, this use of MSM is not clinically proven. Several animal studies have found that MSM appears to protect against cancer; however, these findings have not been replicated in human studies. At moderate levels, MSM helps to maintain healthy skin, nails, and hair.

DEFICIENCY SYMPTOMS

None known.

THERAPEUTIC DAILY AMOUNT

Oral doses of MSM range from 250–2,250 mg per day.

MAXIMUM SAFE LEVEL

MSM is not believed to be toxic. A laboratory study examining doses up to about 250 times the highest dose normally used by humans reported that no toxic effects were observed.

SIDE EFFECTS/CONTRAINDICATIONS

None known.

MGN-3

GENERAL DESCRIPTION

MGN-3 is produced by integrating an extract from the outer shell of rice bran with extracts from three different types of mushroom—shiitake, kawaratake, and suehirotake. In Japan, extracts of these three mushrooms are leading pre-scription treatments for cancer.

ROLE IN ANTI-AGING

MGN-3 strengthens the immune system by **boosting the activity of natural killer cells, T cells, and B cells.** Cancer patients have used MGN-3 both as a treatment and as an adjunct to lessen the toxicity of conventional therapies and improve their effectiveness. MGN-3 also has been used successfully, though to a lesser extent, with AIDS patients and patients with hepatitis B and C.

DEFICIENCY SYMPTOMS

Not applicable.

THERAPEUTIC DAILY AMOUNT

Depends largely upon preparation used. One clinical study gave participants 3 grams per day for six months with no reports of adverse effects.

MAXIMUM SAFE LEVEL

Not established.

SIDE EFFECTS/CONTRAINDICATIONS

None known.

Nicotinamide Adenine Dinucleotide (NADH)

GENERAL DESCRIPTION

NADH, which occurs naturally in meat, is present in all cells and assists in metabolism and in breaking down food.

ROLE IN ANTI-AGING

NADH is effective in treating **chronic fatigue syndrome,** perhaps because it stimulates production of adenosine triphosphate (ATP), which gives the body energy. Santaella et al. (*P R Health Sci J.* 2004;23:89–93) conducted a study to compare the effectiveness of oral therapy with NADH to conventional modalities of treatment in patients with chronic fatigue syndrome. A total of 31 patients fulfilling the Centers for Disease Control criteria for CFS, were randomly assigned to either NADH or nutritional supplements and psychological therapy for 24 months. Results showed that the twelve patients who received NADH had a dramatic and statistically significant reduction of the mean symptom score in the first three months of treatment. However, symptom scores in the subsequent months of therapy were similar in both treatment groups. When metabolism is slowed by cutting calories, NADH is freed up and is able to support a protein that influences the life span of cells. NADH may also be useful for the treatment of **jetlag.** Birkmayer et al. (*Wien Med Wochenschr.* 2002;152:450–454) found that individuals given NADH after an overnight flight performed significantly better on 4 cognitive test measures and reported less sleepiness compared with those who received placebo. The authors concluded that NADH significantly reduced jet lag-induced negative cognitive effects and sleepiness, was easily administered, and did not cause any side effects.

DEFICIENCY SYMPTOMS

NADH deficiency is only known to occur when an individual is deficient in vitamin B_3.

THERAPEUTIC DAILY AMOUNT

The therapeutic dosage for NADH ranges from 5–50 mg daily.

MAXIMUM SAFE LEVEL

NADH appears to have no adverse effects when 5 mg or less is taken over a long period of time. Chronic studies have not been carried out on higher doses.

SIDE EFFECTS/CONTRAINDICATIONS

The safety of supplementary NADH in pregnant and lactating women, and those with kidney or liver disease has not been established.

Polyphenols

GENERAL DESCRIPTION

Polyphenols are potent antioxidants found in both green and black tea. Although most of the research on tea has been done in the laboratory and on animals, there is strong evidence that tea offers positive health benefits to humans. Herbal teas do not contain polyphenols in any significant amount. (*See* entry on Green Tea).

ROLE IN ANTI-AGING

Polyphenols, particularly the flavonoids, are among the most **potent plant antioxidants,** and they **protect and recycle other antioxidants,** such as vitamin E. Many epidemiological studies have found that a high dietary intake of polyphenols is strongly associated with a low incidence of cancer. Results of Lu et al. (*Cancer Res.* 2000;60:6465–6471) found that theaflavin-3'-monogallate (TF-2), a polyphenol found in tea, triggers cell death in cancer cells while leaving healthy cells unharmed, thus suggesting that polyphenols protect against cancer in a number of different ways. They are also known to protect against heart disease. One of the ways by which polyphenols protect the heart is by **lowering the production of the protein endothelin-1**, which causes blood vessels to constrict and reduces the flow of oxygen to the heart. They also **chelate metal ions** such as iron, lead, and copper; this prevents them from being absorbed by the body where they would promote free-radical generation. The polyphenols present in green tea may promote weight loss. Lin et al. (*Obes Res.* 2005;13:982–990) found that epigallocatechin gallate (EGCG) increased apoptosis in mature adipocytes, and inhibited lipid accumulation in maturing preadipocytes in a dose-dependent manner. The authors conclude: "These results demonstrate that EGCG can act directly to inhibit differentiation of preadipocytes and to induce apoptosis of mature adipocytes and, thus, could be an important adjunct in the treatment of obesity."

DEFICIENCY SYMPTOMS
Not applicable.

THERAPEUTIC DAILY AMOUNT
Fruits and vegetables have significant variations in polyphenol content, depending on the part of the plant used (leaves are highest), cultivation and harvesting methods, degree of ripeness, storage conditions, and so on. A flavonoid intake of about 150–300 mg per day would be obtained from eating the recommended five servings of fruit and vegetables each day; thus, supplemental intake should also be in this range. Refer to packaging, as dosages will vary in different preparations.

MAXIMUM SAFE LEVEL
Not established.

SIDE EFFECTS/CONTRAINDICATIONS
None known.

Resveratrol

GENERAL DESCRIPTION
Resveratrol is a naturally occurring antioxidant thought to be responsible for many of the health benefits attributed to red wine. It is found in more than seventy species of plants, including mulberries and peanuts; however, the main dietary source of resveratrol is wine, as the compound is found in the skin of grapes. Both red and white wine are sources of resveratrol, although red wine contains significantly higher concentrations of the compound—mainly because of the way in which red wine is produced. Fresh grape skin contains

roughly 50–100 mcg (micrograms) of resveratrol per gram, while its concentration in red wine ranges from 1.5–3 milligrams per liter. For non-wine drinkers, resveratrol is available as a dietary supplement.

ROLE IN ANTI-AGING

A number of scientific studies have found evidence to suggest that resveratrol is beneficial for cardiovascular health. Results of laboratory and animal studies have shown that it **decreases the "stickiness" of blood platelets,** thus reducing the risk of developing stroke or heart attack-inducing blood clots. Other studies have shown that it may help to **prevent arteries from constricting,** which may help to keep blood pressure under control. Results of both epidemiological and clinical studies also indicate that resveratrol is at least partially responsible for the **cholesterol-lowering effects** of red wine.

As well as reducing the risk of cardiovascular disease, resveratrol is also thought to prevent both the development and progression of **cancer.** Resveratrol has been shown to block the multistep process of carcinogenesis at various stages: tumor initiation, promotion, and progression. It has both antioxidant and anti-mutagenic properties, and several studies have shown that it boosts production of the enzyme quinone reductase, which is known to detoxify carcinogens.

Resveratrol has also demonstrated **anti-inflammatory** effects in laboratory studies. Recent studies suggest that chronic inflammation may play an important role in the development of cardiovascular disease and cancer; thus, regular consumption of an anti-inflammatory compound like resveratrol may help to protect against these diseases.

There is evidence to suggest that resveratrol may promote longevity. Recent research suggests that resveratrol activates Sir2 (sirtuin) enzymes both *in vitro* and *in vivo*. Sir 2 enzymes play a crucial role in many cellular processes including gene silencing, regulation of the p53 gene, fatty acid metabolism, and cell cycle regulation. Furthermore, the apparent lifespan-extending benefits of calorie restriction are thought to be due to Sir2 activation. Borra et al. (*J Biol Chem.* 2005;280:17187–195) report that resveratrol has been shown to increase lifespan in three model organisms through a Sir2-dependent pathway.

DEFICIENCY SYMPTOMS

Not applicable.

THERAPEUTIC DAILY AMOUNT

As with most health-benefiting compounds, it is better to obtain them from the diet; one 8-ounce glass of red wine contains roughly 640 mcg of resveratrol, whereas a handful of peanuts provides about 73 mcg. Packaging on resveratrol supplements generally recommends an intake of 200–600 mcg per day; however, it should be noted that this is significantly less than doses used in animal studies to prevent cancer. The optimal intake level is yet to be established.

MAXIMUM SAFE LEVEL

Not established.

SIDE EFFECTS/CONTRAINDICATIONS

None known.

Saponins

GENERAL DESCRIPTION

Saponins are a group of plant chemicals found in soybeans, chickpeas, asparagus, tomatoes, potatoes, and oats. In nature, saponins appear to act as antibiotics that protect plants from microbes. In humans, saponins might fight cancer and infection.

ROLE IN ANTI-AGING

Several *in vitro* and *in vivo* studies have found evidence to support the belief that saponins have **potent anticarcinogenic properties.** It is thought that saponins protect against cancers via a range of different mechanisms, including an overall antioxidant effect, direct and select cytotoxicity of cancer cells, immune modulation, and regulation of cell proliferation. Research by Zhong et al. (*Zhong Yao Cai.* 2005;28:119–122.) found that saponins from Panax notoginseng appeared to protect choline neurons against pathological lesions in a rat model of Alzheimer's disease. Thus suggesting that saponins may have neuroprotective properties.

Research supports the use of saponins as adjuvants (an additional treatment used to increase the effectiveness of the primary therapy) to enhance the immune response to vaccines.

DEFICIENCY SYMPTOMS

Not applicable.

THERAPEUTIC DAILY AMOUNT

Depends upon preparation. Refer to packaging.

MAXIMUM SAFE LEVEL

Do not exceed recommended dosage, as saponins are highly toxic.

SIDE EFFECTS/CONTRAINDICATIONS

The majority of saponins cause some degree of bloating. They can also cause nausea and diarrhea. Pregnant women and people who are anemic or who have other blood disorders should not take saponins without consulting their doctor.

Transfer Factors

GENERAL DESCRIPTION

Transfer factors were discovered by H. S. Lawrence in 1949, when he found that the immune fraction of an individual's white blood cells was able to transfer immunity to a non-sensitized person. As small messenger molecules, transfer factors conduct immune recognition signals between immune cells. In doing so, they help "educate" young immune cells about present or potential danger. The most abundant source of transfer factors is colostrum, the "first milk" of humans and other animals such as cows.

ROLE IN ANTI-AGING

Transfer factors have been used to **treat bacterial and viral infections, parasites, and fungal disease.** Research has shown that transfer factors are effective in treating chronic sinusitis, viral hepatitis, chronic candidiasis, chronic infection, otitis media, AIDS, and other viral infections. Other conditions that may benefit from treatment with transfer factors include cancer, asthma, allergic conditions, autoimmune disease, vaccination-induced illness, fibromyalgia, and chronic fatigue syndrome.

DEFICIENCY SYMPTOMS

A deficiency of transfer factors causes vulnerability to infection.

THERAPEUTIC DAILY AMOUNT

Standard transfer factors, use for preventive purposes, are balanced preparations with no one factor predominating. Refer to dosage instruction on packaging or use as directed by a physician.

MAXIMUM SAFE LEVEL

Not established.

SIDE EFFECTS/CONTRAINDICATIONS

Transfer factors may cause flu-like symptoms in some individuals.

SECTION FOUR

Longevity Through Lifestyle

Our body is a machine
for living.

—LEO TOLSTOY (1828–1910)

Chapter 14

The Long-Life Diet: Nutrition for Longevity

THE HEFTY CONCERNS OF OVERWEIGHT AND OBESITY

The latest estimates are staggering: 1.7 billion people worldwide are overweight or obese. The London-based International Obesity TaskForce said the revised figure—50 percent higher than previous estimates—reflects a deliberate ignorance on the part of most governments in facing one of the biggest universal risks to health worldwide.

In the United States, obesity is the second leading cause of preventable deaths. According to the American Obesity Association, about 69 million Americans are overweight and 51 million are obese. These numbers have been rising steadily—61 percent of American adults aged twenty years and older are overweight, and 26 percent are obese. Overweight/obesity causes at least 300,000 excess deaths annually in the United States, burdening the nation with a healthcare tab of more than $100 billion each year. The nation's military is not immune to the obesity epidemic sweeping the United States. Despite the rigors of basic training and regular field exercises, 54 percent of military personnel are overweight and 6.2 percent are obese. Obesity affects military performance: obese soldiers have higher risk of heat injury and increased musculoskeletal injuries.

In Europe, an estimated 20 percent of residents are obese and many more are overweight. Professor Andrew Prentice from the London School of Hygiene and Tropical Medicine cites obesity as the single most greatest threat to the gains in longevity made during the last 100 years. He observes that people are getting fatter, not taller, at a much younger age. Thanks to high-fat fast-food diets, exercising less, and spending more time indoors in front of computers and televisions, adolescents are packing on the pounds at younger and younger ages, and are likely to remain overweight/obese into adulthood. As a result, some British nutritionists expect many parents to outlive their children. In Britain, the National Audit Office reports that about 30,000 people die of obesity-related causes each year, cutting short their lives by about nine years.

Newest recommendations from the World Health Organization (WHO) may add another half-billion to the tally of overweight/obese people worldwide. A WHO expert group found that a lower body mass index threshold (23.3, rather than 30 for non-Asian populations) can put Asians at an increased risk for obesity-related health risks. This prompted the group to propose that WHO adopts a revised definition of obesity that is specific to Asian populations to accommodate the body mass index difference. That would mean that of the world's 6.3 billion residents, 2.2 billion—more than one in three—are overweight or obese.

Overweight/Obesity Shortens Longevity

An analysis of data of 3,457 participants in the Framingham Heart Study from 1948 to 1990 found that being overweight at middle-age can dramatically shorten life expectancy. Nonsmokers who were overweight (but not obese) lost an average of three years from their lives. Obese people die even sooner. Obese female nonsmokers lost an average of 7.1 years, while non-smoking obese men lost 5.8 years. As a risk factor, overweight/obesity ranks as deleterious to life expectancy as smoking.

Fortunately, there is some encouraging news for those who are overweight or obese and are trying to lose weight. They may live longer than those who do not try to shed their excess pounds. In a study of 6,000 obese and overweight people aged thirty-five and older who were followed for nine years, Dr. Edward Gregg of the Centers for Disease Control and Prevention (Georgia) found a 24 percent lower death rate in overweight/obese men and women who lost weight intentionally than in people whose weight remained steady during the course of the study. Even people who were trying to lose weight but did not succeed had a lower death rate. Dr. Gregg suggests that even modest attempts at physical activity and improving diet and nutritional intake could be beneficial even if they do not result with weight loss.

No matter the amount of research that scientists do into anti-aging medicine, no matter how skilled physicians become in using these tools, if people will not turn their own attention to changing their diets for the better, there can be no completely successful cases in the realm of longevity medicine. It's just that important.

Proper nutrition must be combined with appropriate exercise (see Chapter 16) and necessary anti-aging medicine tools in order to create a fully lived, long, and healthy life.

DIET: THE LATEST RESEARCH

The biggest health problem facing Americans today is obesity. More than half of us are over our ideal weight and more than one-third are obese enough to significantly raise the risk of disease and premature death.

Nutrition is one of the greatest weapons against disease. Keeping fats below 30 percent of total calories consumed and cholesterol intake below 200 mg will markedly cut your risk of heart disease. Eating five servings a day of fruits and vegetables lowers your chances of getting cancer. And a recent study found that eating nine to ten daily servings of fruits and vegetables along with three servings of low-fat dairy products is as effective as medication in lowering high blood pressure, and can help reduce or eliminate your chances of stroke.

It is established that the risk of several other prominent age-related disorders, including cardiovascular disease, cancer, and diabetes, is influenced by the nutrient value of the food you eat and by the level of food intake—high food intake increases risk, and low food intake reduces risk.

A number of studies indicate that moderate calorie restriction can extend the life span. Dr. Sonntag and colleagues from Wake Forest University School of Medicine in South Carolina conducted a study of lab animals in which they restricted the caloric intake to 60 percent of normal.

The team found that moderate caloric restriction induced a wide range of physiological changes. Of particular importance were adaptive changes within the endocrine system that serve to maintain blood levels of glucose (sugar). Specifically, Dr. Sonntag's team observed that growth hormone secretion increased and plasma levels of IGF-1 decreased. Noting that these adaptive mechanisms to maintain glucose can be induced at any age, the team suggests that these alterations reflect some of the many beneficial aspects of moderate caloric restriction.

Further, Dr. Sonntag notes that numerous studies indicate that growth hormone and IGF-1 decrease with age and that administration of these hormones ameliorates the deterioration of tissue function evident in animals left to eat as they desired. Dr. Sonntag proposes that endocrine compensatory mechanisms induced by moderate caloric restriction decrease the stimulus for cellular replication, resulting in a decline in pathologies and increased life span.

Additionally, dietary restriction may stave off the onset of the neurodegenerative process. Dr. Mattson from the National Institutes of Aging published findings in 2000 indicating that diseases including Alzheimer's disease are precipitated by increased levels of oxidative stress, perturbed energy metabolism, and accumulation of insoluble proteins. Dr. Mattson suggests that dietary restriction may enhance the resistance of neurons in the brain to metabolic, excitotoxic, and oxidative insults that are associated with Alzheimer's disease and other neurodegenerative disorders.

As we age, the nutritional value of dietary intake becomes very important. It has been suggested that the age-associated declines in immune function are similar to that seen by protein-calorie malnutrition. Additionally, many older people live alone and may not give adequate attention to the quality of foods they consume. Many older men and women are deficient in vitamin C, vitamin E, riboflavin, pyridoxine, iron, and zinc.

Several researchers have indicated that proper nutrition can modulate the age-related decline of the immune system. Indeed, Dr. Lesourd and colleagues from the Hopital Charles Foix in France have documented a decline in cell-mediated immunity that is largely responsible for increased rates of infection and cancer in the elderly. Dr. Lesourd's study reinforces the notion that nutritional factors play a major role in the immune responses of older people—and that even the healthy older population can benefit from proper choices in daily nutrition.

THE FRUSTRATIONS OF DIETING

Most people who look to dieting as a means of losing weight consider the whole process a rather Sisyphean experience. Just like old Sisyphus, who was cursed by the ancient gods to roll a rock to the top of a hill only to have it roll back down again, dieters often find that their goal weight rushes away from them. Just when they seem about to lose those last few pounds or maintain their new desired weight, they fall off their diets, begin to gain, and the whole dieting cycle starts all over again. A 1993 issue of *Consumer Reports* put the rate at which this rollercoaster rebounding occurs for dieters at 75 percent. Dr. Xavier Pi-Sunyer of St. Luke's Hospital in New York puts the figure even higher, at about 85 percent.

Nutritionists, scientists, and dieters themselves have long quarreled over why weight should be so hard to lose and so easy to gain, especially after one has already established a certain higher-than-optimal weight. The most persuasive theory speaks about the *set point,* the body's predetermined comfort zone for weight, which represents a complex negotiation of genetic factors, the amount of food available in infancy, and eating patterns as a child and adult. Once the body decides on a set point, however, it mobilizes all of its resources to maintain weight at that level. If weight drops below the set point, the body, fearing starvation, lowers metabolism to burn fat more slowly while at the same time increasing appetite. As weight approaches the set point, metabolism picks up again and appetite decreases.

According to this theory, frequent dieting followed by regular regaining of lost weight confuses the body and causes it to stick ever more stubbornly to its set point. The less food the frequent dieter eats, the lower his or her metabolism drops, so that losing weight becomes extremely difficult and gaining weight seems to take place with virtually any intake of food.

In addition to the frustrations of so-called yo-yo dieting, health professionals have recently raised concerns that frequent weight gains and losses might actually be dangerous to the dieter's health. These fears, however, seem to be largely unfounded. According to a recent survey by the National Institutes of Health task force of forty-three different studies of dieting, "Obese individuals should not allow concerns about hazards of weight cycling to deter them from efforts to control their body weight."

Even if you're not worried about the potential dangers of dieting, what about the more basic problem of finding an effective way to reduce body fat? The bad news is that there is no easy answer. The good news is that with the proper combination of exercise and dietary change, you can alter both your body weight and your chances for a long and healthy life. The dietary changes explored in this chapter aren't so much "diets" as long-term approaches to eating. And the stakes aren't just a slender figure or a chance to wear last year's jeans, but rather a new lease on life.

THE HAZARDS OF FAT

Over the past two decades, our society has become increasingly preoccupied with both health and thinness. The popularity of gyms, health clubs, and personal trainers, along with the extremely svelte silhouettes of beauty queens and fashion models, attests to the ideals of fitness and slenderness.

At the same time, more Americans are obese than ever before. According to the American Obesity Association, 61 percent of the U.S. adult population are overweight, and 26 percent are obese (which is defined as being at least 20 percent over the desirable weight range for one's height, with fat constituting 30 percent or more of the body in women and 25 percent or more in men).

The U.S. obesity figure of 33 percent is up from a rate of 25 percent in 1980 and 24 percent in 1962.

Although no one knows exactly what the health hazards of obesity are, excess weight seems to be implicated in some 300,000 deaths a year.

> Heart disease aside, there is overwhelming evidence that a high-fat diet increases the risk for cancers of the colon, breast, and prostate.

More significantly, excess weight prevents a person from extending his or her life, and contributes to many of the diseases of aging: high blood pressure, heart disease, stroke, diabetes, cancer, digestive disorders, and gallbladder complications. High weight is correlated with high cholesterol, which in turn is a predictor of cardiovascular problems.

Fat in men tends to settle in the stomach, creating the so-called "apple" shape, whereas fat in women most often settles around the hips, giving overweight women a "pear" shape. Men seem to be at higher risk for most obesity-related conditions than are women.

To determine whether your shape is dangerous to your health, measure your waist at its narrowest point and then measure your hips and buttocks at their widest point. Divide the waist measurement by the hip figure. If your waist-to-hip ratio is higher than .8 (for women) or .95 (for men), you probably need to lose weight.

Another way of finding out whether your weight is in a reasonable range is to look at the chart on the following page.

THE BENEFITS OF A PROPER DIET

There truly is no way to overstate the importance of a proper diet. It is not only the source for our life's energy, but also the basis for the concept of longevity. A good diet can make an enormous difference to how quickly or how slowly we age.

Among other benefits, a good diet:

- provides the food, water, and oxygen that your cells need to reproduce, transmit information, and repair damage;

- assures the body a continuous supply of usable fuel, which improves your emotional stability and energy levels;

- helps you to purge toxins and waste products, retention of which can increase your risk of cancer and other degenerative diseases;

Are you at a healthy weight?

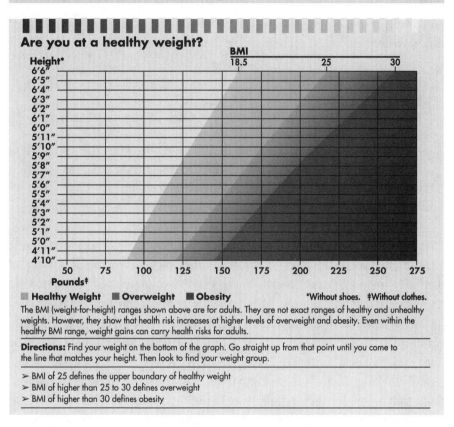

Healthy Weight   **Overweight**   **Obesity**   *Without shoes. ‡Without clothes.

The BMI (weight-for-height) ranges shown above are for adults. They are not exact ranges of healthy and unhealthy weights. However, they show that health risk increases at higher levels of overweight and obesity. Even within the healthy BMI range, weight gains can carry health risks for adults.

Directions: Find your weight on the bottom of the graph. Go straight up from that point until you come to the line that matches your height. Then look to find your weight group.

➤ BMI of 25 defines the upper boundary of healthy weight
➤ BMI of higher than 25 to 30 defines overweight
➤ BMI of higher than 30 defines obesity

Reprinted from USDA, *Dietary Guidelines for Americans,* (2000) p. 11.

- decreases your risk of cancer, arteriosclerosis, hypertension, heart disease, osteoporosis, senility, and depression;

- synchronizes your body rhythms, helping you to function physically, mentally, and emotionally at peak efficiency;

- adds years to your life—and helps make those years more healthy.

Of all the topics covered in this book, diet is probably the most emotionally charged. For most of us, food is much more than just a source of nutrition. It's also a source of comfort, a symbol of love, a recreational pastime, a connection to family and community, and, occasionally, the ground for potent emotions such as anger, fear, anxiety, and depression. Moreover, despite the healthful changes in diet that have become increasingly accepted over the past two decades, many of us have much farther to go before we are able to maintain a true anti-aging regimen. Encountering a long list of "do's" and "don'ts" can be overwhelming, especially where food is concerned.

Less than one-third of Americans meet the U.S. Government's Healthy People 2000 goal of eating two to four servings of fruits and three to five servings of vegetables per day. In October 2000, the U.S. Department of Agriculture Center for Nutrition Policy and Promotion reported that women, ages twenty-five to fifty, ate just 0.8 servings of fruit and 2.0 servings of vegetables daily, whereas men in the same age range ate merely 0.9 servings of fruit and 2.5 servings of vegetables a day.

As you consider your diet, our advice to you is that you take it one step at a time. Once you've understood the basic principles on which our anti-aging diet recommendations are based, you can evolve your own system for making the changes that will be most helpful to you. Some people find it easiest simply to overhaul their eating habits once and for all. Other people are more comfortable making one change at a time. Likewise, some people find that once they give up a "forbidden" food, they never miss it. Others work out a system of allowing themselves occasional tastes of the sweet desserts or high-fat foods that are no longer a regular part of their diets.

Whatever your modus operandi, remember that dietary changes can be both immensely difficult and extremely rewarding. Following the right diet can literally add years to your life.

EATING RIGHT FOR A LONGER LIFE

Basically, the diet that will most support healthy longevity follows these principles:

It's nontoxic. That means it contains hardly any preservatives, additives, pesticides, growth hormones (routinely given to livestock and poultry), antibiotics (likewise), food coloring, chemical flavoring, and other substances that tax your liver, your digestive system, and your heart.

It contains enough nutrients and fuel to satisfy your daily needs. Since most fresh fruits and vegetables lose much of their nutritional value within hours after being picked, you'll probably have to augment even the healthiest diet with vitamin and mineral supplements. Nevertheless, the more you can obtain basic nutrients from natural sources, the healthier your diet is likely to be.

It consists of foods that are easy to digest and eliminate. Evidence dating back to prehistoric times indicates that humans were originally vegetarians. Eating meat developed later, as an acquired taste. Certainly our digestive systems bear this theory out, for they process and eliminate meat and poultry with far greater difficulty than high-fiber foods, complex carbohydrates, and fresh produce. Although occasional consumption of meat—say, twice a week—is probably a key ingredient of a healthful diet, there's mounting evidence that more frequent consumption increases the risk of colon and pancreatic cancers.

In short, your diet should contain the following:

- raw or lightly cooked whole-grain cereals

- raw or lightly steamed vegetables and sprouts

- raw fresh fruit, including the skin (except on citrus fruits) because of the fiber and pectin it contains

Dietary Guidelines

1. Dietary fat intake should be less than 30 percent of total calories.

2. Saturated fat intake should be less than 10 percent of total calories.

3. Polyunsaturated fat should not exceed 10 percent of total daily calories.

4. Cholesterol intake should not exceed 300 mg per day.

5. Carbohydrate intake should represent 50 percent or more total calories with emphasis on complex carbohydrates.

6. Protein intake should constitute the remainder of the calories.

7. Sodium intake should be limited to fewer than 3 grams per day.

8. Alcohol consumption is not recommended, but if consumed, should not exceed 1 ounce a day of hard liquor or 8 ounces of wine or 24 ounces of beer.

9. Total calories should be consumed with the goal of achieving and maintaining a person's recommended body weight.

10. Consumption of a wide variety of foods is encouraged.

- lightly cooked beans, lentils, and peas

- raw nuts and seeds (unsalted)

- a certain amount of non-homogenized dairy products, particularly cultured products like yogurt

- fresh meat, fish, and poultry about two times a week

> A report in the *Journal of the American Medical Association* esti-
> mated that up to 50,000 deaths from heart disease could be pre-
> vented each year if Americans consumed more folic acid. A deficiency
> of folic acid may increase levels of homocysteine, a newly identified
> risk factor for heart disease and stroke.

Along with this healthy diet, you may want to take the vitamin and mineral supplements discussed in this book, if only because it's so difficult, in our
mechanized, nonagricultural society, to find uncontaminated, truly fresh food.
For example, frozen vegetables have 25 percent less of the common vitamins
(A, C, B_1, B_2, and B_3) than cooked fresh vegetables, while canned vegetables
have two to three times fewer vitamins than frozen. (Canned peas, for example, have lost 96 percent of their vitamin C content.) Yet, fresh produce that
sits in a truck or on a grocery shelf for a few days may have even fewer nutrients than frozen food. Bagged vegetables in the supermarket not only stay
fresher longer than unwrapped vegetables, but they also retain vitamin C and
beta-carotene better. Exposure to oxygen, carbon dioxide, heat, cold, moisture,
and light all cause food to degenerate, as does physical damage.

We all need a certain amount of fat, protein, and carbohydrates. Yet the
typical American diet maintains entirely the wrong balance of these essential
nutrients: it's 40 to 45 percent fat, 15 to 20 percent protein, 20 to 25 percent
simple carbohydrates (refined sugar and related foods), and 20 to 25 percent
complex carbohydrates (whole grains, vegetables, and fruits). A healthier
balance would be only 10 to 20 percent fat and a similar amount of protein;
0 to 5 percent simple carbohydrates; and at least 65 percent complex carbohydrates.

You'll notice that some foods are conspicuously absent from the "healthy
diet." Sugar, salt, alcohol, caffeine, and foods high in preservatives, as well as
high-fat foods, will all contribute to making you old before your time. American staples such as presweetened cereals, luncheon meats, bacon and pork
products, white flour, cola and other sweet drinks (even if made with aspar-

FOODS THAT HEAL, FOODS THAT HARM

Top 25 Healing Foods*	Top 25 Foods to Avoid
Apricots	Anchovies
Bananas	Alcohol
Beans (dry and green)	Bacon
Bell peppers (red and green)	Canned, bottled or frozen sweetened fruit
Broccoli	Canned soups**
Cantaloupe	Chocolate
Carrots	Fried foods
Garbanzos	Gravies**
Garlic	Ice cream
Greens (spinach, kale, turnip greens, Swiss chard, curly endive)	Peanuts, salted/roasted Pork**
Kiwi	Pickled eggs
Lamb	Processed cheese products
Oat bran	Processed lunch meats
Onions	Processed/sweetened oatmeal/cereals
Oranges	Saturated fats
Papaya	Soft cheeses
Pasta (whole wheat)	Soft drinks
Potatoes (baked)	Tuna, canned in oil
Soybeans Rice (brown)	Vegetables, canned, frozen with salt/additives
Tomatoes	White, brown or raw sugar
Tuna (water-packed)	White-flour products
Turkey (skinless breast)	White rice
Yams/sweet potatoes	White vinegar
Yogurt (non-fat)	Yogurt with fruit/syrup

*Unless you are allergic.

**Selection based on usual ingredients. Exceptions for low-fat, low-sodium, or other healthful modifications would apply.

tame), sweetened fruit drinks, potato chips and pretzels, roasted nuts and seeds, instant foods of all types, fried foods, coffee, tea, and chocolate all tend to age the body. They put a strain on your organs, digestive system, and cardiovascular system, and in many cases, they actively introduce free radicals into your body.

A HEALTHY WAY TO EAT: THE MEDITERRANEAN DIET

Olive oil has been shown to have numerous health benefits. The traditional Mediterranean diet, rich in olive oil and moderate amounts of wine, is now widely considered to have significant long-life benefits.

The six-year study of 182 rural Greek men and women over age seventy found that those who consumed a diet including olive oil, whole-grain breads, and fresh fruits and vegetables had significantly reduced their chances of dying during the length of the study, as compared with those whose diets were rich in red meat and saturated fats.

The study broke down the Mediterranean diet into four components:

1. a high ratio of monounsaturated to saturated fats;

2. moderate alcohol consumption;

3. high consumption of cereals, fruits, and vegetables;

4. low intake of meats and dairy products.

According to these components, for every unit increase there was an astounding 17 percent reduction in overall mortality.

On the other hand, several types of commonly used fat are relatively dangerous to your system and should be avoided:

- *Hydrogenated fats* (such as margarine and shortening). These are fats created through the process of hydrogenation, which converts a liquid (unsaturated) fat to a solid (saturated) fat by exposing the fat molecules to hydrogen. The unnatural molecules it contains raise your blood cholesterol, (even though margarine itself contains less cholesterol than butter), deposit fats in your arteries, increase the body's exposure to free radicals, and interfere with the body's production of prostaglandin, a substance that helps create a resistance to pain and helps produce healthy cells and tissues.

- *Highly heated or reheated fats*. Unless you're buying cold-pressed oils (available in natural food stores and some gourmet stores and supermarkets), you're buying fat that has already been heated, which oxidizes it and increases its ability to oxidize in the body. Fats heated to more than 300 degrees Fahrenheit are more likely to be highly oxidized.

Here are some additional suggestions for healthy uses of fat in your diet:

- Buy small bottles of oil with narrow necks and tightly closed lids; refrigerate after opening. This will limit the fats' exposure to oxygen.

- Use nonhydrogenated fats, such as butter, olive oil, sunflower oil, or sesame oil, rather than hydrogenated fats, such as margarine or shortening.

THE USES AND ABUSES OF DIETARY FAT

In the current focus on low-fat foods and the dangers of cholesterol (to some extent related to fats in the diet), it's important to remember that the body needs a certain amount of some kinds of fat. Natural fats provide a concentrated form of energy and create the environment in which fat-soluble vitamins, such as A and E, can be digested. They also provide the essential fatty acids (EFAs), which the body uses to maintain its cellular structure. Here are some forms in which fat can be useful to your body:

- Cod liver oil: This form of fat contains EFAs that convert into chemicals that protect your heart.

- Evening primrose oil: Available in health food stores, this substance also contains EFAs, including gamma-linoleic, which lowers cholesterol and blood pressure, heals eczema, eases hangovers and premenstrual tension, and helps to control weight.

- Olive oil: This is probably the most beneficial form of fat to use for cooking, as olive oil lowers LDL cholesterol without affecting HDL cholesterol. It is known as a monounsaturated fat. The best olive oil is extra-virgin and hand-pressed, as hydraulic presses may generate heat that in turn damages the oil.

- Polyunsaturated fats, such as sunflower seed oil and sesame seed oil: Like their cousin, the monounsaturated olive oil, both these fats lower LDL cholesterol, but they also lower HDL cholesterol. They're also more susceptible to turning rancid than olive oil—a process known as "auto-oxidation," which, as the name suggests, introduces those free radicals that antioxidants must then combat.

Fish Oil and Heart Disease

Observations of the diet and lifestyle of Greenland Eskimos show that a high-fat diet composed of Arctic foodstuffs and low in cholesterol results in a population with a very low incidence of heart disease, hypertension, and platelet aggregability.

The reason? Fish oil. Actually, it's because of *eicosapentaenoic acid*, or EPA, which is found in high concentrations in fish and marine life. Unlike the damaging prostaglandins which are found in land animals (like thromboxane, which constricts arteries), when we consume EPA, we experience less vasoconstriction in arteries and less platelet aggregation. Therefore, we reduce chances of blood clots, atherosclerosis, stroke, and heart attack. Consuming fish oil can also help lower serum cholesterol and triglyceride levels.

According to a recent study conducted at the University of Washington in Seattle, eating 5.5 grams of omega-3 fatty acids per month (the equivalent of four 3-ounce servings of salmon) may reduce the risk of cardiac arrest by 50 percent.

However, a word to the weight-conscious: fish oil is not calorie-free. If you want to start taking fish oil daily, you might want to reduce your daily food consumption by about 300 calories, or else you'd be putting on about twenty-five extra pounds per year.

FIBER: THE ANSWER TO FAT

Fiber tends to soak up fat. A high-fiber diet can be an effective anti-aging tool, improving your digestion, relieving the strain on your liver and gall bladder, and reducing your risk of large bowel cancer, gallstones, diabetes, arteriosclerosis, colitis, hemorrhoids, hernia, and varicose veins.

Fiber is the structural material that gives plant cell walls their integrity. Hence, fresh fruits and vegetables, whole grains, nuts, seeds, and legumes are all good sources of fiber. Fiber is also an important part of the human digestive process. It gives volume to the food we ingest, so that our intestines can more easily pass along their contents. Both absorption of nutrients and the elimination of waste are eased by fiber, with consequent benefits to your intestines.

There are many different types of fiber, and your body will benefit from absorbing some of each. Broccoli, green beans, and lettuce contain *cellulose,* which swells to increase the weight of food ingested. A high-cellulose content helps food move more quickly through the intestines, reducing the amount of time that bacteria can breed. It also eases pressure on the colon.

Cereals, brans, and whole grains contain *hemicellulose,* which increases the bulk of fecal matter, relieving pressure on the colon. Hemicellulose

Stop That Fat

Choose	Instead of
breads or muffins, low-fat	cake and doughnuts
Canadian bacon	bacon
cereal, plain whole-grain	granola
cod, flounder or scrod	salmon and mackerel
corn, hot-air popped	microwave/oil popcorn
cottage cheese, low-fat	ricotta cheese
crispbreads or flatbreads	regular crackers
farmer cheese	cream cheese
fish, baked or boiled	breaded and fried fish
frozen yogurt, non-fat	ice cream
fruit spreads or jam	butter and cream cheese
graham crackers/fig bars	chocolate-chips
ground beef, extra-lean	regular ground beef
milk, low-fat or skim	whole milk
mozzarella, part-skim	muenster or cheddar
mustard or ketchup	mayonnaise
pita or bagel	croissant
pretzels	chips and nuts
poultry, skinless light-meat	dark meat w/skin
sirloin tip roast	T-bone or chuck
tomato sauce	cheese sauce
tuna, water-packed	oil-packed fish
turkey or chicken, baked	bologna and salami
turkey ham or smoked ham	hot dogs and sausage
yogurt, low-fat or non-fat	sour cream

reduces the possibility of gallstones, it lowers cholesterol levels, it generally absorbs and neutralizes many harmful toxins, and, by moving food more quickly through the system, it reduces the amount of time that bacteria and carcinogens may breed within it.

Pectin is a type of fiber found in apple peel and carrots. It is known to lower cholesterol and generally to act as an antitoxin. *Mucilage,* found in legumes and seeds, also lowers cholesterol, as well as speeds the process of food through the system. *Lignin,* found in wheat bran and apples, helps bind the heavy metal trace elements in food, preventing their oxidizing effects, as well as producing other antitoxic effects.

However, if you're depending on bran as your major source of fiber, be aware that it can leach calcium, magnesium, and zinc from your system. As with most nutritional elements, it's a good idea to get fiber from many sources, and to avoid "megadoses" of any one type of food.

THE CHOLESTEROL ISSUE

Cholesterol remains a somewhat mysterious term to many health-conscious Americans. We've all heard about the striking dangers of this bodily substance: its relationship with deadly heart disease and other cardiovascular disorders, its dangers to the immune system, and its possible correlation with certain types of cancer. What many people do not know is that more than 90 percent of blood cholesterol is actually manufactured by one's own body. Reducing dietary cholesterol will therefore have relatively little effect on blood cholesterol levels.

This is not to say that your blood cholesterol levels are outside of your control. On the contrary, many factors tend to increase your cholesterol level: smoking, high blood pressure, liver problems (exacerbated by a diet high in toxic additives and preservatives), inadequate exercise, carrying too much body fat, stress, and depression. Because consuming too much fat tends to aggravate these other factors, it will indirectly raise your cholesterol level.

Also, evening primrose oil, cod liver oil, and olive oil actually reduce total and/or LDL cholesterol in your body. Lecithin, carnitine, vitamins C and E, dietary fibers such as oat bran, and deodorized garlic also lower cholesterol and/or triglycerides. In addition, vitamin E, oat bran, and garlic increase your body's level of HDL cholesterol.

In terms of diet, you have many options for reducing your cholesterol level. Try substituting vegetable protein for animal protein (vegetable proteins contain sterols, which block your blood's ability to absorb cholesterol from your intestines and may also help your liver better regulate cholesterol production). Try eating more fiber (fiber blots up excess fat), and make sure you get the EFAs that will regulate your blood fat. Finally, exercise regularly.

A Primer on Cholesterol

What is cholesterol and why do we need it?

Cholesterol is a crystalline substance made up of fats. Naturally, it is found all throughout the body—in the brain, liver, blood, and bile. Produced mainly in the liver, cholesterol is needed for the body to function properly; it is used by the cells to build membranes; it's needed to make bile salts, hormones, and vitamin D; and it aids in digestion. As cholesterol travels through the body, cells take what they need and leave the excess in the bloodstream. It is this excess cholesterol that can "stick" to arteries as plaque and lead to various forms of heart disease.

What are triglycerides?

Triglycerides are fats attached to a glycerol molecule, which are made up of three fatty acids. They are essentially the major transport and storage form for fats in our bodies, but high levels of triglycerides in the body have been associated with heart disease and diabetes.

Can cholesterol be both good and bad?

Researchers have discovered two different types of cholesterol: low-density lipoproteins (LDL "bad" cholesterol) and high-density lipoproteins (HDL "good" cholesterol). Our bodies can't use LDL cholesterol because it's obtained through animal products, and our cells usually reject it. Therefore, LDL cholesterol usually ends up as plaque that clogs our artery walls, while the body produces its own serum cholesterol, which it can utilize. HDL cholesterol, however, actually helps remove excess cholesterol from tissues and the bloodstream. Studies have shown that those individuals who have high levels of HDLs and low levels of LDLs also have a lower risk of heart disease. And if a person has already experienced a heart attack, increasing HDL levels and decreasing LDL levels brings improvement in arterial plaque.

INDIVIDUAL FOODS: THE GOOD AND THE BAD

Having taken a look at food in general, let's turn our attention to some specific foodstuffs, some of which are major tools in our quest for longevity. Others offer both benefits and disadvantages. Then, there is sugar, which we call the "killer" food.

HELPER FOODS

Garlic and Onions: The Miracle Foods

Certainly, along with olive oil, there are no foods more associated with the Mediterranean diet than are garlic and onions. But beyond the Mediterranean, they are two of the most valuable foods on the planet, which can be used as delicious spices in place of salt. For centuries, people have recorded the healing and life-giving properties of these two miracle foods.

> Pyramid builders in ancient Egypt ate garlic daily for endurance and strength.

Since Biblical times, garlic has been used to cure a variety of ailments:

- It lowers blood pressure by dilating blood vessel walls.

- It thins blood by inhibiting platelet aggregation, thereby reducing the risk of blood clots and heart attack.

- It lowers serum cholesterol.

- It aids in digestion.

- It stimulates the immune system.

- It acts as an antibiotic.

The Russians refer to garlic as a natural antibiotic. Garlic actually contains an amino acid derivative called *alliin,* which when consumed, releases an enzyme called *allicin.* Allicin is capable of killing twenty-three kinds of bacteria, sixty types of fungi and yeast, and salmonella. This enzyme has such a powerful antibiotic effect on the body that some say it is equivalent to penicillin.

Garlic has also been reported to protect against certain types of cancer, especially stomach and colon cancers. Studies done at the Memorial Sloan-Kettering Cancer Center found that garlic compounds stifled the growth of cancer cells. John Milner, a garlic researcher at Pennsylvania State University, reported that garlic was found to inhibit cancer in all tissues, including breast and liver.

Garlic was used in treating wounds and infections during World War I to prevent gangrene.

Garlic also has many antioxidant properties. Like vitamins C, E, and A, garlic blocks free radicals from oxidizing LDL cholesterol, so it won't clog arteries. Therefore, it subsequently helps arteries damaged by atherosclerosis heal, and it protects against other forms of heart disease. Studies have shown that a mere clove and a half of garlic daily can reduce cholesterol levels by as much as 9 percent. However, not everyone enjoys the robust flavor (or pungent odor) of a whole clove. In that case, odorless garlic capsules are available as supplements at most health food stores.

The following conversion can be used as a reference if you choose not to eat fresh garlic. Two to three fresh cloves equals:

- one teaspoon garlic powder

- four 1,000 mg garlic tablets

- four gel capsules of concentrated, standardized garlic extract

- one teaspoon of liquid concentrated, standardized garlic extract

Onions play a similar role in fighting against age-related diseases. A close kin of garlic, onions (red and yellow, not white) are full of antioxidants, the most important being *quercetin,* an antioxidant that has been reported to inactivate many cancer-causing agents, especially in the stomach, as well as to inhibit enzymes that spur cancer growth. Quercetin also prevents oxidation of LDL cholesterol. In addition, much like garlic, onions help thin the blood to prevent clotting, boost HDL cholesterol levels, and lower triglyceride and LDL levels, and therefore prevent stroke.

The best way to reap the benefits of these two foods is through your daily diet, and both can be used freely and easily in cooking—in salads and salad dressings, as spices, or in marinades and sauces. And in powder form, they can be added to just about any meal you wish to prepare.

Soybeans: The Ultimate Solution

Acting as one of nature's own antioxidants, the soybean may be one of the most important foods we add to our long-life diet. Some nutritionists call soybeans a natural "anti-aging pill," because they may interfere with free-radical damage and enhance our cells' defenses against aging and age-related diseases.

In a study conducted by Dr. Denham Harman, father of the free-radical theory of aging, laboratory animals that consumed soybean protein drastically reduced free-radical damage to their cells, more so than animals fed casein, a dairy protein. In addition, the animals that ate soybean protein extended their life spans by 13 percent.

The effect soybeans have on longevity is not restrained to laboratory animals, however. It is a known fact that the Japanese, who eat the highest daily amount of soybeans in the world, live longer lives than any other group of people on the planet. The Japanese consume about an ounce of soybeans per day—almost thirty times more than Americans—and they have far fewer cases of heart disease, cancer, diabetes, and osteoporosis.

> Scientists at the University of Pennsylvania School of Medicine found that soybeans contain a protease inhibitor called the Bowman-Birk inhibitor, which is so versatile against various cancers that it has been dubbed "the universal cancer preventive agent."

Perhaps the key ingredient that makes soybeans such a powerful antioxidant food is a substance called *genistein*. Genistein is a rare, vital antioxidant that has immense anti-aging biological activity. Some of genistein's potent anti-aging effects include:

- interfering with cancer activity at every stage, including breast, colon, lung, prostate, skin, and blood (leukemia) cancers;

- reducing plaque buildup in artery walls and reducing the risk of heart attack, stroke, and atherosclerosis.

Exposure to the chemical genistein reduces breast cancer in animals by 40 to 65 percent, according to Dr. Stephen Barnes, professor of pharmacology at the University of Alabama at Birmingham. Japanese women (who eat soybeans regularly) have only one-fourth as many instances of breast cancer as American women, whose soy consumption is extremely low. Soybeans fight breast cancer in two ways: they have a direct anticancer effect on our cells; and they prevent estrogen from causing malignant changes in breast tissue. This phenomenon is seen in both pre- and postmenopausal women.

As with breast cancer, soybeans also help prevent prostate cancer. Observing the differences between Japanese and American males, the power of the soybean is quite evident. While Japanese men are still prone to prostate cancers, their cancers don't grow fast enough to become as deadly as most American cases of prostate cancer do. And according to Finnish researcher Herman Adlercreutz, eating soybeans and soy products has been shown to reduce prostate cancer in laboratory animals.

Other amazing effects of this little bean on the human body include boosting HDL cholesterol levels and lowering triglycerides, keeping blood sugar at healthy levels—thus reducing our risk for adult-onset diabetes (type II) and heart disease—and increasing bone mass by helping our systems retain calcium.

In order to reap the anti-aging benefits of the soybean, you must make sure you are eating the beans' protein (that is, soy sauce or soybean oil contain very little protein, and therefore exhibit very few life-giving properties). According to Dr. Mark Messina, author (with Virginia Messina and Kenneth Serchell) of the book *The Simple Soybean and Your Health* (Avery, 1994), some of the best sources for soy protein are:

- soy flour: $\frac{1}{2}$ cup = 50 mg
- soymilk: 1 cup = 40 mg
- tofu: $\frac{1}{2}$ cup = 40 mg
- soy nuts: 1 ounce = 40 mg
- miso: $\frac{1}{2}$ cup = 40 mg
- tempeh: $\frac{1}{2}$ cup = 40 mg

Obviously, you don't have to eat all of this soy product once a day—Dr. Messina recommends perhaps one cup of soymilk and three to four servings of tofu daily. That would equal what the Japanese normally consume—about 50 to 75 mg per day. It's also important to remember that to see any of these anti-aging effects, you must eat soy every day; studies have shown that chemicals like genistein remain in our bodies only for twenty-four to thirty-six hours at most. Therefore, daily servings are needed to keep our cells fully stocked with the power of soy.

Water: Wetter Is Better

Water is the most essential nutrient for human life. Our bodies are composed of two-thirds water, and the brain alone is made up of 85 percent water! It is present in every cell and tissue of the body and plays a vital role in almost every biological process including digestion, absorption, circulation, and excretion. Water also is the foundation of blood and lymph, regulates body temperature, helps maintain youthful skin and strong muscles, and lubricates our joints and organs to keep them in working order. Yet, despite our need for a constant fresh supply of water, many people—especially the elderly—do not consume and maintain enough of it for good health and long life. In the elderly, the most consistent biomarker of aging is dehydration and one contributing factor may be a loss of thirst sensitivity with age.

When you are dehydrated, your body temperature increases and you lose not only water but also valuable electrolytes such as the essential minerals potassium and sodium. Dehydration can creep up on you especially when exercising. It's a good idea to keep a bottle of water near you at all times. Dehydration warning signs can include:

- dizziness

- headache, heaviness in the head

- flushed skin

- weakness, fatigue

- dry mouth, loss of appetite

Advanced signs of dehydration can include:

- blurred vision

- hearing loss

- dry, hot skin

- rapid pulse, shortness of breath

- unsteady gait

- extremely frequent urination without drinking fluids

You cannot replace the health benefits of drinking water by substituting beverages such as soft drinks, coffee, alcohol, and juices. Many alcoholic and/or caffeinated drinks actually act as diuretics, causing us to urinate more frequently than normal. This can cause a general state of dehydration resulting in urinary tract infections and cellular damage. Everyone should drink at least eight 8-ounce glasses of water per day (64 ounces total), but not just any water. Not all water is the same nor is it all good for you. Which type of water then is best?

- *Steam-distilled water.* The best water a person can drink is pure water—

water that contains nothing but molecules of two hydrogen atoms and one oxygen atom. Pure water is easily energized. It begins to attract other substances that end up destroying its pure state. Therefore, the best state of drinking water we can hope to find in supermarkets is called *steam-distilled water.* Distillation involves vaporizing water by boiling it. As the steam rises, it leaves behind most of the bacteria, viruses, and chemicals. The steam is then condensed and cooled where it becomes distilled water. Drinking steam-distilled water actively removes inorganic and toxic materials that are rejected from our bodies by our cells and tissues. An added benefit is its ability to *chelate* or attach to other toxic molecules and minerals and eliminate them.

It is important to realize that steam-distilled water is devoid of minerals, which over a long period can become a problem if your diet is mineral deficient. Read your supplement labels carefully to see if they include necessary trace minerals and supplement if needed. Additionally, distilled

---

Chlorella

Chlorella is a therapeutic green algae that's been in existence since the Pre-Cambrian period—almost 2.5 billion years. It consists of 60 percent protein, 20 percent carbohydrates, and contains unsaturated (good) fats. In addition, chlorella contains an abundance of vitamins, minerals, and antioxidants including vitamins A, B_2, B_6, C, K, and E, calcium, magnesium, iron, zinc, phosphorus, iodine, and beta-carotene. Proponents of this nutritional superfood speak of its ability to ward off disease and slow the aging process. Chlorella has also been credited with:

- boosting immunity
- reducing high blood pressure
- reducing the risk of diabetes
- helping reduce symptoms of premenstrual syndrome
- reducing the risk of anemia
- reducing symptoms of menopause
- promoting cell growth
- healing wounds

Chlorella contains chlorophyll, which can help speed the cleansing of the bloodstream. And its high content of DNA and RNA has been found to protect against the effects of ultraviolet radiation.

water may contribute to general acidity of the body, which may further deplete the body of necessary essential minerals. Check your body's pH level to avoid chronic acidity and supplement trace minerals if needed. Tip: Adding fresh lemon juice to distilled water improves its taste while preventing mineral depletion.

- *Natural spring water.* Another popular bottled water sold today is termed *spring water.* Natural spring water means that the water has risen to the earth's surface from some type of underground reservoir. Spring water's mineral content is not altered, but it may or may not have been filtered or otherwise treated. Therefore, you may want to read the labels of these bottled waters carefully and find out if what you're drinking really is natural.

- *Tap water.* The worst water you can put in your body is, unfortunately, the most accessible: tap water. Although using a filter can help, this type of water comes out of household faucets and in many communities is highly contaminated with chemicals such as chlorine, flourine, biological poisons, and various pollutants. Tap water has very little benefit to the functioning of our cells and tissues, and it may do more harm to our bodies than good.

QUESTIONABLE FOODS

Protein: A Double-Edged Sword

The right place for protein in a healthy diet is a problematic concept for many Americans to grasp, for virtually all of us have been brought up with the notion that "more is better" where protein is concerned. In a sense, traditional nutritional ideas about protein have been oriented toward an outmoded model of building up muscles and body mass. This was useful for a short-lived people facing the physical dangers of a hunting society or the enormous physical demands of agricultural labor, but it is not particularly useful for the prevention of aging and age-related disease that concerns us now.

The very name *protein* comes from the Greek word for "of first importance." And protein is truly vital for human life itself. Our bodies use the twenty-two amino acids of protein to build muscles, skin, hair, nails, and blood, as well as to nourish the heart, the brain, and other organs.

Yet excessive consumption of protein not only puts an unwarranted strain on our digestive and eliminative systems, but it also reduces our immunity, increases cholesterol levels, and causes calcium to be leached from our bones.

How much protein your body needs depends on your lean body weight, because protein is the substance used to maintain that weight. A number of factors may increase your need for protein. A child's growth requires protein, as muscles, organs, and other parts of the body rely upon that substance for their ability to expand. Exercise and weight training use protein to increase muscle mass. Alternately, stress, serious illness, and wasting diseases deplete the body's protein intake, requiring increased consumption to make up the loss.

Many nutritionists believe that the recommended daily allowance for protein in the American diet is vastly inflated. And, even given these high standards, the average American male eats nearly twice the recommended amount. The American female likewise overconsumes.

Studies of centenarians, on the other hand, show that they tend to have a low intake of protein, and to favor vegetable sources over animal protein. A diet high in rice, beans, and other grains and legumes, supplemented by small amounts of dairy products and fish, is far healthier than one that relies on red meat and chicken for protein.

Sensible Salts

By now, most Americans have heard the warnings about a high-salt intake: it tends to raise blood pressure, increases the risk of prostate problems, heightens premenstrual tension, and contributes to heart attack and stroke. Yet salt is so widely used in American cooking that, unless you cook all your own food from fresh and natural sources, you are likely to be exposed to salt without knowing it.

Here's a list of some common high-sodium foods that a person on an anti-aging diet would do well to avoid:

Beverages: commercial buttermilk, tomato juice, and V8 juice.

Fats: gravy, peanut butter, and prepared salad dressings.

Protein foods: canned salmon and tuna, cheese, luncheon meats, ham, bacon, smoked fish, other cured meats and fishes, and frozen dinners.

Snacks: (unless unsalted) pretzels, potato chips, popcorn, and crackers.

Vegetables: virtually all canned vegetables, sauerkraut, olives, and pickles.

Soups: virtually all canned, dried, or instant soups.

Condiments: virtually all commercially prepared condiments, including ketchup, soy sauce, meat sauce, barbecue sauce, chili, prepared mustard, seasoned salt, MSG, and meat tenderizers.

The following are some healthy alternatives to salt. Even though you should use these substances, too, in moderation, they are likely to be easier on your system than commercial salt:

Sea salt: contains only 75 percent sodium chloride (the basic elements in table salt) and 25 percent trace minerals.

Kelp: contains only 18 percent sodium chloride and many trace minerals.

Miso: a fermented soybean product, contains only 12 percent sodium chloride, 15 to 20 percent protein, 5 to 8 percent fat, and 12 to 22 percent carbohydrates.

THE KILLER FOOD

Sugar: Sweet and Deadly

We've saved the worst news for last: sugar is very bad for you. Whether you take your sweetness in the form of table sugar, brown sugar, turbinado, raw sugar, honey, glucose, dextrose, or corn syrup, it puts an enormous strain on your system and acts as a cross-linking free radical to damage your cells.

One of the most common results of overconsumption of sugar is *hypoglycemia,* or low blood sugar. Some 35 percent of all Americans suffer from some form of this condition, in which a craving for sugar is followed by a swift high and then a painful crash as sweet foods are consumed. Fatigue, trembling, rapid heartbeat, inability to concentrate, memory problems, and emotional instability are only some of the symptoms of this troubling condition, which feel so familiar to many people with hypoglycemia that they don't acknowledge it as a "condition" at all. Only after they have given up or greatly reduced their consumption of sugar do they realize what reserves of energy and calm might routinely be within their reach.

Sugar addicts who drink sweetened caffeinated beverages experience a double rush—and a double crash. Ironically, the very substance that seems to perk you up also drains you, so that you're caught in a vicious cycle of needing coffee to wake up and sugar to keep yourself going. Reducing or eliminating your intake of sugar and caffeine, on the other hand, beside prolonging your life, will enable you to feel more energetic, alert, and productive on the same amount of sleep—or less!

Most Americans consume 22 percent of their calories in sugar, which is added to virtually all prepared and packaged foods, including many vegetables, meats, and whole-grain products as well as the more obvious sweetened cereals and breads. Yet, sugar leads to fat gain, the degeneration of one's muscles, dysfunction of the immune system, cardiovascular problems, arteriosclerosis, and premature aging, as well as diabetes and hypoglycemia.

If you would like to cut down on your sugar consumption, here are a few suggestions:

- Read food labels. Ingredients are listed in the order of amount, with the most plentiful substance listed first, so if "sugar" is anywhere in the top three or four, you know you're eating something far too sweet. Read carefully, as many manufacturers break up their sugar counts by listing "sugar," "dextrose," "corn syrup," and other forms of sweeteners in a single list, making each element look less significant than it really is.

- Increase your consumption of whole grains—they reduce cravings for sweets.

- Pay attention to *when, how,* and *why* you need sweet foods. Sometimes the need for a sugary treat is more psychological than anything else, and you may be able to learn to meet those emotional needs in a way that's gentler to your system and better for your health.

NOURISHING YOURSELF

One of the best ways to change your diet to promote your health and longevity is to listen closely to your body. Pay attention to your cravings and reactions, to the way things taste and feel inside your mouth, and to your sense of hunger or satiety. Sometimes we keep eating long past the point of hunger, just out of habit, or from nervousness or anger. Listening to your body and your emotions can help ease this habit. We often expect foods to be sweet or salty simply because we've forgotten to pay attention to how else they might taste or because we don't take the time to identify what we're craving: a sweet food or simply a soft one? A salty food or just something to crunch between our teeth?

Honoring your appetites and cravings will actually make healthy eating easier, as well as enable you to get more satisfaction out of both your healthy and your "treat" consumption.

The Long-Life Diet may not be easy. But take heart. It will pay off—in more vigorous and exciting years of life and health.

CHAPTER 15

Detoxification Basics

FROM IMMUNITY TO INFINITY

Each of us is in a constant state of war with billions of creatures—bacteria, viruses, fungi, and parasites—on us, around us, and in us—that threaten to give us an infection that can compromise how we feel and quite possibly shorten how long we live. We are in the midst of a huge pandemic that is largely ignored by the traditional medical community. As many as 75 percent of Americans suffer from some form of bacterial, viral, fungal, or parasitic infection, which can manifest as:

- fatigue
- chronic sinus infection
- asthma
- allergies
- skin conditions such as eczema, psoriasis, acne, and rosacea
- ulcers
- sexually transmitted diseases
- urinary tract infections
- frequent colds or flu
- recurring bronchitis and pneumonia
- recurring ear infections
- dental problems, such as gingivitis, bad breath, or abscesses
- food poisoning
- and more!

New research suggests that infections may be a possible mechanism for heart disease and cancer—today's most virulent killers. In short, infections that compromise our immunity may well be the trigger that accelerates the onset and/or progression of the chronic degenerative diseases of aging. Infectious agents may well be the single most important yet undiscovered cause of premature aging and the chronic degenerative disorders of aging that now plague Americans—Alzheimer's disease, arthritis, cancer, fatigue, heart disease, memory loss, and more.

Low-grade, undetected, untreated infections may shave twenty years or more off of your active and productive life span, and rob you of a lifetime of bountiful energy and happiness.

Build super immunity and beat back the bugs! Start with a most basic place—what you eat and how your body does (and does not) process those foods.

THE BOWEL

Connected to the twenty-five feet of the gastrointestinal (GI) tract, where digestion and assimilation of nutrients occurs, lies the colon, the body's disposal system. Although just five feet long, the large bowel is one of the four key human organs (lungs, kidneys, and skin are the others).

"Out of sight, out of mind"—hardly a single one of us thinks about colon health. As a result, most of us have neglected colons, which signal their distress by causing gas, constipation, diarrhea, cramping, and—the dangerous extreme—colorectal cancer.

The colon is, to be direct, the body's garbage disposal. It serves as a temporary holding tank for what the stomach and small intestine does not digest or assimilate. Properly functioning bowels produce painless and effortless bowel movements. It should take about eighteen to thirty-six hours for food to travel the length of the entire GI tract (this is known as transit time). Most of us who eat two to three meals a day should produce one substantial bowel movement every day. The stool (feces) should be formed or semi-formed and of a bulky but soft consistency. It should not regularly contain recognizable undigested food morsels, nor should it be abnormally foul in odor, have a greasy texture, or contain blood.

More than 400 different kinds of microorganisms reside in the large and small intestines. The flora of our intestines must be balanced. That is, we must have healthy quantities of friendly bacteria (*Lactobacillus acidophilus and Lactobacillus bifidus*). These bacteria feed on the fermentable carbohydrates in our diet to help facilitate good, thorough digestion. *Lactobacillus* also inhibit the growth of pathogenic bacteria, such as *E.* coli, H. *pylori, Staphylococcus,* and *Candida albicans.*

Aging Starts at Your Lips; Reverse It at Your Colon

There perhaps isn't a more misunderstood food component than fiber (see page 388), which may be considered as an essential anti-aging nutrient. It may reverse or prevent a multitude of diseases that are frequently experienced as we age. Fiber is a dietary workhorse: it keeps toxins from building up in the intestines, thus promoting the proper absorption of important nutrients from food. The supply of cellular nutrients that fiber helps to release are responsible for many of the biological processes essential to life. Because many of us fail to get our optimal daily dose of fiber, here are some insights that will help you to understand the importance of fiber in your diet and make selections of fiber-rich foods.

With many doctors and nutritionists encouraging people to eat no less than 20–30 grams of fiber a day, the American Dietetic Association reports that most Americans consume only 11 grams daily. Researchers have noted that upward of 35 grams of roughage a day may actually reduce the risk of chronic diseases, such as those involving the heart.

Fiber is composed of complex carbohydrates, and is found only in plant foods. Fiber is categorized as either soluble or insoluble. Sources of soluble fiber include dried beans, oats, barley, apples, citrus fruits, and potatoes. Insoluble fiber may be found in whole grains, wheat bran, cereals, seeds, and the skins of many fruits and vegetables. The human body needs both kinds of fiber. While your doctor or nutritionist may recommend a fiber supplement, you should be aware that many of these products contain only a single type of fiber and thus are less preferable than dietary sources.

Fiber can benefit a number of medical conditions, including:

- *Obesity.* High-fiber foods are often recommended in dietary plans to help those who have extra weight to shed. Fiber functions in a multitude of beneficial ways. Dietary fiber not only can help to enhance weight loss, but also can act to decrease feelings of hunger often felt in reducing caloric intake. Elevated blood pressure, a common and dangerous side effect of excess pounds, can be combated by a diet rich in fruits and vegetables. Roughage provides not only a healthy dose of fiber but potassium as well, which helps even the mildly overweight to lower blood pressure.

- **Heart Disease.** Many types of cardiac conditions may be countered effectively by consuming foods that are high in fiber. A variety of nutritional factors, including total and saturated fat consumption, and fiber intake from fruits and vegetables, impact atherosclerotic cardiovascular disease (ASCVD), which can strike as either coronary heart disease (CHD), cerebral vascular disease, or peripheral vascular disease. Fiber-rich foods such as vegetables, fruits, whole-grain cereals, and legumes are rich sources of nutrients, phytochemicals, and antioxidants that play a beneficial role in heart disease. High-fiber foods contain soluble and insoluble fiber, minerals, vitamins, other micronutrients, and phytochemicals. These same foods often act as rich sources of the "good" fats—monounsaturated fatty acids and omega-3 fatty acids. Legumes (beans) deliver oligosaccharides to our bodies. Just recently, the results from the Nurses' Health Study reported that whole grains can deliver a protective role in CHD. This benefit is suspected as a result of not only the dietary fiber in whole grains, but also vitamins such as folate, vitamin B_6, and vitamin E that are richly present. Earlier reports from the Nurses' Health Study found that women consuming cereal regularly were able to reduce their risk of CHD, mostly as a direct result of the fiber content. The Iowa Women's Health Study likewise found that postmenopausal women eating whole-grain products such as cereal could reduce their risk of ischemic heart disease, through both the fiber and antioxidant vitamins that these foods contain. Fiber also benefits the lipid profile. A variety of studies demonstrate that soluble fiber can be effective in lowering cholesterol by clinically significant amounts. The National Heart, Lung, and Blood Institute Family Heart Study reports that dietary fiber can beneficially impact plasminogen activator inhibitor type 1 (PAI-1), an emerging marker of cardiovascular disease.

- **Cancer.** Fiber increases the mobility of the intestinal tract, which many physicians and scientists believe reduces exposure to potential carcinogens ingested from foods. This is relevant to understanding how fiber can reduce your risk of two leading types of cancer: colon and breast. While consumption of large amounts of fat and animal products is suspected to increase the risk for colon cancer, it is believed that diets high in fiber and low in fat may protect against colon cancer. To reduce colon cancer risk, enjoy a diet that is low in fat, alcohol, and preserved food items, while high in fiber and vitamins A, C, E, and beta-carotene. Beginning at age forty, both men and women should undergo regular colon cancer screenings (digital rectal exam; DRE), and, starting at age fifty, occult blood testing should be administered as well. For women surviving breast cancer, a reduced risk of the recurrence of the disease is now linked to increased blood levels of carotenoids. Raise these through a diet that is high in vegetables, which coincidentally raises fiber intake to reduce the time that cancer-causing agents are in contact with the intestines.

Cancer patients frequently suffer from significant alterations in carbohydrate, protein, and fat metabolism. Animal studies have provided evidence that foods relatively low in simple carbohydrates with moderate amounts of high-quality protein, fiber, and fat (especially fats of the omega-3 fatty acid series) are beneficial for those with, or recovering from, cancer. In the near future, nutritional intervention may become a powerful tool for controlling malignant disease and for reducing toxicity associated with chemotherapy and radiation therapy.

- *Diabetes.* While in both insulin-dependent and non-insulin-dependent diabetic patients, a high-carbohydrate diet does not offer any advantage in terms of blood glucose and plasma lipid concentrations compared with a high-fat (mainly unsaturated) diet, researchers have found that it is the fiber content that plays a key distinguishing role. In diabetics, adverse metabolic effects of high-carbohydrate diets are neutralized when fiber and carbohydrate are increased simultaneously. A number of studies have demonstrated that a high-carbohydrate/high-fiber diet significantly improves blood glucose control and reduces plasma cholesterol levels in diabetic patients compared with a low-carbohydrate/low-fiber diet. In addition, a high-carbohydrate/high-fiber diet does not increase plasma insulin and triglyceride concentrations, despite the higher consumption of carbohydrates. In diabetics, fiber in its soluble form is more beneficial for glucose and fat metabolism purposes. Legumes, vegetables, and fruits are to be encouraged in the diabetic diet. The fiber content, by influencing the accessibility of other nutrients, also promotes proper digestion and absorption. A balanced increase in consumption of fiber-rich foods and unsaturated fat is generally beneficial for diabetics.

EASY STEPS FOR ADDING MORE FIBER TO YOUR DAILY DIET

1. **Know the fiber values in your foods.** The U.S. Food & Drug Administration has recently issued guidelines for claims relating to the fiber content of foods. When you see that a product states that it is "a good source" of fiber, it contains no less than 2.5 grams of fiber per serving (10 percent of the Daily Value based on a 2,000-calorie diet). Likewise, those products

which are "high in," "rich in," or "excellent source of" fiber provide at least 5 grams of fiber per serving (20 percent of the Daily Value).

2. **Use the pyramid as your dietary foundation.** If you follow the recommendations of the U.S. Department of Agriculture's new Food Pyramid, you are eating two to four servings of fruit, three to five servings of vegetables, and six to eleven servings of cereals or grains. By doing so, you will be achieving the optimal 25–30 grams of daily fiber.

3. **Less processing equals more health benefit.** Opt for foods that are as close to their unprocessed state as possible:

   • **Uncooked vegetables:** after thoroughly washing your veggies, why not eat them *au naturale*? During any cooking process, fiber can be broken down into its carbohydrate state, reducing its ability to act as roughage. If you choose to cook your vegetables, try a gentle steaming, so you retain their crunch.

   • **Show a little skin:** enjoy the skin and membranes of foods such as apples, potatoes, and nuts, as they are rich in fiber.

   • **Wholeness:** next time you're grocery shopping, purchase a whole-grain cereal or bread, as these contain grains that retain their nutrient-rich outer husks. Add some variety to your meals by choosing more exotic side dishes such as bulgur, couscous, or kasha.

   • **Cool beans:** to your favorite soup, stew, or salad recipe, add a cupful or two of beans. Take a break from meat-based dinners and put bean burritos or a dish of zesty rice and beans on your table.

   • **Smart snacks:** sometimes, it's those "little treats" that can do the most damage. Instead of reaching for a sugar-packed or fat-laden snack food, choose the fiber-rich, sensation-satisfying crunch of fresh fruit, banana or apple chips, or a handful of dry-roasted nuts.

Through many research studies, fiber is repeatedly demonstrated to be of benefit in conditions such as cancer, heart disease, and diabetes. By making very small changes in our dietary choices, we can empower ourselves with a potent way to fight the most common degenerative diseases of aging. Make fiber a part of your daily routine, and you're on your way to looking and feeling younger.

THE LIVER

The bowel operates in close relation with the liver, one of the most important components of the GI system. The liver may be considered a vast metabolic factory. It processes proteins, carbohydrates, and fats, and synthesizes bile, glycogen, and serum proteins that the body uses for metabolism.

Most important, the liver is the key organ responsible for detoxification. A properly functioning liver protects the individual from both environmental and metabolic poisons.

A toxic liver leaks poisons into the bloodstream. When your bowel fails to perform optimally, the liver has to do extra work. At some point, too many harmful substances will accumulate, and they will escape into circulation in the body, injure tissue, and diminish your health.

Fortunately, the liver is one of the only organs in the human body that can regenerate. It has the capacity to heal itself, particularly when supported by effective therapeutic agents and interventions.

Liver-Cleansing Tips

Certain liver-friendly nutrients and botanicals can be used to periodically cleanse and mildly purge the body of accumulated toxins and potential toxins. This is an ideal way to:

- jump-start a weight-management program

- revitalize a weight-management program when you are hitting a plateau

- jump-start a new fitness program

- revitalize energy

- synergize with a smoking-cessation program

- generally feel better

The liver's role in detoxification is activated through the coordinated effort of two families of enzymes, known as cytochrome p450s and conjugation enzymes. By activating these enzymes, we can assist the liver in its job to detoxify and excrete toxins from our bodies. Common factors that cause a sluggish liver include:

- use of certain drugs, both over the counter (OTC) and prescription (Rx)

- lack of fresh vegetables in the diet

- smoking

- excessive alcohol consumption

- poor diet

- genetics

- chronic stress

- aging

Not only do cytochrome p450s and conjugation enzymes need to be activated, but they have to be balanced as well. The enzymes families work together as a team to progressively detoxify the body. The cytochrome p450s actually generate free radicals in order to accomplish their task. Left unchecked, these can become harmful. The conjugation enzymes capture these free radicals, and inactivate them and prepare them for excretion.

Remember, the liver and the GI tract—specifically the bowel—are closely interconnected in terms of physiology and function. To properly digest and absorb foods, eliminate toxins and undesirable substances, and maintain optimal immunity from germs, each of us needs our total GI tract to perform at its peak.

Collectively, natural liver and GI-assistive nutrients such as those mentioned above can help to:

- gently enhance peristalsis

- absorb and eliminate bile (bile helps to eliminate fatty substances)

- provide healthful probiotics

- provide prebiotics to feed the probiotics

- provide substances to help to eliminate unwanted organisms that can inhabit the intestines

- provide fuel for the functioning of the GI cells

The liver and GI tract are miraculous components of the human body. Safeguard and maintain your body's well-being, reduce your susceptibility to infectious diseases, and regain energy and stamina by employing a simple program to promote the health of these unseen and underemphasized organs.

Natural Botanicals and Nutrients That Aid in Maintaining a Healthy Liver

• *N-Acetylcysteine* is a powerful antioxidant that serves three functions: 1) it helps protect the liver from free radicals, 2) it is the nutritional precursor to the body's own vital glutathione, and 3) it can act as a phase II detoxifier. Glutathione is a phase II conjugation enzyme that helps rid the liver of several potential toxins. As we age, eat poorly, and incur stress and infection, glutathione levels decrease.

• *Schisandra* is a Chinese medicinal herb that has been used for centuries to cleanse and detoxify the liver. It stimulates the body to make more glutathione, and it has several active chemicals in it that have been demonstrated to protect the liver against various toxins and infectious agents.

• Rosemary activates the liver to rid itself of a variety of toxins including excess hormones.

• *Green Tea* extract has numerous antioxidant protectors that protect the liver.

• *Curcumin* is an extract of an Asian spice that has strong phase II conjugation activity. It is also an antiviral and a strong antioxidant.

Natural Botanicals That Assist with the Gentle Enhancement of Natural Peristalsis and Bowel Cleansing

• *Scutellaria* is a Chinese medicinal herb that has strong anti-*Candida albicans* activity as well as other antimicrobial activity.

• *Peppermint* has been shown to be helpful in maintaining a healthy bowel.

Fibers and Probiotics

• *Glutamine* is a restorative amino acid that is used by the GI tract as its source of fuel. Pharmaceutical companies sell it as a medical food for GI healing.

- *Fibersol* (soluble fiber) has been shown to help gently increase peristalsis. A powerful prebiotic, it helps restore healthy bowel flora and helps reduce cholesterol and blood sugar.

- *Soy fiber* helps to reduce cholesterol and blood sugar.

- *Probiotic blend,* at effective levels, helps restore healthy flora in the gut. This blend of six healthful microorganisms is protective against intestinal pathogens, and helps to lower cholesterol, relieve chronic bad breath, and balance GI elimination, among a number of other healthful activities.

CHAPTER 16

Exercises
for Longevity

Until the Industrial Revolution in the early 1800s, strenuous physical activity was an integral part of daily life—in work as well as in religious, social, and cultural expression. With this diminished work-related physical activity, the healers and philosophers of the time questioned whether long life and health could be maintained with a decreased level of exercise.

By 1953, almost 60 percent of American children failed to meet even a minimum fitness standard for health, compared to less than 10 percent in Europe. When John F. Kennedy became president in 1961, he convened a conference on physical fitness and young people and established what would eventually be called the President's Council on Physical Fitness and Sports. In the mid-1970s, popular interest in the benefits of exercise sprouted a widespread enthusiasm for the benefits of physical activity in preventing and treating a variety of conditions that continues to this day.

Despite the government's efforts to educate the public about the benefits of exercise, a report published by the Centers for Disease Control and Prevention (CDC) in March 2001 revealed that just 25 percent of adults met government recommendations for physical activity in 1998.

After age thirty, each of us experiences a decline in functional capacity of 0.75 percent to 1.0 percent per year. However, exercise is an intervention that will help maintain and enhance functional ability as chronological age increases. Without exercise, however, the aging process can take a terrible toll, most especially for those whose lifestyles can be considered "sedentary."

PHYSICAL EFFECTS OF AGING

More than 48 million adults in the United States, who are otherwise healthy and able-bodied, can be classified as sedentary. If you are one of these people, then you need to know that an inactive lifestyle only places extra strain on your body, increasing risk for cardiovascular problems, cancer, diabetes, and many other diseases. A quarter of a million deaths per year are attributable in part to sedentary lifestyles. There is hope, however. A modest change in lifestyle enables every couch potato to reduce their propensity for illness, and can add years to their youthful and productive life span.

More and more, scientists are finding that an adequate exercise program, coupled with a healthy diet, can help you to recapture your youthful vitality by slowing or reversing many of the physiological changes that are associated with aging.

The Aging Metabolism

An aging metabolism is less able to use fatty acids properly, thus burdening your body systems, depressing your immune system, and possibly leading to atherosclerosis. Exercise uses fatty acids for 80 percent of the calories needed to complete an activity, essentially converting them to energy. As we have learned, the production of growth hormone improves the function of your immune system. It also builds your muscles, burns off fat, and generally contributes to your overall well-being. Although your body manufactures less growth hormone as you grow older, accounting for a 40 percent loss with a 30 percent decrease in strength by age seventy, exercise stimulates and increases production of this vital hormone.

Aging and Muscle Strength

Not only does aging result in a reduced ability to function physically, but also the less muscle you have, the less energy you burn while you're resting (your metabolic rate). Therefore, as your metabolic rate and your activity level go down, you need fewer and fewer calories to maintain your body weight. But most people don't decrease their calorie intake to match their declining needs. They just buy new clothing when they gain weight.

Light weightlifting can be an effective method to burn off at least some of these excessive calories. A small study done at Tufts University set twelve volunteers, fifty-six and older, on a twelve-week strength-training program. The group worked out for thirty minutes three times a week. Researchers found that the volunteers' bodies were burning more energy, allowing them to consume an average of 300 additional calories a day without gaining weight.

Aging and Bone Mass

After age thirty-five, there is also a decline in total bone mass of up to 1 percent per year. Women going through menopause may begin to lose their bone density at an even higher rate of up to 3 percent per year. With low bone density, there is an increased risk of breakage and of developing osteoporosis. Victims of osteoporosis have brittle, porous bones that fracture easily and can result in such deformities as the curved spine, known as a "dowager's hump." These conditions are not only debilitating but can also be fatal. Weight-bearing exercise is the key to building maximum bone mass before age forty and in retarding the gradual loss of bone mass after age forty. For women, treatments like estrogen replacement therapy (ERT) can also help overcome bone loss.

Aging and Flexibility

Flexibility is yet another factor that diminishes with age. Older people are more prone to stiffness and orthopedic injury than younger people because of physical inactivity. Over time, muscles become stiffer and joints degenerate, producing less joint-lubricating synovial fluid. Connective tissues gradually lose their elasticity and muscle fibers shorten. This loss in flexibility can make common daily tasks, such as bending over, a chore and fool the mind and body into thinking that it is unable to embark on any exercise. However, about eighty percent of all lower back pain results from poorly conditioned muscles. A simple exercise program can help strengthen the back and eliminate most of these pains, even after a few weeks. By strengthening these joints and muscles, you may eventually be able to participate in other activities and reduce your risk of injury.

Use It or Lose It

As studies have shown again and again, older people begin to lose certain physical and mental abilities because they are not using them. In fact, scientists believe that the decline in strength and muscular endurance is due more to disuse of the neuromuscular system than to aging. Small, gradual decreases in strength take place because of a loss in muscle fiber until about age sixty, when a more marked decline occurs. Yet, elderly people who are put on a program of strength training produce increases in strength, and suffer a loss of strength with age that is considered "hardly noticeable."

HOW EXERCISE FIGHTS AGING

In a study of 6,200 men conducted at the Veterans Affairs Palo Alto Health Care System/Stanford University and published in a 2002 issue of the *New England Journal of Medicine,* physical fitness was determined to be a more important factor in longevity than high blood pressure, sky-high cholesterol levels, or bad habits such as smoking. In fact, researchers found that men with the lowest exercise capacity were roughly four times more likely to die during the study than the fittest participants. Altogether, physical fitness was shown to have a greater impact on the risk of death than all other well-publicized risk factors for heart disease. For example, researchers found that a physically fit man suffering from high blood pressure was approximately 50 percent less likely to die than an unfit man with high blood pressure. These findings, study authors say "confirm the protective role" of exercise.

According to Waneen Spirduso, author of *Physical Dimensions of Aging,* "Chronic resistance strength training enables individuals to maintain high levels of strength for many years and also provides individuals who have not been involved in strength training an opportunity to reverse many of the age-related deterioration processes that are observed in the muscles of sedentary people."

Recent studies have shown that exercise may also fight mental aging as well as physical aging. Tests revealed that highly aerobically fit adults tend to have higher cognitive abilities than sedentary people who are not particularly fit; they seem to process information more quickly and more easily than their inactive counterparts. Researchers speculate that this is because exercise has a beneficial effect on the circulation of blood to the brain, on certain brain chemicals, on the neuroendocrine system (involved in information processing), and on the ability to get restorative sleep.

Because exercise helps normalize brain chemistry and restore mental equilibrium, studies are pointing to regular physical activity as an effective alternative or counterpart to psychotherapy for people who suffer from mild to moderate depression. And unlike many medications, exercise delivers positive side effects. Physical activity calms the nerves of people who feel anxious and agitated, and invigorates those who feel lethargic and tired. It can also improve appetite for people who don't feel like eating, and reduce food cravings in those prone to overeating.

Perhaps the most impressive study demonstrating the life extending benefits of exercise was conducted by the American Cancer Society, which followed more than 1 million American women and men for twenty years. Their conclusion: "Physical exercise lengthens life and wards off heart disease and stroke," particularly for men.

The Cancer Society's findings are supported by a number of other studies. In 1972, T. Khosla of the Department of Medical Statistics at the Welsh National School of Medicine found that exercise had a beneficial effect on his subjects' health. He concluded that because people who exercised were less likely to be obese or to start smoking at an early age, they were not only spared these health hazards but also gained the overall benefits of exercise.

> According to the *American Journal of Clinical Nutrition*, exercising while you diet not only improves your mood and self-confidence, but also may actually help you stick to your regimen. Researchers found that obese women who exercised forty-five minutes per day, three times per week during a twelve-week diet program lost an average of 19.3 pounds of fat, while non-exercisers only lost an average of 13.4 pounds of fat. Those who exercised also reported reductions in anxiety and depression, and an increase in positive feelings.

A study conducted by Dr. Ralph Paffenbarger and his colleagues focused on nearly 17,000 Harvard male alumni with similar demographic characteristics. Men who used fewer than 500 calories a week on exercise were the group with the highest death rate. The men who expended 500 to 1,000 calories a week on exercise (the energy burned in, say, walking five to ten miles) had a 22 percent lower risk of death, while the men who expended up to 3,500 calories a week on exercise (the equivalent of five to ten hours of intense exercise) had a 54 percent improvement in longevity.

Interestingly, both the Paffenberger study and another Harvard alumni study found that while a certain amount of exercise is good, more is not necessarily better. In the Paffenberger study, men who used up more than 3,500 calories a week (more than ten hours of intense exercise weekly) had a slightly lower improvement in longevity than their moderately exercising counterparts. While the moderate exercisers had a 54 percent improvement in longevity over the no-exercise group, the intense exercisers had only a 38 percent improvement.

> If you have high blood pressure and exercise regularly, you'll have a greater life expectancy than if you have normal blood pressure and don't exercise regularly.

A 1977 study of Harvard graduates conducted by Anthony Polednak and Albert Damon compared men who were major athletes (a letter in one or more sports), minor athletes (participation but no letter), and nonathletes. They found that "minor athletes generally and, for the most part, lived significantly longer than major athletes and non-athletic classmates. . . . In percentages of men still alive and in percentages of men reaching ages 70 and 75, minor athletes were consistently and for the most part significantly higher in [life span]."

When you think about exercise that will prolong life and health, your goal should be to find vigorous, demanding physical activity—but not overly intense, highly competitive, or physically abusive patterns of exercise, which can create negative stress, generate excess adrenaline, or divert energy from the body's normal maintenance processes.

Vigorous exercise creates lactic acid, which can greatly benefit the heart, as well as bind and remove toxic metals that accumulate in our bodies. Excess lactic acid, however, can also make our muscles stiff and sore. Therefore, our goal in exercise, as in all aspects of anti-aging, is balance—enough exercise to win the enormous benefits to our health, but not so much as to put undue strain on our bodies or our spirits.

EXERCISE FOR "IMMORTALITY"

As many gerontologists and researchers have found, exercise is the closest thing to an anti-aging pill that exists. People who are physically fit, eat a healthy, balanced diet, and take nutritional supplements can measure out to be ten to twenty years biologically younger than their chronological age—this is what makes an *Immortal*. An Immortal doesn't necessarily live forever, but can be free from mental and physical disease and degeneration for years longer than an unhealthy individual. Exercise is an extremely important part of achieving this "immortality."

If you're a sedentary person, any regular exercise of moderate intensity—even if it's mowing the lawn, gardening, or climbing the stairs—will allow you to live longer. Even if you're sixty or seventy, it's important to realize that it's never too late.

The CDC and the American College of Sports Medicine recommend that you exercise thirty minutes a day in addition to your normal daily activities—and it doesn't have to be thirty minutes consecutively. People who have busy schedules often have to exercise intermittently. The *Journal of the American Medical Association* lists brisk walking, cycling, swimming or calisthenics, racket sports, golf (if you pull your cart or carry your clubs), housecleaning, and raking leaves as some of the options of moderate-intensity physical activities. Thirty minutes a day of exercise is what is recommended for a significant improvement in life expectancy.

To improve your fitness and quality of life, you need to perform at least twenty minutes of sustained aerobic exercise that increases your heart rate at least three days a week.

It takes twelve weeks of regular exercise to become "fit"—meaning that your oxygen capacity has improved. It takes only one brisk walk, however, to improve your health, that is, to lower indicators such as blood pressure, blood sugar, and triglycerides. Exercise reduces the risk for stroke, lowers LDL cholesterol and raises HDL cholesterol, lowers the risk for sleep disorders, improves mood, boosts creativity, preserves mental acuity, and maintains muscular strength, flexibility, and balance. Regular stimulation of the immune system may have a cumulative effect.

Remember, it doesn't matter if you were once physically active in your younger years; if you're not currently engaged in a physical activity program on a regular basis, your body is not receiving the innumerable health-related benefits of exercise.

When pursuing any kind of physical fitness, always obtain medical clearance from your doctor, especially if you have preexisting cardiovascular disease or cardiac problems, chronic obstructive pulmonary disease (emphysema, asthma, chronic bronchitis), uncontrolled diabetes, osteoporosis, or arthritis. Always start out slowly and increase your level of exercise gradually. You should never feel any strange discomfort. It's also a good idea, especially for those with osteoporosis or arthritis, to exercise on a mat or padded floor to protect against serious injury.

GETTING PREPARED

Before beginning a regular exercise program, we recommend the following tests to determine your level of fitness and heart rate. However, if you're over age thirty-five, haven't exercised for a year or more, or have any type of heart trouble, *be sure to consult your physician* before giving yourself this test.

Test #1: The Step Test

1. Find or build a step that is eight inches high.

2. Practice until you can step up and then down with each foot—two "up-down" cycles—in five seconds. (You might want a partner to help time you.)

3. For three minutes, step up and down with alternate feet, at a rate of two cycles per five seconds. Then wait thirty seconds and take your pulse for thirty seconds.

4. Check the following table to find out how to rate yourself.

Classification Age	20–29	30–39	40–49	50+
Men		Number of beats/30 seconds		
Excellent	34–36	35–38	37–39	37–40
Good	37–40	39–41	40–42	41–43
Average	41–42	42–43	43–44	44–45
Fair	43–47	44–47	45–49	46–49
Poor	48–59	48–59	50–60	50–62
Women		Number of beats/30 seconds		
Excellent	39–42	39–42	41–43	41–44
Good	43–44	43–45	44–45	45–47
Average	45–46	46–47	46–47	48–49
Fair	47–52	48–53	48–54	50–55
Poor	53–66	54–66	55–67	56–66

Score

Poor or Fair: You are at increased risk for cardiovascular disease and need an aerobic exercise program. Find the exercise that best fits your lifestyle or seek out a personal trainer. Remember, always start at a beginning level.

Average: You need to exercise more regularly to gain the full anti-aging benefits. Make sure you exercise for at least twenty minutes a day three times a week.

Good: You are in good shape, but there is still room for improvement. Increase the intensity or duration of your aerobic workouts.

Excellent: Congratulations! You're in the top of your class based on age range. Your time is best spent focusing on body contouring and increasing your flexibility and balance. There is always room for improvement.

Test #2: Determine Your Target Heart Rate

Generally, you should aim for raising your heart rate during exercise to about 70 to 85 percent of its maximum capacity. Subtract your age from 220 and multiply the result by .70 (or 70 percent), then also multiply the result by .85 (85 percent). This is your *target heart rate zone,* which will give you the greatest benefits available while not straining your heart or depleting the life energy necessary for maintaining your system. For example, if you are forty years old, your maximum rate is 220 minus 40, which equals 180. Your target heart rate zone, then, is 70 to 85 percent of 180, or 126 to 153.

APPROXIMATE TARGET HEART RATE ZONES BY AGE

Age	Beats Per Minute	Age	Beats Per Minute
20	140–170	50	119–145
25	137–166	55	116–140
30	133–166	60	112–136
35	130–157	65	109–132
40	126–153	70	105–128
45	126–153		

You should aim for raising your heart to its target rate and keeping it there for thirty minutes at a time, for a minimum of about two hours a week. In other words, you're looking for four half-hour sessions of vigorous exercise per week.

Work Up Gradually

However, if you haven't exercised in a while, plan on working up to this ideal rate gradually, over a period of three or four months. To determine your level of vigor, try talking while exercising. If you're so out of breath that you can't talk, you're working too hard. Slow down. And don't start with half-hour workout sessions—try ten or even five minutes at first—until your stamina increases.

Keep It Regular

If possible, though, try to exercise at least four times a week, even if for only five minutes at a time. Repeated attempts at exercise will build up your muscles as well as strengthen your heart and lungs. The more often you exercise, the more easily exercise will come to you.

Don't Get Discouraged

Although building your strength and stamina is a gradual process, most people experience fitness as a series of quantum leaps. One day you can barely drag yourself around the block—the next day, jogging seems so easy and natural, you feel like you're floating. Exercise can also vary so that after that "floating" day, you may again experience one or two days of difficulty before moving back up to your new, higher plateau. You'll soon find that regular, appropriate exercise will help you create a new sense of power and well-being that is well worth any times of difficulty or frustration.

PLANNING AN EXERCISE PROGRAM

There are different types of exercise, each of which brings its own benefits, each with its own demands. Therefore, as you begin your exercise program, it is important that you experiment with different ways of moving, different types of exercise. But, whatever program you choose, there are some basics of exercising that will always remain the same.

Warm Up

It is very important to warm up before embarking on any physical activity to lessen the chances of pulling a muscle, ligament, or tendon. The warm up can be compared to a balanced breakfast that fuels your body and mind in the morning, preparing it for a hard day of work. A proper warm up will take a good ten to fifteen minutes and will loosen muscles that, left tight, can cause injury.

An easy way to warm up is to mimic the exercise you are planning to engage in. For example, low-level walking may be the precursor leading to more demanding brisk walking. Slow, light stretching of the arms over the head and to the sides can eventually lead into a vigorous game of tennis.

Never overexert yourself during the warm up since it can cause fatigue by building up an oxygen debt. This is called an *anaerobic* state, which can end up tiring you out before you've even begun to really exercise. Remember, treat the warm up like a slow-motion exercise, a light, essential step that can make planned exercise a safer and more enjoyable activity.

If you've been inactive for a long time, however, we recommend beginning with just daily light stretching exercises to help you regain functional range of motion in certain joints and to avoid risk of injury.

> Older people have a low percentage of body water and are more susceptible to dehydration. Therefore, it is important to drink water regularly before, during, and after exercise.

Add Aerobics

After you feel ready to exert yourself more, start with an exercise that is aerobic in nature—one that requires a high use of oxygen. (You'll find examples of aerobic exercises listed in the chart below, under "Endurance and cardio-respiratory function.") Swimming and other water exercises are excellent starters because they don't place a lot of stress on the joints. Similarly, stationary

Is Walking Your Workout?

Walking is an excellent exercise in itself. It not only improves health and aerobic fitness, but is also one of the safest ways to exercise. Studies have shown that walking decreases risk of coronary heart disease by raising HDL cholesterol levels and increases maximal oxygen consumption. Dr. Kenneth Cooper of the Aerobics Institute in Dallas ranks walking as one of five top aerobic activities—along with jogging, cycling, swimming, and cross-country skiing. It is the perfect initial step for the beginning exerciser, which can eventually lead to other higher endurance exercises. Don't underestimate the power of walking though, as very fast walking can actually be more beneficial aerobically than jogging or slow running at the same speed.

1. Try to walk at least once every day.

2. Walk to your favorite music. Many studies have shown that when people exercise to music, they exercise harder, longer, and better.

3. Walk faster, farther, and more frequently, and those extra calories will start to burn off.

4. Walk wherever and whenever you can. Don't sit when you can stand or walk around.

5. Keep a walking journal. Jot down not only what you eat, but also each mile you walk. This will help you chart your progress and give you an idea of how many calories you are using.

6. Set goals for yourself, both short and long term. Goals give us something to shoot for and keep our motivation high.

7. Reward yourself with non-food rewards for making these goals— a new piece of clothing for a small goal, or a weekend trip when you complete a long-term goal.

8. Walk with a friend. The support is not only comforting, but it also helps people stay focused and motivated.

9. Practice moderation. Exercise should be enjoyable, not a hassle or an obsession. If you can't walk one day, don't punish yourself. There's always tomorrow.

10. Practice positive thinking during your walks. Use walking time as personal time for yourself. Meditate. Think about how good you feel when you exercise, and about how much healthier you are mentally and physically. You'll end your walk with a positive and upbeat attitude.

cycling places less stress on the joints than other activities and is recommended for beginners over outdoor cycling because of the hazards of the road. You'll see that many exercises contribute toward two or three different aspects of fitness.

THE SIX ASPECTS OF FITNESS

1. Endurance and cardio-respiratory function
brisk walking, hiking, jogging, running, bicycling, aerobics classes, cross-country skiing, swimming, rowing, and jumping on a trampoline.

2. Strength and muscular development
weight training, sprinting, swimming, rowing, tennis, yoga, isometrics, martial arts, squash, and basketball.

3. Speed and reaction time
sprinting, tennis, Ping-Pong, racquetball, baseball, handball, martial arts, Frisbee throwing, soccer, and football.

4. Coordination and balance
dancing, golf, squash, sailing, tennis, jumping on a trampoline, bowling, horseback-riding, baseball, tai chi, basketball, football, badminton, billiards, skating, martial arts, and yoga.

5. Flexibility
dancing, stretching, tai chi, meditation, and yoga.

6. Neuromuscular relaxation
gardening, golf, Frisbee throwing, kite flying, martial arts, tai chi, and yoga.

Find a way of working different types of physical activity into your week, as well as choosing an exercise that affords more than one fitness benefit. For example, you might jog or walk briskly four times a week for a half hour, followed by a session of light, strength-oriented weight training. On the weekend, you might go dancing, throw around a Frisbee, or play a game of golf.

Alternatively, try combining different exercises for even better all-over body conditioning. For example, if your favorite exercise is jogging, try something completely different like yoga to trigger head-to-toe relaxation. Do both workouts and you get the *yin* and the *yang* (opposites) of exercise benefits: a strong heart and a limber body combined with a calmer outlook. Another combination might be to look on popular hobbies such as gardening and bicycling as part of your workout. The options are so endless that you could literally turn the great outdoors into your own personal gymnasium.

Cool Down

All exercise programs, no matter how light or hard, need an adequate cool-down period that includes stretching and relaxation. Not doing so can cause discomfort and in some cases, cardiac abnormalities. The cool-down allows the body to return to a resting state. Take at least five minutes to walk around at a slow pace, swinging your arms back and forth. Breathe deeply and release everything from your mind, except for how good you feel from exercising.

Warning Signs to Stop Exercising

- nausea or vomiting

- chest pain

- excessive fatigue during or after exercise

- pain in the neck or jaw area

- palpitations (irregular heartbeats)

- shortness of breath

- severe, unrelenting pain in muscles and joints

GETTING STARTED: EXERCISES FOR GROWING YOUNG

There are many components of physical fitness. Health-related components include cardiovascular endurance, muscular strength and endurance, muscular flexibility, and body composition. Skill-related components include agility, balance, coordination, power, reaction time, and speed. It is very important to gradually work on all of these areas in order to achieve the anti-aging benefits of exercise as well as all-round physical conditioning.

Too often people and personal trainers buy into the aging myth and accept that becoming weaker, slower, and clumsier with age is inevitable. Essentially, we give up on ourselves and assume that our bodies aren't capable of taking great strides or even small strides. Older people get stuck doing only low-aerobic activities such as walking (not to say walking isn't a great way to exercise), and ignore other vital areas. It is important to realize that no matter what your age or current condition, it is likely that your body can reach new, higher limits of performance.

Here is a full range of ten "anytime/anywhere" exercises that will help get you started on the path to "immortality." Each of these exercises has been included here because they have been found to have a healing impact upon those who use them regularly. Individually, each is an excellent exercise. However, if they are used together, combined with one another in different ways on different days (while still always using exercise #1 as your warm up), they make for a fully rounded program of exercise for the beginner.

When the exercises included here have become a part of your everyday life and when they no longer present the same challenge they once did when you were just getting up off your couch to begin exercising, consider adding the Power Exercises that begin on page 433 to your daily exercise program.

TEN HEALING EXERCISES

1. The Tai-Chi Circle of Life

This fluid breathing exercise is adapted from Daniel Reid's book *The Tao of Health, Sex and Longevity*. It incorporates your body and mind with the four distinct stages of breathing: inhalation, retention, exhalation, and pause. Breathing exercises help relax the nerves, calm the heart, boost circulation, and enhance energy reserves.

1. Stand with your heels together and toes splayed at a forty-five degree angle, knees bent and spine erect. Bring your hands together in front of you, below the navel, palms up, with the right hand cupped in left.

2. Empty your lungs, then slowly inhale. As you inhale, slowly raise your hands out to the sides, palms up, and make as wide a circle as possible with your arms as you raise them above your head. At the same time, slowly straighten your knees, with your hands still raised above your head and

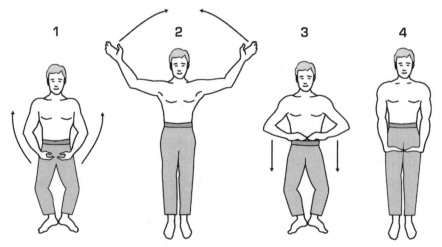

FIGURE 16.1. The Tai Chi Circle of Life. A four-stage breathing exercise, for energizing, relaxing, and calming.

your lungs full. Tuck in your pelvis, retain briefly, and swallow audibly. Be sure to try to keep your neck as stretched as possible.

3. Slowly exhale through your nose. At the same time, gradually lower your hands, palms down, in a straight line back down to the starting position, while bending your knees into a semi-squat position.

4. Empty your lungs with a final contraction, pause to relax your abdominal wall, then turn your palms upward, cup them, and begin another inhalation. Repeat 10–20 times.

2. Walk, Push, Pull, Jump

If you spend a lot of time at home, this exercise is perfect. Use a sturdy piece of furniture such as a sink, immovable table, or heavy sofa.

1. Place your hands on the sink or furniture, head down, elbows out, and walk in place. It should look as if you are trying to move the sink.

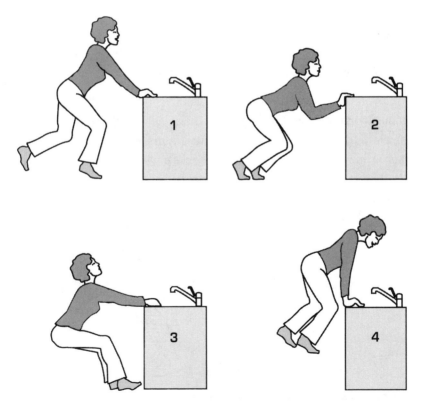

FIGURE 16.2. Walk, Push, Pull, Jump. You can use your kitchen to get fit just as easily as you can use it to get fat.

2. In the same position, really push the sink with all your strength while still walking in place. You should feel the backs of your shoulders down to your forearms really working.

3. Holding on to the sink, pull back on the sink so that your ankles are touching the ground and your toes are pointing upward. You will feel the backs of your shoulders and arms supporting your weight.

4. Lean forward, transferring all your weight on top of the sink and onto your forearms and calf muscles. Jump up off the ground. Repeat 10–20 times.

3. Mountain Out of a Molehill

This stretching exercise will help alleviate sore muscles and joints and improve muscle tone in the upper body.

1. Lay facedown on the floor. Place your hands, palms down against the floor, and your toes in a flexed position, spaced about two feet apart; your arms and legs should be kept straight.

2. Start with your arms perpendicular to the floor and arch your spine, so that your body is in a sagging position. Bring your head back as far as possible. Feel the stretch in your neck and pectoral muscles.

3. Bring your chin forward, tucking it against your chest. With your feet flat on the floor, raise your buttocks up in the air, while bringing your body into an inverted "V" position. Return to your original position, and start all over again. You will feel the stretch in the backs of your thighs, legs, and calves. Breathe in deeply as you raise your body and breathe out fully as you lower it. Repeat 10–20 times.

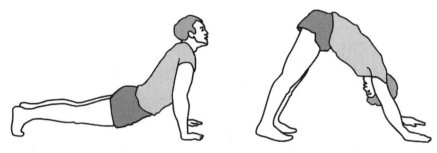

FIGURE 16.3. Mountain Out of a Molehill. A stimulating stretch to relieve soreness and invigorate muscles.

4. Pelvic Push-Up

This yoga-like exercise not only benefits the spine and many other inner organs, it also effectively releases muscular tension in the shoulders.

1. Lie on your back with your hands by your sides, knees bent, and feet about hip-distance apart and flat on the floor.

2. Inhale and press down on your feet and raise your pelvis slightly upward, squeezing your buttocks.

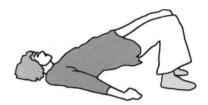

FIGURE 16.4. Pelvic Push-Up. A center-body toner and shoulder relaxer.

3. While maintaining this position, raise the rest of your torso off the floor as far as is comfortable.

4. Keep pressing down with your feet as you hold the pose. In addition to releasing tension in your pelvic region, you will also feel the front of your thighs working. Repeat 10–20 times.

5. Cat-Man-Do!

This hyperextension exercise strengthens the lower back, allowing increased flexibility of the neck, shoulders, and spine.

1. Kneel on all fours.

2. Inhale as you lean your head back slowly.

3. Exhale as you bring your head down and slowly arch your spine. As you become fluent in this exercise, try to make the movement rhythmic. Repeat 10–20 times.

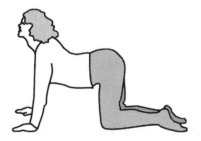 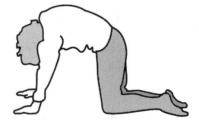

FIGURE 16.5. Cat-Man-Do! Copy cats' sinuous stretches for lower-back strength, and more.

6. Symphony No. 5

This exercise combines physical movement with either humming or counting. Vocalization will increase concentration and help you warm up, just as an orchestra tunes its instruments before a performance.

1. Start humming or counting. Let your imagination guide you as you select your musical tone. Try different melodies, and different rhythms as you do this exercise.

2. Standing with your feet slightly apart, arms out, and elbows high and out to the side, trace two C's that are back to back with your forearms. Repeat this motion as many times as possible, being careful not to overstrain your arms. This exercise increases mobility in the elbow joints as well as works the entire arm. (Try holding light weights or unopened cans of soda while doing this exercise to help build upper arm strength. Gradually increase the weight.)

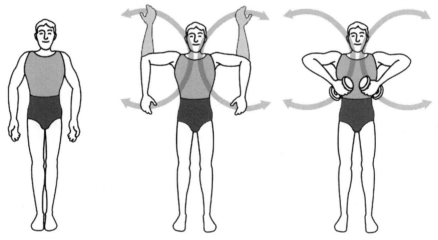

FIGURE 16.6. **Symphony No. 5.** Tune up with a harmonious hum.

7. Towel Tug of War

This is an exercise of stressing muscles and then releasing. And since you are on both sides of the tug of war, there is no way you can be anything but the victor!

1. Grasp a hand towel firmly at both ends, pulling it taut. Wrap it around your forehead, holding one side with your left hand. Forcefully, but carefully, pull your head in the opposite direction, against the towel, while still grasp-

ing on tightly. Change sides and repeat. Do the same exercise with your head going backward and forward. This position works all of the neck muscles and helps release accumulated stress and tension.

2. A variation on this exercise involves keeping the taut towel parallel to the floor. You then pull it slowly to the left while resisting with your right hand. Then pull the towel slowly to your right while resisting with your left hand. Start with six pulls in each direction and gradually increase repetitions.

3. Now, keeping the towel taut, take a deep breath and start with your

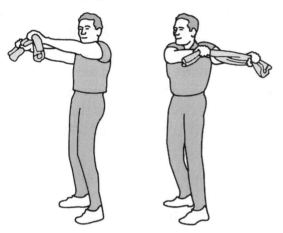

arms in front of you. Move your arms in a huge circle stretching them over your head and down again, and exhale slowly. Inhale and repeat. You will feel your shoulders rotating and your entire upper body working together in every direction. Make sure to maintain a good range of motion. Repeat 10–20 times.

FIGURE 16.7. Towel Tug of War. You're on both sides of this contest, so you can only win, with stress release as the prize.

8. Flamingo Dance

Most falls in older people are due to weak ankles. This exercise builds strength in the ankles for increased support. The ultimate goal is to gain maximum balance and equilibrium, while reducing risk of injury.

1. Stand on a hard floor, wearing shoes, with your legs slightly apart. Raise yourself up on your tiptoes and then come back down to standing position. Do this until you don't feel wobbly and your balance is secure.

2. Now, raise both arms over your head while standing on your tiptoes. Still on your tiptoes, raise only one of your arms, lower it, then raise only the other arm. Continue doing this until you feel that your balance is secure.

3. Keeping your left leg firmly planted on the floor, raise up your right leg on

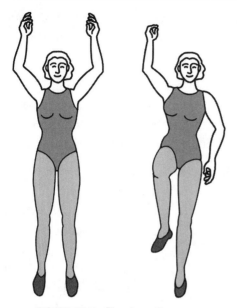

FIGURE 16.8. Flamingo Dance.
Balancing tips from the birds.

tiptoes and lift your right arm. Hold for five to ten seconds. Then, switch sides. Repeat 5-10 times. Close both eyes while you are on your tiptoes. Then close one eye.

This exercise can be done in a variety of combinations. After mastering it in shoes on a hard floor, move up to shoes on plush carpet or another uneven surface. Next, try the exercise with bare feet on floor and carpet. For safety precautions, you may want to place a cushioned chair on either side of you. Repeat 5–10 times.

9. Leg Drops

This exercise is beneficial for the lower abdomen, the hip flexors, and front thigh muscles.

1. Find a heavy, sturdy chair and place it against a wall. Sit forward on the chair, gripping the sides and lean your shoulders backward.

2. With your left foot remaining on the floor, lift your right leg into the air, keeping it as straight as possible. Lower it, then raise your left leg. Repeat about four times and gradually work your way up to ten times.

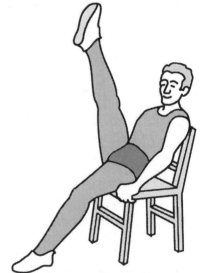

3. Once you are proficient with this movement, try lifting up both of your legs at the same time, then set them down together. You will feel your arms working along with your

FIGURE 16.9. Leg Drops. Keep at this exercise and see the payoff in a tighter abdomen and more powerful legs.

stomach muscles, which tighten as you do this exercise. Remember, just because you may not be able to straighten your legs all the way doesn't mean you aren't getting the benefits of the exercise. Repeat 5–10 times.

10. Sock 'em, Knock 'ems

Sock 'em, Knock 'ems are a great way to get out extra frustration while building up your upper body and cardiovascular system.

1. Stand erect with your feet shoulder-width apart. Flex your knees slightly and visualize a punching bag in front of you.

2. Clench your right fist and punch the invisible bag with all your might, then punch with the left fist. Move your arms in a complete motion, bringing them all the way forward and all the way back. Use your whole body. Breathe deeply. Alternate right and left twenty times.

3. Try doing the same exercise overhead by aiming the punches toward the ceiling, bringing the elbow down toward the floor with each punch. This position is especially good for posture and arms. Try alternating positions. Start out slowly and increase speed to burn off even more calories. Repeat 5–10 times.

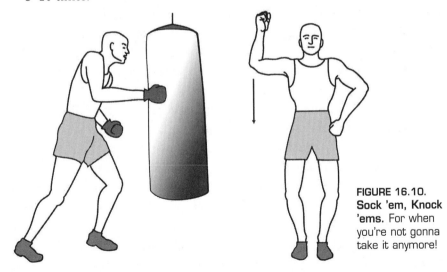

**FIGURE 16.10.
Sock 'em, Knock
'ems.** For when
you're not gonna
take it anymore!

POWER EXERCISES

There is no doubt that the exercises in this section are more challenging than those explained above. But because they are more difficult, they have more to offer in terms of health benefits.

Vigorous endurance exercise training in older people, where the challenge of exercise is progressively increased, elicits a proliferation of muscle capillaries and an increase in oxidative enzyme activity. Likewise, progressive resistance training in older individuals results in muscle growth and increased strength. From these observations, researchers suggest that older people can, indeed, adapt to resistive and endurance exercise training similar to young people. Decline in the muscle's metabolic and force-producing capacity can no longer be considered an inevitable consequence of the aging process. Rather, the adaptations in aging skeletal muscle to exercise training may enhance the ease of carrying out the activities of daily living and exert a beneficial effect on such age-associated diseases as type II diabetes, coronary artery disease, hypertension, and obesity.

Also, exercise can increase the mineral content of bone, raising the expectation that exercise programs may be effective therapy for the treatment of osteoporosis, and the prevention of hip and spinal fractures. Specifically, a program primarily consisting of weight-bearing exercise prevents the age-related decline in the trunk of the body and, in some instances, increases bone mineral content. Dr. Birge and colleagues from Washington University School of Medicine in Missouri reviewed published studies on physical activity in the elderly and found that neither hormonal status nor age appears to preclude the skeletal benefits of exercise. Indeed, Dr. Birge's team states that physical activity is a major and dynamic determinant of skeletal integrity. Therefore, it is important to promote and preserve gains in skeletal mass achieved through exercise in the older population.

Short-duration, high-intensity exercise, such as strength-training activities, exerts a powerful effect on the hormones of the brain and the endocrine system and have been proven to boost human growth hormone (HGH) release into the bloodstream raising IGF-1 levels by 200 to 400 percent.

In 1994, Dr. Maria Fiatarone of the Human Nutrition Research Center on Aging of Tufts University, conducted an exercise therapy experiment on a group of men and women between the ages of sixty-three and ninety-eight. In spite of the fact that 83 percent required a cane, walker, or wheelchair, and 66 percent had fallen during the past year, each underwent a high-intensity weight-training program including leg presses three times per week. Over the course of this ten-week training session, the results were remarkable with significant increases reported in muscle growth and strength improvements in stamina and stability. Many of the subjects were able to put aside their walkers entirely, or at least improve so much as to need only a cane.

High-intensity exercise is a wakeup call to the pituitary. Just starting an exercise program can stimulate your pituitary gland to produce more HGH, and will help your body to make the best use of the HGH it has in the circulation.

The following are samples of strength-training exercises that are of benefit in stimulating HGH release. The lower extremities and pelvis account for nearly 70 percent of the muscle mass within you, so to achieve maximum stimulation of the neuroendocrine system lower extremity exercise is key. If you are over age forty, a sports and cardiac physical exam is a prudent first step before beginning any new strenuous physical-training program.

FIVE POWER EXERCISES

While the exercises explained below call for either a weight machine or free weights, it is important to note that you can substitute many things for professional free weights. In fact, sealed canned goods, from peas to tomato sauce, are excellent substitutes for weights, as are unopened bottles of water. As you become stronger, you can then turn to manufactured weights for your exercise program.

Basic Principles of a Weight-Resistance Workout

- To increase *muscular strength* and *build up muscle mass*, use more weight and do fewer repetitions.

- To increase *muscular endurance*, perform exercises that take the muscle through its full range of motion. Use less weight and perform more repetitions.

- For best results, weight-resistance exercises should include both *positive and negative contractions:*

  - a *positive* (concentric) contraction is when you flex and contract the muscle to overcome resistance, the muscle shortens (for example, performing a bicep curl, pulling the weight toward your body).

  - a *negative* (eccentric) contraction is when a group of muscles are forced to extend to a fully outstretched position (for example, when a bicep curl is complete, lowering the weight away from your body extends the bicep to its full length).

1. Hack Squat

1. If you are using a weight machine, position yourself beneath the machine pressing bar so that the handlebars rest across the backs of your shoulders. Place your hands on the handlebars in a comfortable position. If you are

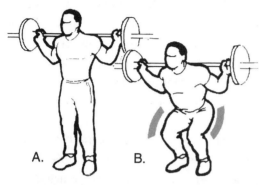

using free weights, such as a barbell, place the barbell behind your neck and across the tops of your shoulders. Stabilize the weight by placing your hands on the bar near your collarbones in a comfortable position. Stand erect, head up, back straight, with your feet about sixteen inches apart.

FIGURE 16.11. Hack Squat Exercise. Works upper thighs.

2. Inhale deeply, then exhale as you squat down until your thighs and lower legs are at about a 120-degree angle. Slowly return to the starting position and inhale. Repeat 5–10 times.

2. Dumbbell Squat-to-Bench

1. Hold a dumbbell in each hand, at arms' length, with your palms facing your thighs. Position yourself at the end of a workout bench so that your heels are aligned with the end of the bench. Stand erect, back straight, and head up. Keep your feet flat on floor, about sixteen inches apart.

2. Inhale deeply, then exhale as you squat down until your buttocks touches the bench. Do not take tension off your thighs by actually sitting on the bench. Return immediately to the starting position and inhale. Repeat 5–10 times.

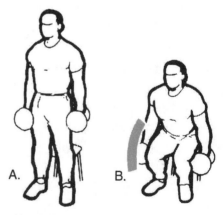

FIGURE 16.12. Dumbbell Squat-to-Bench Exercise. Works upper thighs.

3. Squat-to-Bench Close

1. Position yourself at the end of a workout bench so that your heels line up with the end of the bench. Stand erect with your arms crossed over your chest. Keep your head up, back straight, and feet flat on floor about eight inches apart (close stance).

2. Inhale deeply, then exhale as you squat down until your buttocks touch the bench. Do not take tension off your thighs by actually sitting on the bench.

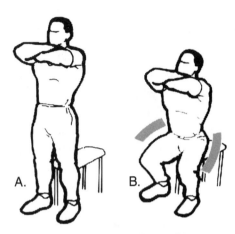

FIGURE 16.13. Squat-to-Bench Close Exercise. Works outer thighs.

Return immediately to the starting position. Be sure to keep your head up and back straight throughout the motion. Repeat 5–10 times.

4. Front Lunge

1. Stand erect with your hands on your hips. Keep your head up, back straight, and stand with your feet about fourteen inches apart.

2. Inhale and step forward as far as possible, until your leading leg is parallel with the floor and your trailing leg is extended as straight as possible. Push yourself back to the starting position and exhale. Repeat this movement with your other leg. Repeat the full-cycle (alternate leg) movement 5–10 times.

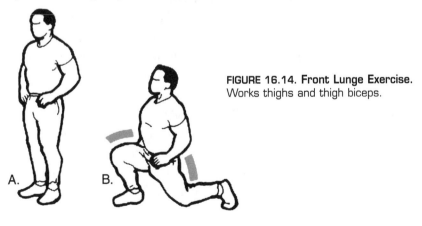

FIGURE 16.14. Front Lunge Exercise. Works thighs and thigh biceps.

5. Side Lunge

1. Stand erect with your hands on your hips. Keep your head up, back straight, and stand with your feet about fourteen inches apart.

2. Inhale and step to the side as far as possible until the thigh of your leading leg is parallel to the floor and your trailing leg is extended as straight as possible. Push yourself back to the starting position and exhale. Repeat this movement with your other leg. Repeat the full-cycle (alternate leg) movement 5–10 times.

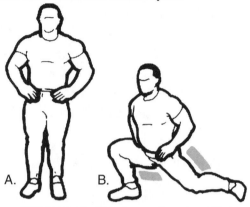

FIGURE 16.15. Side Lunge Exercise. Works inner thigh and thigh biceps.

MAKING THE MOST OF YOUR EXERCISE PROGRAM

Experts agree that older people especially should check with their physicians before embarking on any exercise program. Once you've been given the go ahead, the key is to get moving and have fun doing it. Give yourself feedback. For example, wear a pedometer, which will measure the number of footsteps you've taken, so you can chart a progress report and reward yourself for the effort.

If you do exercise but look upon it as one more miserable chore that an unfair world demands of you in order to prevent the effects of aging, you may become somewhat more fit, but the added emotional stress of this "unpleasant task" may well wipe out any possible anti-aging benefits that you might expect. If, on the other hand, you view exercise as a time of joyous communion with your body, a time of testing your limits, or of experiencing your physical place in the world, the sense of fitness that you can expect will be enhanced by a new sense of empowerment and accomplishment that can virtually take years off your age.

It may take you a while to find the type and routine of exercise that's right for you—but once you grasp it, you'll discover that exercise is not only the most effective anti-aging medicine you can acquire, but also a pleasure in its own right. After all, why bother living 100 years or more if you can't have a positive mental outlook and an active lifestyle?

CHAPTER 17

Secrets of "The Immortals"

Johnny Kelley finished his sixtieth Boston Marathon
at age eighty-three.

Ada Thomas started jogging after she retired at age sixty-five.
At age sixty-eight, she ran her first marathon; at age sixty-nine,
she finished first in her age group in the women's division.
At age seventy-two, she was still running five miles
during the week and playing tennis on the weekends.

Ivor Welch didn't start his athletic activity until he was eighty-three.
Five years later, at age eighty-eight, he had run in five marathons.
At age ninety, he ran in two half-marathons.

In 1991, Ruth Rothfarb and Ida Mintz, both over age eighty,
ran the Boston Marathon in a little over five hours.

Most of us may not match the athletic feats of these senior athletes—no matter what our age. The remarkable accomplishments of these athletes, however, are not just personal triumphs; they are also tributes to the amazing resilience of the human body. They demonstrate that whether you start your exercise program early or late in life, you can still enjoy the physical strength and vigor that most people attribute only to the young.

A MAN AHEAD OF HIS TIME: JACK LA LANNE

Jack La Lanne is truly a testament to the virtues of lifelong exercise. Born September 26, 1914, La Lanne grew up as a sickly child. By age sixteen, he suffered from failing health: he was underweight, ridden with acne, and a sugarholic. After his mother took him to a seminar given by Dr. Paul Bragg, one of the founding fathers of the natural health movement, La Lanne was "reborn." After speaking with Dr. Bragg, La Lanne began his lifelong quest to promote good nutrition, diet, and proper exercise throughout his community and the world.

In 1931, La Lanne opened a spa in his home—actually, it was on his front lawn and in his basement—where he began working with local policemen and firemen in order to train them for physical tests. It was this spa, named "Jack La Lanne's," that started it all.

By 1936, La Lanne had opened the first commercial health club in Oakland, California. This was just the first of many firsts. La Lanne was the first to put weights in the hands of women. He was the first to invent sectionized weight machines. He was the first to put men and women together in the gym. He was the first to turn the gym into a comfortable, pleasant place where anyone could work out, opening the concept of a gym visit to the general public.

Even though La Lanne began his healthy lifestyle early in life, as the years have gone by, the rewards of physical fitness do not ever seem to leave him. In fact, the more La Lanne ages, the more amazing his athletic feats become:

- At age sixty, La Lanne swam from Alcatraz Island to Fisherman's Wharf, with handcuffs on his wrists and shackles on his feet, while towing a thousand-pound boat. "Why did you do that?" people asked. La Lanne's response: "To give the prisoners hope."

- In 1976, at age sixty-one, La Lanne wanted to do something special to commemorate the Spirit of '76 for the country's bicentennial celebration. He did this by swimming the length of Long Beach Harbor, approximately one mile, handcuffed and shackled, towing thirteen boats, one for each of the original colonies, containing the appropriate number of people—seventy-six.

- At age sixty-two, La Lanne swam the length of the Golden Gate Bridge underwater, against treacherous tides. This time, he towed a 2,000-pound boat.

- By age sixty-five, La Lanne was swimming in Lake Ashinoko, Japan, handcuffed and shackled, towing sixty-five boats, which, coincidentally, were loaded with 6,500 pounds of Louisiana wood pulp!

- Again, at age seventy, once again handcuffed and shackled, and fighting blustery winds and currents, La Lanne hit the water and succeeded in towing seventy boats and seventy people—one person on each boat—for an unbelievable one and one-half miles.

So how does a seventy-year-old tow seventy boats through rough waters? La Lanne's daily regimen consists of about 450 nutritional supplements, including liver and yeast, which, he believes, help him build strength. He eats natural foods in their natural states, being sure to avoid red meats, but includes fresh poultry, such as turkey. And of course, everything he eats is low in fat.

La Lanne does not live on diet alone, however. He trains two and a half hours daily, combining both weights and aerobics. In fact, when training for a swimming feat, La Lanne has been known to practice treading water against the weight of a harness in his pool for up to five hours at a time.

Today, at the ripe age of eighty-nine, La Lanne is currently training for yet another amazing athletic feat to take place within the next few years: a twenty-six-mile underwater swim—literally an underwater marathon—from Los Angeles to Catalina Island.

And with La Lanne's incredible track record, it looks as if his next feat will not be his last.

BOB DELMONTEQUE: A MAN STILL IN HIS PRIME

At age sixteen, Bob Delmonteque stood six feet tall and weighed 195 pounds. Today, at age eighty-four, nothing has changed. Delmonteque still boasts the same toned, muscular, athletic frame he sported in his teenage years.

His commitment to exercise and good health began in childhood, growing up on a Texas ranch. He remembers running back and forth to school— eight miles each way. These daily "sprints" sparked Delmonteque's interest not only in track and field, but also in a variety of other sports, including basketball and football. His initial reasoning for buying a set of barbells was not to bulk up, but rather to improve his athletic abilities and simply "be the best athlete in Texas." He achieved this remarkable goal, gaining all-star status in every varsity sport he played throughout school.

At age eighty-one, Delmonteque is still considered one of the greatest athletes in the country, let alone Texas, with one of the most impressive physiques of his generation. In 1996, Delmonteque ran the Sante Fe Marathon in an amazing five hours and twenty-three minutes—and he did this without heavy training. When really training seriously, he has finished marathons in as little as three hours and nineteen minutes!

When asked for his secret for maintaining amazing physical and mental health, Delmonteque said that he believes it's all a person's mindset. In fact, meditation and yoga-inspired breathing exercises are a large part of his daily routine. For twenty minutes every morning, noon, and evening, he meditates, during which he practices both deep breathing and self-hypnosis exercises. These sessions, he feels, help him release any negativity, stress, or toxic bodily poisons, while supercharging him physically, spiritually, and mentally.

Aside from his daily meditations, Delmonteque doesn't believe in obsessive or regimented exercising. Instead, he does "whatever he feels like doing," be it jogging, skiing, weight lifting, or sprinting. He does, however, believe in a basic three-faceted longevity exercise program, consisting of the following:

- aerobic activity to strengthen the cardiopulmonary system and build endurance;

- weight training to build lean muscle mass and reduce the risk of osteoporosis;

- stretching to build pliability of the tendons and ligaments.

Delmonteque eats the same way he trains, insisting that an individual should not get too fanatical or obsessive. Instead, he opts to "eat things as close to nature as possible," and he firmly believes in the famous old adage, "you are what you eat." His daily goal is to keep his weight at 195 and his waist at thirty-two inches. If he goes above or below these markers, he works to regain his goal.

Delmonteque is a true role model for other men and women looking to get back into shape and regain some of the spirit and vitality of youth. His advice? "Well," he says, "there's a saying: man who sit on bottom get up on bottom." The best thing to do is to just do it.

The following six profiles are based on stories that appear in *Growing Old Is Not for Sissies 2: Portraits of Senior Athletes* by Etta Clark (Corte Madera, CA: Pomegranate Calendars and Books, 1995), an inspiring text-and-picture survey of senior athletes.

BODYBUILDING FOR LIFE: BILL PEARL

Looking at Bill Pearl today, it is difficult to believe that he actually retired from competitive bodybuilding almost thirty years ago. A four-time Mr. Universe, at age seventy-two he's still in the fabulous shape he was in during his competitive years, and his training schedule is definitely not that of a weary old man.

Since age ten, Pearl has worked out four to five times every week. That's sixty-two years of exercise—and proof that weight training has some serious implications for extending human life, both in years and in quality of health.

Currently living on a farm in Oregon, Pearl still religiously continues to bodybuild. Following the advice of the old adage, "Early to bed, early to rise, makes a man healthy, wealthy, and wise," Pearl credits his good shape to his sleep schedule. Being in bed by 8:00 P.M. each night allows Pearl the freedom to do what he loves most: train hard and train early. He'll wake at 2:30 in the morning and start his workout with thirty to forty-five minutes on the stationary bike, stair climber, or rower. He then proceeds to weight train from about 4:15 until 6:00. One hundred and twenty minutes of serious training, four to five times per week, is a workout not many twenty-five-year olds can keep up with.

Pearl's philosophy on life is one for which we all should strive. Several years ago he stated, "At sixty-five, my goal is to have a productive lifestyle. I want to put in seventeen to eighteen waking hours, all of which are productive."

SWIMMING AGAINST THE TIDE: TOM RICE AND GEORGE FARNSWORTH

Like Jack La Lanne before them, Tom Rice and George Farnsworth are proof of the benefits of long-term exercise. Both men are lifelong athletes: Farnsworth, a competitive swimmer; and Rice, a professional wrestler once known as "The Masked Marvel." In 1966, they began swimming together virtually every day, inside San Francisco Aquatic Park and out into the bay. Farnsworth has continued his vigorous physical regimen into his early seventies and Rice into his late seventies. When wrestling injuries forced Rice into the water to strengthen his legs, he found he liked water sports. He continued to use swimming as a bodybuilding exercise, occasionally towing boats attached to a belt around his torso. Once he even towed a 200-ton ship some 400 yards as a publicity stunt!

Both Rice and Farnsworth have suffered health problems that might have kept less dedicated athletes out of the water. At age sixty-eight, Farnsworth had a triple bypass; a year later, Rice had a quadruple bypass. Nevertheless, they both found their way back to health and continue to swim together. Rice says that swimming is one of the best ways to fight off the physical miseries of age:

"If you work out in the water—even if you just walk in a swimming pool—you can beat whatever ailments you have."

POWERLIFTING: HELEN ZECHMEISTER

At age eighty-one, Helen Zechmeister could lift weights that men and women several decades younger might find themselves unable to budge. The national age-group power-lifting records she has held include 245 pounds for the dead lift, 94.5 pounds for the bench press, and 148 pounds for the squat. The only reason that Zechmeister's scores were not considered world records was because the International Power Lifting Federation had no age classification for senior citizens. This means that Zechmeister was, in effect, competing against women in their thirties.

Even women in their thirties, however, would be proud to match Zechmeister's strength and endurance. At age eighty-one, she was working out in a daily regimen of running, swimming, and lifting. She even competed in a men's thirty-five-years-and-older contest. And, guess what? She won.

OVERCOMING ADVERSITY: A.J. PUGLIZEVICH

Sometimes people begin athletic activities in response to illness or physical hardship. A.J. Puglizevich had a known life-threatening illness as early as age thirteen, when a doctor told A.J.'s mother that he would be dead within the year. He survived, however, but only to be told at age thirty-five that a hip problem would take away his ability to walk unaided within a matter of months.

Fortunately, Puglizevich did not accept these prophecies. He went on to become a renowned senior athlete who at age seventy-six was competing in the International Senior Olympics. Puglizevich's events are sprinting, the shot put, the discus, and javelin throws. He has also won several Senior Olympic boxing competitions.

GRACEFULLY DEFYING GRAVITY: KENT DIEHL

You wouldn't expect a fine-arts appraiser and the owner of a successful antiques business to be a world-record trick roper—but Kent Diehl has been roping since he was only nine years old. At age sixty-nine, ten years ago, he still called himself "a part-time cowboy." About his roping, he comments, "With plenty of business pressures, it is most gratifying to pick up a length of rope and spend some time with a good clean sport. The concentration required to keep a limp rope in the air going at full speed clears the head and muscles of everything but the job of rope spinning."

In fact, Diehl is living proof that fitness at an older age not only is physically rejuvenating, but can be mentally stimulating, as well. Sports such as rope spinning not only get the blood flowing, but can also hone concentration, precision, and overall mental agility.

At age sixty-three, Diehl held a world record for five years in a difficult roping event: the largest loop ever thrown and spun while lying down. In the course of his rope-spinning career, Diehl has met such personalities as Will Rogers, Tom Mix, and President Franklin D. Roosevelt. He speaks of his rope-spinning the way a dancer might speak of body movement, as a physically demanding art form that requires immense stamina, skill, concentration—and grace:

"People are fascinated with trick roping because to take a very limp length of rope and keep it going smoothly, defying gravity with graceful flowing loops suspended in the air, inanimate but seemingly endowed with life—to perform intricate figures, mystic patterns of flowerlike arrangements in ever-changing sizes and designs at will—all of this takes consummate skill."

DIVING IN: LUELLA TYRA

As we look forward to growing old, many of us hope to feel physically healthy into our seventies, even into our eighties. But imagine staying physically active into your nineties.

At age ninety-two, Luella Tyra was still engaged in competitive swimming. At the 1984 Nationals in Mission Viejo, she entered several races, diving into the water and swimming 100-meter courses in the backstroke, breaststroke, butterfly, and freestyle. Although her coaches had to help her out of the water at the end of every race, she completed every contest by herself. She was the oldest competitor that day at Mission Viejo—perhaps giving some of the other swimmers something to look forward to.

FIGHTING FOR THE LEAD: "MASTERS" ATHLETICS

In the last few decades, a new category of athlete has been developed: "masters" athlete. *Masters* are active athletes who exceed the age limit that's considered necessary for world-class success in a particular sport: in swimming, twenty-five; in track and field, thirty-five; in race-walking, forty. Various masters' competitions have sprung up over the years, including the National Senior Sports Classics (formerly the Senior Olympics), which is open to top athletes over age fifty, and the World Veterans' Games, a track-and-field event for men over age forty and women over age thirty-five. As the baby boomers grow older, we can expect a growing interest in masters' athletic events.

SENIOR ATHLETES: BREAKING THE BARRIERS

Senior athletes are so inspiring because they allow us to realize what the human body is capable of achieving. They are pushing the limits of what is possible. In most athletic events, there's a kind of "barrier of the possible"— the utmost boundary that one can imagine. Runners, for example, thought for years that the four-minute mile was the *ne plus ultra* of athletic achievement. However, once Roger Bannister broke through that time barrier, several runners suddenly began turning in lower times. Our physical limits seem to be just as much a function of the imagination as of the body.

Senior athletes help us redefine what we expect of our bodies with age. Of course, there are huge genetic variations among us, plus environmental factors (pollution, bright sunlight, and high levels of noise) and lifestyle choices (smoking, high-fat diet, and sedentary life), which are all relevant deciding factors to future physical health. But overall, the healthier your choices in youth, the greater your reserves in age. And, as the athletes profiled in this chapter demonstrate, these reserves can be much greater than we're used to thinking.

You may not break a world weight-lifting record or run the Boston Marathon at age eighty, but perhaps you will discover a regimen of healthy eating, a regular exercise program, and nutritional supplementation that will allow you to enjoy physical longevity for many years to come. These senior athletes prove that such a choice is possible, at any age, for anyone who chooses to make it.

CHAPTER 18

Sleep:
"The Revitalizer"

Sleep is a necessary and integral state that permits mental and physical restoration. Adequate restful sleep, like diet, exercise, and supplement habits, is critical to good health. Insufficient restful sleep can result in mental and physical health problems.

Sleep is one of the most basic and universal activities in which we all engage. Sleep is a necessary and integral state that permits mental and physical restoration. Adequate restful sleep, like diet and exercise, is critical to good health. Insufficient restful sleep can result in mental and physical health problems. Yet, getting to sleep, staying asleep, and waking refreshed can be highly elusive to most of us some of the time, and to many of us all of the time. The National Sleep Foundation reports (2002) that America is on the verge of a poor sleep epidemic. Results of their latest national poll revealed: 63 percent of American adults get less than the eight hours of sleep that experts recommend to maintain optimal physical, mental, and emotional health; one-third of the U.S. population says they get less sleep now than they did five years ago; one-half of all Americans have experienced insomnia; and drowsiness due to a lack of a proper night of sleep interferes with the daily activities of 37 percent of all adults. More than 70 million people suffer from sleep deprivation caused by poor or interrupted sleep and about 50 million suffer negative health effects as a result. The nationwide sleep debt, resulting in fatigue, has been reported to cost the American economy about $120 million annually in both health expenditures, lost worker productivity, and property destruction.

Making sure you get enough sleep each night appears to have a wide range of benefits. Clinical trial results suggest that a good night's sleep can give the immune system a boost and reduce the risk of heart disease, heart attack, and type II diabetes. There is also evidence to suggest that getting adequate amounts of good quality sleep may increase longevity!

A study conducted by Japanese researchers involving men aged forty to seventy-nine uncovered an important connection between sleep and heart attacks. They found that men who worked sixty-one hours or more a week in the year preceding the heart attack were twice as likely to have a heart attack as men who worked forty hours or less. And the men who slept five hours or less on average each working day during the year preceding the heart attack were two to three times more likely to have a heart attack. Meanwhile, research by Ayas, et al. (*Arch Intern Med.* 2003;163:205–209) revealed a link between heart disease and sleep. Their results showed that compared with women who slept for eight hours each night, women who slept less than five hours a night had an 82 percent greater risk of heart disease, those who slept six hours a night had a 30 percent increased risk, and those who slept nine hours or longer had a 57 percent increased risk.

Research published in 2001 found that people who slept for less than six hours each night were more likely to gain weight, and were therefore at higher risk of type II diabetes. Meanwhile, Mander, et al. also reported in 2001 that healthy men and women (aged twenty-three to forty-two) who got less than six and a half hours of sleep a night for eight consecutive nights displayed far lower insulin sensitivity than those who slept seven to eight hours a night. Mander suggests that chronic sleep shortage in healthy adults impairs the ability of insulin to function properly, thereby creating a risk for future onset of diabetes. Results of a study by Ayas, et al. (*Diabetes Care* 2003;26:380–384) published in 2003 supports early studies linking sleep to diabetes risk. Results showed that people who got too little sleep (fewer than five hours each night) and too much sleep (nine or more hours each night) were 1.5 times more likely to be diagnosed with type II diabetes than people sleeping between six and eight hours each night.

Sleep deprivation appears to have a profound deleterious effect upon the immune system (see Chapter 15). Vgontzas, et al. (*Metabolism.* 2002;51:887–892) found that healthy men and women in their twenties and thirties experienced a 40 to 60 percent increase in the levels of the inflammatory protein IL-6—a blood marker associated with heart disease and other chronic medical conditions—when they got only six hours of sleep a night for eight consecutive nights. This is supported by Moldofsky, et al., who found that sleep deprivation reduces both the production and activity of immune cells. Disrupted sleep also was found to increase IL-6, along with levels of cortisol (the hormone responsible for our stress response).

The human brain is just as active during sleep as it is during wakefulness.

It must maintain the temperature of the body, as well as breathing and circulatory functions. The active state of the brain during sleep is what enables us to wake from a snooze in a noisy public place when our name is called.

The structure of sleep is composed of five distinct stages. Normal sleep contains REM (rapid eye movement) and NREM (non-REM) segments. NREM sleep is divided into stages 1 through 4, where sleep deepens until stages 3-4 (delta sleep). REM sleep, also known as stage 5, is where dreaming occurs.

SLEEP LOSS AND AGING

Dr. Eve Van Cauter from the University of Chicago reports that biological signs of accelerated aging appear in healthy young men after less than a week in which they slept no more than four hours a night. Dr. Van Cauter also found that by reversing the sleep loss through twelve hours of bed rest for several consecutive nights, the elevated cortisol release that had transformed the physiological patterns of the twenty-year-old study participants into that of middle-aged adults was also reversed. Commenting on this study, Harvard Medical School's neurophysiology lab director J. Allan Hobson suggests that serious sleep loss "might predispose you to getting diseases that are known to be genetic."

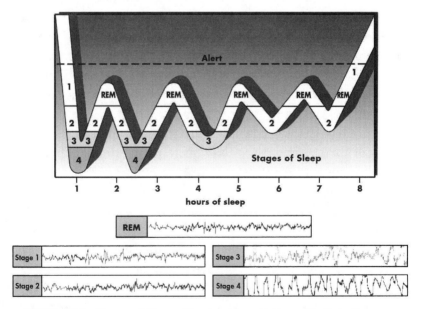

FIGURE 16.1. Stages of Sleep. [Reprinted from Goldman, R. *Brain Fitness*, Doubleday Books, 1999.]

In Van Cauter's research published in the *Journal of the American Medical Association* in August 2000, her team elucidated on the changes in the type of sleep as well as hormone changes observed from youth to later life. Van Cauter's research suggests that, as we age, the average percentage of deep, slow-wave sleep decreases, somewhere between young adulthood (ages sixteen to twenty-five) and midlife (ages thirty-six to fifty). The research also shows that slow-wave sleep is replaced by lighter sleep (stages 1 and 2) without significant increases in sleep fragmentation or decreases in rapid eye movement (REM) sleep. While the transition from midlife to late-life years (ages seventy-one to eighty-three) involves no further significant decrease in slow-wave sleep, the team did observe an increase in time awake that reduced light, non-REM sleep.

Interestingly, Van Cauter and her colleagues observed that the decline in slow-wave sleep from early adulthood to midlife was paralleled by a major decline in growth hormone (GH) secretion. From midlife to late life, GH secretion further declined. Concurrently, increasing age was associated with an elevation of evening cortisol levels that became significant only after age fifty, when sleep became more fragmented and REM sleep declined. Thus, age-related changes in slow-wave sleep and REM sleep occur and are associated with specific hormonal alterations.

University of Chicago researchers report that four hours of sleep for several consecutive nights causes blood sugar (glucose) to spike much higher after breakfast, versus levels after receiving nine hours of sleep. To compound this problem, the rate at which glucose cleared the bloodstream was 40 percent slower in the sleep-deprived state. This sluggish sugar metabolism causes physiological signs of aging, most likely as a result of elevations in the stress hormone cortisol present with lack of sleep.

Additionally, it has been established that the human immune system takes advantage of the period of sleep to promote its infection-fighting actions. Sleep-deprived rats are shown to be more susceptible to viruses and bacteria of an otherwise innocuous nature.

Dr. Robert Stickgold at Harvard Medical School/Massachusetts Mental Health Center has discovered a new link between sleep and memory. Dr. Stickgold reports on experiments demonstrating that performance of a newly acquired skill does not improve until the person has had more than six, and preferably eight, hours of sleep. The research supports a new hypothesis that memory formation is a function of the two stages of sleep (REM and NMREM), during which the brain undergoes physical and chemical changes that produces or strengthens memory traces. Without adequate sleep, skills—as well as new factual information—may not be properly encoded into memory.

In October 2001, the United Kingdom Sleep Council called on the country's employers to create flexible-hour workdays, so that employees could take midday naps. The Council's global Internet survey indicated that the Mediterranean siesta—a snooze taken during the middle of the day—could help to promote employee productivity in the afternoon.

Another study carried out in 2001 found that people who slept for fewer than six hours each night were more likely to gain weight and were therefore at higher risk of type II diabetes. When you are asleep, your parasympathetic nervous system (PNS) is in control and your nervous system is being rejuvenated. Many important immune system processes occur as you sleep, which is why "getting a lot of rest" is prescribed as a treatment for so many illnesses.

New research suggests that seniors who find it difficult to get to sleep and those who get little sleep are more likely to die than those who sleep well. Dew, et al. (*Psychosomatic Medicine* 2003;65:63–73) found that people between ages fifty-nine and ninety-one years old who were apparently healthy but who spent more than thirty minutes each night trying to get to sleep were more than twice as likely to die within the next thirteen years than people who nodded off more quickly. Furthermore, people who spent the least or the most time in the REM (rapid eye movement), or dream phase of sleep, were almost twice as likely to die, compared with those spending an average amount of time in REM. Dew believes that sleep problems may serve as a "subtle indicator" that apparently healthy people may have undetected problems that could affect their health in the future.

Given their apparent simplicity, bed rest and deep sleep are perhaps the two most underestimated therapeutic interventions that deliver the greatest benefit for the time spent.

SLEEP NEEDS AND AGING

How much sleep do you need? The general rule of thumb has been eight hours per night. However, research published in 2002 found that people who slept for eight hours were 12 percent more likely to die within the study's time span of six years; those who slept six to seven hours a night lived longer. Furthermore, results of another study, also published in 2002, found that 14 percent of people who said they slept for more than eight hours a night had a history of stroke or transient ischemic attacks (TIAs), whereas less than 6 percent of those who slept for just six hours a night had a stroke history. Together, these findings suggest that six to seven hours may be the optimum amount of sleep for adults.

A person's need for sleep does not decline with age. Researchers have demonstrated that sleep needs (typically seven to nine hours) remain constant throughout adulthood. However, changes in the stages of sleep directly alter the deepness of sleep that is achieved. Middle-aged and older people tend to spend less time in deeper sleep than younger people do. By age sixty or seventy, the period of delta sleep is much shorter. Across all ages, the percentage of REM sleep remains largely constant.

A number of factors commonly associated with aging may interrupt, delay, or shorten sleep. As we age, nighttime sleep is likely to be disturbed for a number of reasons:

- lifestyle changes

- decreased secretion of melatonin

- changes in body temperature cycle

- decrease in exposure to natural light

- dietary changes

- decreased mental stimulation during daytime

- aches and pains

- diseases and/or medications to treat them may disrupt sleep (A 1996 National Sleep Foundation Gallup Poll found that 30 percent of all nighttime pain sufferers experience arthritis pain at night; the number rises to 60 percent for people aged fifty and over, to which the loss of approximately two hours of sleep for a little over ten nights a month per person is attributed.)

- hot flashes in menopausal women

- psychological changes or conditions including depression and anxiety

- frequent waking at night to go to the bathroom

- accentuated sensitivity to light or sound

- stress or bereavement

While insomnia affects men and women across all age groups, it is more common in postmenopausal women and in the elderly. Insomnia results in daytime tiredness, lack of energy, difficulty concentrating, and irritability.

Dr. Ira Shapira, Assistant Professor at Rush-Presbyterian-St. Luke's Medical Center Sleep Disorder Clinic in Chicago, is a highly respected sleep expert. He is widely sought for his valuable insights into the diagnosis and effective treatment of sleep apnea (attacks of loss of breath) and has lectured on the subject to promote awareness among anti-aging physicians.

Dr. Shapira recommends, "If your sleep has been disturbed for more than a month and interferes with the way you feel or function during the daytime, you should seek the advice of your physician. You may be referred to a sleep disorders specialist, who may be a general practitioner or specialist in neurology, pulmonary medicine, dentistry, psychiatry, or psychology."

SLEEP IS A LONGEVITY ESSENTIAL

In 350 B.C., Aristotle wrote that "All animals are clearly observed to partake in sleep . . . Nutrition and growth are then especially promoted." Modern-day science has uncovered many of the biological and physiological underpinnings of sleep. We now know that sleep is vital to every body system, organ, and cell of the body. Sleep is also highly correlated to longevity. Compromised sleep can lead to compromised quality or quantity of life. Achieving a refreshing, restorative, and rejuvenative sleep should be the goal for each and every one of us.

In today's 24/7, stimulus-overloaded, stress-filled society, many of us need to make a deliberate effort to achieve the best sleep we can get. An anti-aging approach to sleep is one that supplements with a regimen that aims to boost daytime hormone levels, the changing gentle evening trends of which promote the ability to fall and stay asleep. Consider selecting a product containing nutrients for which scientific evidence suggests sleep promotion, such as the following sleep-assistive nutrients:

SLEEP-ASSISTIVE NUTRIENTS

Nutrient	Reviewed on	Nutrient	Reviewed on
Melatonin	page 103	Lemon balm extract	page 322
Jujube extract	page 319	Hops extract	page 318
Passionflower	page 334	Chamomile flower extract	page 288
Mucuna pruiens extract	page 345		
Valerian root extract	page 343	Magnesium	page 220

REVITALIZE WHILE YOU SLEEP

A frequent overseas traveler, coauthor Dr. Bob Goldman has devised a practical, tried and true program that often helps him and others to boost the quality of sleep. While Dr. Goldman's complete program appears in *Brain Fitness* ([New York]: Doubleday Publishing, 1999), these are some of the highlights:

1. **Practice good sleep hygiene.**
   - Where you sleep directly impacts how well you sleep. Create a sleeping environment that is comfortable in temperature, absent of distracting lighting and sounds, and serene.
   - Don't become overstimulated: television emits full-spectrum lighting and electromagnetic fields that can cause wakefulness and/or agitation.
   - If you have allergies to airborne agents, remove plants and humidifiers (both can be sources of mold), don't let pets into your bedroom (sources of dander), and encase your mattress, boxspring, blankets, and pillows (havens for dust mites) in allergy barrier covers.

2. **Eat for sleep.** Starchy foods like breads, pastas, potatoes, and dairy products help promote sleep. They prompt your brain to generate the sleep-inducing neurochemical serotonin.

3. **Herbs help.** For some people, a modest dose orally ingested of valerian root, kava kava, chamomile, or a few drops of lavender oil inhaled, speeds the trip to dreamland.

4. **Avoid certain medications.** Check with your physician to verify whether any prescription and/or over-the-counter products you take may cause you difficulty in falling asleep. Blood pressure medicines, decongestants, nicotine, caffeine, diet pills, and some cold/cough remedies are frequent culprits.

5. **Lower your body temperature.** You reach sleep once your body temperature dips. A warm bath or shower before bedtime makes it easier for your body to cool down and the time to reach dreamland shorter.

6. **Take two.** Try taking two baby aspirins (non-caffeinated) at bedtime.

7. **Power nap.** Just twenty minutes of restful slumber during a hectic day not only rejuvenates your thinking, but also can make it easier for you to sleep at night.

Chapter 19

Mind Over Matter: Antistress Tips for Anti-Aging

Throughout this book, we've looked at the aging process and factors that can contribute to it. We've also explored a range of nutritional supplements, lifestyle choices, and hormonal treatments that can slow, ease, or even reverse the aging process. But perhaps the most powerful anti-aging weapon that you have is your mind.

> A hormone produced by the body when under stress, *cortisol*, is associated with a dozen or more serious degenerative diseases and has been found in some studies to be present in elevated levels in the last days of life.

Numerous studies have shown that your health is greatly affected by how you react to stressful events in life—setbacks or deadlines at work, conflicts, and losses at home. By the same token, changing your reactions, learning to meditate or to do other relaxation techniques, and generally committing to a positive, open attitude toward life can help make you younger, reducing your biological age and expanding your abilities to maintain a vigorous and energetic lifestyle.

WHAT IS STRESS?

More than half a century ago, Dr. Hans Selye recognized the mind-body connection involved with stress, as all of his patients had similar physiological and psychological characteristics. Two of which were loss of appetite and increased blood pressure. Further studies found that rats exhibited these same physical responses when they were put under stress. Selye concluded that stress is "the non-specific response of the body to any demand placed upon it." However, according to Selye, it is not stress that harms us but distress. Distress occurs when we prolong emotional stress and don't deal with it in a positive manner.

Dr. Selye referred to our bodies' response to stress—or distress—as the general adaptation syndrome (GAS). GAS consists of three different stages: alarm, resistance, and exhaustion. The alarm stage is comparable to the well-known "fight or flight" response, during which the body releases the hormone cortisol and prepares either to battle whatever is threatening it or to retreat from it.

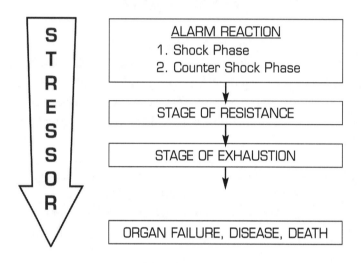

FIGURE 17.1. Diagram of the general adaptation syndrome.

However, since many modern-day stressors are not physical things we can run from and escape from immediately, the alarm stage is lengthened, leading up to the next phase, the stage of resistance. This stage allows us to adjust our bodies to counteract the physiologic changes that occur in response to the stress. However, if the stress factor does not disappear, the third stage occurs, exhaustion. It is during exhaustion that the body creates a situation of distress, and responses can range from extreme fatigue to disease and possibly death.

STRESS AND AGING

Stress in itself is not necessarily a negative thing. The term stress simply refers to any situation—physical, emotional, or both—that requires any bodily response more active than equilibrium. A slight change in temperature is experienced by the body as stress, that is, a demand from nature to mobilize the body's resources and raise or lower body temperature. A new love affair is stressful even while it is blissful, as it evokes your intense attention to a new person and creates powerful emotions that demand a new kind of attention to yourself. Playing tennis, negotiating a big deal, planning a birthday party for your child, even reading an exciting mystery novel are all sources of stress in that they demand physical or emotional responses from you, pleasurable though these activities may be.

Where stress becomes negative is in our responses to it. If your reaction to negotiating a big business deal is not pleasurable suspense, but a killing anxiety, then your body will probably respond with a headache or stomachache, and your immune system may become weaker as well. If the daily commute to work is the occasion for a hundred little explosions of temper, you are creating a level of negative stress that will affect your body quite differently than if you enjoy the challenge of driving skillfully through crowded city streets.

This type of negative stress creates a number of ailments, from mental frustration, anxiety, and depression to headaches, allergies, ulcers, and heart disease. In the long run, negative responses to stress can wear down the immune system, potentially leading to cancer and other diseases traditionally associated with aging.

> Doctors at King's College Hospital in London found that out of 100 women diagnosed with early stage breast cancer, 50 percent had experienced at least one severe adverse event (for example, the breakup of a marriage or the death of a close family member) in the past year.

Many studies have been done on the physical stress response in the elderly, and it was found that when placed under stress, elderly people experienced loss of appetite, weight loss, a lowered lymphocyte count—which impairs immune function—and an increase in psychological distress and in cholesterol levels.

Moreover, negative stress increases our bodies' production of free radicals. In response to a stressful situation, the hypothalamus releases neuropeptides that keep the body in a perpetual state of excitement. This, in turn, causes the pituitary to stimulate the adrenal glands, which, in turn, produce the stress hormones: cortisol, epinephrine, and norepinephrine. It's as though our cells' furnaces were stoked, causing them to burn energy at a higher rate—with free radicals as a kind of polluting byproduct. These chemical reactions set off a chain reaction resulting in still more free radicals.

Stress is now recognized as a major risk factor for heart disease. Results of one study showed that men under constant stress at work are more likely to develop atherosclerosis. Results of a study published in 2002 revealed that stress can triple a heart disease patient's risk of death. Stress has also been shown to slow wound healing and has been implicated in the development of a whole range of illnesses, including rheumatoid arthritis and stomach ulcers.

Studies carried out on rats have revealed that chronic stress during early life can significantly impair memory. The study found that young rats who were injected with the stress hormone corticotropin-releasing hormone (CRH) had 10 to 18 percent fewer cells in the hippocampus by the time they were twelve months old compared with rats who had not been given CRH—thus suggesting that chronic stress during the first weeks of life can alter brain chemistry on a permanent basis.

Meanwhile, other studies have shown that adult rats placed under chronic stress suffer memory loss and are less able to learn new things. Researchers in a new field called psychoneuroimmunology are exploring the links between the immune system and feelings and thoughts. In several classic studies linking immune system response to stress, researchers found that people under psychological stress were more likely to develop a cold when injected with a respiratory virus, more likely to have heart attacks and strokes, and less likely to produce antibodies when given a flu vaccine. Therefore, reducing stress can improve overall health and well-being, boost the immune system, and reduce the risk of heart disease.

Cortisol may be a particularly dangerous catabolic hormone as far as aging is concerned. In "Stress Cortisol, Interferon, and Stress Diseases," an article for *Medical Hypotheses,* Dr. Sapse cites studies that point to the increased presence of cortisol some two to seven days before death. High cortisol levels, according to Dr. Sapse, are associated with many of the degenerative diseases of aging: hypertension, ulcers, myocardial infarction, diabetes, infections, arthritis, cerebral vascular accidents, psychosis, psoriasis and other skin conditions, Parkinson's disease, multiple sclerosis, and Alzheimer's disease. Studies have also shown high levels of cortisol to inhibit muscle growth. In addition, acne, alcoholism, and obesity are also to some degree associated with elevated levels of cortisol.

Apparently, high cortisol levels, generated by negative responses to stress, interfere with the immune system as well as actively encourage disease. Cortisol not only interrupts our bodies' production of antibodies, it may actually destroy antibodies already in circulation, as well. Although stress-induced cortisol levels affect people of all ages, the loss of cortisol receptors in the brain—a sign of aging—may be responsible for the generally higher levels of cortisol among the elderly, and consequently their heightened vulnerability to diseases. Furthermore, laboratory studies have shown that the duration of the stress reaction is longer in older animals, possibly explaining the decreased rate of cortisol elimination with age.

> Researchers at Harvard Medical School interviewed 1,623 heart attack victims four days after the attack and discovered that angry episodes doubled their risk of a heart attack—which often occurred a mere two hours after the outburst.

There are a number of ways we can combat the destructive effects of a negative response to stress. Diet and exercise play a large part in our responses. The B vitamins in particular help our minds and bodies to cope with stress, while regular exercise, particularly aerobic exercise, enables us to meet life's challenges with a more relaxed and healthy attitude—and fewer symptoms of negative physical stress.

HOW TO DETERMINE
YOUR LEVELS OF STRESS

In order to determine your current stress level, we've come up with a quick and simple life stress quiz (pages 460–462) that you can take on your own. It is based on both external and internal stress factors and events that affect us daily. The first part of the test examines external events that may affect your personal stress index. The second part of the test deals with thoughts and emotions. Follow the instructions provided with each part.

Part I. External Stress Index

Circle each of the events that have occurred in your life during the past six months, add up the appropriate values, and write your total below.

Life event	Value	Life event	Value
Death of a spouse	100	Change in number of arguments with spouse	31
Divorce	73		
Marital separation	65	Change in responsibilities at work	29
Jail or imprisonment	63	Son or daughter leaving home	29
Death of close family member	63	Trouble with in-laws	29
Serious personal injury or illness	53	Outstanding personal achievement	28
Marriage	50	Spouse begins or stops work	26
Fired at work	47	Begin or end school	26
Marital reconciliation	45	Change in living conditions	25
Retirement	45	Trouble with boss	23
Change in health of family member	44	Change in work hours or conditions	20
Pregnancy	40	Change in residence	20
Sex difficulties	39	Change in schools	20
Business readjustment	39	Gain of new family member	39
Significant change in financial state	38	New mortgage or significant loan	17
Death of a close friend	37	Change in sleeping habits	16
Change to a different line of work	36	Weight gain or loss over ten pounds	15
Foreclosure of mortgage loan	30		

Total score of external stress events: _____

Add up your values to determine your external stress index:

0–50 points: Clean, virtually stress-free living.

51–99 points: Average stress index for modern life.

100–149 points: Warning! Take steps such as the strategies discussed later in the chapter to limit stress-related illness.

150 points or more: Danger! Real problems in your home and work environment may be taking their toll on you and placing you at a genuine risk for premature illness and accelerated aging. Don't be brave—GET HELP. Your longevity is at stake.

PART II. INTERNAL STRESS INDEX

This index deals more with thoughts and emotions, rather than external events. Read each of the following statements and mark the response that best describes yourself.

1. I feel unhappy or depressed.
   a) seldom   b) sometimes   c) usually

2. I don't lead a full life.
   a) seldom   b) sometimes   c) usually

3. I'm losing weight without trying.
   a) seldom   b) sometimes   c) usually

4. The things I once did easily, I now have difficulty doing.
   a) seldom   b) sometimes   c) usually

5. I have more energy early in the day.
   a) seldom   b) sometimes   c) usually

6. Constipation is often a problem.
   a) seldom   b) sometimes   c) usually

7. I am hyperactive.
   a) seldom   b) sometimes   c) usually

8. I feel I have no purpose in life.
   a) seldom   b) sometimes   c) usually

9. I find myself crying spontaneously.
   a) seldom   b) sometimes   c) usually

10. The future seems hopeless.
    a) seldom   b) sometimes   c) usually

11. I don't seem to enjoy the same things I once did.
    a) seldom   b) sometimes   c) usually

12. I have trouble sleeping at night.
    a) seldom   b) sometimes   c) usually

13. My thoughts are not as clear as they were last year.

    a) seldom   b) sometimes   c) usually

14. Lately, I am more irritable.

    a) seldom   b) sometimes   c) usually

15. I feel I have no contribution to make to society.

    a) seldom   b) sometimes   c) usually

16. I sometimes think I need professional help.

    a) seldom   b) sometimes   c) usually*

17. I use alcohol, drugs, food, and/or tobacco to help me
feel better about life.

    a) seldom   b) sometimes   c) usually*

18. I have thoughts of suicide.

    a) seldom   b) sometimes*   c) usually*

For each question you answered (a) give yourself one point; for each question you answered (b) give yourself two points; and for each question you answered (c) give yourself three points. Now add up your score for your final internal stress index. Rate yourself as follows:

18–26 points: Internal stresses seem well under control.

27–36 points: Something is missing, and you may want to take a closer look at how you handle some of the internal stress-related events in your life. Try to incorporate some of the strategies for coping with stress discussed in this chapter.

37–54 points (or any answers marked*):   There are some real stress-related problems involved here. You should seek outside help immediately. After all, what's the point of living beyond 100 if you feel that life is miserable? If we allow the affects of stress-related illness and aging to go unchecked, we allow stress to control and destroy our lives. Life is a precious gift, and it is meant to be enjoyed. There are answers out there, and help is available if you need it.

TWENTY-FIVE STRATEGIES FOR COPING WITH STRESS

Now that you've identified your strengths and weaknesses in dealing with stress, what other options do you have for responding to frustration and anxiety? We've already discussed diet and exercise as great stress-busters. You're probably also aware of simple but effective things you can do for yourself, like making time to relax each day, giving yourself frequent treats and positive reinforcement, and finding new ways of expressing and asserting your feelings with loved ones and living companions.

Besides these daily changes, however, there are some long-term habits and practices that can generally lower the level of stress in your life. The following twenty-five stress-relieving, anti-aging strategies can help you to function at a biological age that is far lower than your chronological age, so that you can live longer and enjoy life more:

1. **Get a regular medical checkup.** Not only can checkups be comforting if the doctor confirms that you're in good health, but they are also an indispensable method of preventing any minor health problems from becoming worse. Your annual life extension physical exam should be thorough and inclusive, paying particular attention to the very early detection of cancer, heart disease, diabetes, stroke, and metabolic disorders.

2. **Tie the knot!** Studies show that married people are healthier than single people. In fact, married people have been reported to reduce their risk of illness, accidents, and death by up to 50 percent!

3. **Take a siesta—that is, a short nap.** These twenty- to thirty-minute naps are best taken midday, since it is at this time that the body's metabolism is at its lowest. Taking afternoon naps also fits in with your body's natural circadian rhythm.

4. **Don't ever assume that your children's success or failure is completely the result of your parental influence.** By not accepting our children for who they are, a stressful burden is placed not only on you as a parent but also on the entire family unit.

5. **Spend high-quality time with friends.** Social relationships are not only fun, they're necessary for good mental health, as well. When our internal resources are depleted, the comfort of close friends can help lessen our worries and burdens.

6. **Become more spiritual, either through an organized religion or through your own personal meditations.** People who are affiliated with religious or spiritual groups are usually tapped into three powerful stress reducers: forgiveness, hope, and understanding.

7. **Adopt a pet.** Various studies have shown pet owners to live not only longer lives, but happier, more fulfilled lives as well, and like human friends, a pet can show devotion and bring necessary companionship, closeness, and comfort to anyone's life.

8. **Take up a hobby or develop a new interest.** If you truly enjoy doing something, stress will evaporate on its own.

9. **Use of time-management techniques.** A daily planner or a daily list of "things to do" cannot only be very productive but can relieve stress as well. By listing what we need to accomplish, we reduce our risk of trying to do too many things at once, thus burning ourselves out physically and mentally.

10. **Examine your surroundings.** If you feel the source of your stress is coming from where you live, for example, a major city or urban area, you might want to consider moving to a calmer, quieter place of residence. However, if moving is not an option, perhaps forming a closer sense of community with your neighbors may help ease some of the stresses related to your living situation.

11. **Think outside the box.** Sometimes something as simple as a mere change in the way we think about things can help reduce stress in our lives. For example, start perceiving your commute to work—be it by train, plane, or automobile—as an opportunity to relax, reflect, prepare, or meditate, rather than as an aggravation.

12. **Keep a careful check on your finances.** Money, whether we have too little or too much, can become a huge emotional strain. Be prudent and be smart. Try to realize that you have value and quality as a human being. More important, the quality of your life is not determined by how much money you have. Ultimately, material items become a burden, and many wealthy people find they are slaves to their possessions.

13. **Practice the art of meditation and relaxation** (discussed later in this chapter). Studies have shown that people who take time out of the day to

devote to these activities have lower blood pressure and a reduced risk of heart disease.

14. **Smile!** Scientists have actually discovered a connection between the facial muscles used when smiling and an area of the brain that releases "feel-good" neurochemicals.

15. **Communicate clearly.** By improving your communication skills, you cannot only reduce stress but also unneeded frustration, anger, and resentment in your life. Mixed signals are never pleasant to give or to receive. It is not only important to be a better communicator, but a better listener as well.

16. **Get moving.** Exercising more will not only lower your anxiety levels, but will also decrease any feelings of depression and low self-esteem. It is probably one of the most essential elements of any stress-reducing program (see Chapter 19).

17. **Change your diet.** Perhaps the extra pounds you're carrying around is adding to the extra internal or mental pounds you've been carrying as well. A healthy change of diet will help you feel more alive, more energized, and happier overall.

18. **Cut back on alcohol consumption.** While many people view alcohol as a way to escape from stress, it never reduces it. In reality, drinking more than two ounces of alcohol daily has been shown to raise blood pressure, inflame tempers, damage brain cells, and eventually increase stress levels.

19. **Say no to that second cup.** Caffeine is one of the most agitating substances your body can consume. By substituting a decaffeinated beverage for that usual cup of coffee, you'll remain much calmer and reduce the jitters associated with caffeine.

20. **Stop smoking!** By quitting right now, you can significantly improve your current state of health and live a longer life. Quitters can expect to notice improved lung function within days, a decreased risk of coronary heart disease within a year, and a diminished risk for cancer within three years.

21. **Think positive.** You may not want to be an eternal optimist, but do try to avoid being a perpetual pessimist. For maximum stress control, try being a little bit of both, so as neither to overextend yourself nor to

become a total cynic. Negative thinking can cost you added years of a healthy life span.

22. **Don't second-guess past mistakes or failures.** By dwelling in the past, we only end up harboring feelings of guilt and remorse that should be let go. If you're going to remember past mistakes, try to evaluate them in a positive way. Life is an education. Sometimes negative events are our best learning experiences.

23. **Learn to assert yourself positively.** Speak from your own point of view and help others understand what you are trying to convey.

24. **Learn to express your anger positively and respectfully.** Don't scream or act hostile. Positive anger can actually help us change stress into strength; destructive anger, on the other hand, when turned inward can lead to stroke, high blood pressure, and heart disease.

25. **Feel good about yourself.** Convert feelings of low self-esteem, not into forms of stress but into forms of strength. Everyone experiences personal defeats and losses, and a key element to stress reduction is not to allow these setbacks to control our lives.

MEDITATION

Perhaps the single most effective way of coping with stress—and a true anti-aging technique—is meditation. Transcendental Meditation in particular, founded by the Maharishi Mahesh Yogi, has been the subject of numerous studies that have validated its amazing physiological and emotional effects. Transcendental Meditation, or TM, must be learned from a practitioner, but it is relatively easy and inexpensive to do. Most cities now have people who will gladly teach you this life-enhancing practice. (If you're not sure where to find a teacher, ask at your local health store or health restaurant.)

We are all familiar with three states of consciousness: waking, sleeping, and dreaming. Meditation apparently creates a fourth state of consciousness, in which the mind is awake, but still. During meditation, muscles relax, the metabolism of red blood cells slows down, breathing and heart rate are lowered, and the blood flow to the brain increases.

Daily meditation seems to have the long-term benefit of lowering anxiety, improving mental functioning, and, in the long run, reducing a person's biological age. According to a literature review conducted by Dr. Kenneth Eppley,

TM lowered anxiety more than twice as much as any of the other relaxation techniques studied by researchers. Studies conducted by Dr. Hari Sharma and his colleagues at Ohio State University and the Maharishi International University at Fairfield, Iowa, found that lipid peroxides (indicators of free radicals in the blood) were significantly lower in elderly people who meditated regularly. Comparing meditators with non-meditators, with both groups maintaining a similar fat content in their diets, meditators aged sixty to sixty-nine had 14.5 percent fewer lipid peroxides in their blood, while meditators aged seventy to seventy-nine had 16.5 percent fewer. According to Dr. R. Keith Wallace's study of meditators, people who had meditated for more than five years had a biological age averaging twelve years younger than a control group who did not meditate. In some cases, the meditator's biological age was actually younger than his or her chronological age on the day he or she learned to meditate.

PROGRESSIVE RELAXATION

Progressive relaxation, intended to create deep muscle relaxation, was originally developed by E. Jacobson, and is currently a very popular method used in most physical and occupational therapy programs. This technique works by combining tension and gradual relaxation in a series of muscle groups. For example, you would begin by contracting the biceps muscles for five seconds, then gradually relaxing them for the next forty-five seconds. This would be followed by the same contraction and relaxation of the triceps muscles. The complete sequence of muscle groups starts at the head and continues downward to the feet, or vice versa. Once the technique is learned, you will be able to recognize which muscle groups need relaxing, and can then progress more quickly through the sequence to those specific muscles that need attention.

SELECTED AWARENESS

Selected awareness involves utilizing the biological limitations of people to respond to a small number of stimuli simultaneously. This means that by directing ourselves to concentrate on just a few selected stimuli, relaxation is induced. There are several selected awareness techniques currently used today:

- *Hypnosis:* With hypnosis, a therapist can induce relaxation by providing you with either a mental task or a repetitive stimulus. By doing so, your perception is altered, allowing the hypnotist to restrict your awareness. Hypnosis can be learned by the patient, and once learned, this state can be achieved without the aid of a hypnotist.

- *Autogenic training:* This method is similar to hypnosis in its use of a therapist to help direct awareness. However, instead of focusing on a mental image or task, autogenic training concentrates on physical stimuli—sensations of the relaxation response. You are taught how to imagine physiological sensations, such as warmth or heaviness, which evoke relaxation.

- *Guided imagery:* This method concentrates solely on your imagination. The place can be anything, from an exotic island to one's own bedroom, real or fantasy. The relaxation response evoked from this image can then be retrieved whenever needed.

BREATH CONTROL

Breath control originated as an essential component of yoga, and ranges from simple to complex. This technique can be employed anytime, anywhere—if you're stuck in traffic or even when you're in a board meeting.

Simple breath control consists of a modification of the breathing pattern. By lengthening the expiration phase of breathing, relaxation occurs. During breath control, you should think of something positive or calming, which will enhance the overall feeling of relaxation.

According to Dr. Neil Schachter, pulmonologist at Mount Sinai Medical Center in New York City, taking a full, deep breath every now and then throughout your day can reduce the risk of getting stress headaches and muscle tension.

EXERCISE AND PHYSICAL ACTIVITY

While exercise has always been recommended for overall health (see Chapter 16), recently many researchers and physicians have been recognizing it as a powerful way to relieve stress. Exercise helps the body eliminate the metabolic byproducts of stress on our systems, and it lessens our response to any new stressors. It makes us feel good about ourselves, instills a sense of accomplishment, and improves our appearance. However, if you plan to use an exercise program as a stress-reducing method, be sure to choose a noncompetitive activity, since a competitive activity itself may be a stressor and only aggravate your tensions.

MASSAGE

If you've ever had a massage, you probably remember it as a soothing, relaxing experience. However, you may not have been aware of its potential long-term benefits in lowering stress and combating aging.

Marian Williams, a nurse at the California Pacific Medical Center, states that massage has proven enormously effective as a means of treating a wide range of hospital patients. Megan Carnarius, a nurse who worked at a nursing home, found that massage also improved the cognitive skills of her elderly patients, as well as provided them with more youthful, elastic skin. Massage can help in combating depression, and even in stimulating the growth of premature babies, suggesting that it may have some ability to encourage the release of growth hormone.

Therapeutic massage involves the manipulation of the soft tissue structures of the body to prevent and alleviate pain, muscle spasm, and stress. There are several different types of therapeutic massage available, including Swedish massage, deep-tissue massage, and craniosacral massage. Therapeutic massage is carried out by a suitably qualified practitioner.

Research suggests that medical massage can strengthen the immune system as well as relieve acute and chronic pain, reduce the level of damaging stress hormones, and alleviate symptoms of depression and anxiety. Massage also has been linked to reducing acute and chronic inflammation, helping people with asthma breathe easier, the alleviation of chronic fatigue and migraines, and ease the symptoms of irritable bowel syndrome. Scientists speculate that massage accomplishes all this by improving circulation, boosting the flow of lymph, flushing out lactic acid, and stimulating the release of endorphins.

THINK YOUNG, LIVE LONG

All the techniques described in this chapter have one thing in common: each requires a commitment to a full and happy life, taking time for pleasure in the day as well as using hours for achievement and obligation. In the final analysis, the best way to stay young and live long is to love your life, filling it with a wide variety of challenges and joys that nourish your mind, body, and spirit. We end this chapter at a place you might begin: with the suggestion that you listen to yourself, discover what you need, and find a self-loving way to achieve it.

CHAPTER 20

Skin: Your Anti-Aging Survival Suit

Skin is the body's largest organ and performs three critical functions:

1. to serve as the first-line of the body's immune defenses in keeping germs out

2. to maintain water and salt balance within the body

3. to cushion delicate internal organs

Our skin and our immune system (see Chapter 15) maintain an intimate biological connection. The health of our skin and its ability to perform its immunoprotective function are critical to our well-being. Equally as important to many of us is how our skin looks, which is actually a significant biological subject. This chapter orients readers on the science of skin, why and how skin changes over time, and what we can do to regain our timeless beauty.

SKIN BASICS

Skin is composed of an integrated set of three distinct layers, each of which performs key functions for the body:

- **Epidermis.** With a total of fifteen to forty layers of flattened skin cells, the epidermis is the skin's outermost layer and the body's first-line physical barrier against bacterial, viral, fungal, and parasitic invasions, as well as other environmental insults such as sun exposure. The epidermal layer includes corneocyte cells, which are filled with keratin and a fatty lipid that keeps skin cells hydrated. Melanocytes in the epidermis are responsible for producing the pigment melanin, which protects the skin from UV radiation and also promotes tanning. The corneum stratum ("horny layer") of the epidermis is the very most topical level of skin cells and the layer targeted by most skincare products.

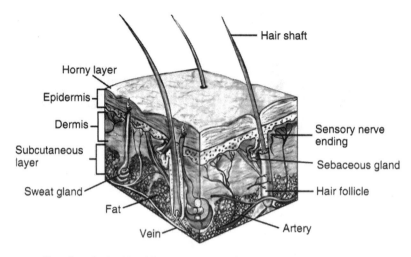

Figure from Gordon M and Fugate E. *Complete Idiot's Guide to Beautiful Skin*, 1998.

- **Dermis.** A layer rich in collagen and elastin, giving youthful skin its suppleness.

- **Subcutaneous fat.** Home to structures with functional purposes. Sebaceous glands secrete oils to lubricate skin and help retain water. Hair follicles, surrounded by a network of nerves, give skin its tactile sensitivity. Eccrine glands produce sweat to cool the body. Capillaries shuttle nutrients to the dermis and epidermis, transport waste products away, and dispel body heat.

HOW SKIN AGES

Present scientific evidence indicates five major mechanisms for skin aging:

1. Our skin is at the mercy of *free-radical damage*. Free radicals are highly charged molecules that steal electrons from other molecules, a cycle that results in the production of reactive oxygen species, the accumulation of which in cells is associated with more than 100 human clinical conditions, including autoimmune diseases, heart disease, and cancers. While skin possesses an extremely efficient and unique antioxidant activity level that surpasses that of other tissues, scientists have observed that skin releases low molecular weight antioxidants (LMWA) from its surface in an age-dependent fashion. When subjected to oxidative stress and aging, LMWA release is decreased and levels of free radicals rise. An important mechanism that may also contribute to free-radical damage in skin is microinflammation,

which can cause inelasticity and thinning of the skin. Scientists have observed that surface peroxides form when the turnover of macromolecules in the dermis is imbalanced, and this peroxide accumulation can be reversed by the application of topical antioxidants. (Kohen R, Gati I. Skin Low Molecular Weight Antioxidants and Their Role in Aging and in Oxidative Stress. *Toxicology.* 2000;148:149–157; Giacomoni PU, Declercq L, Hellemans L, Maes D. Aging of human skin: review of a mechanistic model and first experimental data. *IUBMB Life.* 2000 Apr;49[4]:259-63.)

2. *Hormonal declines.* DHEA, estrogen, progesterone, testosterone, and androstenedione are hormones produced in women and men, youthful levels of which are associated with supple skin (see figures on page 474).

    Dr. Karlis Ullis from the University of California School of Medicine/Los Angeles (USA) has explained that "Aging produces aberrations of sex hormone ratios and changes in target tissue receptors and skin." According to Dr. Ullis, by the time age-related changes in skin are noticed, hormonal declines have already affected other functions of the body.

    The importance of hormones in the healthy, extended human life span is discussed further in Section Two of this book, and in *Human Growth Factors: Advanced Anti-Aging Science Optimizes Your Peak Performance* (Goldman and Klatz, 2003).

3. *Sun exposure leads to photoaging.* Even the most minimal unprotected sun exposure is damaging to the skin. The sun will target your skin when you are walking to your car, hanging your arm out the car window, driving with the sunroof open, and so on: cumulatively over the years, these tiny doses of sun exposure set the stage for wrinkles, discolorations, and—at worst—skin cancer. Ultraviolet (UV) radiation accounts for 90 percent of the symptoms of premature skin aging. UV radiation can result in:

    • lines and wrinkles

    • lentigos (brown freckles)

    • telangiectases (dilated capillaries)

    • blackheads and whiteheads (senile comedones)

    • dry complexion

    UV radiation comes in two forms—UVA and UVB. Until relatively recently, it was believed that most of the changes in aging skin were the result of UVB damage, but now there is commanding evidence that implicates UVA as a major pathophysiological factor in photoaging. UVA rays

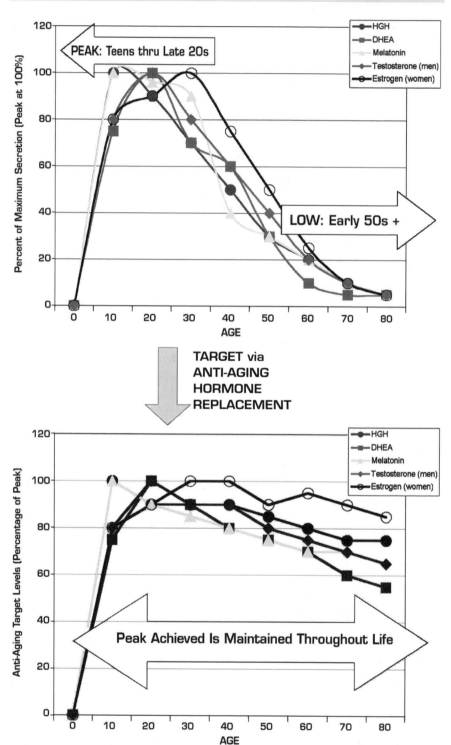

cause induction of the skin's metalloproteinases. These enzymes stray from their normal stimulatory function for collagen reformation, instead causing collagen degradation after sun exposure. The result is an uneven matrix of disorganized collagen fibers, called solar scars. In repeating this process of imperfect skin rebuilding due to sun exposure, wrinkles result. (Leyden J. What is photoaged skin? *Eur J Dermatol.* 2001 Mar;11[2]:165-7; Varani J, Warner RL, Gharaee-Kermani M, et al. Vitamin A Antagonizes Decreased Cell Growth and Elevated Collagen-Degrading Matrix Metalloproteinases and Stimulates Collagen Accumulation in Naturally Aged Human Skin. *J Invest Dermatol.* 2000;114:480–486; Chung JH, Kang S, Varani J, Lin J, Fisher GJ, Voorhees JJ. Decreased Extracellular-Signal-Regulated Kinase and Increased Stress-Activated MAP Kinase Activities in Aged Human Skin In Vivo. *J Invest Dermatol.* 2000; 115:177-182.)

4. *Cigarette, cigar, and pipe* smoking, compounding photoaging damage (see number 3 above). Skin of smokers is typically pockmarked and characterized by deep vertical lines around the mouth. In a study by Kings College (London, Britain), the researchers found that matrix metalloproteinases were even higher in the study's eleven smokers than the nineteen nonsmokers, before they were exposed to UV light. It was found that the study's smoker participants incurred such extensive damage to the skin's collagen protein that it resembled scar tissue, and the research team could not determine any nonsurgical means to reverse this damage. ("New wrinkle on a bad habit," *Popular Science,* Sept. 2001, p. 41.)

5. The *Maillard reaction* also factors prominently into skin aging. In collagen, relatively high levels of the advanced glycation end product (AGE) pentosidine accumulate with age. With age, scientists have found that the cross-linking of tissue proteins caused by the Maillard reaction causes pentosidine levels in skin cells to rise, leading to skin browning and collagen changes. (Verzijl N, DeGroot J, Oldehinkel E, Bank RA, Thorpe SR, Baynes JW, Bayliss MT, Bijlsma JW, Lafeber FP, Tekoppele JM. Age-related accumulation of Maillard reaction products in human articular cartilage collagen. *Biochem J.* 2000 Sep 1;350 Pt 2:381-7.)

Signs of Skin Aging

As we age, distinct changes occur in skin, which impact both its functional abilities and visual appearance ("Clinical Update: Skin Aging On the Cellular Level," *Anti-Aging Medical News,* Spring-Summer 2001).

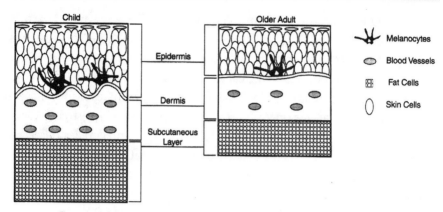

Figure from Gordon M and Fugate E. *Complete Idiot's Guide to Beautiful Skin*, 1998.

- Skin cells divide more slowly causing the dermis layer to **thin**.

- Fat layer beneath the dermis begins to atrophy; underlying network of elastin and collagen fibers, responsible for supporting the surface layers, loosen and unravel. Skin loses its elasticity and becomes **rough**, prone to **sags and furrows**.

- Sweat- and oil-producing glands begin to atrophy, depriving skin of their protective secretions. Skin becomes dry, yet also can become **acne-prone** and **pores become clogged**.

- Ability of skin to repair itself diminishes with age. Wounds become slower to heal, with healed skin **duller** than uninjured skin.

- Frown **lines** (between the eyebrows) and crow's feet (lines radiating from the corners of the eyes) develop due to permanent small muscle contractions. Habitual facial expressions form early **wrinkles**, which worsen with gravity.

- Aberrations in skin pigmentation emerge, causing a variety of **skin discolorations**.

SKIN BEAUTY—A PRIZED FLOWER

Think "flower power" when you consider how to maintain the youthful look and feel of your skin. We propose that there are seven "petals" to the perfect flower of human skin. If one of these petals is left untended, the flower's total beauty suffers. You need not be a gardener extraordinaire, but we suggest that

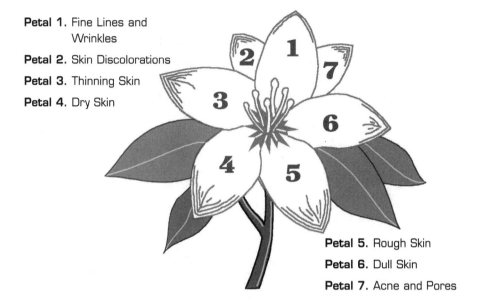

Petal 1. Fine Lines and Wrinkles

Petal 2. Skin Discolorations

Petal 3. Thinning Skin

Petal 4. Dry Skin

Petal 5. Rough Skin

Petal 6. Dull Skin

Petal 7. Acne and Pores

you understand these basics in order to attain a "green thumb" with which you can tend to your skin's beauty!

We have identified seven of common aging-related skin problems. Depicted in our flower power analogy, we then will review the impact of each of these factors on your skin.

✿ Petal 1. Fine Lines and Wrinkles

Humans express feelings, and as such, these emotions become the fine lines seen with aging. Squinting leads to crow's feet (lines radiating from the corners of the eyes), frowning causes frown lines (furrows between the eyebrows), and laughing leads to laugh lines (arc-shapes around the mouth). In addition, any other habits that cause small muscle contractions will produce additional places for fine lines and wrinkles to take hold.

Wrinkles are a result of age-related weakening of the skin's collagen and elastin, the fibers that keep the skin firm in youth. Skin becomes loose and lax, loses fat, becomes thinner (see petal 3 below), and thus looks less plump and smooth. Lastly, gravity pulls at the skin to cause it to sag. Factors that increase fine lines and wrinkles include:

- Sun exposure (see "How Skin Ages," number 3 above). Sun exposure as a child can start you on the road to wrinkles.

- Cigarette smoking (see "How Skin Ages," number 4 above)

- Genetics—the tendency to wrinkle is inherited. Take a good look at your parents and then take a thorough close-up look at yourself in the mirror.

Some of the more reliable line and wrinkle preventers include:

- Always wear sunscreen with a sun protection factor (SPF) of 15 or greater, no matter if you intend to be in the sun for five minutes or fifty minutes.

- Wear a hat with a large brim.

- Avoid sun exposure between 10 A.M. and 3 P.M., when UV rays are at their strongest.

Before and after being out in the sun, drink plenty of water (we recommend distilled). It will make its way through your system and into your cells—including those in the skin, hydrating them. The better hydrated the skin cells are, the smoother the skin will appear.

Remember, every part of the body wrinkles. While 62 percent of women use skincare products to fight signs of aging on the face, the legs, arms, neck, and chest often go untended. Again, flower power reminds us to take care of all the signs of skin aging, wherever they may be!

❀ Petal 2. Skin Discolorations

Blotches in which small patches of skin appear to have a different color than the main skin area become common as we age. It is important for you and your dermatologist to watch your skin discolorations carefully. Most skin discolorations will likely be harmless—warts and liver spots (also known as age spots), and others will be temporary—such as melasma, caused by hormonal fluctuations during pregnancy or taking birth control pills. But some skin discolorations can be harmful: a small flat brown spot can become cancerous, especially if its shape changes or it starts to itch—early signs that signal melanoma, a deadly form of skin cancer. Most aberrant skin discolorations are caused by years of sun exposure, so wearing sunscreen is again a number-one defense.

The amount of melanin, the pigment responsible for your skin tone, determines the propensity for your getting dark circles around the eyes ("periorbital"). If your skin is fair (not a lot of melanin), the blood vessels underneath may be easier to see. Wearing sunglasses and SPF 30 sunscreen (made for the face) can be helpful. On the other hand, if you have a lot of melanin (darker skin), dark circles will be more pronounced when you rub your eyes or are sleep-deprived. Try to get adequate sleep and reduce your exposure to allergens.

With age, however, a circulatory condition called "varicosity" becomes an issue. Most of us have heard of varicose veins, which are enlarged leg veins that appear blue and bulging, and sometimes are twisted and swollen. A faulty valve that returns blood to the heart is usually the cause. Varicose veins that appear on the face are called spider veins, the size and nature of which are typically smaller than non-facial varicosities. Both varicose and spider veins are seldom dangerous, but some individuals experiencing them consider them unsightly. Improving the blood flow, specifically by seeing your physician to rule out a medical disorder that can restrict circulation—such as arteriosclerosis, hypertension, or diabetes mellitus—is recommended. In addition, do not smoke, and keep hydrated.

❀ Petal 3. Thinning Skin

The skin of older people becomes papery thin: specifically, while the stratum corneum thickens, the epidermis and dermis thin and suffer a decrease in oil gland activity. This is largely a function of hormonal decline. Primarily, the age-related decrease in human growth hormone (see Chapter 4) is at fault. In the landmark study by Dr. Daniel Rudman of the Medical College of Wisconsin and published in the *New England Journal of Medicine* in July 1990, six months of HGH therapy enabled improvement in skin texture, skin thickness, and skin elasticity, while 61 percent observed fewer wrinkles. Patients started to notice changes within a few weeks of treatment. Fine lines vanished, deeper wrinkles receded, and facial fat decreased so that puffs of fat under the eyes evaporated, while the facial muscles that lift and hold the skin became stronger.

HGH also increases the synthesis of new proteins that lie underneath skin structure. In animal experiments, HGH increases the strength and collagen content of the skin, thereby enabling the skin to retain its turgor (bounciness) that is characteristic of young skin.

Countering the age-related decline of sex hormones in both men and women is an integral facet of an anti-aging skincare regimen. Doing so helps to maintain skin elasticity and firmness, decrease wrinkle depth, and maintain proper skin sebum production. Finally, an age-related loss of DHEA causes skin to bruise and rip easily.

❀ Petal 4. Dry Skin

As we age, skin becomes drier. Actually, "xerosis," the medical name for dry skin, affects only the very outermost layer of the epidermis—the stratum corneum (see "Skin Basics" above). It causes the skin to become flaky, itchy, or "tight," and discomfort is often the prevailing complaint. Genetics, disease, lifestyle, and the environment can all cause the skin to become dry, which can lead to dull skin (see Petal 6) and dry skin.

Normal, healthy skin is kept moist and supple by the sebaceous glands, which secrete an oily substance known as sebum. Sebum, other lipids, and natural moisturizing factors (NMFs) produced by the skin combine to form a barrier known as the hydrolipid system. This barrier has dual purposes; it acts to prevent foreign substances from gaining entry into the body via the skin, and it helps to prevent a process called transepidermal water loss (TEWL) and thus works to keep water inside the body for as long as possible.

The most common causes of dry skin are:

1. Inadequate transepidermal water supplied to the skin cells. Originating from the deeper dermal tissues, transepidermal water hydrates and nourishes the stratum corneum. Thus, TEWL occurs when the transepidermal water in the epidermis evaporates into the environment. TEWL is a normal bodily process; however, if the skin's hydrolipid system is damaged in any way, the rate at which TEWL occurs is increased. This increased rate of moisture loss eventually results in dry skin.

2. Dry skin is more prevalent among older people simply because the sebaceous glands are less efficient at producing the natural oils required to maintain the hydrolipid system. Similarly, babies and young children are also susceptible to the condition because their sebaceous glands are not fully developed.

3. Genetics are thought to play a role in the development of dry skin; thus, some people have an inherent disposition to the condition.

4. Winter is a particularly bad time of year for people who are prone to dry skin. Cold, windy weather, reduced humidity, and the effects of indoor artificial heating all combine to dehydrate the skin by increasing the rate of TEWL. Thus, flare-ups of dry skin are especially common at this time of year, and people already suffering from the complaint are likely to see it worsen.

5. Frequent showering or bathing in very hot water, swimming, or exposure to harsh detergents can also deplete the skin's protective oil layer.

6. Poor nutrition, particularly vitamin-A and vitamin-B deficiencies, can contribute to dry skin.

7. Medications, such as diuretics, antispasmodics, and antihistamines, may also aggravate the condition.

It is important to seek medical advice if no obvious cause of dry skin can be identified, as the complaint may be caused by an underlying medical problem. Dry skin may arise as a direct result of another dermatological problem, for example dermatitis, eczema, or psoriasis, however it can also be a sign of hypothyroidism (an underactive thyroid gland). Diabetics should always consult their doctor if they develop signs and symptoms of dry skin (or any other skin complaint), as diabetes can cause serious skin conditions.

❀ Petal 5. Rough Skin

Rough skin is commonly caused by the accumulation of dead skin cells on the skin's surface. These dead cells are usually discarded by the body via a natural process called exfoliation, where newer cells push older skin cells to the surface and the uppermost layer of dead cells flake off to reveal the newer cells underneath. However, for some reason, exfoliation does not always happen. The resulting buildup of dead skin cells causes the skin surface to appear bumpy and rough in texture, and the complexion often looks dull (see Petal 6).

Surface roughness can also be caused by a common, harmless skin condition known as keratosis pilaris, which is characterized by rough, "goosebumpy" patches of skin that often resemble chicken skin. Keratosis pilaris typically affects the backs of the arms and outer thighs but it can present itself on any part of the body where hair grows. Aside from being a cosmetic problem, keratosis pilaris is totally harmless. Some people may find that the affected skin is itchy and possibly inflamed; however, if this does become a problem, it is easily treatable with a short course of a topical steroid. Believed to be caused by a buildup of keratin around hair follicles—keratosis pilaris typically affects people who suffer from eczema or atopic dermatitis. The condition tends to run in families, and most commonly plagues children and teenagers—50 to 80 percent of adolescents are sufferers. The good news is that most people grow out of the condition by the time they reach their twenties or thirties.

There are other dermatological conditions that can cause rough skin. However, these are much less common than keratosis pilaris. Additionally, overexposure to the sun's harmful UV rays can cause damage to the skin that can make the skin appear rough. So, one of the easiest ways to safeguard against rough skin is, once again, protection against sun exposure.

Generally, rough patches of skin are only a problem from a cosmetic point of view. Gentle exfoliation can do wonders to make rough skin a thing of the past.

Petal 6. Dull Skin

Up to age fourteen, the skin on the face exfoliates naturally every fourteen days. This quick rate of renewal leaves the youngster with a healthy-looking glowing complexion. However, as we get older, the rate of natural exfoliation slows down. By age twenty-five and over, the skin will exfoliate every twenty-eight days or so. The resulting buildup of dead skin cells can leave the skin looking dull or gray.

Other factors can also contribute to surface dullness. Smoking has a negative effect on the circulation. As a result, the skin is often starved of the nutrients required to keep it healthy and give it a youthful glow. A lack of exercise also has a negative effect on skin health for the same reasons. Altogether, today's fast-paced lifestyle, which often results in little sleep and a fast-food diet, is a perfect recipe for dull-looking lifeless skin.

Petal 7. Acne and Pores

Acne

Acne is caused by a disorder of the sebaceous glands (glands in the skin that produce oil) (see "Skin Basics" above) that blocks pores, thus producing an outbreak of skin lesions we've nicknamed zits, pimples, and other less-flattering names.

Acne is America's number-one skin disease, with an estimated 17 million citizens suffering from it at any given time. Roughly 85 percent of twelve to twenty-four year olds develop acne. However, the condition usually clears up of its own accord with age—typically by the time a person reaches their late twenties. Statistics show that acne affects men and women almost equally. However, men tend to develop more severe and longer lasting forms of the disease. Women are more likely to suffer from intermittent outbreaks, which have been linked to monthly changes in hormone levels associated with the menstrual cycle. While acne is not a threat to health, it often makes people feel miserable about themselves and can cause permanent disfigurement and psychological problems if severe.

Doctors and dermatologists refer to acne as a disease of the pilosebaceous units. Pilosebaceous units consist of a sebaceous (oil-producing) gland connected to a hair follicle, they can be found over most of the body, but are present in particularly high numbers on the face, neck, shoulders, upper back, and chest—places most commonly affected by acne. Sebaceous glands are responsible for the manufacture of an oily substance called sebum, which usually passes through the hair follicle and empties onto the surface of the skin.

Acne occurs when a change takes place in the inner lining of the hair follicle. What triggers this change is unclear; however, it causes cells that line the hair follicle to be shed too quickly and clump together, ultimately blocking the follicle and preventing the exit of sebum. The resulting mixture of sebum and clumped cells causes a bacterium called *Propionibacterium acnes* (*P. acnes*), which usually lives on the surface of the skin, to grow inside the blocked follicle. The spots, or pimples, characteristic of acne develop because the skin becomes irritated by inflammation-promoting chemicals produced by *P. acnes*.

If you ever take a close look at the skin of someone suffering from acne, you may notice that not all pimples are the same. Acne can produce many different types of pimples, the most common of which is called a comedo or comedone. Comedos are simply enlarged follicles filled with oil and bacteria. Because they cannot be seen with the naked eye, comedos are often called microcomedo. If the comedo stays beneath the skin's surface, it is called a closed comedo or a whitehead. However, if the comedo reaches the skins surface it is called a blackhead because of its black appearance. Other types of pimples caused by acne include:

- papules—small pink bumps on the skin

- pustules—inflamed pus-filled lesions, commonly known as pimples

- nodules—large, painful, and solid lesions

- cysts—deep, inflames, pus-filled lesions that are painful and can cause scarring

The exact cause of acne is still a mystery to scientists; however, changing hormone levels and genetics are known to contribute to the disease:

• Rising levels of a class of hormones called androgens (sex hormones) can cause the sebaceous glands to enlarge and produce more sebum, thus increasing the risk of acne. This may explain why adolescents are particularly prone to the condition. Fluctuations in hormone levels are also thought to be responsible for the outbreaks of acne women may experience two to seven days before their menstrual period, during pregnancy, when starting or stopping using the contraceptive pill, or when they reach menopause.

• There is some evidence to suggest that acne may be a hereditary condition. Several studies have found that people with close relatives who suffered from acne are significantly more likely to develop the disease.

Several other factors are also known to cause or aggravate acne:

• Some prescription drugs, especially androgens, lithium, and barbiturates can cause acne, while stress may worsen the condition.

• A study carried out in 2001 revealed that smoking is a risk factor for acne. The study of nearly 900 people revealed that 40.8 percent of smokers suffered from acne compared with just 25.5 percent of nonsmokers. The study also found that smokers are significantly more likely to develop more severe cases of the disease.

• While the volley continues as to whether greasy foods and acne are connected, the latest research conducted by Colorado State University and announced in April 2003 suggests that highly refined carbohydrates can promote acne. Lead Researcher Dr. Loren Cordam reports that "in parts of the world where people don't eat refined carbohydrates, acne is almost nonexistent, so the evidence against carbohydrates is pretty compelling." When high-glycemic foods (like white flour, potatoes, and sugar) raise the blood's insulin levels, testosterone also rises, promoting acne.

Pores

Pores are tiny openings in the skin, which provide a way for oils secreted by the sebaceous glands to reach the skin's surface.

During puberty, the sebaceous glands begin to produce greater quantities of oil; this makes the pores enlarge so that they can handle the increased amount of oil passing through them. However, real problems occur if the pore becomes clogged due to the excessive amount of oil passing through it—this is when pores start to become very noticeable. The glands don't stop producing oil and the clogged pore gets bigger and bigger if left to its own devices. If left unattended, the oil will harden and cause blackheads (see "Acne" above).

The size of our pores is determined genetically and is nonnegotiable. Pores cannot be shrunk or otherwise minimized. Pores do not have muscles that can be promoted to open or close; pores are simply openings in the skin. Their primary function is to discharge oil and perspiration from the body. We are born, live, and die with the same number of pores for our entire life (barring injury or surgery to the skin). Pores perform an important function: they modulate the skin's hydration levels.

However, pore size is variable. Genetically, some people have small pores (generally those with fairer skin) and others have larger pores (those with darker skin). There are also more pores on the center of your face, and fewer at the side of the cheeks and at the forehead. Pores can become more prominent due to the cumulative exposure to sun: sun-damaged skin looks more bumpy and that is because the pores become more prominent.

People prone to dry skin are unlikely to have a problem with enlarged pores, as they tend to be a problem for those with oilier skin. They are most apparent in the T-zone—the area of the face that comprises the forehead, nose, and chin. However, on people who have very oily skin, they may also be visible on the cheeks and temples. Enlarged pores are typically most noticeable on the nose, simply because the skin that covers the nose has more sebaceous glands per square inch than any other part of the body.

Sadly, enlarged pores are not just a teenage curse. Once the pores enlarge at puberty, they usually remain enlarged until middle age, when they shrink back to their previously unnoticeable size. However, the pores of people of any age will enlarge if they become clogged. Dead skin cells, makeup, dirt, perspiration, and excess oil all contribute to clogged pores—thus emphasizing the importance of regular cleansing. Some blame can also be directed at the sun—enlarged facial pores can become a problem for people who commit the ultimate skin sin and irresponsibly forgo the sunblock, as UV light weakens support structures that exist around the pores thus causing them to dilate.

CUTTING-EDGE DERMATOLOGICAL INGREDIENTS TARGET TIMELESS BEAUTY

To protect and beautify your anti-aging survival suit, we have identified fifty-five of the most cutting-edge, advanced anti-aging skincare ingredients, and how they can help you maintain your petals of skincare beauty.

ALLANTOIN

Botanical extract said to be healing and soothing. Considered an excellent temporary anti-irritant and is believed to aid in the healing of damaged skin by stimulating new tissue growth. Appropriate for sensitive, irritated, and acne skins. Found in the comfrey root, it is considered non-allergenic.

Petal 3 (Thinning), **Petal 5** (Rough)

ALOE BARBADENSIS GEL

The mucilage obtained from aloe vera leaves, it is a popular botanical recognized for centuries, regarded as an emollient with hydrating, softening, healing, antimicrobial, and anti-inflammatory properties. Widely recognized for moisturizing ability, aloe vera penetrates the skin, supplying moisture directly to the tissue. Other properties include moisture regulation and an apparent ability to absorb UV light. Has slightly relaxing effect on the skin, making it beneficial for sensitive, sunburned, and sun-exposed skins. Found to be effective component in emulsions formulated for regulating dry skin. Apparently has a synergistic effect when used in conjunction with other anti-inflammatory substances. Constituted 99.5% of water, but more important includes minerals, polysaccharides, amino acids, and carbohydrates.

Petal 1 (Lines/Wrinkles), **Petal 4** (Dry)

ASCORBYL PALMITATE (VITAMIN C)

Preservative and antioxidant in cosmetic creams and lotions to prevent rancidity. Facilitates the incorporation of ingredients such as vitamins A, D, and C into cosmetic formulations. No known toxicity.

Petal 1 (Lines/Wrinkles), **Petal 2** (Discoloration),
Petal 3 (Thinning), **Petal 4** (Dry), **Petal 5** (Rough)

BISABOLOL

Botanical claimed to be anti-inflammatory and soothing. Derived from chamomile and/or yarrow.

Petal 5 (Rough)

BROMELAIN (ENZYME)

Enzyme found in pineapple. Theoretically, bromelain breaks down the connecting structure that holds surface skin cells together, to result with exfoliation.

Petal 7 (Acne/Pores)

CAMELIA SINENSIS EXTRACT

aka Green Tea extract. Journal of Photochemistry and Photobiology (Dec 31, 2001) stated the polyphenols "are the active ingredient in green tea and possess antioxidant, anti-inflammatory, and anticarcinogenic properties . . . Studies conducted on human skin have demonstrated that green tea polyphenols prevent Ultraviolet-B induced skin cancer induction." April 2003—Dr. Stephen Hsu and colleagues at Medical College of Georgia found that green tea's most abundant polyphenol, EGCG reactivates skin cells. At Day 20 (a week before the normal time of death of skin cells), when the cells sit atop the surface of the skin, topical EGCG from green tea was applied and found to make the cells begin to redivide, make DNA, and produce energy. Topical EGCG from green tea was absorbed only at the epidermal layer, and are purported to work by eliminating free radicals.

Petal 3 (Thinning)

CERAMIDES

Ceramides are the major component of the stratum corneum, accounting for 30–40% of the stratum corneum lipids by weight and are composed of at least seven molecular groups. Together with cholesterol and fatty acids, ceramides form extracellular lamellae that are responsible for the epidermal permeability barrier. Act primarily in the uppermost skin layer, affecting the intercellular spaces of the corneum layer where they form a protective barrier and reduce the natural transepidermal water loss of the skin. Ceramides repair the corneum layer in cases of dry skin, improve skin hydration, and increase the feeling of softness. They are also protective, particularly for stressed, sensitive, scaly, rough, and dry skin, as well as in the cases of elderly skin which exhibits a ceramide deficiency, and skin damaged by sun exposure. Ceramides are naturally present in the skin, playing an essential role in the structure of superficial epidermal layers, and forming an integral part of f the intercellular membrane network. The topical preparation could benefit the stratum corneum if the ceramides manage to fill the intercellular spaces and if they are hydrolyzed by the correct extra-cellular enzymes on the skin. Assuming everything works properly, topically applied ceramides can play a role in maintaining the skin's barrier function, especially when considered in regard to the stratum corneum's moisture requirements. If the stratum corneum's hydration is maintained, then it functions more normally in terms of flexibility and desquamation. Ceramides have been documented to deliver emollients into the epidermal layer, thereby suggesting that ceramides containing lipids may improve skin conditions involving transepidermal water loss (TEWL) such as erythema.

Petal 5 (Rough)

CETEARYL ALCOHOL (AND) CETEARETH-20

Cetearyl Alcohol: Emulsifying and stabilizing wax produced from the reduction of plant oils and natural waxes. Also used as an emollient and to give high viscosity to a finished product. Cetearyl alcohol is a mixture of fatty alcohols consisting primarily of cetyl and stearyl alcohols. Ceteareth 12: Used for their emollient, emulsifying, antifoaming, and/or lubricant properties in cosmetic formulations. Ceteareth is obtained from a combination of cetyl alcohol and stearyl alcohol.

Petal 5 (Rough)

CETYL DIMETHICONE COPOLYOL

Emulsifier and emollient used in cosmetic preparations to form water-in-oil emulsions that have viscosity but also rub out easily. Used in sunscreen formulations where good spreadability and waterproofing are valued characteristics. In moisturizers, provide good moisture barrier and reduce speed of transepidermal water loss.

Petal 2 (Discoloration)

CHAMOMILE (ANTHEMUS NOBILUS) OIL

Considered as a capillary wall constrictor, antiallergenic agent, antiseptic, cooling, analgesic, and healing. Found good for treating burns and skin inflammations, as well as dermatitis. Emollient properties. Good for use with acne, dry, or supersensitive skin. Active principles are a pale blue volatile oil (which can turn yellow with keeping) a little anthemic acid, tannic acid, and a glucoside. The volatile oil obtained through distillation is lost in the preparation of the extract. The whole plant is odiferous, but the flower heads are primarily credited with therapeutic benefits. Because the chief botanical virtue of the plant lies in the central disk of the yellow florets and in the cultivated double form of the white florets, it is considered that the botanical properties of the single, wild chamomile are the most powerful.

Petal 1 (Lines/Wrinkles), **Petal 2** (Discoloration),
etal 4 (Dry), **Petal 6** (Dull), **Petal 7** (Acne/Pores)

COLLAGEN (AND) ADENOSINE TRIPHOSPHATE (ATP NUCLEOTIDES)

Collagen: very popular in skincare formulations for great hydration potential and ability to bind and retain many times its weight in water. This water-binding and retention ability makes collagen effective for use in skin moisturizers as a skin protecting agent. It does not leave a feeling of tackiness or dryness, especially when used as hydrolyzed or soluble collagen. As a film former, collagen aids in reducing natural moisture loss, thereby helping hydrate the skin. Increases the humectancy of a topical product, contributes sheen, builds viscosity, and leaves skin smooth and soft. Collagen is not water-soluble. Today's collagen is considered "commercially pure" protein found in animal connective tissue, and is similar to the collagen produced by the body in the skin and bones. Also considered an anti-irritant, collagen does not cause allergic reactions when used on the skin. It is very stable, bland in odor, and light in color. One of the most effective and economical proteins available to cosmetic formulators.

Adenosine Triphosphate (ATP Nucleotides): A nucleotide (building blocks of nucleic acid) added to skincare products to bind water and moisture and may affect cellular energy.

Petal 1 (Lines/Wrinkles), **Petal 4** (Dry)

CYCLOMETHICONE

Provides silky, smooth feel to skincare products. Considered a noncomodogenic emollient. A form of silicone that can deliver active ingredients and also serve as a vehicle for delivering fragrance.

Petal 4 (Dry)

DHEA

A French study involving 280 subjects found that DHEA improved skin epidermal thickness, sebum, skin hydration, and pigmentation.

Petal 2 (Discoloration), **Petal 3** (Thinning), **Petal 4** (Dry)

DIMETHYL MEA (DMAE)

2-dimethyl-amino-ethanol, has been available in Europe under the product name Deanol for over 3 decades. DMAE is chemically similar to choline, so applied topically it is thought to have similar cell-membrane protective properties.

Petal 3 (Thinning), **Petal 4** (Dry), **Petal 5** (Rough)

EXTRACT OF PINE BARK, GREEN TEA AND GRAPE SEED

Excessive collagen cross-linking leads to wrinkles and sagging. Oligomeric proanthocyanidins (OPCs)—complex (dimer- and trimer-) extracts of botanicals including grape seed, pine bark, and green tea—bind to collagen and enable it to become more resistant to age-related breakdown. Additionally, elastin in the skin is supported by OPCs. As we age, skin becomes less supple due to an increase in the release of an elastin-degrading enzyme. Oxidative damage of the skin is accelerated by exposure to ultraviolet (UV) rays present in sunlight. OPCs have also been found to reduce skin redness and water loss caused by sun exposure. [A complete discussion on OPCs is available in our work *OPCs: Harvesting Nature's Anti-Aging Bounty* (Goldman and Klatz, 2003)]. In new research reported in April 2003, Dr. Stephen Hsu and colleagues at Medical College of Georgia reported that green tea's most abundant polyphenol, EGCG reactivates skin cells. At Day 20 (a week before the normal time of death of skin cells), when the cells sit atop the surface of the skin, the researchers applied EGCG from green tea topically, and observed that the cells begin to redivide, make DNA, and produce energy. Topical EGCG from green tea was absorbed only at the epidermal layer, and the researchers purported they worked by eliminating free radicals. Recently, a commercially-developed grapeseed-shell extract 50 times more potent than any other antioxidants, was coupled with pine bark extract as a time-releasing ingredient, and remained active topically for 20 hours.

Petal 4 (Dry)

FRUCTOSE 1,6 DIPHOSPHATE

Fructose is a member of a group of carbohydrates known as monosaccharides (simple sugars). Phosphate derivatives of fructose (for example, fructose-1-phosphate, fructose-1, 6-diphosphate) are important in the metabolism of carbohydrates. Fructose-1,6-diphosphate offers a high-energy source directly without oxygen: this technology has demonstrated utility in organ preservation and the ability to reverse free radical damage associated with aging. The mechanism of activity operates on direct dermal stimulation, as determined by human cell culture and validated by clinical testing.

Fructose-1,6-diphosphate, a natural substance, is prepared by the action of yeasts on glucose, mannose, fructose or sucrose, or by enzymatic conversion from precursors. Fructose-1,6-diphosphate and its derivatives, precursors, and mixtures thereof are generally soluble in water. Since topical application to affected sites of epidermal or mucosal damage requires that the active ingredient be in a form permitting such use, it generally will be the case that the diphosphate or precursor or derivatives be employed in association with a carrier, and particularly one in which the active ingredient is soluble per se or is effectively solubilized (such as an emulsion or microemulsion). It is necessary that the carrier be inert, so as not to deactivate the diphosphate or its derivative or precursor, and also avoid any adverse effect on the skin or mucosal areas to which it is applied. Fructose-1,6-diphosphate functions as a topical anti-inflammatory in epidermal and mucosal tissues and its utilization is being extended to anti-aging objectives. This compound aids the skin's ability to improve its barrier function and integrity, while reducing irritation and inflammation.

Petal 1 (Lines/Wrinkles), **Petal 2** (Discoloration), **Petal 4** (Dry),
Petal 5 (Rough), **Petal 6** (Dull), **Petal 7** (Acne/Pores)

GERANIUM MACULATUM OIL

Botanical properties are described as refreshing, anti-irritant, mildly tonic, and astringent. Although good for all skin types, it is of particular benefit to oily and acne skins, and those with inflammatory tendencies. The cell regenerating activities claimed for geranium also would make it useful for aging skin.

Petal 1 (Lines/Wrinkles), **Petal 4** (Dry), **Petal 5** (Rough),
Petal 6 (Dull), **Petal 7** (Acne/Pores)

GLYCERIN

Humectant used in moisturizers due to its water-binding capacities that allow it to draw and absorb water from the air. Glycerin helps the skin retain moisture, and has been studied extensively for that ability. Associated skin benefits are attributed to the ability to facilitate enzymatic reactions in the skin which enhance comocyte desquamation. Based on data available, glycerin has definitely been established as a good skin moisturizing agent. Glycerin also improves the spreading qualities of creams and lotions. It is a clear, syrupy liquid made by chemically combining water and fat that is usually derived from vegetable oil. While glycerin has not been shown to cause allergies, in concentrated solutions it may be comodogenic and irritating to the mucous membranes.

Petal 5 (Rough)

GLYCERIN (AND) WATER (AND) SODIUM PCA (AND) UREA (AND) TREHALOSE (AND) POLYQUATERNIUM-51 (AND) SODIUM HYALURONATE (ADVANCED MOISTURE COMPLEX)

Glycerin: Humectant used in moisturizers due to its water-binding capacities that allow it to draw and absorb water from the air. Glycerin helps the skin retain moisture, and has been studied extensively for that ability. Associated skin benefits are attributed to the ability to facilitate enzymatic reactions in the skin which enhance comocyte desquamation. Based on data available, glycerin has definitely been established as a good skin moisturizing agent. Glycerin also improves the spreading qualities of creams and lotions.

Sodium PCA: High-performance humectant due to its moisture-binding ability. Derived from amino acids. Sodium PCA also exists naturally in the skin as a component of the natural moisturizing factor. Considered noncomodogenic, nonallergenic raw material recommended for dry, delicate, and sensitive skins.

Urea: Increases absorption of other active ingredients, relieves itchiness, and helps leave skin feeling soft and supple. Regarded as a "true" moisturizer rather than a humectant, since it attracts and retains moisture in the corneum layer. Has a desquamating action as it dissolves intercellular cement in the corneum layer. Can act as an antimicrobial, by including water in its crystal structures. Can regulate the hydrolipid mantle, considered a buffering action. Properties include enhancing the penetrating abilities of other active substances. Anti-inflammatory, antiseptic, and deodorizing actions allow it to protect the skin's surface against negative changes and help maintain healthy skin. Studies show that urea does not induce photoallergy, phototoxicity, or sensitization.

Sodium Hyaluronate: Used as a moisturizing agent, viscosifier, and emulsifier, sodium hyaluronate is capable of binding 1,800 times its own weight in water. It is the sodium salt of hyaluronic acid, a glycosaminoglycan component.

Hyaluronic acid: Occurs naturally in the dermis. Its water-absorption abilities and large molecular structure allow the epidermis to achieve greater suppleness, proper plasticity, and turgor. When applied to the skin, hyaluronic acid forms a viscoelastic film in a manner similar to the way it holds water in the intercellular matrix of dermal connective tissues, suggesting that hyaluronic acid makes an ideal moisture base, allowing for the delivery of other agents to the skin. Ability to retain water gives immediate smoothness to rough surfaces and significantly improves skin appearance.

Petal 5 (Rough), **Petal 6** (Dull)

GLYCERYL STEARATE

May be used as a skin lubricant and imparts a pleasant skin feel. Mixture of mono-, di-, and tri-glycerides of palmitic and stearic acids, and is made from glycerin and stearic fatty acids. Derived for cosmetic use from palm kernel or soy oil, it is also found in the human body. Mild with a low skin-irritation profile.

Petal 4 (Dry)

GLYCERYL STEARATE (AND) PEG-100 STEARATE

Glyceryl Stearate: May be used as a skin lubricant and imparts a pleasant skin feel. Mixture of mono-, di-, and tri-glycerides of palmitic and stearic acids, and is made from glycerin and stearic fatty acids. Derived for cosmetic use from palm kernel or soy oil, it is also found in the human body. Mild with a low skin-irritation profile.

PEG 100 Stearate: Stabilizer and emulsifier for creams and lotions. The polyethylene glycol ester of stearic acid containing 100 moles of PEG. A cleansing agent and surfactant utilized in skincare products.

Petal 5 (Rough)

GLYCOLIC ACID (HYDROXYACETIC ACID)

Reduces corneocyte cohesion and corneum layer thickening where excess skin cell buildup can be associated with many common skin problems. Glycolic acid acts by dissolving the internal cellular cement responsible for abnormal keratinization, facilitating the sloughing of dead skin cells. Improves skin hydration by enhancing moisture uptake, as well as increasing the skin's ability to bind water. Hyaluronic acid is known to retain an impressive amount of moisture and this capacity is enhanced by glycolic acid. As a result, the skin's own ability to raise its moisture content is increased. Glycolic acid is the simplest alpha hydroxy acid (AHA). It also is the AHA that scientists and formulators believe has greater penetration potential because of its smaller molecular weight. Glycolic acid proves beneficial for acne-prone skin as it helps keep pores clear of excess keratinocytes. It is also used for diminishing the signs of age (liver) spots. A popular anti-aging cosmetic ingredient due to its hydrating, moisturizing, and skin normalizing abilities, leading to a reduction in the appearance of fine lines and wrinkles. Regardless of skin type, glycolic acid use is associated with a softer, smoother, healthier, and younger-looking skin.

Petal 2 (Discoloration), **Petal 3** (Thinning), **Petal 4** (Dry), **Petal 7** (Acne/Pores)

GLYCOSAMINOGLYCANS (MDI COMPLEX)

Skin is comprised of a complex matrix of molecules including collagen, elastin, proteoglycans, fibronectin and other glycoproteins. Deterioration of this matrix is implicated in skin aging, with enzymes such as the collagenases destructively impacting the firmness, elasticity and maintenance of the skin's extracellular matrix (ECM).

Glycosaminoglycans, in general, refer to a group of chemically related polysaccharides that are major components of the ECM and of connective tissues. They are used in cosmetics for their ability to increase hydration and the elasticity and pliability of the skin. Glycosaminoglycans are credited with moisturizing and firming properties. They reportedly leave the skin smooth and with a pleasant, velvety softness and evenness, and minimize wrinkle appearance. They are easily accepted by the skin due to their high charge and affinity.

MDI Complex is a novel type of glycosaminoglycans, an enzymatic inhibitor that can potentially control the protein-related declines seen in aging skin. Clinical trials have demonstrated the MDI Complex inhibits the enzymes that destroy the skin's collagen network. As a result, MDI Complex has the potential to improve the protective functions of the skin, reduce skin irritation, decrease skin redness, reduce the appearance of dark eye circles, increase skin firmness and elasticity, retard appearance of the skin sagging and fine lines, and reduce damage caused by sun exposure.

Petal 1 (Lines/Wrinkles), **Petal 2** (Discoloration), **Petal 3** (Thinning),
Petal 4 (Dry), **Petal 5** (Rough), **Petal 6** (Dull)

GRAPEFRUIT (CITRUS GRANDIS) OIL

Used as a fragrance and also as an active component with anti-irritant properties. Grapefruit oil is believed to help control the liquid process, and as such, is indicated for work with the lymphatic system.

Petal 5 (Rough)

HYDROLYZED DNA

(DNA not hydrolyzed) Surface film-forming protein with moisturizing action. DNA's large macromolecules do not enable it to penetrate the skin. In addition, its affinity with the corneum layer keeps it anchored to the skin's surface where it serves to protect and retain skin moisture.

Petal 4 (Dry)

HYDROLYZED RNA

(Ribonucleic acid not hydrolyzed) Surface film-forming agent with moisturizing action. The polyribonucleotide found in both the nucleus and cytoplasm of cells.

Petal 4 (Dry)

JOJOBA OIL

A moisturizer and emollient, jojoba oil was traditionally held in high regard by Native Americans of the Sonora Desert for its cosmetic properties. Mystical properties have been attributed to it for its apparent ability to heal the skin. Jojoba oil reduces transepidermal water loss without completely blocking the transportation of water vapor and gases, providing the skin with suppleness and softness. Gives cosmetic products excellent spreadability and lubricity. Studies indicate rapid penetration ability by means of absorption by the pores, where it diffuses into the corneum layer and acts with intercellular lipids to further reduce loss. Jojoba oil is now commercially produced, and, in general, is not considered a skin irritant and does not promote sensitization.

Petal 3 (Thinning)

LACTIC ACID

aka Sodium Lactate. A multipurpose ingredient used as a preservative, exfoliant, and moisturizer, and to provide acidity to a formulation. In the body, lactic acid is found in the blood and muscle tissue as a product of metabolism of glucose and glycogen. It is also a component of the skin's natural moisturizing factor. Studies indicate lactic acid increases the water-holding capacity of the corneum layer. They also show the pliability of the corneum layer is closely related to the absorption of lactic acid: that is, the greater the amount of lactic acid, the more pliable the corneum layer.

Petal 6 (Dull)

LAVENDER (LAVANDULA ANGUSTIFOLIA) OIL

Fragrance. Lavender oil is considered an all-purpose oil credited with many medicinal and folklore properties—including antiallergenic, anti-inflammatory, antiseptic, antibacterial, antispasmodic, balancing, energizing, soothing, healing, tonic, and stimulating. In addition, it is said to help clean minor wounds, regulate skin functions, and repel insects. Lavender oil works well on all skin types and produces excellent results when used for oily skin, as well as in the treatment of acne, burns, dermatitis, eczema, and psoriasis. Its benefit to the dermis is immediate since it is easily and rapidly absorbed by the skin. Lavender oil is said to normalize any skin type, and stimulate cellular growth and regeneration. Lavender is also claimed to help relieve stress, and as such, is believed useful in treating skin problems caused or aggravated by stress. It is generally considered nontoxic, nonsensitizing, and nonirritating.

Petal 1 (Lines/Wrinkles), **Petal 4** (Dry), **Petal 5** (Rough),
Petal 6 (Dull), **Petal 7** (Acne/Pores)

LECITHIN (LIPOSOMES)

Natural emollient, emulsifier, antioxidant, and spreading agent. Lecithin is a hydrophilic ingredient that attracts water and acts as a moisturizer.

Petal 1 (Lines/Wrinkles), **Petal 2** (Discoloration), **Petal 3** (Thinning),
Petal 4 (Dry), **Petal 5** (Rough), **Petal 7** (Acne/Pores)

LEMON (CITRUS MEDICA LIMONUM) OIL

One of the most versatile essential oils in aromatherapy, it is considered a counterirritant, antiseptic, depurative, and lymphatic stimulant.

Petal 5 (Rough)

PANTHENOL (VITAMIN B$_5$)

Acts as a penetrating moisturizer. Panthenol appears to stimulate cellular proliferation and aid in tissue repair. Studies indicate that when topically applied, panthenol penetrates the skin and is converted into pantothenic acid, a B-complex vitamin. Such action could influence the skin's natural resources of pantothenic acid. It imparts a nonirritant, nonsensitizing, moisturizing, and conditioning feel and promotes normal keritinization and wound healing. Panthenol protects skin against sunburn, provides relief for existing sunburn, and enhances the natural tanning process. Its humectant character enables panthenol to hold water in the product or attract water from the environment, resulting in a moisturizing effect. As a skin softener, it provides suppleness, and claims are that is also acts as an anti-inflammatory agent. Considered noncomodogenic.

Petal 1 (Lines/Wrinkles), **Petal 4** (Dry), **Petal 7** (Acne/Pores)

PAPAIN (ENZYME)

Papaya enzyme with the ability to dissolve keratin. Papain is used in face masks and peeling lotions as a very gentle exfoliant. Considered noncomodogenic.

Petal 7 (Acne/Pores)

PHENYL TRIMETHICONE

Serves as a barrier protecting the skin from excessive water loss. Leaves skin feeling soft and smooth, adds emolliency to the formulation, and reduces feeling of tackiness.

Petal 2 (Discoloration), **Petal 4** (Dry)

PREGNENOLONE

Corticosteroid, acts as anti-inflammatory and anti-itch agent. When applied topically, it may work as a water-binding agent.

Petal 2 (Discoloration), **Petal 4** (Dry)

PROGESTERONE

Combat the intrinsic skin-aging processes, increase elasticity and firmness, decrease wrinkle depth and pore size, and maintain skin sebum production.

Petal 1 (Lines/Wrinkles), **Petal 2** (Discoloration), **Petal 4** (Dry), **Petal 7** (Acne/Pores)

PYRIDOXINE HYDROCHLORIDE (VITAMIN B$_6$)

Skin-conditioning agent.

Petal 3 (Thinning)

PYRUS MALLUS EXTRACT

Technical name for apple. The pectin derived from it is used as a thickener.

Petal 6 (Dull)

RETINYL PALMITATE (VITAMIN A)

Skin conditioner. Considered to be a milder version of retinoic acid due to conversion properties. Once on the skin, it converts to retinol, which in turn, converts to retinoic acid. Physiologically, it is credited with increasing epidermal thickness, stimulating the production of more epidermal protein, and increasing skin elasticity. Cosmetically, retinyl palmitate is used to reduce the number and depth of fine lines and wrinkles, and prevent skin roughness resulting from UV exposure. Low incidence of redness, dryness, or irritation. Gains more effectiveness when used in combination with glycolic acid because it achieves greater penetration.

Petal 1 (Lines/Wrinkles), **Petal 4** (Dry), **Petal 5** (Rough)

ROSEMARY (ROSMARINUS OFFICINALIS) OIL

Credited with antiseptic properties, is considered beneficial for acne, dermatitis, and eczema. Some reports indicate that rosemary oil may stimulate fibroblast growth with a possible increase in epidermal cell turnover. This would make it useful in products for aging skin.

Petal 3 (Thinning), **Petal 7** (Acne/Pores)

SACCHAROMYCES LYSATE EXTRACT (DRF)

Healing and protecting properties. Extract is credited with the ability to protect against infection and boost immunodefenses. Constituents include polysacccharides d-mannan and d-glucan.

Petal 4 (Dry)

SAFFLOWER OIL

Carrier oil also considered hydrating to the skin. Consists primarily of linoleic acid triglycerides. Noncomodogenic, obtained from plant seeds.

Petal 3 (Thinning), **Petal 4** (Dry)

SALICYLIC ACID (BETA HYDROXY ACID)

aka Beta Hydroxy acid. Keratolytic activity when used in proper concentrations, helping to dissolve the top layer of corneum cells to improve the look and feel of the skin. Excellent ingredient in acne products because it reduces sebaceous follicle blockage and has antimicrobial action.

Petal 5 (Rough), **Petal 7** (Acne/Pores)

SANDALWOOD (SANTALUM ALBUM) OIL

Credited with astringent, anti-inflammatory, antibacterial, tonic, stimulant, cooling, and soothing properties. Considered a good antiseptic in cases of acne and as an astringent for oily skin. Some indications that sandalwood oil may promote epidermal cell turnover as some report it may stimulate fibroblast growth.

Petal 1 (Lines/Wrinkles), **Petal 5** (Rough), **Petal 6** (Dull), **Petal 7** (Acne/Pores)

SHEA BUTTER (BUTYROSPERMUM PARKII)

Protects skin from dehydration and other climatic influences. Restores skin suppleness, increases moisturization, and can improve the appearance of irritated dry skin. Natural fat obtained from the fruit of the karite tree.

Petal 1 (Lines/Wrinkles), **Petal 4** (Dry)

SODIUM CARBOXYMETHYL BETAGLUCAN

Beta glucans are said to stimulate the formation of collagen and aid in the reduction of appearance of fine lines and wrinkles.

Petal 1 (Lines/Wrinkles), **Petal 3** (Thinning)

SODIUM HYALURONATE

Used as a moisturizing agent, viscosifier, and emulsifier, sodium hyaluronate is capable of binding 1,800 times its own weight in water. It is the sodium salt of hyaluronic acid, a glycosaminoglycan component. Hyaluronic acid occurs naturally in the dermis. Its water-absorption abilities and large molecular structure allow the epidermis to achieve greater suppleness, proper plasticity, and turgor. When applied to the skin, hyaluronic acid forms a viscoelastic film in a manner similar to the way it holds water in the intercellular matrix of dermal connective tissues, suggesting that hyaluronic acid makes an ideal moisture base, allowing for the delivery of other agents to the skin. Ability to retain water gives immediate smoothness to rough surfaces and significantly improves skin appearance.

Petal 1 (Lines/Wrinkles), **Petal 2** (Discoloration),
Petal 3 (Thinning), **Petal 4** (Dry), **Petal 6** (Dull)

SODIUM PCA

High-performance humectant due to its moisture-binding ability. Derived from amino acids, the building blocks of proteins. Sodium PCA also exists naturally in the skin as a component of the natural moisturizing factor. Recommended for dry, delicate, and sensitive skins. Considered noncomodogenic, nonallergenic.

Petal 3 (Thinning), **Petal 4** (Dry), **Petal 6** (Dull)

SOY ISOFLAVONE AGLYCONE (PHYTO-ESTROGEN)

Isoflavones have an apparent ability to inhibit sebaceous gland activity and reduce oil formation and flow. Properties make it excellent for oily and acne skin, as a newcomer ingredient it is being studied for such applications.

Petal 2 (Discoloration), **Petal 7** (Acne/Pores)

SQUALANE

Excellent moisturizer and lubricant. Compatible with skin lipids, since human sebum is comprised of 25% squalane.

Petal 1 (Lines/Wrinkles), **Petal 4** (Dry)

SUPEROXIDE DISMUTASE

Enzyme that can serve as an inhibitor of free-radical production and a free-radical scavenger. In cells, it constitutes a natural defense system against activated oxygen species. SOD converts superoxide radical into hydrogen peroxide, which is then changed into harmless molecules of oxygen and water.

Petal 4 (Dry)

TOCOPHERYL ACETATE (VITAMIN E)

Vitamin E is considered the most important oil-soluble antioxidant and free-radical scavenger. Studies indicate that vitamin E performs these functions when applied topically. It is also a photoprotectant, and it helps protect the cellular membrane from free radical damage. In addition, vitamin E serves a preservative function due to its ability to protect against oxidation. As a moisturizer, vitamin E is well-absorbed through the skin, demonstrating a strong affinity with small blood vessels. It is also considered to improve the skin's water-binding ability. Vitamin E emulsions have been found to reduce transepidermal water loss, thereby improving the appearance of rough, dry, and damaged skin. Vitamin E is believed to help maintain the connective tissue. There is also evidence that vitamin E is effective in preventing irritation due to sun exposure. Many studies show that vitamin E topically applied prior to UV irradiation is protective against epidermal cell damage caused by inflammation. This indicates possible anti-inflammatory properties. Vitamin E appears to counteract age-dependent, decreased functioning of the sebaceous glands and also may reduce aberrant skin pigmentation.

Petal 1 (Lines/Wrinkles), **Petal 2** (Discoloration),
Petal 3 (Thinning), **Petal 4** (Dry), **Petal 5** (Rough)

TOCOTRIENOLS

Super-potent forms of vitamin E that are considered stable and powerful antioxidants.

Petal 3 (Thinning), **Petal 5** (Rough)

TYROSINE

An amino acid. Cutaneous applications may produce an extra reserve of tyrosine in the skin, which may assist in melanin synthesis. This in turn may increase and prolong the effect of the tanning process. Tyrosine's effect is improved if the product contains vitamin B_2 (riboflavin) plus ATP.

Petal 5 (Rough)

YEAST EXTRACT (NAYAD®)

Constituents include enzymes, vitamins, sugars, and mineral substances.

Petal 4 (Dry)

CHAPTER 21

Emerging Environmental Hazards

Humankind is at the most important crossroads between environmental influences and health that it has ever faced. History is replete with examples where health hazards demonstrating an association with an external, controllable exposure have been raised based on what seemed, at the time to be unconvincing and inadequate scientific study. Years later, such hazards become well-recognized triggers for disease, robbing thousands of people of their lives or compromising the quality of the lives of those exposed.

Asbestos and lung cancer; lead paint and stunted intellect and behavior in children; contaminated beef and mad cow disease; smoking and lung cancer and heart disease—all of these associations received dubious skepticism and rejection initially, only to be proven true in the final analysis. This chapter is designed to give you a better understanding of many everyday exposures that can put the length and quality of our lives at risk.

THE BIG BAD WORLD

The majority of us have an immune system that enables us to ward off many of the more common pathogens that are out to make us sick. Many of the microbes you encounter every day are relatively harmless. In fact, they are useful because they force your immune system to react, thereby keeping it healthy and robust. This reaction is called antigenic stimulation.

Nevertheless, the World Health Organization estimates that one in every four incidents of death or disease in the world is due to an environmental problem. The number of chemicals introduced into our lives since World War II is staggering. With them arrives an alarming increase in autoimmune diseases, allergies, and infections. Of the 100,000 chemicals now in common use, 25 percent are thought to be toxic. Your body fat may contain residue from hundreds of different chemicals. A toxic overload can cause life-threatening diseases like cancer and central nervous system disorders. Chemicals also weaken the immune system, inviting bacteria, viruses, fungi, and parasites to take command.

HOME SWEET HOME

Research by the University of Arizona at Tucson reported in May 2000 warns that germs frequently lurk among household objects. Here are some of the observations:

- *Salmonella,* which can thrive in human stools, is frequently spread through mutual contact with an object in the home. If a tiny amount of contaminated stool touches the hand of an infected person who then uses a phone, the next person handling it will come in contact with about 107,000 *Salmonella* cells, of which as many as one-third will survive long enough to enter the unwitting person by transmission through the membranes of the eyes, nasal passage, or mouth.

- *Rotavirus,* in as small a quantity as 10,000 virus cells, can lead to infection. Telephone receivers are a preferred spot: contact by an unwitting person can expose them to about 6,600 *Rotavirus* cells—with 200 descending on a single fingertip.

- The common cold gravitates toward kitchen faucets. If nasal secretions on the hands of someone with a cold comes in contact with a faucet, the next household member to handle the faucet can expect more than 1,000 cold viruses to hitch a ride.

- Make a gracious, germ-reduced exit from the bathroom. While the faucet is running, wipe your hands dry, then use a clean paper towel to turn off the faucet and open the bathroom door to exit, then discard the towel at the first chance you get.

COMMON HOUSEHOLD HAZARDS

Below are some of the most common hazards of the household, and tips on minimizing your exposures.

Bedroom

Inhaling dust mite allergens (body parts and fecal matter) aggravates—and may even cause—allergies and asthma. Dust mites thrive in the damp environment created by perspiration on sheets and have plenty of human skin scales to eat.

RECOMMENDATIONS

- Cover your mattress, box spring, pillows, and comforter with a dust mite barrier.

- Wash your sheets regularly.

- Try sleeping with a fresh towel placed over your pillow, and change the towel nightly.

- Use an electrostatic air cleaner with the air aimed at your face.

Kitchen

Research shows that kitchens—namely, kitchen sponges, sinks, and counter-tops—are far more contaminated than bathroom sinks and toilets.

Cleaning solutions contain harmful chemicals such as crystalline silica (in cleaning powders), which can cause cancer, and butyl cellosolve (in glass cleaners), which can damage kidneys and liver, compromising your body's ability to fend off invasion from germs.

RECOMMENDATIONS

- Maintain smart food-handling practices and keep "cleaning products" clean.

Laundry Room

Pathogens can be present in undergarments if fecal matter remains. The pathogens can then be swished around from garment to garment during the washing and drying process. If the moisture is not completely removed from the garment, germs will be encouraged to multiply.

A word of caution to those who use public laundering facilities: a study in New York demonstrated that people who share washing machines with others are more likely to get diarrhea or the common cold. Before loading the washer, run an empty cycle of $\frac{1}{2}$ to 1 cup of bleach set at hot wash/hot rinse.

RECOMMENDATIONS

- To prevent transmitting bacteria from garments to yourself, always wash your hands after handling wet laundry

- To avoid cross-contamination, separate items that may harbor disease-causing bacteria (undergarments and baby diapers, in particular) and wash and dry in a separate batch. Remember, just because the germs aren't visible to the naked eye does not mean they're not aboard the garment.

- To disinfect the washing machine, run an empty wash cycle with some bleach added to the water at least once a week.

Garden

In September 2000, two cases of Legionnaires' disease, a frequently fatal form of pneumonia, were reported to have been contracted from potting soil. A third case a few months earlier, in which the man died, is also linked to the soil. A rare bacterial strain was found in soil used by the infected people ten days prior to their reporting symptoms. Potting soil has been blamed for outbreaks in Australia and Japan.

RECOMMENDATIONS

- Garden in a well-ventilated area. Repot indoor plants outside.

- Avoid inhaling particulate that frequently swirl up from soil during handling.

Pesticide Use

Pesticides contain chemicals in sufficient levels to cause physical distress in humans, including weakening of the immune system. A company in Nashville, Tennessee is working on a new line of people-friendly insecticides, composed of oils from cloves, cinnamon, blueberries, and other fruits and spices to attack bugs. The oils interfere with a key enzyme found only in insects. According to preliminary studies, people and animals will be able to swallow the concoction without harm.

Car

What's that funny smell in your car when you turn on the air conditioning? It could be bacteria and fungi that can trigger allergies.

RECOMMENDATIONS

- Let your engine run for a few minutes with only the ventilator on to dry up trapped moisture. You can also have the system flushed with an antimicrobial to help alleviate the problem.

"BACTERIAL WILDERNESS" HAZARDS

Below are just a few of the hundreds of everyday contacts that, quite literally, can make us sick.

"Sick House" Syndrome

Exposure to formaldehyde in low doses can cause burning of the eyes, nose, and throat; tearing; nausea; dizziness; cough; chest pain; and shortness of breath. Chronic exposure has been associated with memory loss, menstrual irregularities, and certain cancers. Formaldehyde is used extensively in building materials and furnishings. It is also in fresh latex paint, new paper and plastic, new clothing, and some cosmetics.

RECOMMENDATIONS

- Test the formaldehyde concentration in every room with a home-testing kit.

Daycare Center

Daycare children are sick almost twice as much as children cared for at home. There is so much fecal bacteria at a daycare center, children usually end up with diarrhea or a stomachache sooner rather than later. Children in full-time daycare are at greater risk for upper respiratory tract infections and ear infections than children who don't attend daycare.

RECOMMENDATIONS

- Choose a daycare center that separates children still in diapers from those who aren't.

- Impress upon the staff how important you believe it is that they wash their hands after changing a diaper and that they teach children to wash their hands after using the bathroom.

- Ask the staff to keep your child out of the wading pool. In addition, staff members who change diapers should not handle food.

"Sick Building" Syndrome (Offices)

Ozone from photocopying machines and printers irritates lungs and triggers allergies. Markers, highlighter pens, and correction fluid emit xylene, which causes headaches and, in extreme cases, nerve damage. "Sick building" syndrome is a cluster of symptoms, including lethargy, sore throat, stuffy nose, eye irritation, impaired memory and concentration, dizziness, nausea, skin irritation, and shortness of breath, caused by volatile organic compounds and bioaerosols (bacteria, mold, and fungi circulating in the air supply).

RECOMMENDATIONS

- Place office equipment as far away as possible from workspaces and be sure ventilation is adequate.

Healthcare Settings

Studies have shown that infectious microbes are often present on stethoscopes. More than 10 million people undergo surgical procedures involving endoscopes yearly. Flexible scopes are difficult to clean and can harbor biological debris—dried blood, feces, and mucus. Unclean endoscopes have been responsible for the spread of infection such as tuberculosis.

RECOMMENDATIONS

- Ask your doctor, nurse, or other healthcare provider to swab his/her stethoscope before your examination.

- Insist that your healthcare provider *sterilize* your endoscope. Disinfectant alone does not offer enough protection from infection.

Gym

Athlete's foot fungus can contaminate shower floors. Moreover, the bacteria *Pseudomonas* often thrive in hot tubs and Jacuzzis. Additionally, a rare but deadly amoeba (*Naegleria fowleri*) thrives in warm water (hot tubs and heated pools).

RECOMMENDATIONS

- Wear rubber sandals in the shower.

- Foam is a sign of unclean hot tubs. Examine a glass of water from the tub. If it is cloudy or discolored, stay out.

Swimming Pool

In 1997 and 1998, the water in public pools made more than 2,000 people sick. Swimming pools can easily become contaminated with the feces of young children. Chlorine does not kill all microbes!

RECOMMENDATIONS

- Do not swim if you have diarrhea.

- Do not allow your children to swim if they have diarrhea.

- Do not change diapers poolside.

- Never swallow swimming pool water.

Hotel

It is estimated that only about half of all hotels provide adequately clean air. In a *Wall Street Journal* test of air quality in nine major hotels, four had higher bacteria counts than found in a typical suburban home. Mold counts were abnormally high in some of the hotels. Contaminated air can cause burning eyes, headaches, and dizziness and can trigger allergic reactions.

RECOMMENDATIONS

- Check for telltale signs of dampness and stuffiness before accepting a hotel room.

- Avoid hotels that use vinyl wallpaper; it doesn't breathe and traps pathogens.

- Look for hotels that position themselves as "environmentally smart."

- Frequent travelers and companies that require employees to travel can hire an environmental consultant to assess the hotels.

CELLULAR PHONE RADIATION

Ring, ring . . . no it's not your mom, its irradiation calling. The notion that cellular phone radiation emissions might result with adverse health effects is the twenty-first century's first great environmental challenge. By most admissions from experts and advocates on both sides of the issue, the introduction of broad-scale public exposure to radiofrequency and microwave radiation by the use of cellular phone technology represents uncharted territory.

In our work, *Cellular Phones/RF Radiation: Medical Menaces of a Modern-Day Convenience* (Goldman and Klatz, 2002), it was our goal to make available to interested readers a survey of the scientific literature relating to the possible health effects of exposure to cellular phone radiation. On this subject, we recognize that studies to date are equivocal; there is a minimal proactive involvement by the government and regulatory agencies, and that the media tends to incite public frenzy and confusion. Thus, we also include a tempered discussion of these issues with the regard to their possible unintended influences on the public perception of the risks involved in cellular phone use.

We are firm believers that knowledge is power. The public and those who they trust with their health—their physicians—have, by and large, been left to scramble up a coherent review of this subject. Consumers should be given the opportunity to know what potential health consequences they may experience as a result of using cellular phones and, by all rights, should have the opportunity to make informed judgments as to whether they wish to continue such risk-related use. In the words of Dr. George Carlo, public health expert, "We're now in a gray area that we've never been in before with this. When we're in a gray area, the best thing to do is let the public know about the findings so that they can make their own judgment."

According to the wireless industry's trade association, Cellular Telecommunications & Internet Association, at the time of this writing, 137,458,902 Americans were cellular phone subscribers. This number has skyrocketed since the advent of low-priced phones and service plans became widely available to the general public in the mid-1990s. Some estimates report that there are 1 million new subscribers every month.

Worldwide, it is estimated that more than 400 million people now use cellular phones. Global cellular phone subscribership outstrips the sales of cars and PCs combined. Cellular phones are more popular in European countries than they are in the United States: more than 60 percent of Europeans own a cellular phone, compared with 40 percent of Americans. By the year 2005, it is projected that 1.3 billion people will use cellular phones.

Because of the immense numbers of present and future users, some scientists and public health experts are worried that even if only a small percentage of the population are adversely affected by radiofrequency (RF)/electromagnetic (EM) waves emitted by cellular phones, this could still equate to a public heath issue of epidemic proportions.

There is a sufficient body of evidence that suggests possible adverse effects of exposure to cellular phone radiation on the human brain, and other studies link these emissions and general malaise, immune system dysfunction, sexual and reproductive issues, changes in the central nervous system and cardiovascular system, elevations in blood pressure, skin damage, and changes in red blood cells, possibly leading to kidney stones or heart disease.

Electromagnetic emissions fall into two types: ionizing, having energy levels high enough to strip electrons from atoms and molecules (resulting in "ionization"); and non-ionizing, having insufficient energy to cause ionization. Cellular phone radiation falls into the non-ionizing category.

However, non-ionizing radiation is not without its biological effects. Cellular phone use can heat up brain structures. This thermal biological effect is characterized by irreversible damage to the most basic components in cells of living organisms. Raising the temperature of brain cells by as little as a fraction of one degree Fahrenheit can be "genotoxic"—that is, cause damage to cellular genetic material. This DNA damage may show up as mutations that can be replicated and passed on to other cells, a mechanism that is suspected to contribute to cancer.

Yet, the main biological effect of cellular phone radiation may be in non-thermal biological effects. Such mechanisms have been suggested to factor into diseases from cancer, respiratory ailments, and infertility.

One of the most important non-thermal effects of cellular phone type radiation involves the blood-brain barrier. No matter how long a cellular phone was in use, the blood-brain barrier opened up at once upon exposure. This increased permeability has been suggested to permit certain proteins found in the blood to cross into the brain, causing autoimmune diseases such as multiple sclerosis, damage nerve cells that can lead to dementia or Parkinson's disease, and cause an increased or unexpected exposure of brain cells to medications not designed to come into contact with cells in the brain.

Non-thermal effects of cellular phone radiation also have raised questions about potential damage caused by heat shock proteins (HSPs) present in the brain. Heat shock protein responses, when activated frequently and extensively, can cause the mechanism to malfunction and make the brain susceptible to cellular damage.

Taken collectively, scientific studies to date have been equivocal. In the lab setting, in human volunteer studies, and in surveys involving large populations, some researchers have found cellular phone emissions to stimulate responses, but other times there was no effect. This may be a result of variability from person to person of how susceptible he or she may be to cellular phone radiation emissions. Just like how a cold does not equally and completely affect all of the family members in a household, some researchers suggest that physical and biochemical differences from person to person influence how our bodies respond to cellular phone radiation.

Additionally, there has been some speculation that cumulative lifetime radiofrequency/microwave exposure may be identified in the future as the greatest determinant of our susceptibility to possible cellular phone radiation health effects. In addition to cellular phones and their base stations and other transmission equipment, today people are exposed to a wide and diverse range of radiofrequency/microwave emissions. Our environment is saturated with transmissions of radio, television, and paging devices, as well as cellular phones. Exposures of individuals to each of these sources of RF radiation may be well below established guidelines, but it is yet to be determined whether the collective, cumulative exposure over a lifetime translates into changes in our health.

Yet, the sheer numbers of current and future cellular phone users creates great cause for worry. Even if only a small percentage of cellular phone users are adversely affected, that could still equate to a public health issue of epidemic proportions. Adjusting for latency of disease states to the initial triggering exposure, it may be 2020 before a full-scale epidemic hits. Or it might not happen at all.

There are a number of ways in which to minimize your exposure to cellular phone radiation, and we discuss these in *Cellular Phones/RF Radiation: Medical Menaces of a Modern Day Convenience* (Goldman and Klatz, 2002). Heed the wisdom of Thomas John Watson, Sr. (1874–1956), American industrialist and founder of the International Business Machines Corporation (IBM) who remarked: "Follow the path of the unsafe, independent thinker. And on issues that seem important to you, stand up and be counted at any cost."

SECTION FIVE

Living Longer, Living Better

When you have eliminated the impossible,
Whatever remains, however improbable,
Must be the truth.

—SIR ARTHUR CONAN DOYLE (1859–1930)

Chapter 22

Personal Secrets of Longevity

Imagine if you could gather the greatest minds in the area of anti-aging medicine and ask them what they do in their own lives to make sure that they live the longest and healthiest lives possible. Imagine if you could find out just what these experts do in their own homes to enrich their own lives—what exercises they do, what daily supplements they take, and so on. Just that information is gathered here for your use—so that you can adapt this information for your own life, and for your own personal anti-aging protocol.

A word of caution: While much of the information presented in this chapter and throughout this book will allow you to treat yourself, you must learn to use this information appropriately and safely. Other chapters concern products that you must obtain through your doctor, such as HGH. Our point is this: the therapies of anti-aging medicine are serious business and, although most are inherently safe, they must be used carefully and appropriately. We strongly urge you to work with a qualified physician on your own anti-aging program. If your own doctor is not interested in these new developments, find one who is. Although you can do much on your own to increase your longevity, you need a qualified professional who will be better able to analyze your problems, chart your course to optimum health, and follow your programs with objective lab tests and medical intuition.

PIONEERS OF ANTI-AGING MEDICINE
SHARE THEIR SECRETS

Here are the personal life-extension programs of twenty pioneers in the new science of anti-aging medicine. These hardy souls are the founders, the leaders, the educators, the discoverers, and the promoters who over the past forty years have created the basis for the next age of health care in the new millennium.

Jeffrey S. Bland, Ph.D.

(Gig Harbor, Washington) is an international authority and lecturer on human biochemistry, nutrition, and health. He earned his doctoral degree in chemistry from the University of Oregon and was a research associate to Dr. Linus Pauling at the Linus Pauling Institute of Science and Medicine. Dr. Bland conducts an annual series of seminars for health professionals on the latest developments in nutrition and functional medicine focusing on assessment and early intervention. Hundreds of physicians and researchers subscribe to his monthly audio magazine, *Preventive Medicine Update* (PMU).

Personal Longevity Program:

Exercise: Aerobic exercise program with weight training, forty-five minutes, six times per week, uses stair climber and stationary bike.

Daily Supplements: Multivitamin with minerals in addition to

1,000 mg of vitamin C	400 IU of vitamin E
5,000 IU of vitamin A	400 mcg of folic acid
400 mg of magnesium	100 mcg of selenium
20 mg of beta-carotene	100 mcg of chromium
20 mg of zinc	

Dietary protocol: Predominately vegetarian, high-fiber, low-fat diet. Five servings of fresh fruits per day.

Alcohol: Minimal amount.

Sleep: Six hours.

Relaxation and stress relief: Reading and listening to music at least 1 hour per day; exercise.

Personal secret: Great marriage.

Best habit to cultivate: Time management.

Jeffrey Blumberg, Ph.D.

(Boston, Massachusetts) is a professor in the School of Nutritional Science and Policy and the associate director and chief of the Antioxidants Research Laboratory at the USDA Human Nutrition Research Center on Aging at Tufts University. He received his doctoral degree in pharmacology from Vanderbilt University School of Medicine. He received post-doctoral training in cyclic nucleotide metabolism at the Tennessee Neuropsychiatric Institute and the University of Calgary. Dr. Blumberg has published more than 100 scientific articles and serves on several professional editorial boards.

Personal Longevity Program:

Exercise: Stair climbs twenty minutes per day; walks one mile.

Daily supplements: Multivitamin with minerals in addition to:

500 mg of vitamin C	400 mcg of folic acid
18 mg of iron	400 IU of vitamin D
600 mg of calcium	15 mg of zinc
15 mg of beta-carotene	CoQ_{10} occasionally

Dietary protocol: High-fiber, low-fat diet with moderate protein; five glasses of juice; three to four pieces of fresh fruit. Occasionally eats fried foods, red meat, and shellfish. No coffee or carbonated beverages.

Alcohol: One to two glasses of wine per day.

Sleep: Six hours.

Relaxation and stress relief: Listens to music.

Mental exercise: Work and problem solving.

Personal secret: Enjoy your work.

Best habit to cultivate: Regular exercise.

Bob Delmonteque, N.D.

(Malibu, California) is an athlete, author, editor, writer, and is America's premier "senior fitness" consultant. He earned his advanced degree from Midwestern College in Columbus, Missouri. Mr. Delmonteque is a former bodybuilder and was the personal trainer to many noted movie stars in the mid-1940s, including Clark Gable, Joan Crawford, and John Wayne. From 1962 to 1968, he was NASA's personal trainer for the astronauts including Alan Shepherd, John Glenn, and Gus Grissom. He has had ownership of more than 500 health clubs and counseled and helped set up personal training programs for more than 100,000 people. Mr. Delmonteque is the senior fitness editor with Weider Publications for *Muscle and Fitness* magazine and authored the best-selling book *Lifelong Fitness: How to Look Great at Any Age.*

Personal Longevity Program:

Exercise: Strenuous workout forty-five minutes, three to five times per week, includes aerobics, weight training, and stretching exercises, plus 100 sit-ups before bed nightly. Trains for six weeks and participates in an annual marathon.

Daily supplements: High-potency multivitamin with minerals and B-complex in addition to:

2,000 mg of vitamin C	30,000 IU of vitamin A
25 mg of folic acid	450 mg of ginkgo biloba
wheat grass occasionally	

Dietary protocol: 25 to 30 percent protein, 50 to 55 percent carbohydrate, 15 to 20 percent fat; six pieces fresh organic fruit; 100 ounces of distilled water, plus one cup each of sassafras, chamomile, and fenugreek tea.

Alcohol: Seldom.

Sleep: Five hours.

Relaxation and stress relief: Meditates twice daily for twenty minutes.

Mental exercise: Problem-solving and reading.

Personal secret: Good genetic background and passion for life.

Best habit to cultivate: Know you can accomplish whatever you want and have self-confidence and self-respect.

Eric Braverman, M.D.

(New York, NY) received his medical degree with honors from New York University and did research at Harvard University, Massachusetts General Hospital, and New York University Medical School. He is the founder and director of the Place for Achieving Total Health (PATH Medical), a clinical practice that is devoted to mind and body wellness. Additionally, he conducts research on diagnosing and treating brain illness and the general prevention of medical illness and aging. Dr. Braverman has authored seven books including *The Healing Nutrients Within*.

Personal Longevity Program:

Exercise: Exercises one to two hours, three times per week, includes tennis, swimming, jogging, and weight lifting.

Daily supplements:

290 mg of vitamin C	12,233 IU of beta-carotene
100 IU of vitamin E	50 mg of magnesium
4 mg of zinc	40 mg of molybdenum
200 mg of taurine	500 mg of niacin
56.7 mcg of selenium	60 mg of niacinamide
0.35 mg of boron	200 mg of odorless garlic
50 mg of vitamin B_6	135 IU of vitamin D
6.7 mg of potassium	6.7 mcg of chromium

| 1.5 mg of magnesium choline | CoQ$_{10}$, tryptophan or melatonin, borage oil, fish oil, and saw palmetto occasionally. |

Dietary protocol: High-protein, low-fat, complex carbohydrate diet. Protein source is mainly fish, chicken with an occasional steak; two to three pieces of fresh fruit and vegetables per day; one pitcher of water. No fried foods.

Alcohol: Red wine on weekends.

Relaxation and stress relief: Cranial electrical stimulation, prayer, and meditation.

Sleep: Seven hours.

Personal secret: Higher power as a guide to health care.

Best habit to cultivate: Harmony of body, mind, and spirit.

Robert Goldman, M.D., D.O., Ph.D.

(Chicago, Illinois) has spearheaded the development of numerous international medical organizations and corporations. Dr. Goldman has served as Senior Fellow at the Lincoln Filene Center at Tufts University and as an Affiliate at Harvard University's Graduate School of Education. He is a professor of medicine at the University of Central America Health Sciences, Department of Internal Medicine. He is a Fellow of the American Academy of Sports Physicians, a Board Diplomate in Sports Medicine and Board Certified in Anti-Aging Medicine. Dr. Goldman is the recipient of honors bestowed by Ministers of Sports and government health officials of numerous nations. In 2001, Excellency Juan Antonio Samaranch awarded Dr. Goldman the International Olympic Committee Tribute Diploma for contributions to the development of sport and Olympism. A black belt in karate, Chinese weapons expert, and world champion athlete with more than twenty world strength records, Dr. Goldman's strength and fitness achievements are documented in the Guinness Book of World Records.

Personal Longevity Program:

Exercise: Aerobic exercise one hour per day with light resistance training six times per week.

Daily supplements: Multivitamin in addition to:

2,500 IU of vitamin A	63 mg of thiamin
425 mcg of folic acid	700 mg of calcium
150 mcg of chromium picolinate	3 capsules of odorless garlic
400 mg of ginseng	3,000 mg of vitamin C
65 mg of riboflavin	120 mg of niacin

100 mg of magnesium	325 mg of feverfew
200 IU of vitamin E	250 mcg of vitamin B_{12}
200 IU of vitamin D	5 mg of black currant oil
400 mcg of selenium	

Dietary protocol: High-protein, low-fat diet; meat source mainly fish and poultry; three pieces fresh fruit per day, six glasses of purified water per day. Seldom eats fried foods, red meat, or shellfish.

Alcohol: Minimal red wine.

Sleep: Four to five hours.

Relaxation and stress relief: Aerobic exercise.

Personal secret: Good genes, positive attitude: "I chose my ancestors wisely."

Best habit to cultivate: Regular exercise and a "proper" diet.

Denham Harman, M.D., Ph.D.

(Omaha, Nebraska) earned his doctoral degree in chemistry from the University of California–Berkeley, and his medical degree from Stanford University. He is an educator, clinician, researcher, writer, editor, and administrator. He is a professor at the University of Nebraska School of Medicine. Dr. Harman developed the free-radical theory of aging and expanded this theory to include the possibility that life span was determined by the rate of aging of the mitochondria. He is one of the founders of the American Aging Association, in addition to being a delegate to the White House Conference on Aging.

Personal Longevity Program:

Exercise: Runs two to three times per week.

Daily supplements: Multivitamin with minerals in addition to:

| 1,500 mg of vitamin C | 400 IU of vitamin E |
| 29,000 IU of beta-carotene every other day | 1 aspirin daily |

Dietary protocol: High-fiber low-fat diet with fresh fruit three times per day; five to six glasses of water. Seldom eats fried foods or red meat. No caffeine and seldom drinks carbonated beverages.

Alcohol: Red wine occasionally.

Relaxation and stress relief: Reads, listens to music, and runs.

Sleep: Eight hours.

Mental exercise: Work.

Best habit to cultivate: Keep working at something you enjoy and never retire.

Ronald Hoffman, M.D.

(New York City, New York) is trained in internal medicine and specializes in nutrition. He is the medical director of the Hoffman Center in New York City. Dr. Hoffman practices immunotherapy, focusing on the treatment of allergies and chemical sensitivities. An author of many books, including *Tired All the Time* and *Seven Weeks to a Settled Stomach,* he is a leading authority on nutrition and alternative medicine and the host of *Health Talk,* a radio show on WOR that originates in New York City.

Personal Longevity Program:

Exercise: Aerobic exercise forty-minutes per day, including stationary bike, stair master, treadmill, and running; strength trains three times per week.

Daily supplements: Multivitamin with multimineral with antioxidants in addition to:

L-glutamine   Ginseng   Melatonin

Dietary protocol: Salad and salmon diet that is high in phytonutrients with lean protein and monounsaturated fats; one piece of fruit per day; eight cups of water; three to six cups of green tea daily.

Alcohol: Organic wine and microbrewery beers.

Relaxation and stress relief: Reads novels and short stories, surfs the Internet, radio broadcasting; and uses kava kava.

Mental exercise: Writes books and articles, reads journals.

Personal secret: Diversification.

Best habit to cultivate: Adapt to new circumstances.

Gwen Ivy, Ph.D.

(Toronto, Ontario) is an internationally published researcher and educator. She received her doctoral degree in psychobiology from the University of California at Irvine. In addition to her work on the mechanisms of aging, she has done research on longevity and on health drugs, most notably l-deprenyl. Dr. Ivy is a widely published researcher who appears frequently on television and radio as an authority on longevity issues.

Personal Longevity Program:

Exercise: Works out major muscles while protecting lower back, one and a quarter hours, three times per week; swims a half hour, three times per week.

Daily supplements: Multivitamin with minerals in addition to:

500 mg of vitamin C	400 IU of vitamin E
200 mcg of chromium	100 mcg of selenium
10,000 IU of beta-carotene	ginseng
odorless garlic	green tea

Dietary protocol: High-fiber, low-fat diet with plenty of fresh vegetables and seafood; fruit juices. No fried foods.

Alcohol: Moderate amount of red wine.

Relaxation and stress relief: Reads mysteries and exercises.

Mental exercise: Reads and conducts research.

Personal secret: Learn to reduce stress and watch your diet.

Dharma Singh Khalsa, M.D.

(Tucson, Arizona) is the president and medical director of the Alzheimer's Prevention Foundation/Brain Longevity Institute in Tucson, Arizona. Board certified by the American Academy of Pain Management, he earned his medical degree from Creighton University School of Medicine and is a graduate of the UCLA Medical Acupuncture for Physicians Program. His principal research interest is the effects of stress, conscious relaxation, nutrition, and exercise on the performance, health, and longevity of the brain and nervous system.

Personal Longevity Program:

Exercise: Works out aerobically, one hour, three to four times per week when possible, includes stair master and circuit training; plays tennis, swims, practices advanced yoga and meditation, one and a half hours per day.

Daily supplements: High potency multivitamin with minerals in addition to:

3–6 g of vitamin C	400 mcg of folic acid
400 mg of vitamin E	25,000 IU of vitamin A
Carnitine	Ginkgo biloba
Ginseng	Astragalus
Blue-green algae	Spirulina
Wheat grass	

Pharmaceutical: 50 mg of DHEA every other day

Dietary protocol: Vegetarian with protein supplementation, fresh fruit twice day; little fried food, no meat, fish or eggs; one cup of tea per day.

Alcohol: None.

Sleep: Usually seven hours.

Relaxation and stress relief: Practices advanced Kundalini yoga, meditation, and prayer daily; goes to movies; takes a day off.

Mental exercise: Memorizes things for cognitive exercise.

Personal secret: I love life and love the life I live. Relax and see what God has in store for you.

Best habit to cultivate: Develop a relationship with your spiritual self.

Kenichi Kitani, M.D.

(Tokyo, Japan) is an eminent educator, clinician, editor, and researcher. Dr. Kitani received his medical degree from the Faculty of Medicine, University of Tokyo, where he is currently professor and director of radioisotopic research. For twenty years, Dr. Kitani served as director of the clinical physiology department at the Tokyo Metropolitan Institute of Gerontology. His main research interests have been the functional alteration of the liver during aging, the effects of deprenyl on antioxidant modulation, and life prolongation in animals.

Personal Longevity Program:

Exercise: Walks two hours per day; swims and snorkels when possible.

Daily supplements:

Gingko biloba	Ginseng
Blue-green algae	Odorless garlic

Dietary protocol: High-fiber, very low-fat and high seafood diet with little to no red meat, includes a lot of miso soup; drinks green tea.

Alcohol: Moderate red wine with meals.

Relaxation and stress relief: Walks; meditates thirty minutes per day.

Personal secret: Learn how to manage stress and take stress-free vacations.

Best habit to cultivate: Manage stress and follow a healthy diet.

Ronald M. Klatz, M.D., D.O.

(Chicago, Illinois) is a physician, surgeon, and the founder of the new clinical science of anti-aging medicine. For more than a decade, Dr. Klatz has been integral in the pioneering exploration of new therapies for the treatment and prevention of age-related degenerative diseases. In his capacity as President of the American Academy of Anti-Aging Medicine (A4M), the world's leading nonprofit medical organization dedicated to the exploration and application of innovative diagnostics and therapeutic interventions that aim to detect, prevent, and treat aging-related diseases, Dr. Klatz oversees AMA/ACCME-approved continuing medical education programs for more than 50,000 physicians, health practitioners, and scientists from over 100 nations annually. Dr. Klatz is a professor at the University of Central America Health Sciences, Department of Internal Medicine. He is Board Certified in the specialties of Family Practice, Sports Medicine, and Anti-Aging Medicine. Dr. Klatz is the inventor, developer, or administrator of 100-plus scientific patents relating to organ transplant, human resuscitation, and life extension technologies. A bestselling author, Dr. Klatz serves on the editorial boards of numerous international medical and health publications. A consultant to the biotechnology industry and a respected advisor to several members of the U.S. Congress and others on Capitol Hill, Dr. Klatz devotes much of his time to research and to the development of advanced biosciences for the benefit of humanity.

Personal Longevity Program:

Exercise: thirty-minute aerobic workout that includes walking, stair climbing, and weight training, five times per week.

Daily supplements:

2,000 mg of vitamin C

10,000 IU of vitamin A

900 mg of niacin

1 gram lysine

90 mg of CoQ$_{10}$

10 mg of melatonin (two times per week as a sleep aid)

800 mg of vitamin E

400 mcg of selenium

400 mcg of chromium picolinate

500 mg of l-acetyl-carnitine

gingko biloba

15 g of blue-green algae and chlorella

Pharmaceuticals:

0.50 grain of thyroid hormone every other day

50 mg of DHEA every other day

5 mg of deprenyl (eldepryl) at bedtime

$\frac{1}{2}$ tablet of aspirin

Dietary protocol: Primarily vegetarian diet with limited amount of red meat and fried food; fresh fruit two times per day; eight glasses of distilled water with lemon (for detox).

Sleep: Six to eight hours per night; rest: thirty-minute midday nap.

Relaxation and stress relief: Aerobic exercise.

Personal secret: Lead a full, robust, and meaningful life. Do what you love and it transforms from work to joy.

Best habit to cultivate: Positive mental expectation of health and longevity.

Hans Kugler, Ph.D.

(Redondo Beach, California) earned his doctoral degree in organophosphorus chemistry from the State University of New York at Stony Brook. He is the president of the International Academy of Alternative Health and Medicine. The author of six books on health and aging, including *Tripping the Clock,* a practical guide to anti-aging and rejuvenation, Dr. Kugler is the editor of *Preventive Medicine Update,* senior science advisor to the *Journal of Longevity Research,* and does research on fitness work and immune enhancement at Health Integration Center in Torrance, California. Dr. Kugler is widely published and appears frequently on television and radio as an authority on longevity, health, and nutrition issues.

Personal Longevity Program:

Exercise: Alternates aerobics and weights, one and a half hours, three times per week; horseback rides at cowboy events, two hours two times per week; swims.

Daily supplements: B-complex, multiminerals, and antioxidant complex in addition to:
1,000 mg of vitamin C
200 IU of vitamin E
100-200 of mcg selenium (nightly)
1 tablet of calcium/magnesium
Vanadium, glutathione, and omega fatty acids occasionally and Phycotene, DMG, echinacea, goldenseal, and specialty nutrients

Pharmaceuticals:
30 mg of DHEA
GH-3
Prostat
Oral thymus (three days on, two to three weeks off)
Oral cell therapy (two weeks, two times per year) using cell extracts from specific organ tissues for revitalization

Dietary protocol: Low-fat, high-complex carbohydrate diet with protein at every meal; extra protein between meals and before going to bed.

Alcohol: Extremely little; some beer or red wine.

Sleep: seven hours.

Relaxation and stress relief: Meditates; takes twenty-minute rest period in the late afternoon.

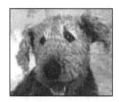

Lex, the Wonder Dog

(Chicago, Illinois) champion Airedale, mascot of the American Academy of Anti-Aging Medicine. He was featured on numerous television news shows and has been the subject of magazine articles. The average life span for Airedales is about eleven years. At age ten, Lex's health was starting to fail. Dr. Ronald Klatz placed Lex on the regime below and saw startling anti-aging effects. Within six months, Lex had apparently de-aged to the condition of an eight-year-old dog. He was able to jump three-foot fences, his coat returned to a dark black-brown from his senescent gray. His eyes became bright and animated, where before the therapy they were cloudy and dull. Lex ran and played vigorously with dogs five years his junior. Lex suffered a stroke at age sixteen; although he made a good recovery, he developed a weakness in his hindquarters at age sixteen and a half, which limited his activity and the quality of his existence. Rather than have Lex suffer the infirmity of aging, he was put to sleep at an equivalent of human age 116 years.

Personal Longevity Program:

Exercise: Walks, fifteen to twenty minutes, two to three times per day; stair climbs ten minutes daily.

Daily supplements: Because Lex was sixty-five pounds, he received one-half the dose of daily supplements normally prescribed for humans. Pediatric vitamin with meal two times per day in addition to:

.4 mg of vitamin C	400 IU of vitamin E
10,000 IU of vitamin A	vitamin B complex formula
100 mg of niacin	200 mcg of chromium picolinate
1 mg of folic acid	5,000 IU of beta-carotene
100 mcg of selenium	100 mg of CoQ_{10}
Ginkgo biloba extract	Ginseng
Hydergine	Garlic
green tea extract	

Pharmaceuticals:

PBN (mitochondrial antioxidant shown to extend lives of laboratory animals)
5 mg of Eldepryl every other day　　　　DHEA
10 mg of melatonin nightly

Dietary protocol: Science Diet for senior dogs; two Kosher hot dogs per week with sauerkraut and mustard; one slice low-fat pizza per week.

Ralph Merkle, Ph.D.

(Palo Alto, California) is a pioneering researcher in computational nanotechnology at Xerox PARC and was the manager of the Language Group at Elxsi. He received his doctorate in electrical engineering from Stanford University. Dr. Merkle is the author of numerous publications and the holder of six patents. He is a researcher, educator, author, and administrator.

Personal Longevity Program:

Exercise: Stair climbs, thirty minutes, five times per week; bikes twenty miles once a week.

Daily supplements: Multivitamin with minerals, no iron, additional chromium picolinate.

Pharmaceuticals:
1 mg of melatonin
½ tablet aspirin

Dietary protocol: Average American diet; fresh fruit daily; four glasses of water a day.

Alcohol: None.

Sleep: Eight hours.

Relaxation and stress relief: Works, browses the Internet, bikes, and plays video games.

Personal secret: Enjoy life.

Best habit to cultivate: Thinking.

Steven Novil, Ph.D.

(Chicago, Illinois) earned his doctoral degree in nutritional sciences from the Missouri College of Health Sciences. He is a clinical consultant in nutritional science to the Evanston Health Center and Director of the Evanston Nutrition Center. Dr. Novil is a nationally and internationally published author of articles relating to metabolic and eating disorders as well as weight management. His research on longevity, low blood sugar, allergies, asthma, and Eastern and American Indian medicinal herbs has been published in numerous professional journals.

Personal Longevity Program:

Exercise: Walks, thirty minutes, three times per week; yoga-like exercises, forty minutes seven times per week; calisthenics, twenty minutes, three times per week; jogs thirty minutes once a week.

Daily supplements: Multivitamin with minerals in addition to:

6,000 mg of vitamin C	800 IU of vitamin E
25,000 IU of beta-carotene	500 mg of proline
500 mg of lysine	400 mg of folic acid
100 mg of pantothenic acid	100 mg of niacin
300 mcg of chromium picolinate	9 mg of vanadyl sulfate
50 mg of zinc	100 mcg of selenium
1,000 mg of magnesium	1,500 mg of calcium
9 mg of boron	100 mg of CoQ_{10}
Ginkgo biloba	4 tablets of blue-green algae
150 mg of cinnamon	6 capsules of odorless garlic

Pharmaceuticals:

25 mg of DHEA (every other day)

0.5 mg of melatonin (every other night)

Note: One day each week, he does not take any supplements.

Dietary protocol: 90 percent vegetarian with no shellfish, seldom eats fried foods; three to four pieces of fresh fruit daily; four to six glasses of distilled water daily.

Relaxation and stress relief: Meditates, fifteen minutes, three times per day; cabalistic study and physical exercise.

Personal secret: Care for others and keep a positive mental attitude.

Best habit to cultivate: Try to find something good in all situations.

Brian Rothstein, D.O.

(Baltimore, Maryland) is a graduate of the University of Osteopathic Medicine and Health Sciences in Des Moines, Iowa. He is the medical director of the Rothstein Center for Health and Healing, which provides the largest chelation preventive medicine facility in Maryland. He is a diplomate of the American Academy for Advanced Medicine in Chelation Therapy. Dr. Rothstein served as a physician in the United States Army in human biologic research.

Personal Longevity Program:

Exercise: Walks, two to four miles daily; bike rides, hikes, and plays with children on weekends.

Daily supplements: High-quality multivitamin with minerals in addition to:
3–5 g of vitamin C

Dietary protocol: Whole grain, low-meat diet with a lot of filtered water.

Alcohol: Three to four times per week.

Relaxation and stress relief: Prays, sixty to ninety minutes per day; walks and uses the hot tub; mental exercise and cabalistic study.

Personal secret: Chose parents wisely and looks to God for help.

Best habit to cultivate: Balance.

Joan Smith Sonneborn, Ph.D.

(Laramie, Wyoming) a leading gerontologist, was educated at Bryn Mawr College and earned her Ph.D. at Indiana University in Biochemistry/Zoology. She did postdoctoral research at Brandeis University, University of California–Berkeley and the University of Wisconsin–Madison. Presently, she is professor and chair of the Program of Aging and Human Development at the University of Wyoming. Dr. Smith Sonneborn has been on the Executive Board and is a Fellow of the Gerontology Society of America. She was the first woman to chair the Biology of Aging at the prestigious Gordon Conference and has given more than 100 presentations nationally and internationally to both the public and private sector. She has been on the Advisory Board for government agencies and the Alliance for Aging Research, as well as international and national scientific journals. She is an administrator, an educator, researcher, scholar, and grandmother, with a love of life and humankind.

Personal Longevity Program:

Exercise: Performs Schopp aerobic weight-lifting circuit, forty minutes, three times per week; jogs, forty minutes, three times per week in fall, spring, and summer; practices contour exercises, one hour, one to two times per week.

Daily supplements: Multivitamin in addition to:

20,000 IU of vitamin A	15 mg of thiamin
17 mg of riboflavin	18 mg of pantothenic acid
21 mg of pyridoxine	15 mcg of cyanocobalamin
400 mcg of folic acid	500 mg of vitamin C
600 IU of vitamin E	100 mcg of iodine
25 mcg of selenium	1 mg of cobalt
15 mg of zinc	100 mg of potassium
18 mg of iron	3 mg of copper
1.5 mg of manganese	800 mg of calcium
400 mg of magnesium	30 mg of CoQ_{10}

500 mg of carnitine 750 mg of glucosamine sulfate

Pharmaceuticals:

Estradiol for HRT Dietary protocol: High-carbohydrate, low-fat, low-protein (mostly chicken, buffalo, wild meat, or salmon and orange roughy), diet—sixteen ounces of low-fat yogurt daily; eight glasses of water per day. No fried foods.

Alcohol: Minimal; champagne or red wine, if any.

Relaxation and stress relief: Scuba dives, watches movies and TV, dances, attends football and basketball games, hunts, fishes, also reserves "quiet time" for spiritual renewal and positive thinking.

Mental exercise: Prepare lectures, read journals, attends scientific meetings, takes new classes to keep current in new areas of expertise.

Personal secret: Be happy. I see the "good" in myself and in all those around me. I try to bring some pleasure to those I touch during the day. I grow and learn from my interaction with my students.

Best habit to cultivate: Self-discipline.

Stephen Sinatra, M.D., F.A.C.C.

(Manchester, Connecticut) is an author, clinician, educator, editor, inventor, and administrator. He is board certified in internal medicine and cardiology and is chief of cardiology and director of medical education at Manchester Memorial Hospital in Connecticut and is an assistant clinical professor of medicine at the University of Connecticut School of Medicine. Dr. Sinatra has special expertise in utilizing behavior modification and emotional release as tools for healthy living particularly in heart disease with emphasis on preventive cardiology. Trained in Gestalt and Bioenergetic psychotherapy, he is a certified bioenergetic analyst. He is the author of the books *Lose to Win, Heartbreak and Heart Disease, Optimum Health, The CoEnzyme Q_{10} Phenomenon*, and *Heart Sense for Women.* He just finished his latest book, *Eight Weeks to Lowering Blood Pressure.*

Personal Longevity Program:

Exercise: forty minutes, five times per week, includes aerobic fast walk/arm swing; back and abdominal strengthening exercises; light resistance training with ten pound dumbbells; and snow skiing and fly fishing as often as possible.

Daily supplements: Antioxidant multivitamin with minerals in addition to:

400 mcg of folic acid 90 mg of CoQ_{10}

30 mg of Pycnogenol 600 mg of choline

500 mg of inositol 180 mg of taurine

180 mg of methionine 180 mg of betaine

75 mg of l-carnitine

Enzymes:

Papain Bromelain

Aloe vera Acidophilus

Herbs and spices:

250 mg of cayenne pepper 100 mg of ginger

Gotu kola Hawthorn berry Fenugreek

Chamomile Hyssop

Fennel Astragalus

1–2 cloves of garlic 1,000 mg of omega-3 oil

600 mcg of melatonin with valerian root

three to four times per week at night

Dietary protocol: Mediterranean diet that is high-fiber (greater than 30 grams per day), low-fat (less than 30 grams per day), grains, pastas, fruits, and vegetables daily, fish one to two times per week; occasionally red meat and poultry; eight to ten glasses of water per day.

Alcohol: one to two glasses of red wine every other day.

Relaxation and stress relief: Prays, cooks, reads, and fly fishes, plays with dogs, emotional release (laughter, express anger, give myself permission to cry).

Sleep: Four to five hours.

Mental exercise: Writes books and newsletters.

Personal secret: Be able to "surrender" and listen to the "messengers" around us. Listen to your body.

Best habit to cultivate: Open your heart to love, avoid negative thoughts, create emotional support systems, and maintain connections with people you care about and who care about you.

Ben Weider, C.M., Ph.D.

(Montreal, Canada) is the founder and president of the International Federation of Body Builders (IFBB) in Montreal, Canada. IFBB now represents more than 160 countries and is a member of the General Association of International Sports Federations. Since 1945, Ben Weider and his brother Joe have operated Weider Sports Equipment Co., Ltd., and Weider Health and Fitness in Canada and the United States. He was instrumental in developing the vitamin, mineral, protein, and sports nutrition industry and has been the recipient of numerous awards for outstanding leadership in the promotion of health and fitness.

Personal Longevity Program:

Exercise: Works out one hour, three times per week; thirty minutes on treadmill; thirty minutes using various exercise equipment.

Daily supplements:

2,000 mg of vitamin C	1,000 IU of vitamin E
10,000 IU of vitamin A	100 mg of vitamin B complex
200 mg of folic acid	200 mg of CoQ_{10}
1,600 mg of niacin	500 mg of pantothenic acid
1,000 IU of vitamin D	1,000 mg of calcium
99 mg of potassium	200 mcg of chromium
500 mg of magnesium oxide	100 mcg of selenium
6 mg of iron	25,000 IU of beta-carotene
0.66 mg of copper	60 mg of ginkgo biloba
150 mg of ginseng	280 mg of odorless garlic
1,500 mg of either flaxseed or borage oil	

Pharmaceuticals:

3 mg of melatonin

Dietary protocol: High-fiber, low-fat, medium protein diet plentiful in fresh vegetables with four pieces of fresh fruit. Seldom eats fried foods and red meat; main meat source is poultry (white meat only), no shellfish. Four glasses of water daily; minimal caffeine and carbonated drinks.

Alcohol: Red wine occasionally.

Sleep: Six to seven hours.

Relaxation and stress relief: Reads; watches historical videotapes; listens to music nearly one and a half hours per day; exercises; and naps.

Mental exercise: Reading.

Personal secret: Keep a positive outlook.

Best habit to cultivate: Healthy lifestyle.

Grace H. W. Wong, Ph.D.

(South San Francisco, California) is a noted researcher in the area of gene regulation. She earned her doctorate from the Walter and Eliza Hall Institute of Medical Research, Royal Melbourne Hospital, Victoria, Australia. She has received numerous research awards. In July 1994, Dr. Wong gave one of the invited presentations on mitochondrial disease at the Nobel Symposium 90.

Personal Longevity Program:

Exercise: Aerobics, one hour, seven times per week; runs a half hour every evening.

Daily supplements: Multivitamin with minerals in addition to:
800 mg vitamin C   400 IU vitamin E
40–80 mcg folic acid

Dietary protocol: Grazes throughout day on high-fiber foods and proteins such as fish and poultry; plenty of fresh fruit (always three oranges and two lemons a day); water with added lemon. Avoids fried foods, tea, and coffee.

Alcohol: None.

Relaxation and stress relief: Exercise and work.

Personal secret: Think and work hard.

Best habit to cultivate: Be happy and keep a positive attitude.

A LAST WORD

Having read this far, you now know more about the science of anti-aging medicine than most doctors on the planet. The real answer to aging without disease and disability starts with education—learning all you can about anti-aging science. Your destiny and health is in your hands. It means taking action—the time to start your own anti-aging program is now. And anti-aging takes determination. You must say "No" to aging.

Although for centuries humankind has dreamt of long life and eternal youth, for most people, these dreams were perpetually out of reach. Now we know much and are learning more about how to prolong and maintain youth.

As you explore your own anti-aging program, your path will be shaped by your needs and wishes, biological inheritance, environmental circumstances, and personal preferences in diet and lifestyle. It may take some time before you find the anti-aging treatment that is right for you. But keep trying. The rewards will be far more valuable than the cost and the effort. Remember, old age is for the "other" guy. You know better, so why take it lying down? The choice is yours: whether to be a diseased and decrepit victim or an ageless and vital "immortal."

After all, as we asked at the beginning of this book, who wants to live to be 150? You will—the minute after you celebrate your 149th birthday.

CHAPTER 23

Arrival of the Triple-Digit Life Span: Biotech-Human Enhancement/Augmentation

THE HUMAN GENOME PROJECT: MICROSCOPIC DISCOVERIES LEADING TO MACROSCOPIC APPLICATIONS

The Human Genome Project (HGP) is an international research program designed to construct detailed genetic and physical maps of the human genome, to determine the complete nucleotide sequence of human DNA, to localize the tens of thousands of individual genes within the human genome, and to perform similar analyses on the genomes of several other organisms used extensively in research laboratories as model systems. The scientific products of the HGP will comprise a resource of detailed information about the structure, organization, and function of human DNA, information that constitutes the basic set of inherited "instructions" for the development and functioning of a human being. Successfully accomplishing these ambitious goals will demand the development of a variety of new technologies. It will also necessitate advanced means of making the information widely available to scientists, physicians, and others in order that the results may be rapidly used for the public good. Improved technology for biomedical research will thus be another important product of the HGP. The acquisition and use of such genetic knowledge has momentous implications on the future of preventive medicine.

On April 14, 2003, the International Human Genome Sequencing consortium, led in the United States by the National Human Genome Research Institute (NHGRI) and the Department of Energy (DOE), announced the successful completion of the Human Genome Project.

Proudly completed more than two years ahead of schedule and under budget, the international effort sequenced the 3 billion DNA letters in the human genome, considered by many to be one of the most ambitious scientific undertakings of all time. NHGRI Director Dr. Francis Collins remarked,

"The Human Genome Project has been an amazing adventure into ourselves, to understand our own DNA instruction book, the shared inheritance of all humankind."

As of the spring 2003, the finished sequence produced by the Human Genome Project covers about 99 percent of the human genome's gene-containing regions, sequenced to an accuracy of 99.99 percent. Thanks to the HGP, more than 1,400 disease genes have now been identified, up from the handful identified in 1990 when the HGP first began.

LEARNING ABOUT OURSELVES
AT THE MOST BASIC BIOLOGICAL LEVEL

"The completion of the Human Genome Project should not be viewed as an end in itself, rather it marks at the start of the era of genome in medicine and health," states Dr. Collins. He continues, "we firmly believe the best is yet to come." Over the next fifteen or twenty years, the Human Genome Project will develop tools to identify the genes involved in both rare and common diseases. Such discoveries, in turn, are likely to bring improvements in the early detection and treatment of disease and new approaches to prevention. Some of these applications are already coming into actual use.

Among the most potent practical applications of this new field of genomic medicine is customized DNA screening analyses. DNA is a helical ladder consisting of paired blocks of chromosomes, but scientists have detected subtle variations called single nucleotide polymorphisms (SNPs) that involve base-pair changes in DNA. SNPs may play an important role in defining your own genetic code, offering the opportunity to begin a more targeted approach to your health and longevity. Indeed, the U.S. Health and Human Services' "Healthy People 2000" project has established an initiative for scientists to discover and score single nucleotide polymorphisms to develop predicative testing to identify early the risks of cancer, heart disease and stroke, diabetes, and chronic disability conditions, as well as prenatal testing and maternal screening.

BETTING ON A BRIGHT FUTURE

The prospect of the extension of the human life span well past the centenarian mark is receiving rapid adoption by some of the world's most renowned forecasters. The Global Business Network (GBN), a worldwide membership organization engaging in a collaborative exploration of the future, discovering the frontiers of knowledge, and creating innovative tools for strategic action, predicts that:

Science and medicine will not only extend more people's lives to their full Hayflick span, 120 years, but advances in biology will lengthen human life even beyond that. If we look at the current work on stem cells and phenomena like telomerase . . . we find we're learning a great deal about the control mechanisms for aging. It's very likely that over the next 25 years, society will see serious and effective medical intervention in the aging process—people undergoing such therapy will keep looking and feeling and acting younger than their calendar age. The prospect of individuals living significantly longer than the current norm will begin to open up. In fact, looking at historical trends, one finds that over the past century, we nearly doubled our lifespan, the average having gone from about 45 to 85. There's no reason to imagine that we won't do at least as much in the next century. If you double 85, you're at 170—so [this] bet is actually conservative.

Indeed, GBN is so certain of the accuracy of this prediction that it has placed a wager with the Long Bets Foundation speculating that at least one human born in the year 2000 will still be alive in 2150. At the time this article first went to press, the bet remained without a challenger.

Perhaps the wager goes unchallenged because the number of people who subscribe to the notion of a limited human life span are on the decline. After all, it is difficult to ignore the leaps in medicine and health care that have resulted from discoveries in biotechnology. According to the Biotechnology Industry Organization:

- More than 250 million people worldwide have been helped by the more than 117 biotechnology drug products and vaccines approved by the U.S. Food and Drug Administration.

- There are more than 350 biotech drug products and vaccines currently in clinical trials targeting more than 200 diseases, including cancers, Alzheimer's disease, heart disease, diabetes, and arthritis.

- Biotechnology has produced hundreds of medical diagnostic tests that have advanced the accuracy of predicting diseases.

- The biotechnology industry has more than doubled in size since 1993, with revenues increasing from $8 billion in 1993 to $22.3 billion in 2000.

The future prospects for the quality and quantity of the human life span are bright. Biotechnology generates a cascade of benefits that improve the human condition. The A4M envisions a future in which the worldwide population is free of the diseases that presently ravage old age. This may be achieved as scientists continue to make discoveries in biotechnology and apply them to preventive healthcare.

THE TOP FIVE BIOTECHNOLOGIES LEADING TO PRACTICAL IMMORTALITY

Clearly, we are experiencing the dawning of an exciting new era in medicine, one which will result with longevity intervention orders of magnitude greater than any other advancements made in medicine to-date. Advancement in these five key biotechnologies will undoubtedly impart a vast wealth of knowledge about the most basic cellular mechanisms of aging and sickness, and such discoveries, taken collectively, are the single most important contribution which will enable mankind to overcome its oldest, most debilitating, and most elusive disease—old age. As a result of the quantum leaps in biotechnology, it is within reason to expect that Practical Immortality—human life spans of 120+ years—may well be achieved by the year 2029.

1. Stem Cells

Generally speaking, stem cells are self-renewing primitive cells that can develop into functional, differentiated cells. They have the unique ability to be manipulated by genetic engineering to give rise to specific cell types.

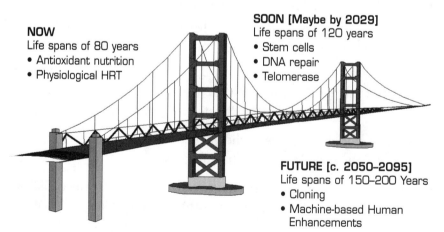

Practical immortality may be achieved if we employ anti-aging therapeutics as the bridge between now and the immediate future.

With regard to human immortality, the focus is on human pluripotent stem cells (hPSCs), which are unique because they can develop into all cells and tissues in the body. "Pluripotent" is a term that means the cells have the capacity to form into the three types of cellular layers: gut epithelium (endoderm); cartilage, bone, and smooth and striated muscle (mesoderm); and neural epithelium, embryonic ganglia, and stratified squamous epithelium (ectoderm). There are two types of hPSCs: human embryonic stem (hES) cells, which are derived from donated *in vitro* fertilized blastocysts (very early stage embryos); and human embryonic germ (hEG) cells, which are derived from donated fetal material.

The pluripotency of human stem cells creates the vast potential for humans to grow cells, tissues, and even organs—in a controlled laboratory setting, for use in applications from acute emergency care to treatment of chronic, debilitating disease. The culmination of stem cell research is to achieve a plentiful source of human cells for transplantation.

2. Cloning

The process of making genetically identical copies became science-fact when in early 1997, Dr. Ian Wilmut and his colleagues at the Roslin Institute unveiled Dolly the sheep. Dolly demonstrated that the nucleus of an adult cell could be successfully transferred to an enucleated egg to create cloned offspring. The birth of Dolly was significant because it demonstrated the ability of egg cytoplasm (the portion of the cell outside of the nucleus) to "reprogram" an adult nucleus. Reprogramming enables the differentiated cell nucleus to express all the genes required for full embryonic development of the adult animal. When cells differentiate—develop from embryonic cells to produce functionally defined adult cells—they lose the ability to express many genes; instead, they express only those genes specific for the cell's differentiated function.

Following Dolly's creation, cloning has been used to replicate mice, goats, and cattle from donor cells obtained from adult mice, goats, and cattle, respectively. These examples of cloning normal animals from fully differentiated adult cells demonstrate the universality of nuclear reprogramming. Using nuclear transfer, multiple identical copies of animals can be produced that express only the genetic traits of the animal whose cells were used as the nuclear donors. While the frequency of success is currently low, it is expected to improve as the fundamental mechanisms of nuclear reprogramming by egg cell cytoplasm become better understood.

The current scientific focus of cloning experts is to successfully confer the reprogramming capability normally found in the egg cell cytoplasm to the cytoplasm of a somatic cell in order to eliminate reliance on harvested eggs. In this way, experts expect that transplantable genetically matched cells could be derived from pluripotent stem cells generated through nuclear transfer using adult cells taken from the intended transplant recipient. Such cells would not trigger immune rejection because they would exactly match the tissue antigens of the transplant recipient. This technology is expected to produce genetically matched cells for use in repairing organs damaged by degenerative disease. Gene engineering and nuclear transfer techniques could be used to produce cloned animals with uniform genetic traits to produce consistent organs, tissues, and proteins for biomedical use in humans.

3. Nanotechnology

Employing nanodevices—high-tech, miniaturized devices on the scale of billionths of a meter, nanomedicine manipulates human biology at its most basic levels. These tiny tools enable scientists to play on the size scale of biology itself, just as a mechanic works on a car's engine using tools that are on the same scale as the engine.

Nanotechniques may be our best armament in treating—and even curing—stubborn diseases such as cancer and diabetes. Researchers have now designed clever ways to power nanomachines with biologically based components. Nanomotors, as well as nanotweezers—the mechanical and energy aspects of which are completely built from DNA—are revolutionary innovations that will enable scientists to unleash microscopic robots within the human body on missions to correct the ravages of age.

4. Artificial Organs

The medical makeover is just a few years away. Forget the tummy tuck; we're talking about checking in to a clinic near you and checking out with new body parts. Advanced prototypes of nearly every single body part already exist in research laboratories. Not farfetched, tomorrow's body part shop is an extension of work that began in the mid-twentieth century. Dr. Willem Kolff, inventor of the kidney dialysis machine, emigrated to the United States from the Netherlands, in the mid-1950s, and became known as the "father of artificial organs" after he developed the artificial heart at the Cleveland Clinic, and created the nation's first artificial organ research program at the University of Utah in the 1960s.

Research teams from around the world are working on projects to produce mechanical body parts that would vanquish many diseases and disabilities with which thousands of people struggle. Replacement parts for worn out or damaged human organs, along with applications of genetic engineering and stem cell research, hold great promise both today and in the not-so-distant future for extending the healthy human life span.

5. Nerve-Impulse Continuity

Today, both the young and old can succumb to serious medical conditions that are caused by the brain's failing to communicate properly with the rest of the body. The majority of these cases are due to spinal cord injury (SCI), which occurs when a traumatic event results in damage to cells within the spinal cord or severs the nerve tracts that relay signals up and down the spinal cord, usually leaving the patient with limited, if any, movement of the body and limbs. In addition, some individuals suffer from damaged brain circuitry, causing them to have cognitive problems, most notably memory difficulties.

In the not-so-distant future, machine enhancements in the form of various types of implants may help these individuals to regain nerve-impulse continuity.

With regard to SCI, in January 2002, researchers at Good Samaritan Regional Medical Center (Phoenix, AZ USA) report that, after implanting a quadriplegic with an electronic stimulator for the spinal cord, combined with four months of treadmill therapy, the patient regained impressive walking ability. At Brown University, in March 2002, it was reported that scientists were developing a neural prostheses that aims to give paralyzed patients control over computers that would then enable commands to be given to the paralyzed parts of their bodies. Additionally, in May 2002, scientists at State University of New York (USA) demonstrated the ability to control the movements of a live rat by using a laptop computer, a radio, and brain implants. The team was able to guide five equipped rats through a complex maze, stimulating electrodes with impulses that functioned as navigational cues.

Repair of damaged brain circuitry is also a key research focus in public, private, and university settings. In the fall of 2003, researchers from University of Southern California hope to demonstrate that they can restore the signals responsible for memory in humans. Their current tests, being conducted in a rat model, suggest that their prototype memory-restoring chip will mimic the processing duties of thousands of neurons, serving to complete an otherwise damaged circuit.

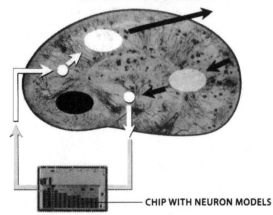

HEALTHY HIPPOCAMPUS

Signals out

CA1

Signals in

DG

CA3

DAMAGED HIPPOCAMPUS

CHIP WITH NEURON MODELS

When the hippocampus area of the brain is damaged, memory loss occurs. The University of Southern California hopes to implant a chip into the hippocampus of a human brain to restore memory.

TOWARD AUGMENTATIVE MEDICINE

To summarize the important potential biotechnological advancements in medicine, we cite the speculations produced in a study of the next fifty years of cardiology, released by the American College of Cardiology at its annual meeting of 2000. Their prediction:

It is the year 2024. You are 75 years old, and you discover that a man next to you on an airplane has a pig heart, and his arteries are swarming with "smart dust" that sends continuous reports on his condition to his doctor's computer. That's not so strange, because you have a pig heart, too. And by 2049, when you are 100, many of your organs will be replaced. Plus you'll feel better than you did at 50 because "nanolabs" in your blood can manufacture and supply drugs whenever they are needed.

Collectively, these five biotechnologies also pave the way for human enhancement/augmentation—whereby healthy men and women enhance mental and/or physical performance. By doing so, our capacity for preserving and enhancing our minds and bodies is seemingly limitless.

Returning full-circle to Chapter 1 of this book, when we first introduced you to the anti-aging phenomenon and how Dr. Marvin Minsky sparked more than 1,000 scientists and academicians to strive to live to a ripe young age of 150 years, Dr. Minsky separately commented that:

> Everyone wants wisdom and wealth. Nevertheless, our health often gives out before we achieve them. To lengthen our lives, and improve our minds, in the future . . . we must imagine ways in which future replacements for worn body parts might solve most problems of failing health. We must then invent strategies to augment our brains and gain greater wisdom. Eventually we will entirely replace our brains—using nanotechnology. Once delivered from the limitations of biology, we will be able to decide the length of our lives—with the option of immortality—and choose among other, unimagined capabilities as well.

According to a report jointly issued by the US Commerce Department and the National Science Foundation, America's leading researchers are already designing and perfecting technological advancements to boost peak mental and physical performance, such as:

- brain-computer assisted interfaces to allow individuals to control artificial or paralyzed limbs simply by thinking about moving them

- for healthy men and women, enhanced coordination and reflexes to attain physical edge and increase cognitive acuity

- a digital cerebral interface for augmented reality

The U.S. Commerce Department-National Science Foundation concludes their report that "new paradigms in communication (brain-to-brain, brain-machine-brain) could become reality in 10–20 years."

The value of biotechnology and its application to human health and longevity is best stated by the Board of Editors of *Scientific American*. In the magazine's March 2001 issue, the editors remark that "Thanks to modern technology and medicine, people have taken much more control over their differential survival. . . . ills are not the barriers they once were. Our technology may exert the greatest influence."

INTERNET RESOURCES

www.worldhealth.net The World Health Network, to keep updated on the latest advancements that can help you lead a productive, vital, healthy life. Sign up for the free Biotech E-Newsletter, featuring longevity news you can use.

www.worldhealthnet.tv View videos of the world's top doctors and longevity experts as they share their secrets for your maximum lifespan

www.mylonglife.com Take the state-of-the-art Cyber Longevity Test to see how many more years you can live.

CHAPTER 24

The Longevity Test

People age *biologically* and *chronologically*. Chronological age measures the amount of time that has gone by since birth. Most of us can distinguish an elderly person from a young person. We can even categorize what age range a person might fall into. But what about a person who is sixty-five but looks as if he's only forty-five? Or a person who is eighty but functions as well as a sixty year old?

This is biological age or *functional* age. We all age biologically at different rates.

As we have seen throughout this book, age changes affect different parts of our bodies at different times. These age changes occur in the DNA, tissues, organs, and hormone levels, as well as in every component of the human body. This variance in our biological "clock" can help explain why one eighty-year-old may be able to work during the day, go bicycling in the afternoons, and garden on the weekends, exerting more youthful qualities than another eighty-year-old who may, biologically, be eighty or even ninety years old.

A comprehensive battery of metabolic tests and complex laboratory analyses is necessary to accurately determine your individual biological age, a procedure that is beyond the scope of this book. However, this procedure is available at most anti-aging diagnostic and treatment centers listed in the Appendix of this book. Established anti-aging centers perform extensive measurements of individual biomarkers that establish aging rates for each organ system through molecular and DNA analysis.

The purpose of this chapter is to emphasize how extremely useful and important it is to recognize some of the basic markers and risk factors for premature aging. Through the test presented in this chapter, you will be able to detect what changes you need to make for longevity—the period of time we can expect to live, given the best of circumstances.

BUILDING ON YOUR NEW KNOWLEDGE

Average life expectancy in the world's advanced countries is rapidly approaching eighty years (eighty-five if you are a woman recently born in Japan). A recent issue of *Science* magazine reported that, with the currently expanding life spans of modern man, all it would take for the average life span to reach approximately ninety-nine years is the elimination of heart disease, cancer, and diabetes.

We now know what causes the majority of age-related disease. We know what mechanisms lead to almost all cases of atherosclerotic heart disease, and how to prevent it. For those with heart disease too advanced to treat by diet and lifestyle adjustment, modern methods of heart bypass, laser-created collateral blood flow, coronary sinuses, balloon angioplasty, artificial hearts and other highly developed techniques now offer a second chance for life and a healthy heart.

Cancer is slowly yielding to modern medical innovation. Ninety percent or more of all cancers are fully curable (not just five-year survival rates, but a total cure) if detected at stage I—usually the size of a pea or smaller. Even better, new analysis of cancer etiology shows that 80 percent of all cancers are environmental in origin. Therefore, your chances of cancer are only one in five if you don't smoke, avoid cancer promoters in food (nitrosamines and fats), and limit exposure to radiation and other environmental toxins. As you learned in previous chapters, your chances for avoiding cancer also greatly improve by supplementing your diet with antioxidants and DNA-repairing nutrients.

Diabetes, especially adult-onset diabetes, is also coming under control thanks to improved methods of early detection and endocrine stabilization and repair. Artificial pancreas and islet cell implants have already cured dozens of people with severe insulin-dependent diabetes. In fact, new glucose control medications should soon eliminate this disease as a major overall risk factor.

Is the possibility of a 120-year life span far behind? The new reality for those age thirty-five and younger is a healthy life span of 120 and beyond (assuming current advances in biotechnology, genetic engineering and medicine continue at their present rate). And 100 years is an expected average lifespan for those fifty-five and younger. For those over fifty-five, researchers are cautiously only predicting an eighty-five-year advanced life span (average life span is interpreted as meaning that 50 percent will die before the specified age and the other half will live beyond that age).

Therefore, it is not unreasonable—and history may ultimately prove us somewhat conservative in our projections—for those who live the healthiest of lives and lifestyles to score a potential maximum expected life span of 150 on this test. We recommend taking the entire test now, then taking it again in three months, when you've had a chance to integrate some of the suggestions in this book into your own anti-aging program. You can continue retaking the test every three months, as an incentive to keep yourself on the path to longevity and to see what changes you've made overall.

TAKING THE TEST

Allow yourself from thirty minutes to an hour to take this test. Don't mull over each question, but don't rush through anything either. Be completely honest. This is a self-test for you to learn which of your habits work toward your longevity and which do not.

The Longevity Test is an educational experience, not cold, hard, objective, scientific analysis. Regardless of what you score, chances are you can do better with simple modifications to your diet, lifestyle, environment, and mental attitude. The rewards are very significant in terms of a longer, healthier, happier, and more vibrant life. Remember, it's never too early or too late to stop the clock on the aging process.

TEST TIP: If you aren't sure about an answer or just don't know, the answer most likely is "no."

THE LONGEVITY TEST

Gender:	Male		−5
	Female	+6	
Age:	0–29	+10	
	30–54	+5	
	55–64	+1	
	65 or older		−10
Heredity:	Any grandparent lived to be over 80 (limit 4)	+1	
	Average age all four grandparents lived to:		
	60–70	+3	
	71–80	+4	
	Over 80	+6	
Family history:			
	Either parent had stroke or heart attack		
	before age 50		−10
	−2 for a family member (grandparent, parent, sibling)		
	who prior to age 65 has had any of the following:		
	Hypertension	−___	
	Cancer	−___	
	Heart disease	−___	
	Stroke	−___	
	Diabetes	−___	
	Other genetic diseases	−___	
SUBTOTAL A:		___ + ___ = ___	

Family income:

0–$9,000		–10
$10,000–$18,000		–5
$19,000–$30,000	+1	
+1 for each additional $20,000, up to $200,000	+____	

Education:

Some high school (or less)		–7
High school graduate	+2	
College graduate	+4	
Postgraduate or professional degree	+6	

Others would best describe your general mood/ temperament as follows:

Calm yet alert	+3	
Laid-back and passive		–3
Angry and easily perturbed or annoyed		–10

Occupation (Choose one):

Professional	+3	
Self-employed	+3	
In healthcare field	+2	
Over 65 and working	+3	
Clerical or support		–1
Shift work		–2
Unemployed		–3
Probability of career advancement	+1	
Regularly in direct contact with pollutants, toxic waste, chemicals, radiation, or carry a firearm to work.		–10

Where you live:

Large, congested urban industrial center		–4
Rural or farm area	+2	
Area with air-pollution alerts		–5
High-crime area		–3
Little or no crime area	+2	
Home has tested positive for radon		–2
Total commuting time to and from work:		
0–½ hour	+1	
½ hour–1 hour	0	
–1 for each ½ hour over 1 hour		–____
Within 30 miles of major medical/trauma center	+1	
No major medical/trauma center in area		–1

SUBTOTAL B: ____ + ____ = ____

Health Status Present overall physical health:

Excellent—almost never ill, feel great most of the time	+6
Good—sick 10 days or less/year, feel good most of the time	+4
Fair—sick 11 days or more/year, feel okay but low energy	–2
Poor—sick 20 days or more/year, feel average to low energy	–10

What is your blood pressure (if measured within the last year):	
Normal: below 140/90 mmHg	+3
Borderline: between 140/90 and 160/95	–5
High: Top (systolic) reading was above 160 and/or bottom (diastolic) reading was above 95	–10
Don't know	–5

Low cholesterol (under 200)	+5
Moderate cholesterol (200–240)	–2
High cholesterol (over 240)	–10
Don't know	–5
HDL cholesterol 29 or less	–10
HDL cholesterol 30–45	0
HDL cholesterol over 45	+8
Don't know	–5

Do you or close family member have diabetes?	
Yes	–4
No	0

Have comprehensive medical insurance coverage	+2
Able to use physicians of your choice	+2
Insurance limits your physician choices	–5
Have no insurance	–7

Tobacco (1 pipe = 2 cigarettes / 1 cigar = 3 cigarettes):

Never smoked	+7
Quit smoking	+3
Smoke up to one pack per day	–7
Smoke one to two packs per day	–10
Over two packs per day	–20
Pack-years smoked (number of packs smoked per day, times number of years smoked):	
7–15	–5
16–25	–10
Over 25	–20

Alcohol (Daily consumption of 1 beer or 1 glass of wine = 1.25 oz. alcohol)

No alcohol consumption	0	
1.25 oz. per day or less	+6	
Between 1.25 and 2.5 oz. per day		–4
–1 more for each additional 1.25 oz. per day		–___

Exercise (20 minutes or more moderate aerobic exercise)

5 or more/week	+10	
4 times per week	+6	
3 times per week	+3	
2 times per week	+1	
No regular aerobic activity		–10

How many flights of stairs (of about 12 steps)
do you climb each day?

1–5	0	
6–10	+1	
More than 10	+2	

Work requires regular physical exertion

or at least two miles walking per day	+3	
+1 more for each additional mile walked per day	+___	
Sedentary work/not much walking or stair climbing		–6

After taking a brisk walk or a slow jog, do you feel any of these
symptoms: racing heart, irregular heartbeat or chest pain?

Yes*		–15
No	0	

__Note:__ See your doctor before continuing any exercise program.

Need more than two pillows to sleep comfortably because of discomfort or breathing while lying on back		–12

Weight:

Maintain ideal weight for height	+5	
5–10 lbs. over ideal		–6
11–20 lbs. over ideal		–10
21–30 lbs. over ideal		–22
–1 more for each additional 10 lbs.		–___

Underweight

5–10 lbs.	+5	
11–20 lbs.		–15

Determine your waist-to-hip ratio as follows:
Measure your waist (W) and hip (H) in inches.
Divide your W measure by your H measure. W/H = ratio

Women:

Your ratio is 0.80 or greater		–5
Your ratio is 0.79 or less	+3	

Men:

Your ratio is 0.96 or greater		–12
Your ratio is 0.95 or less	+2	

Nutrition:

Eat a well-balanced diet	+3	
Don't eat a well-balanced diet		–3
Regularly eat meals at consistent times	+2	
Don't regularly eat meals at consistent times		–2
Snack or eat meals late at night		–2
Eat a balanced breakfast	+2	
Eat fish or poultry as primary protein source (almost replacing red meat, once/week or less)	+5	
Eat at least 5 servings of green leafy vegetables/week	+3	
Eat at least 5 servings of fresh fruit or juice a day		
Yes	+2	
No		–1
Try to avoid fats	+2	
Don't try to avoid fats	–5	
Fifty percent of meals consist of fried take-out foods, prepackaged or precooked foods		–8
Eat some food every day that is high in fiber (whole-grain bread, fresh fruits and vegetables)	+2	
Do not eat some food every day that is high in fiber		–3
Take a daily multivitamin or mineral supplement that includes at least the following: Vitamin A/beta-carotene (5,000 IU), Vitamin E (400 IU), Vitamin B-complex (50 IU), Zinc (30 mg), Selenium (100 mcg), and Vitamin C (500 mg)		
Yes	+10	
No		–10
Women:		
Take calcium supplement	+3	
Do you get colds or other infections more than once every eight weeks?		
Yes		–6
No	0	
Does it take a long time to get over a bad infection? (For example, do your colds typically last longer than two weeks?)		
Yes		–6
No	0	
Do you need antibiotics three times/year or more?		
Yes		–8
No	0	

Are your lymph nodes often enlarged?

Yes		–4
No	0	

Regularly use sunscreen and avoid excessive sun	+2	
Subscribe to health-related periodicals	+2	
Actively involved in a life-extension, prevention or comprehensive wellness program	+5	

SUBTOTAL C: ____ + ____ = ____

Accident control:

Always wear a seatbelt as driver and passenger	+6	
Don't always wear a seat belt as driver and passenger		–6
Never drink and drive or ride with a driver who has been drinking	+2	

–10 for each arrest for drinking while under the influence of alcohol in the past 5 years   –____

–2 for every speeding ticket or accident in the past year   –____

–1 for each 10,000 miles per year driven over 10,000		–____
Primary car weighs over 3,500 lbs.	+10	
Subcompact		–5
Motorcycle		–10

–2 for every fight or attack you were involved in, or witness to, in the past 3 years.   –____

Smoke alarms in home   +1

Preventive and therapeutic measures:

Comprehensive physical exams and blood tests
(every 3 to 4 years before 50,
or every 1 or 2 years over 50)   +3

Women:

Yearly gynecological exam and Pap smear	+2	
Monthly breast self-exam	+2	
Mammogram (35–50, every 3 years; over 50, every year)	+2	
What is your menstrual status?		
Still menstruating	+3	
Went through natural menopause at 41 or older	+1	
Went through natural menopause at 40 or younger		–5
Underwent total hysterectomy before 41		–8
Underwent total hysterectomy at age 41 or older		–4
Postmenopausal and take oral estrogen supplements	+5	

Men:

Genital self-exam every 3 months	+1	
Rectal or prostate exam (yearly after age 30)	+2	

All:

Rectal exam and tested for hidden blood in stool (over 40, every two years; over 50, every year)	+2	
No rectal exam and test by age 50		–4
Well-formed bowel movements 1 or 2 times per day without difficulty	+3	
Constipation and bowel movement less than once per day		–10
Irritable bowel disorder or other problems with elimination	–7	

If over 50:

Sigmoidoscopy of the lower bowel every 3 years	+2	
Have a suspicious skin lesion that hasn't healed in six weeks or that keeps growing		–10

SUBTOTAL D: ____ + ____ = ____

Changeable Psychosocial Factors

Married or in long-term committed relationship	+10	
Not in any long-term relationship		–6
Satisfying sex life twice/week or more	+4	
Unsatisfying sex life		–10
Children under 18 living at home	+2	
–1 for each 5-year period living alone		–____
No close friends		–10
+1 for each close friend (up to 3)	+____	
Active membership in a religious community or volunteer organization	+2	
Have a pet	+2	
Regular daily routine (an orderly day, for example, wake up at 7:00, breakfast at 7:30, work by 8:00, etc.)	+3	
No regular daily routine		–10
Hours of uninterrupted sleep/night:		
Fewer than 5		–5
5–8	+5	
8–10	–7	
No consistent sleep time		–5
Regular work routine	+3	
No regular work routine		–5
–2 for every for every 5 hours worked over 40 in a week		–____
Take a yearly vacation from work (at least 6 days)	+5	
No yearly vacation in past two years (at least 6 days)		–5
Regularly use a stress management technique (yoga, meditation, music, etc.)	+3	
No stress management program		–4

SUBTOTAL E: ____ + ____ = ____

Changeable Emotional Stress Factors

N = Never   **R** = Rarely   **S** = Sometimes   **A** = Always (or as much as possible)

	N	R	S	A
Generally happy	−2	−1	+1	+2
Have and enjoy time with family and friends	−2	−1	+1	+2
Feel in control of personal life and career	−2	−1	+1	+2
Live within financial means	−2	−1	+1	+2
Set goals and look for new challenges	−2	−1	+1	+2
Participate in creative outlet or hobby	−2	−1	+1	+2
Have and enjoy leisure time	−2	−1	+1	+2
Express feelings easily	−2	−1	+1	+2
Laugh easily	−2	−1	+1	+2
Expect good things to happen	−2	−2	+1	+2
Anger easily	+2	+1	−1	−2
Critical of self	+2	+1	−1	−2
Critical of others	+2	+1	−1	−2
Lonely, even with others	+2	+1	−1	−2
Worry about things out of your control	+2	+1	−1	−2
Regret sacrifices made in life	+2	+1	−1	−2

SUBTOTAL F: _____

SUBTOTALS A–F: **A** _____

         + B _____

         + C _____

         + D _____

         + E _____

         + F _____

GRAND TOTAL = _____ x 0.333 = **SCORE:** _____

Scoring

After you've added all of the subtotals together, divide the grand total by 3 or multiply by 0.333. This is your *score*.

Follow the chart for the next step:

If age:					
(1–30)	Age + 30	+	(score x 2.0)	=	_____
(31–46)	Age + 20	+	(score x 1.5)	=	_____
(47–61)	Age + 10	+	(score x 1.2)	=	_____
(62–73)	Age + 5	+	(score x 1.0)	=	_____
(74–82)	Age + 3	+	(score x .50)	=	_____
(83+)	Age + 1	+	(score x .20)	=	_____

This final number is your potential estimated life span.

How did you do? Did you learn something about factors in your life that might be making you "old before your time" or that are sapping your youthful energy, health, and vigor?

Remember, there are no "right" or "wrong" answers to these questions. We're not suggesting that you move to the country or give up your high-powered job. And a life without at least some of the "life-stress" elements we listed would be an empty life indeed. The point is not to judge yourself, but rather to become aware of the things that may be placing a strain on your system. Then you can choose which risk factors or stressors are worth keeping and which need to be corrected.

We now know a great deal about the physical and emotional conditions for staying healthy and vigorous well into a lengthy old age and we hope you have gained a greater appreciation of how your life span can be significantly extended through the application of the therapeutics discussed in this book. Of course, not all the factors determining your biological age, your health, and your life span are within your control. But of those that are, you now have the knowledge you need to make the choices that are right for you.

THE CYBER LONGEVITY TEST

Take the state-of-the-art Cyber Longevity Test to see how many more years you can live: **www.mylonglife.com**

SECTION SIX

Endnotes

The only thing about the future
is that it will surprise even those
who have seen furthest into it.

—E. J. HOBSBAWM (1917–   )

Glossary

acidophilus (*Lactobacillus acidophilus*). Bacterium, part of the normal bacterial flora that help the absorption of food; enhances the immune system.

acromegaly. Disorder characterized by progressive enlargement of peripheral parts of the body, especially the head, face, hands, and feet, due to excessive circulating blood levels of human growth hormone.

adrenaline. Also known as epinephrine, a "fight or flight" hormone released in times of physical stress to increase heart rate and contraction; causes vasodilation (blood vessel widening) and other transient metabolic changes.

amino acid. One of twenty-two known organic acids that serve as building blocks for protein production. The body can make eleven of them; these are called *nonessential amino acids*. The remaining amino acids are called *essential amino acids* because they must come from the diet.

anabolism. Manufacture of complex chemical compounds from smaller simpler compounds (for example, proteins from amino acids), usually with the use of energy.

andropause. Male version of menopause; gradual decline in testicular function and testosterone production.

anthropometric characteristics. Body composition.

antibody. Protein created by the immune system, in response to the presence of a foreign organism or toxin, that is capable of destroying or neutralizing the invader.

antioxidant. Substance that prevents cellular damage due to oxidation; exposure to unstable molecules called free radicals.

arginine. Nonessential amino acid that can stimulate the release of growth hormone; may be an effective immune enhancer; may have benefit in nutritional treatment of male infertility.

arteriosclerosis. Hardening of the arteries, a condition in which the walls of the arteries become stiff and thick impairing circulation.

ascorbic acid (vitamin C). Potent water-soluble antioxidant that appears to be effective in preventing diseases caused by cellular damage from free radicals, for example, heart disease, cancer, and cataracts; may be an important factor in strengthening and maintaining the immune system.

aspirin (salicylic acid). Functions as an anticlotting agent; may help to prevent heart disease, stroke, and certain forms of cancer when taken in small doses.

astragalus. Chinese herb that enhances the immune system; can lower blood pressure and may help prevent heart attack.

atherosclerosis. Type of arteriosclerosis caused by deposits of fatty plaques on the inner lining of the arteries.

basal metabolic rates (BMR). Rate at which cells convert food to energy.

basophils. Type of white blood cell that consumes bacteria, foreign particles, and other cells.

beta-carotene. Vitamin A precursor, an antioxidant that functions in neutralizing free radicals; may help prevent cervical cancer and atherosclerosis; is an immune-system booster; appears to protect against respiratory diseases and environmental pollutants.

betaine. Helps digest fatty acids and is used in the production of RNA and DNA.

bilberry. Herb that may improve vision, particularly night vision; may aid in the prevention of vascular disease.

bioavailability. Quantity of a substance that is active and ready for utilization by the body.

bioflavonoid. Potent group antioxidant compounds found in most fruits and vegetables, usually next to the peel, that have anti-inflammatory and antiviral effects; are used to treat allergies and asthma; may be effective against heart disease and cancer.

black currant oil. High in gamma-linolenic acid, an essential fatty acid; involved in the synthesis of prostaglandin type 3; may protect against cancer and heart disease.

blue-green algae. Single-cell aquatic plants that contain trace minerals; may have neurostimulatory effects.

body fat. Where fat is stored in the body.

borage oil. Contains a linoleic acid that reduces the risk of atherosclerotic heart disease.

boron. Trace mineral that aids in the synthesis of steroids, particularly estrogens and testosterone; may help prevent osteoporosis and maintain strong bones; may help prevent memory loss.

bromelain. Enzyme found in fresh pineapple that helps break down protein; has anti-inflammatory and antiallergenic properties.

calcium. Mineral that has beneficial effects on bone and tooth maintenance; may protect against colorectal cancer and high blood pressure. Note: vitamin D helps facilitate calcium absorption.

carbohydrates. Organic compound composed of carbon, hydrogen, and oxygen that serves as the body's major source of energy.

carnitine. Amino acid that is a cofactor in mitochondrial energy production by transporting activated fatty acids across the mitochondrial membrane in cardiac and skeletal muscles; has a beneficial effect on the heart and muscles; improves stamina and endurance during exercise; may be effective in slowing down the progression of Alzheimer's disease; may help burn fat.

catabolism. Breakdown of complex chemical compounds into simpler ones (such as sugars to CO_2 and H_2O), often accompanied by the liberation of energy.

cayenne pepper (capsaicin). Compound that prevents oxidation of low-density lipoprotein cholesterol; may help prevent cardiovascular disease; aids in digestion by stimulating the production of saliva and gastric acid; stimulates the release of endorphins (mood enhancers).

centenarian. Person 100 years of age and older.

chelation. Type of treatment in which a chemical agent (usually ethylenediaminetetraacetic acid, or EDTA) is injected into the bloodstream where it binds to toxic minerals and metals, allowing the body to excrete them in the urine.

chlorophyll. Plant compound that appears to stimulate nucleic acid (DNA and RNA) production; has well-documented detoxification and antibiotic actions; may help in the production of hemoglobin.

cholesterol. An important constituent in cell walls and a precursor of certain hormones that also aids in the transport of fatty acids from the body.

choline. Member of the vitamin B complex family essential for neurotransmitter production; aids in maintaining cell membranes; may slow down memory loss and help learning ability.

chromium picolinate. Trace mineral that protects the pancreas; a necessary cofactor with insulin to assist in the break down of sugar and metabolism of fat; may help in increasing muscle mass; helps prevent heart disease and diabetes.

clinical trial. Study in which human subjects receive treatment.

chronic. Description of the extent of time during which a condition takes place. The U.S. National Center for Health Statistics defines a chronic condition as one of three months' duration or longer.

cinnamon. Herb that neutralizes acidity and helps regulate blood sugar.

cobalamin (vitamin B$_{12}$). Aids in the production of red blood cells, essential for the normal functioning of the nervous system; aids in the metabolism of protein and fat.

coenzyme Q$_{10}$ (ubiquinone). Cellular lipid that is effective at the mitochondrial level with the production of energy; helps prevent free-radical formation by inhibiting lipid peroxidation; increases stamina and may reduce heart disease.

controlled trial. Study in which at least two groups are compared.

cortisol. Hormone secreted by the adrenal gland in reaction to stress.

crossover trial. Study in which each patient receives both the treatment and the placebo (an inactive pill or procedure).

cyanocobalamin (vitamin B$_{12}$). Helps maintain a healthy nervous system and prevents anemia.

cysteine. Protects against various toxins and pollutants.

cytokine. Chemical messenger that activates immune cells.

degradation. Change of a chemical compound into a less complex compound.

deprenyl. Pharmaceutical approved for use in Parkinson's disease; acts as a neuroprotective agent and enhances mental function, mood, and libido; has been reported in animal studies to extend both length and quality of life.

DHEA (dehydroepiandrosterone). Hormone produced by the adrenal glands, which the body converts into other hormones; appears to aid in the regulation and production of steroidal hormones; appears to help in reducing cholesterol levels and body fats; seems to be involved in increasing muscle mass.

diabetes (adult-onset diabetes/type II). Disorder that most often occurs in overweight people, age forty or older, which is characterized by insufficient or defective production of insulin, a hormone produced by the pancreas that plays an essential role in the metabolism of carbohydrates.

diuretic. Herb or drug that cause kidneys to produce more urine.

dong quai. Anti-aging herb particularly effective in women; presumed to assist in the regulation of female steroidal hormones; may aid in the regulation of blood glucose levels; may aid in lowering blood pressure in men and women.

dopamine. Neurotransmitter (chemical that transmits nerve signals) critical in central nervous system activity.

double-blind study. Study in which neither the researchers nor the subjects know whether they are receiving the active treatment or placebo.

dysmotility. Inability of, or difficulty in, movement.

echinacea. Herb that may stimulate the production of white blood cells; may enhance the immune system; appears to have antiviral and antifungal properties.

epidemiology. Study of patterns of disease in large populations and the factors that influence those patterns.

epinephrine. Also known as adrenaline, a "fight or flight" hormone released in times of physical stress to increase heart rate and contraction; causes vasodilation (blood vessel widening) and other transient metabolic changes.

fat. Also known as adipose tissue, connective tissue consisting chiefly of fat cells and supporting fibers, arranged in lobe-type groupings along or near a blood vessel.

fatty acid synthesis. Chemical process by which acids are manufactured from fats by the process of hydrolysis (breakdown of a complex compound into simpler compounds with uptake of water molecule).

fenugreek. Herb that has been used to treat impotence in men; may aid in regulating estrogens and progesterone levels particularly during menopause; helps expel excess mucus from the respiratory and digestive systems; may help control blood sugar levels. *Caution:* Do not use during pregnancy.

feverfew. Herb possessing anti-inflammatory properties.

flavonoids. *See* bioflavonoids.

flax oil. High in alpha-linolenic acid, protective against heart disease; contains twenty-seven anticancer compounds that may help lower the risk of breast and colon cancer.

folic acid. B vitamin that assists in the formation of red blood cells and in nucleic acids (RNA and DNA); may help prevent heart disease by controlling levels of homocysteine; may help prevent colon, rectal, and cervical cancer.

fo-ti (ho shou wu). Longevity herb used in China to help maintain hair color; may help protect against heart attack by lowering blood cholesterol levels and improving blood flow to the heart.

free radical. A molecule that has at least one unpaired electron, making it highly unstable and easily able to attack cells and cause damage to the body at the cellular level.

gamma-linolenic acid (GLA). Omega-6 fatty acid extracted from the seeds of evening primrose or borage plants; may help prevent cardiovascular disease by lowering cholesterol levels and inhibiting blood clot formation; may help provide relief for rheumatoid arthritis through its anti-inflammatory properties.

garlic (odorless). Has a high concentration of allium (a sulfur-containing compound), selenium, and germanium; possesses broad-spectrum antimicrobial properties; appears to reduce total cholesterol and low-density lipoproteins; due to its ability to increase natural killer cell activity, appears to be an immune stimulator and to have anticancer properties.

genistein. Isoflavone in soy and soy-based products; appears to inhibit the growth of new blood vessels and may indirectly prevent tumor growth; may aid in the prevention of heart disease.

gerontology. Study of aging.

GH3/procaine. Analog of procaine amine; was popularized by Dr. Ana Aslan of Romania in the 1940s; believed to have diverse anti-aging effects on the cardiovascular system, the nervous system, and the skin.

ginger. Spice/herb containing high amounts of geraniol, which may be a potent cancer fighter; may act as an immune stimulant by helping to lower cholesterol; may prevent cardiovascular disease by inhibiting platelet aggregation; has anti-inflammatory activity.

ginkgo biloba. Herb rich in antioxidants; appears to increase the level of dopamine, producing an increase in memory retention and mental alertness; may improve circulation by inhibiting plaque deposition in arteries; appears to inhibit coagulation in blood vessels.

ginseng. Herb that may help improve mental performance; contains antioxidants that prevent cellular damage due to free radicals; may inhibit the growth of cancer cells; increases and enhances energy; appears to help the body cope with stress by normalizing body functions.

glucose. Simple sugar that is the principal source of energy for the body's cells.

glucose tolerance factor (GTF). Water-soluble complex containing chromium needed for normal glucose tolerance.

glutamine. Nonessential amino acid useful for intestinal problems.

glutathione. Body's most abundant antioxidant enzyme; appears to aid in the functioning of the immune system; appears to have anti-inflammatory properties that may be effective as treatment for allergies and arthritis.

glycogen. Complex carbohydrate that is the primary form in which glucose is stored in the body. It is converted back into glucose as needed to supply energy.

glycosylation. Formation of linkages with glycosyl groups, as between D-glucose and the hemoglobin chain to form the fraction hemoglobin A1c, whose level rises in association with the raised blood D-glucose concentration in poorly controlled or uncontrolled diabetes mellitus.

goldenseal. Herb, antifungal and antibacterial agent, effective in urinary infections.

gonadotrophin. Hormone promoting gonadal growth and function.

gotu kola (centella). Herb with antifatigue properties; stimulates memory; strengthens and tones blood vessels and may help prevent circulatory problems.

grape seed extract. Contains proanthocyanidins, unique bioflavonoids that work together with ascorbic acid; potent antioxidant and free-radical scavenger; contains bioflavonoids that may inhibit the release of enzymes that promote inflammation; may aid in the maintenance of small blood vessels.

green tea. Rich source of phytochemicals that appear to help prevent cancer and heart disease; may help reduce cholesterol levels when drunk with meals.

hawthorn berry. Herb rich in bioflavonoids; appears to reduce blood pressure during exertion; has anticholesterol properties; has been reported to increase the contractility of the heart.

homocysteine. Amino acid formed when other amino acids are broken down. Elevated levels appear to be a risk factor for heart attack.

hormone. Chemical messenger produced by one of the endocrine glands to regulate specific functions in the body, including growth, blood pressure, heart rate, glucose levels, and sexual characteristics.

Human Growth Factors (hGf). Chemicals within the human body that help to regulate growth modulation and repair, so that cells may retain their youthful function.

human growth hormone (somatropin). Hormone secreted by the pituitary gland that is involved in the growth and repair of body tissues.

hypoglycemia. Abnormally low concentration of glucose in the circulating blood (less than the minimum of the normal range).

hypogonadism. Condition resulting from abnormally low levels of testosterone.

hyposomatotropism. Age-related impairment in growth hormone secretion.

hypothyroidism. An underactive thyroid.

ideal body weight (IBW). Calculation of an individual's suggested weight based on factors, including height and body frame size.

immunoglobin. Protein manufactured by white blood cells that function as antibodies as part of the body's immune response.

in vitro. Made to occur in a laboratory vessel or other controlled environment.

in vivo. Occurring or made to occur within a living organism or natural setting.

inositol. Phospholipid that is a constituent of cell membranes; may work with biotin and choline to control male pattern baldness; reported to metabolize serum lipoproteins to lower cholesterol; appears to aid in the maintenance of cell membranes.

insulin. Hormone produced by the pancreas needed for the metabolism of carbohydrates, especially sugar.

insulin-like growth factor 1 (IGF-1). Peptides whose formation is stimulated by growth hormone, IGF-1 promotes peripheral tissue effects of GH.

interleukin. Responsible for mobilizing neutrophils and lymphocytes in the immune system.

involution. Gradual shrinkage of the thymus.

iron. Metal essential for red blood cell formation and vitamin E metabolism. Caveat: in excess, iron may be a strong catalyst in free-radical production and may aid in the deposition of plaque in blood vessels.

kava kava. Herb acting primarily as a sedative; may be used for pain control.

letpin. Molecule made in fat cells that is important in the feedback regulation of energy expenditure, in food intake, and in the creation of fat.

licorice root. Major Chinese herb used to invigorate the functions of the heart, spleen and pancreas; contains glycyrrhizic acid that appears to block tumor growth; reported to have anti-inflammatory properties that may be helpful in treating arthritis; contains carbendoxolane, which seems to be effective in treating stomach ulcers.

lipofuscin. Metabolic waste product that occurs when fat binds to protein; excess causes "age spots."

lymphocyte, also known as *T cell* **or** *B cell.* Type of white blood cell that produces antibodies and is crucial for proper immune response.

lysine. Essential amino acid needed for proper growth, enzyme production, and tissue repair; may help stimulate the immune system; appears to have antiviral properties and may inhibit herpes virus.

macrophage. Type of white blood cell that engulfs invading infection or disease, and is crucial for proper immune response.

melatonin. Hormone made by your pineal gland during sleep; appears to be vital for the maintenance of normal body rhythms.

menarche. Onset of menstruation.

menopause. Cessation of menstruation caused by a decrease in the production of the sex hormones estrogen and progesterone.

metabolism. The physical and chemical processes inside the body's cells that create energy.

methionine. Sulfur-containing amino acid that protects against cardiovascular disease.

mineral. One of many inorganic substances necessary for proper functioning of the body.

miso soup. Macronutrient soup; natural alkaline pH balancer; has a high concentration of iodine.

mitochondria. Small, rod-shaped structures in cells that help convert glucose to energy.

mitogen. Any substance that stimulates mitosis (cell division) and lymphocyte transformation into large, blast-like forms (immunoblasts).

mucosa. Mucous tissue lining various tubular structures of the body.

nephron. Tubular structure characterizing the kidney.

neuropeptide. Any of a variety of peptides such as endorphins and enkephalins found in neural tissue.

neurotransmitter. Chemical that transmits impulses between nerve cells in the brain and nervous system.

neutrophil. Type of white blood cell that provides frontline defense for immune system; is first to arrive at site of infection or disease.

niacin (vitamin B$_3$). Potent vasodilator; may help potentiate the effects of chromium; enhances energy production and the normal functioning of the nervous system; helps lower cholesterol; appears to function in promoting healthy skin and nerves.

noradrenaline. Also known as norepinephrine, a hormone secreted in response to hypotension and physical stress; has strong vasoconstrictive (blood vessel narrowing) effects.

norepinephrine. Hormone secreted by the adrenal gland in reaction to stress.

nutraceutical. Food or nutrient-based product or supplement designed to be used for a specific therapeutic purpose.

OKG. Combination of the amino acids ornithine and glutamine; enhances the body's release of muscle-building hormones such as growth hormone and insulin, and increases arginine and glutamine levels in muscle.

omega-3 fatty acids. Contain two polyunsaturated fats; may help prevent the formation of blood clots leading to heart attacks; appear to be protective against cancer. *Caution:* Do not take omega-3 supplements if you are taking a blood thinner or using aspirin daily without first consulting your physician. Excessive amounts may cause bleeding.

OPCs (oligomeric proanthocyanidin complexes): Proanthocyanidins are a specific category of flavonoids, which only are produced by plants and offer them defense against invasions from funguses, toxins, and environmental stress. Oligomeric proanthocyanidins are particularly important to human health because the complex molecular structure makes them very active and potent antioxidants. OPCs are most plentiful in food sources including red wine, blueberry, cranberry (red bilberry), lingonberry, barley (and beer), and other foods. As a nutritional supplement, OPCs are extracted from botanical sources including grape seed (*Vitis vinefera*), white pine (*Pinus maritima, Pinus pinaster*), and other plants.

pantothenic acid (vitamin B₅). Precursor to cortisone in the adrenal gland; appears to aid in steroid synthesis; aids in energy metabolism; an antistress and antioxidant vitamin; may help inhibit hair color loss.

percutaneous. Absorbed through the skin into the bloodstream.

perimenopause. Reduction in the production of estrogen—a transitional phase that begins about three to five years before the final menstrual period.

phytocompounds. Contain trace compounds that may be protective against major diseases.

plasma. Fluid (noncellular) portion of the circulating blood.

proline. Nonessential amino acid; enhances fat metabolism and aids in the production of connective tissue.

protein. Nitrogen-containing compound that is essential part of all animal and vegetable tissues required to growth and repair.

pyridoxine (vitamin B₆). Aids in metabolism of amino acids, synthesis of nucleic acids, and formation of blood cells; appears to be an important cofactor in many cellular reactions. Caution: Toxic in high doses; use should be monitored by a physician.

"rate of living" theories. First version was introduced in 1908 by German physiologist Max Rubner, who made discoveries into the relationship among metabolic rate, body size, and longevity. Rubner's theory purports that we are each born with a limited amount of energy. If we use this energy slowly then our rate of aging is slowed. If the energy is consumed quickly aging is hastened. Other rate-of-living theories focus on limiting factors such as amount of oxygen inhaled or number of heartbeats spent.

red blood cells. Blood cells that contain hemoglobin and transport oxygen and carbon dioxide.

riboflavin (vitamin B$_2$). Has antioxidant properties; works with other substances to metabolize carbohydrates, fats, and proteins for energy; works with glutathione reductase to protect against oxidative damage during exercise; appears to aid in the formation of T lymphocytes, enhancing immunity; seems to help prevent damage to the cornea.

sarcopenia. Age-related loss in skeletal muscle mass.

saw palmetto. Herb that appears to aid in preventing testosterone from binding to cells in the prostate gland; may help treat the symptoms of benign prostate hypertrophy; may be useful in treating genitourinary tract problems in both sexes.

selenium. Mineral that works with glutathione peroxidase to prevent damage by free radicals; appears to be involved in the metabolism of prostaglandins; seems to protect cell membranes from attack by free radicals, giving it anticancer properties; may protect lipids from oxidation, which helps to prevent cardiovascular disease; appears to aid in the production of thyroid hormones; may protect against environmental pollutants.

senescence. Signs of aging.

serum. Fluid portion of the blood.

somatotrope. Type of cell located in the pituitary gland that produces growth hormone.

somatotropin. *See* human growth hormone.

subclinical disease. That which exhibits some or all of the positive findings of a specific disease, but does not necessarily meet the minimum measurement levels considered relevant to make the diagnosis for that disease.

subcutaneous. Absorbed under the skin into the bloodstream.

suppressor T cells. Immune system's "cease fire" switch; keeps B cells and helper T cells under control.

systolic blood pressure. "First" number in the blood pressure reading; a measurement of the contraction of the heart.

T cells. White blood cells, also known as lymphocytes, that consists of helper T cells, natural killer (NK) cells, and suppressor T cells.

taurine. Modulates neurotransmitters; aids in maintaining clear blood vessels; aids in stabilizing heart rhythm.

thiamine (vitamin B$_1$). Involved in the metabolism of carbohydrates to glucose; appears to be necessary for the normal functioning of the nervous system, heart, and muscles; aids in energy production; appears to help alleviate symptoms of stress.

thymocyte. Type of cell that develops in the thymus; a precursor of the thymus-derived lymphocyte (T lymphocyte) that effects cell-mediated (delayed type) sensitivity.

thyroxine. Hormone made in your thyroid gland.

tocopherol (vitamin E). Fat-soluble potent antioxidant that works synergistically with selenium; appears to reduce the propensity of low-density lipoproteins to oxidize; may prevent the formation of blood clots; appears to help maintain normal blood glucose levels; appears to help prevent cancers of the gastrointestinal tract by inhibiting the conversion of nitrates to nitrosamines (carcinogens).

triglyceride. The form in which fat is stored in the body; also the primary type of fat in the diet.

tumor necrosis factor. Hormone produced by activated macrophages (white blood cell), shown to break up tumor cells *in vitro,* and induce hemorrhagic necrosis (death) of certain transplantable tumors *in vivo.*

valerian root. Herb with effective antispasmodic properties; a nerve tonic.

vanadium. Trace mineral that aids in the regulation of insulin metabolism.

vitamin. One of approximately fifteen organic micronutrients needed by the body that must be obtained through diet.

wheat grass. Used to protect against pollutants; excellent source of chlorophyll.

white blood cells. Group of blood cells that fight infection.

zinc. Essential trace mineral; seems to increase the level of T cells in individuals over age seventy; appears to be involved in cellular division, growth, and repair; may help prevent prostate gland dysfunction in older men; may help prevent vision loss due to macular degeneration and cataracts.

Animal and Human Models Demonstrating Advancements Toward Extending and Enhancing the Human Life Span

ANIMAL MODELS

In the short three years from 2000 to 2002, scientific researchers have made remarkable progress in life span research in animal models. These projects have tremendous implications for near-term application to humans. In animal models of longevity, researchers have extended healthy life spans by 30 to 300 percent depending on the species and the degree of intervention.

MAY 2000: Lexicon Genetics Inc. of Texas published research in *Molecular and Cellular Biology* describing a **gene that controls how quickly mice age, and its relationship to a pathway of cancer suppression in humans.** In knocking out the Ku80 gene in mice (mouse and human Ku80 are 85 percent identical and have the same biochemical function), researchers produced mice that aged more than twice as fast as normal mice, manifesting age-related problems triggered by loss of the gene's normal function. The team determined that the Ku80 gene functions as part of a cellular senescence pathway controlled by the p53 tumor suppression gene—one of the most commonly mutated genes in human cancers. ("Lexicon Genetics Discovers Gene Controlling Onset of Aging in Mice" Press Release, Lexicon Genetics Inc., May 10, 2000)

SEPTEMBER 2000: Researchers from the University of Ottawa (Canada) published findings in *Journal of the National Cancer Institute* resulting from studies of the effect of vitamin E on cancer-cell mutations in laboratory mice. The team found that, as **an antioxidant, vitamin E protects against cell mutations through two mechanisms:** one, by scavenging nitric oxide free radicals (previously shown to cause mutations) and two, by reducing the infiltration of white blood cells into tumors (which may generate free radicals and lead to further cancer cell mutations). (Sandhu JK, Haqqani AS, Birnboim HC, "Effect of dietary vitamin E on spontaneous or nitric oxide donor-induced mutations in a mouse tumor model," *J Natl Cancer Inst.*, 2000 Sept. 6; 92[17]; 1429-33)

SEPTEMBER 2000: The Buck Institute for Age Research publishes findings in *Science* demonstrating the use of a drug in lengthening an animal's normal life span. Mimicking enzymes found in most animals, Eukaryon Inc. of Massachusetts developed two drugs—**synthetic forms of the natural enzymes catalase and superoxide dismutase—that could, like their natural counterparts, defuse free radicals and counter their deleterious effects on DNA, thereby extending the life span** of worms by more than 50 percent. Except in very high doses, the drugs did not have any adverse effects in mice or worms. Remarks lead researcher Dr. Melov on his study, "It was only 5 years ago that I heard a very prominent gerontologist at a major aging meeting say there would never be any drug that extends lifespan in any organism." (*Science News.* Oct. 7, 2000, Vol. 158, p. 238)

SEPTEMBER 2000: Researchers at the Massachusetts Institute of Technology report in *Science* that caloric restriction in yeast by physiological or genetic means showed a substantial extension in life span. The team identified that **activation of the protein Sir2p** by the oxidized form of nicotinamide adenine dinucleotide induced by calorie restriction **results in the increased longevity.** (Lin SJ, Defossez PA, Guarente L, "Requirement of NAD and SIR2 for life-span extension by calorie restriction in Saccharomyces cerevisiae," *Science.* 2000 Sep 22; 289(5487); 2126–8)

OCTOBER 2000: Scientists at Massachusetts General Hospital and Department of Genetics, Harvard Medical School in Massachusetts, experimented with two genes—daf-2 and age-1—present in nerve, muscle, and intestine cells. Publishing their findings in *Science,* Dr. Wolkow and colleagues removed and then replaced these genes in each of the various cell types in worms. Replacing either gene in nerve cells restored the long life span of worms. Restoring the gene activity in muscle or intestine cells overcame certain functional defects in the cells, but failed to increase the life span of the worm. Further experiments showed that higher levels of the genes prolong life by activating certain pathways in nerve cells. The team proposes that **activation of these gene pathways controls the health of nerve cells that secrete a variety of hormone signals, some of which regulate the life span of other tissues.** Dr. Wolkow and colleagues conclude that because animals from worms to mammals probably share a common system for controlling life span, "these findings point to the nervous system as a central regulator of animal longevity." (Wolkow CA, Kimura KD, Lee MS, Ruvkun G, "Regulation of C. elegans life-span by insulinlike signaling in the nervous system," *Science.* 2000 Oct 6; 290[5489]; 147–50)

DECEMBER 2000: Researchers from University of Guelph (Canada) report that fruit flies **lived 40 percent longer when given a healthy human gene that fights oxidative cell damage.** Reactive oxygen species metabolism—as results from oxidation—has significant impact on aging and life span determination. Dr. Parkes and colleagues inserted the human SOD1 gene—vital for cells to fight free-radical damage—into nerve cells of the fruit fly. The human gene and the fruit flies' version combined to offer super-protection against oxidation. (Phillips JP, Parkes TL, Hilliker AJ, "Targeted neuronal gene expression and longevity in Drosophila," *Exp Gerontol.* 2000 Dec; 35[9–10]); 1157–64)

DECEMBER 2000: Research conducted by a team from University of Connecticut Health Center and reported in *Science* reveals that **mutations in a metabolism-related gene called "Indy" can double the life span** of the fruit fly. In addition, the flies retained the majority of their physical faculties (determined by their ability to fly and successfully breed). The "Indy" gene, which is involved in nutrient transport, is expressed in both fruit flies and mammals. Study co-author Robert A. Reenan believes that Indy mutations increase life span by altering the metabolism and "mimicking calorie restriction." He also speculated that it might be possible to develop a drug that limits the effect of the Indy gene, thereby extending the human life span. (Rogina B, Reenan RA, Nilsen SP, Helfand SL, "Extended life-span conferred by cotransporter gene mutations in Drosophila," *Science.* 2000 Dec 15; 290[5499]: 2137–40)

APRIL 2001: Brown University researchers report in *Science* that female fruit flies with **defective copies of insulin-like receptor (InR) live up to 85 percent longer** than wild-type controls. Treatment with a juvenile hormone analog restores life span to normal. Dr. Tatar's research shows that juvenile hormone deficiency, which results from an InR mutation, is largely responsible for extended longevity in InR mutants. Dr. Tatar believes the insulin signaling system is likely to regulate aging in humans and may act through secondary hormones such as growth hormone, thyroid hormone, or insulin growth factor. (Tatar M, Kopelman A, Epstein D, Tu MP, Yin CM, Garofalo RS, "A mutant Drosophila insulin receptor homolog that extends life-span and impairs neuroendocrine function," *Science.* 2001 Apr 6; 292[5514]; 107–10)

APRIL 2001: Scientists from Andrus Gerontology Center at University of Southern California in Los Angeles report that a mutation in the gene Sch9 in yeast allows it to live up to three times its normal life span. The mammalian analog of the Sch9 gene is the protein kinase Akt/protein kinase B, which is implicated in insulin signaling and functions in a pathway that regulates longevity and stress resistance in worms. Comments lead researcher Dr. Longo, **Akt/PKB "may be a candidate for gene-based manipulations to improve health [in humans]."** (Fabrizio P, Pozza F, Pletcher SD, Gendron CM, Longo VD, "Regulation of longevity and stress resistance by Sch9 in yeast," *Science.* 2001 Apr 13; 292[5515]; 288–90)

AUGUST 2001: Researchers from the University of Texas Health Science Center report in the *Proceedings of the National Academy of Sciences* that **oxidative stress increases in age.** Dr. Hamilton and team observed significant increase in levels of 8-oxo-2-deoxyguanosine (oxo8dG) in DNA isolated from tissues of older rodents. **Dietary restriction was shown to significantly reduce the age-related accumulation of oxo8dG levels in DNA** in all tissues of the mice studied. (Hamilton ML, Van Remmen H, Drake JA, Yang H, Guo ZM, Kewitt K, Walter CA, Richardson A, " Does oxidative damage to DNA increase with age?," *Proc Natl Acad Sci USA.* 2001 Aug 28; 98[18]; 10469-74)

AUGUST 2001: Scientists from Jefferson Medical College in Philadelphia report in the *Proceedings of the National Academy of Sciences* on the successful use of gene therapy to prevent cancer in mice. Dr. Croce and colleagues targeted the FHIT gene, which is damaged in many forms of cancer: FHIT causes damaged cells to terminate before they can start the uncontrolled growth of cancer. Cells in which this gene is damaged (by carcinogens, for example) do not die the way they normally would. When mice were engineered to lack a working copy of the FHIT gene, they became vulnerable to conditions leading to cancer. The researchers conclude that **"FHIT may be a one-hit tumor suppressor gene in some tissues."** (Zanesi N, Fidanza V, Fong LY, Mancini R, Druck T, Valtieri M, Rudiger T, McCue PA, Croce CM, Huebner K, "The tumor spectrum in FHIT-deficient mice," *Proc Natl Acad Sci USA.* 2001 Aug 28; 98[18]: 10250–5)

SEPTEMBER 2001: Researchers from University of California at Riverside published findings in *Nature* indicating that elderly mice fed a **low-calorie regime demonstrated reversals of changes in several genes that were altered in aging animals.** Furthermore, 70 percent of the anti-aging effects of long-term caloric restriction also occurred in old mice put on a short-term low-calorie diet. (Cao SX, Dhahbi JM, Mote PL, Spindler SR, "Genomic profiling of short- and long-term caloric restriction effects in the liver of aging mice," *Proc Natl Acad Sci USA.* 2001 Sep 11; 98[19]; 10630–5)

SEPTEMBER 2001: Researchers from University of Illinois at Chicago College of Medicine report in the *Proceedings of the National Academy of Sciences* that in aging mice they could promote expression of the **Forkhead box M1B (FoxM1B) gene,** a ubiquitously expressed member of the Fox transcription factor family whose expression is restricted to proliferating cells and that mediates hepatocyte entry into DNA synthesis and mitosis during liver regeneration. By promoting the increased expression of FoxM1B, then removing a portion of the liver, the mice rapidly **regenerated new tissue**—unlike typical aged mice. The DNA in the regenerating liver cells replicated normally, and cells divided as they do in livers of injured young mice. Furthermore, lab studies showed that increasing expression of FoxM1B **restored the activity of numerous other genes involved in cell division.** Importantly, lead researcher Dr. Costa notes that the FoxM1B gene **controls exit from cell division,** without which cells would retain too many copies of DNA—a defect commonly seen in cancer. Because in humans the FoxM1B gene exists not only in the liver but also throughout the body, the team believes their discovery might one day be used in **gene therapy to replace old cells and organs in the elderly.** (Wang X, Quail E, Hung NJ, Tan Y, Ye H, Costa RH, "Increased levels of forkhead box M1B transcription factor in transgenic mouse hepatocytes prevent age-related proliferation defects in regenerating liver," *Proc Natl Acad Sci USA.* 2001 Sep 25; 98[20]; 11468–73)

NOVEMBER 2001: In ongoing research, Dr. Melov and colleagues from the Buck Institute for Age Research report that treatment of mice with antioxidant drugs quadrupled their life span. The study shows for the first time that antioxidant drugs are capable of extending mammalian life span, specifically by reversing oxidation that typically arises in the aging process. The **antioxidant drugs mobilized into cell mitochondria to counter the aging effects of free radicals.** Says Melov, "these new findings suggest **novel therapeutic approaches to neurodegenerative diseases associated with oxidative stress,** such as . . . Alzheimer's and Parkinson's diseases, in which chronic oxidative damage to the brain has been implicated." (Melov S, Doctrow SR, Schneider JA, Haberson J, Patel M, Coskun PE, Huffman K, Wallace DC, Malfroy B, "Life span extension and rescue of spongiform encephalopathy in superoxide dismutase 2 nullizygous mice treated with superoxide dismutase-catalase mimetics," *J Neurosci.* 2001 Nov 1; 21[21]; 8348–53)

JANUARY 2002: Researchers from Baylor College of Medicine in Houston report in *Nature* that a critical protein that protects animals from cancer in their early years appears, in later life, to cause much of the deterioration associated with aging. Conducting their research on mice, the team mutated the animals to demonstrate enhanced resistance to spontaneous tumors; as these altered mice aged, they displayed an early onset of reduced longevity, osteoporosis, organ atrophy, and a diminished stress tolerance. The team concluded that **the p53 protein—integral in the cancer-fighting armament of animals including humans—eventually shuts off the body's ability to renew its organs and tissues, producing bone and muscle deterioration and other hallmarks of aging.** According to lead researcher Dr. Donehower, the results "raise the shocking possibility that aging may be a side effect of the natural safeguards that protect us from cancer." (Tyner SD, Venkatachalam S, Choi J, Jones S, Ghebranious N, Igelmann H, Lu X, Soron G, Cooper B, Brayton C, Hee Park S, Thompson T, Karsenty G, Bradley A, Donehower LA, "p53 mutant mice that display early ageing-associated phenotypes," *Nature* 2002 Jan 3; 415[6867]; 45–53)

JANUARY 2002: Researchers at the University of California Los Angeles report in *Science* that they more than doubled the life span of worms by simply depriving them of a micronutrient called coenzyme Q. Drs. Pamela L Larsen and Catherine F Clarke found that adult worms fed on a coenzyme Q diet lived 59 percent longer than those fed a normal diet. Coenzyme Q is an antioxidant that helps to transport electrons during cellular respiration; however, Larsen and Clarke say that their results suggest that the substance may also have a "pro-oxidant" effect. If this is true, **reducing the animals' consumption of coenzyme Q may extend life span by lowering oxidative damage to cells.** (Larsen PL, Clarke CF, "Extension of life-span in Caenorhabditis elegans by a diet lacking coenzyme Q," *Science.* 2002 Jan 4; 295[5552]; 120–3)

JANUARY 2002: Researchers from the University of California San Francisco report in *Science* that stem cells may play an important role in determining how long we live. Researchers studying germ-line stem cells in nematode worms discovered that the **stem cells appear to regulate a system that speeds up aging.** Dr. Nuno Arantes-Oliveira were already aware that germ-line cells had an impact on life span; however, in their most recent study, they found that they could extend the worms' life span by destroying specific germ-line precursor cells that develop from stem cells. Destroying these cells has also been shown to have the same effect on fruit flies. (Arantes-Oliveira N, Apfeld

J, Dillin A, Kenyon C. "Regulation of life-span by germ-line stem cells in Caenorhabditis elegans," *Science.* 2002 Jan 18; 295[5554]; 502-5)

JANUARY 2002: Scientists from the U.S. National Institute of Neurological Disorders and Stroke, a division of the National Institutes of Health, report in the *Proceedings of the National Academy of Sciences* that feeding fruit flies throughout adulthood **with the drug 4-phenylbutyrate (PBA) can significantly increase life span, without diminution of mobility, stress resistance, or reproductive ability.** Moreover, treatment for a limited period, either early or late in adult life, was also found to be effective. PBA extended the maximum life span of fruit flies by over 50 percent and their average life span by one-third. (Kang HL, Benzer S, Min KT, "Life extension in Drosophila by feeding a drug," *Proc Natl Acad Sci USA.* 2002 Jan 22; 99[2]: 838–43)

APRIL 2003: A research team at BioMarker Pharmaceuticals (Campbell, CA, USA) reports that **metformin,** a drug used to treat diabetes, has been found to produce anti-aging effects similar to those of caloric restriction (CR), an experimental method touted to retard aging, prevent aging-related diseases, prolong youth, and extend life span in animals. Metformin mimics changes in gene expression found in CR-mice, **extending the life span by 20 percent.** This is the first instance where a clinical drug has been found to produce genetic effects similar to those of CR for life extension. ("Scientists Discover Anti-Aging Effects of Diabetes Drug," *PRNewswire,* April 23, 2003)

MAY 2003: University of California San Francisco (USA) report in *Science* magazine the discovery of a class of molecules found in both *C. elegans* (roundworms) and humans that can prolong life and prevent the harmful accumulation of "heat shock proteins," which form undesirable aggregations that accumulate with age and may cause aging-related diseases. Diseases presently thought to be caused by protein aggregation include Alzheimer's, Huntington's, Parkinson's, and prion diseases, collectively suggesting that **heat-shock proteins may be a molecular link between aging and age-related diseases.** ("Researchers discover common cause for aging and age-related disease," *Eurekalert,* May 15, 2003)

HUMAN MODELS

As with animal models for longevity, a number of recent advances suggest that we are close to practical medical interventions to modify the metabolism of aging in humans.

AUGUST 2001: A team from Howard Hughes Medical Institute at Children's Hospital/Harvard Medical School report in the *Proceedings of the National Academy of Sciences* that they have identified a group of genes that appears to determine an individual's life span. Scientists examining the genetic code of 308 siblings of people who had lived until they were at least ninety years old discovered that many of the siblings had inherited a **specific set of genes on chromosome 4**. The region that the scientists have identified contains approximately 500 genes; thus, the team is now trying to pinpoint the gene that grants longevity. Although anyone has yet to attempt to alter human life span by genetic modification, scientists have already extended the life span of lower-organisms such as nematode worms and fruit flies using genetic techniques. The researchers believe that people who live to a ripe old age have had the fortune to inherit genes that extend the life span but, possibly more important, have also managed to avoid inheriting genes that are associated with diseases such as cancer, heart disease, and Alzheimer's disease. Study leader Professor Louis Kunkel said: "It is clear to us that longevity has a genetic component." (Puca AA, Daly MJ, Brewster SJ, Matise TC, Barrett J, Shea-Drinkwater M, Kang S, Joyce E, Nicoli J, Benson E, Kunkel LM, Perls T, "A genome-wide scan for linkage to human exceptional longevity identifies a locus on chromosome 4," *Proc Natl Acad Sci USA.* 2001 Aug 28; 98[18]; 10505–8)

JANUARY 2002: Scientists from Johns Hopkins University report in the *Proceedings of the National Academy of Sciences* that they discovered a gene that appears to have an important role in determining a person's life span. The gene, which has been named Klotho after the Greek Fate who spun the thread of life, was discovered when the scientists were studying the genes of adults aged sixty-five and above and comparing them with those of infants. Results showed that 3 percent of the infants had the Klotho gene variant, compared with just 1 percent of those aged sixty-five and older. According to the researchers, these findings suggest that **infants possessing two copies of the Klotho gene variant are more than twice as likely to die before they reach age sixty-five.** (Arking DE, Krebsova A, Macek M Sr, Macek M Jr, Arking A, Mian IS, Fried L, Hamosh A, Dey S, McIntosh I, Dietz HC, "Association of human aging with a functional variant of klotho," *Proc Natl Acad Sci USA.* 2002 Jan 22; 99[2]; 856–861)

FEBRUARY 2002: Icelandic biotechnologists announce they have isolated a gene that they believe could lead to the development of drugs enabling people to live longer. Scientists at DeCode Genetics have given the gene the name of the Methuselah gene, for which they know the location and soon they predict to discover the exact DNA sequence and how it works in the body. The researchers discovered that **those who lived longer appeared to have inherited a single gene that protected them against old age,** rather than being born into families that did not inherit genes that made them vulnerable to illnesses. (Dalton A, "Scientists find key to eternal life," *The Scotsman,* Feb. 4, 2002)

OCTOBER 2002: Results of a recent study presented at the annual meeting of the American Neurological Association in New York City suggest that the food supplement **coenzyme Q$_{10}$ could slow down the progression of Parkinson's disease.** Lead researcher Professor Clifford Shults of the University of California in San Diego and his colleagues enrolled eighty Parkinson's patients for the trial. All exhibited early-stage Parkinson's, and did not yet need levodopa. After eight months of treatment with coenzyme Q$_{10}$, patients who had received the highest dose of Q$_{10}$ exhibited a 44 percent reduction in disease progression, compared with the placebo group. Even patients treated with the lowest dose the supplement were more able at carrying out simple daily activities—for example, dressing and washing—and demonstrated better mental functioning and mood. The authors conclude that their findings "are supportive of the view that mitochondrial dysfunction does play a role in the pathogenesis of sporadic Parkinson's disease." (*Archives of Neurology* 2002; 59:1541–1550)

OCTOBER 2002: Blood pressure drugs called **ACE inhibitors,** which help diabetics to lower their risk of developing complications, have been suggested to be of value in **developing drugs that delay the effects of aging.** Part of the reason why diabetics tend to age faster than non-diabetics is that their high-blood sugar levels encourage the body to produce complex proteins called advanced glycation end products (AGEs). These proteins interfere with cell functioning, accumulate in skin making it look wrinkly, and stiffen blood vessels. Now researchers at the Baker Institute in Melbourne, Australia, have found that ACE inhibitors appear to exert their anti-aging effects by preventing the buildup of AGEs. ACE inhibitors work by blocking the production of the enzyme angiotensin II, which is thought to encourage the production of cell-damaging free radicals that stimulate the production of AGEs. According to the New Scientist, "ACE inhibitors are unlikely to become an elixir of youth because they cause unpleasant side effects such as coughing and irregular heartbeat." However, there is hope that drugs designed to have a similar effect on AGEs without the adverse effects of current ACE inhibitors could provide us with a new class of age-delaying drugs. (reported by www.bbc.co.uk on October 2, 2002)

APRIL 2003: The Progeria Research Foundation (PRF) announced the discovery of the gene that causes progeria, a rare, fatal genetic condition characterized by an appearance of accelerated aging in children. Children afflicted with progeria typically die from complications of cardiovascular disease or arteriosclerosis at an average of thirteen. As reported in *Nature* magazine, Dr. Francis Collins, director of the National Human Genome Research Institute and senior study author, mutations to the gene Lamin A cause progeria. Because heart disease and stroke are the first and third leading causes of death in the United States, accounting for more than 40 percent of all mortalities, it is hoped that the PRF discoveries will shed insight into interventions for these adult diseases. ("Identification of Gene Gives Hope to Children with Progeria, May Shed Light on Phenomenon of Aging," The Progeria Research Foundation, April 16, 2003)

Anti-Aging Resources

The following list of resources is provided to improve your use of the information presented in this book. Neither the authors nor the Academy of Anti-Aging Medicine (A4M) endorse any physicians, practitioners, products, services, or vendors listed here. This compilation is a representative sampling of individuals and companies involved in anti-aging medical care, and should be considered as a reference and educational resource only. It is the reader's responsibility to use caution and investigate all therapies mentioned in this book as many of them are new and experimental. Please be aware that street addresses, websites, and phone numbers are subject to change.

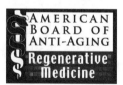

ABAARM PHYSICIANS

The American Board of Anti-Aging/Regenerative Medicine (ABAARM) was founded in 1997 as a professional, physician certification and review board for individuals with a degree as a doctor of medicine (M.D.), a Bachelor of Medicine/ Bachelor of Science (MBBS), and/or doctor of osteopathic medicine (D.O.). ABAARM offers board certification to these medical professionals in recognition of their specialty knowledge and clinical practice of anti-aging medical care.

A written examination assesses proficiency in several key areas of anti-aging clinical care. Passing examinees are designated as diplomates of anti-aging/regenerative medicine. Board certification candidates who pass the written examination may enroll for the oral examination. Passing oral examinees are awarded status as Board Certified in Anti-Aging/Regenerative Medicine.

For more information about the ABAARM program, please contact: Board Coordinator, ABAARM at (773) 528-4333 or by e-mail at exam@worldhealth.net. More than 2,000 physicians are now ABAARM diplomates or board certified.

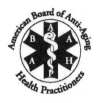

ABAAHP HEALTH PRACTITIONERS

The American Board of Anti-Aging Health Practitioners (ABAAHP) was founded in 1999 to provide advanced education, representation, and specialty recognition to healthcare professionals, including doctors of chiropractic (D.C.), dentistry (D.D.S.), naturopathy (N.D.), podiatric medicine (D.P.M.), registered pharmacists (R.Ph.) and nurses, nurse practitioners, physician assistants, and scientists (Ph.D.).

The ABAAHP program, the first certification program of its kind, raises the standard of professional care and recognition offered by practitioners, as well as allied health professionals, delivering integrative, complementary, and alternative health care. By completing the ABAAHP process, examinees receive specialty certification as a diplomat practicing anti-aging medicine. For more information about the ABAAHP program, please contact: Board Coordinator, ABAAHP at (773) 528-4333 or by e-mail at exam@worldhealth.net.

More than 300 health practitioners are now ABAAHP diplomates.

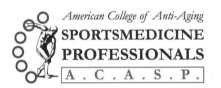

AMERICAN COLLEGE OF ANTI-AGING SPORTS MEDICINE PROFESSIONALS

The American College of Anti-Aging Sports Medicine Professionals (ACASP) Certificate and Workshop programs are a specialized Certificate program in conjunction with medical organizations to allow health professionals to learn the latest in preventative medicine, integrative medicine, anti-aging medicine and longevity medicine and integrate this into their sports medicine practice.

For more information about the ACASP program, please contact: Board Coordinator, ACASP at (773) 528-1000 or by email at: sports@worldhealth.net.

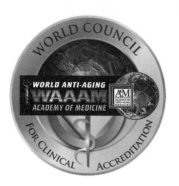

WCCA ANTI-AGING CLINIC/ MEDICAL SPA ACCREDITATION PROGRAM

In 2007, the A4M, in conjunction with the World Council for Clinical Accreditation (WCCA), launched the WCCA Anti-Aging Clinic/Medical Spa Accreditation Program. Accredited facilities meet high standards of quality, service, safety, and efficiency as set forth by the A4M and WCCA, and are committed to ongoing improvements in the facility and its medical programs. To locate an WCCA-accredited anti-aging clinic or medical spa, visit www.worldhealth.net.

USEFUL INTERNET WEBSITES

The following is a representative listing of websites providing useful information on aging, preventive health, and anti-aging medicine.

Resource	Website Address
American Academy of Anti-Aging Medicine (A4M)	www.worldhealth.net
Online Locator Directories of: Anti-Aging Physicians and Health Practitioners; Anti-Aging Clinics and Medical Spas; and Anti-Aging Products and Services	www.worldhealth.net/p/51.html
Anti-Aging Certification and Certificate Programs for Physicians and Health Practitioners	www.worldhealth.net/p/100,360.html
A4M Special Information Center (Publishing & Media Showcase)	www.a4minfo.net
National Academy of Sports Medicine	www.nasm.org
View videos of the world's top doctors and longevity experts as they share their secrets for your maximum lifespan	www.worldhealthnet.tv
Take the state-of-the-art Cyber Longevity Test to see how many more years you can live	www.mylonglife.com

The American Academy
of Anti-Aging Medicine

OUR MISSION

The American Academy of Anti-Aging Medicine, Inc. (A4M) is a non-profit medical organization dedicated to the advancement of technology to detect, prevent, and treat age-related disease and to promote research into methods to retard and optimize the human aging process. A4M is also dedicated to educating physicians, scientists, and members of the public on anti-aging issues. A4M believes that the disabilities associated with normal aging are caused by physiological dysfunction which, in many cases, are ameliorable to medical treatment such that the human life span can be increased and the quality of one's life improved as one grows chronologically older. A4M seeks to disseminate information concerning innovative science and research as well as treatment modalities designed to prolong the human life span. Anti-aging medicine is based on the scientific principles of responsible medical care consistent with those of other healthcare specialties. Although A4M seeks to disseminate information on many types of medical treatments, it does not promote or endorse any specific treatment nor does it sell or endorse any commercial product.

Our objectives are to:

- make available life-extending information about the multiple benefits of anti-aging therapeutics to practicing physicians;

- assist in developing therapeutic protocols and innovative diagnostic tools to aid physicians in the implementation of effective longevity treatment;

- act as an information center for valid and effective anti-aging medical protocols;

- assist in obtaining and disseminating funding for scientifically sound and innovative research in anti-aging medicine;

- assist in the funding and promotion of critical anti-aging, clinically based research; and

- provide government outreach, education, and advocacy for anti-aging medicine.

Founded in 1992, A4M membership now includes 20,000-plus physicians, healthcare practitioners, scientists, researchers, and laypersons from more than 100 countries.

THE WORLD HEALTH NETWORK

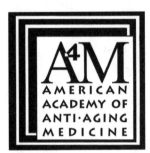

www.worldhealth.net—Internet's Leading Site for Aging Intervention Research & Education

The official website of the American Academy of Anti-Aging Medicine, World Health Network (www.worldhealth.net) provides over 100,000 pages of informative content on health, wellness, and longevity.

FEATURES include:

- EXTENSIVE LIBRARY of news in anti-aging medicine, sports medicine, and biotechnology

- INTERACTIVE LOCATORS to find anti-aging physicians, practitioners, and clinics, as well as products and services

- Information on BOARD CERTIFICATION in anti-aging medicine

- FREE E-NEWSLETTER highlighting the latest advancements in aging intervention, delivered to your desktop

References

DEDICATION

Golden, F., "Day 3: Living to 1,000?" Time Inc., http://www.time.com/time/health/print-out/0,8816,421979,00.html, accessed March 21, 2003.

Magalhaes, J.P., "Winning the war against aging," *The Futurist,* March–April 2003; 48–50.

World Population Prospects: The 2000 Revision-Highlights, United Nations, February 28, 2001.

INTRODUCTION

Gleckman H., "Social Security isn't the only surplus-buster," *Business Week,* May 21, 2001.

McCauhey Ross, B., "Almost a fountain of youth," *U.S. News & World Report,* April 12, 1999.

CHAPTER 1

"Funding First." *Mass High Tech* 2000 Jul; 18(28): 1.

Hendler, S.S., *The Complete Guide to Anti-Aging Nutrients.* New York: Simon & Shuster, 1984.

Klatz, R.M. (ed), *Advances in Anti-aging Medicine,* vol.1. New York: Mary Ann Liebert Publishers, Inc., 1996.

Klatz, R.M. and Goldman, R.M., *7 Anti-Secrets for Optimal Digestion and Scientific Weight Loss.* Chicago: ESM Publications, 1996.

"Validating the Facts and Science of Anti-aging Medicine: Report on the State of the Clinical Specialty." *Medical Committee for Aging Research and Education* 2002; 1: 11.

CHAPTER 2

Bjorksten, J. "Crosslinkage and the Aging Process," in Rockstein, M. (ed), *Theoretical Aspects of Aging.* New York: Academic Press, 1974; p. 43.

Bjorskten, J. "The Crosslinkage Theory of Aging: Clinical Implications." *Compr Ther* 1976; II: 65.

Campanelli, Linda, C., Ph.D. "Theories of Aging." *Theories and Psychosocial Aspects of Aging* (1) 3–13.

Finch, Caleb, E. *Longevity, Senescence, and the Genome.* Chicago: University of Chicago Press, 1990.

Hayflick, L. "Theories of Aging," in Cape, R ., Coe, R., and Rodstein, M. (eds), *Fundamentals of Geriatric Medicine.* New York: Raven Press, 1983.

Hayflick, L. *How and Why We Age.* New York: Ballantine Books, 1994; pp. 222–262.

Kotulak, Ronald, and Gorner, Peter. "Calorie restriction: Taking the lifespan to its limit," in *Aging on Hold.* Tribune Publishing, 1992; pp. 52–57.

Martin, G. M., Sprague, C.A., and Epstein, C.J. "Replicative Lifespan of Cultivated Human Cells." *Lab Invest* 1970; 23: 26.

Medvedev, Z. "Possible Role of Repeated Nucleotide Sequences in DNA in the Evolution of Lifespans of Differential Cells." *Nature* 1972; 237: 453.

Rosenfeld, Albert. *Prolongevity II.* New York: Alfred A. Knopf, Inc., 1985; 247–267.

Rothstein, M. (ed). *Review of Biological Research in Aging,* vol. 4. New York: Wiley-Liss, 1990.

Sharma, Ramesh. "Theories of Aging," in *Physiological Basis of Aging and Geriatrics.* Florida: CRC Press, 1994; 37–44.

Sonneborn, T. "The Origin, Evolution, Nature, and Causes of Aging," in Behnke, J., Fince, C., and Moment, G. (eds), *The Biology of Aging.* New York: Plenum Press, 1979; p. 341.

Wilmoth, J.R., Deegan, L.J., Lundstrom, H., Horiuchi, S., "Increase in maximum life-span in Sweden, 1861–1999," *Science,* September 29, 2000; 2366–2368.

CHAPTER 3

Allen, R.H., Lindenbaum, J., Stabler, S.P. "High prevalence of cobalamin deficiency in the elderly." *Trans Am Clin Climatol Assoc* 1995; 107: 37–45; discussion 45–47.

Anawalt B.D., Merriam G.R., "Neuroendocrine aging in men: Andropause and somatopause." *Endocrinol Metab Clin North Am* Sep 2001; 30(3): 647-69.

Arvat, E., Broglio, F., Ghigo, E. "Insulin-like growth factor I: implications in aging." *Drugs Aging* 2000; 16: 29–40.

Asthana S., Baker L.D., Craft S., Stanczyk F.Z., Veith R.C., Raskind M.A., Plymate S.R., "High-dose estradiol improves cognition for women with AD: Results of a randomized study." *Neurology* Aug 28 2001; 57(4): 605-12.

Badano. L., Carratino, L., Giunta, L., Calisi, P., Lucatti, A. "Age-induced changes in the cardiovascular system in normal subjects." *G Ital Cardiol* 1992; 22:1023–34.

Barak, Y., Levine, J., Glasman, A., Elizur, A., Belmaker, R.H. "Inositol treatment of Alzheimer's disease: a double blind, cross-over placebo controlled trial." *Prog Neuropsychopharmacol Biol Psychiatry* 1996; 20: 729–35.

Barbieri, M., Rizzo, M.R., Manzella, D., Paolisso, G. "Age-related insulin resistance: Is it an obligatory finding? The lesson from healthy centenarians." *Diabetes Metab Res Rev* 2001; 17:19–26.

Bartke, A. "Growth hormone and aging." *Endocrine* 1998; 8:103–108.

Basaria S., Dobs A.S., "Hypogonadism and androgen replacement therapy in elderly men." *Am J Med* May 2001; 110(7): 563-72.

Beharka, A.A., Paiva, S., Leka, L.S., Ribaya-Mercado, J.D., Russell, R.M., Nibkin Meydani, S. "Effect of age on the gastrointestinal-associated mucosal immune response of humans." *J Gerontol A Biol Sci Med Sci* 2001; 56: B218–23.

Bernard, M.A., Nakonezny, P.A., Kashner, T.M. "The effect of vitamin B_{12} deficiency on older veterans and its relationship to health." *J Am Geriatr Soc* 1998; 46: 1199–206.

Bhasin S., Woodhouse L., Storer T.W., "Proof of the effect of testosterone on skeletal muscle." *J Endocrinol* Jul 2001; 170(1): 27-38.

Biedert, S., Stuckstedte, H. "Normal and frequent neurologic findings in elderly patients." *Fortschr Neurol Psychiatr* 1993; 61: 27–32.

Bild, D.E., Fitzpatrick, A., Fried, L.P., Wong, N.D., Haan, M.N., Lyles, M., Bovill, E., Polak, J.F., Schulz, R. "Age-related trends in cardiovascular morbidity and physical functioning in the elderly: the Cardiovascular Health Study." *J Am Geriatr Soc* 1993; 41: 1047–56.

Burns, E.A., Leventhal, E.A. "Aging, immunity, and cancer." *Cancer Control* 2000; 7: 513–22.

Capurso, A., Panza, F., Solfrizzi, V., Torres, F., Capurso, C., Mastroianni, F., Del Parigi, A. "Age-related cognitive decline: Evaluation and prevention strategy." *Recenti Prog Med* 2000; 91: 127–34.

Chan, K.M., Raja, A.J., Strohschein, F.J., Lechelt, K. "Age-related changes in muscle fatigue resistance in humans." *Can J Neurol Sci* 2000; 27: 220–8.

Chauhan, J., Hawrysh, Z.J., Gee, M., Donald, E.A., Basu, T.K. "Age-related olfactory and taste changes and interrelationships between taste and nutrition." *J Am Diet Assoc* 1987; 87: 1543–50.

Cocchi, D. "Age-related alterations in gonadotropin, adrenocorticotropin and growth hormone secretion." *Aging (Milano)* 1992; 4: 103–13.

Cunha, U.G., Rocha, F.L., Peixoto, J.M., Motta, M.F., Barbosa, M.T. "Vitamin B_{12} deficiency and dementia." *Int Psychogeriatr* 1995; 7: 85–8.

Curcio, C.A. "Photoreceptor topography in ageing and age-related maculopathy." *Eye* 2001; 15 (3): 376–83.

Dawson, R. Jr., Pelleymounter, M.A., Cullen, M.J., Gollub, M., Liu, S. "An age-related decline in striatal taurine is correlated with a loss of dopaminergic markers." *Brain Res Bull* 1999; 48: 319–24.

Dawson, R., Jr., Liu, S., Eppler, B., Patterson, T. "Effects of dietary taurine supplementation or deprivation in aged male Fischer 344 rats." *Mech Ageing Dev* 1999; 107: 73–91.

Delion, S., Chalon, S., Guilloteau, D., Lejeune, B., Besnard, J.C., Durand, G. "Age-related changes in phospholipid fatty acid composition and monoaminergic neurotransmission in the hippocampus of rats fed a balanced or an n–3 polyunsaturated fatty acid–deficient diet." *J Lipid Res* 1997; 38: 680–9.

Di Carlo, A., Baldereschi, M., Amaducci, L., Maggi, S., Grigoletto, F., Scarlato, G., Inzitari, D. "Cognitive impairment without dementia in older people: prevalence, vascular risk factors, impact on disability. The Italian Longitudinal Study on Aging." *J Am Geriatr Soc* 2000; 48: 775–82.

Di Perri, R., Coppola, G., Ambrosio, L.A., Grasso, A., Puca, F.M., Rizzo, M. "A multicentre trial to evaluate the efficacy and tolerability of alpha-glycerylphosphorylcholine versos cytosine diphosphocholine in patients with vascular dementia." *J Int Med Res* 1991; 19: 330–41.

Ebly, E.M., Schaefer, J.P., Campbell, N.R. "Folate status, vascular disease and cognition in elderly Canadians." *Age Ageing* 1998; 27: 485–91.

Evans, W.J. "What is sarcopenia?" *J Gerontol A Biol Sci Med Sci* 1995; 50: 5–8.

Fabris, N., Mocchegiani, E., Muzzioli, M., Piloni, S. "Recovery of age-related decline of thymic endocrine activity and PHA response by lysin–arginine combination." *Int J Immunopharmacol* 1986; 8: 677–85.

Fahle, M., Daum, I. "Visual learning and memory as functions of age." *Neuropsychologia* 1997; 35: 1583–1589.

Flanigan, K.M., Lauria, G., Griffin, J.W., Kuncl, R.W. "Age-related biology and diseases of muscle and nerve." *Neurol Clin* 1998; 16: 659–69.

Fleg, J.L. "Alterations in cardiovascular structure and function with advancing age." *Am J Cardiol* 1986; 57: 33C–44C.

Funfgeld, E.W. "A natural and broad spectrum nootropic substance for treatment of SDAT—the Ginkgo biloba extract." *Prog-Clin-Biol-Res* 1989; 317: 1247–60.

Gale, C.R., Martyn, C.N., Cooper, C. "Cognitive impairment and mortality in a cohort of elderly people." *BMJ* 1996; 312: 608–11.

Gambineri, A., Pelusi, C., Vicennati, V., Pagotto, U., Pasquali, R. "Testosterone in ageing men." *Expert Opin Investig Drugs* 2001; 10: 477–92.

Gill, H.S., Darragh, A.J., Cross, M.L. "Optimizing immunity and gut function in the elderly." *J Nutr Health Aging* 2001; 5: 80–91.

Hirokawa, K., Utsuyama, M., Kasai, M., Kurashima, C. "Aging and immunity." *Acta Pathol Jpn* 1992; 42: 537–48.

Hirokawa, K., Utsuyama, M., Kasai, M., Kurashima, C., Ishijima, S., Zeng, Y.X. "Understanding the mechanism of the age-change of thymic function to promote T cell differentiation." *Immunol Lett* 1994; 40: 269–77.

Hoffman, H.J., Ishii, E.K., MacTurk, R.H. "Age-related changes in the prevalence of smell/taste problems among the United States adult population. Results of the 1994 disability supplement to the National Health Interview Survey (NHIS)." *Ann N Y Acad Sci* 1998; 855: 716–22.

Jama, J.W., Launer, L.J., Witteman, J.C., den Breeijen, J.H., Breteler, M.M., Grobbee, D.E., Hofman, A. "Dietary antioxidants and cognitive function in a population-based sample of older persons. The Rotterdam Study." *Am J Epidemiol* 1996; 144:275–80.

Jeglinski, W., Pepeu, G., Oderfeld–Nowak, B. "Differential susceptibility of senile and lesion-induced astrogliosis to phosphatidylserine." *Neurobiol Aging* 1997; 18: 81–6.

Kamel H.K., Perry H.M. 3rd, Morley J.E., "Hormone replacement therapy and fractures in older adults." *J Am Geriatr Soc* Feb 2001; 49(2): 179-87.

Kalmijn, S., Feskens, E.J., Launer, L.J., Kromhout, D. "Polyunsaturated fatty acids, antioxidants, and cognitive function in very old men." *Am J Epidemiol* 1997; 145: 33–41.

Klatz, R.M. "30 Years to Immortality: Ushering in the Ageless Society." *International Journal of Anti-Aging Medicine* 1998.

Kline, D.W. "Ageing and the spatiotemporal discrimination performance of the visual system." *Eye* 1987; 1: 323–329.

Lakatta, E.G. "Changes in cardiovascular function with aging." *Eur Heart J* 1990; 11 (Suppl C): 22–9.

Lal, H., Forster, M.J. "Autoimmunity and age-associated cognitive decline." *Neurobiol Aging* 1988; 9: 733–42.

Lord, J.M., Butcher, S., Killampali, V., Lascelles, D., Salmon, M. "Neutrophil ageing and immunesenescence." *Mech Ageing Dev* 2001; 122: 1521–35.

Lovat, L.B. "Age related changes in gut physiology and nutritional status." *Gut* 1996; 38: 306–9.

Mariani. E., Pulsatelli, L., Meneghetti, A., Dolzani, P., Mazzetti, I., Neri, S., Ravaglia, G., Forti, P., Facchini, A. "Different IL–8 production by T and NK lymphocytes in elderly subjects." *Mech Ageing Dev* 2001; 122:1383–95.

McNerlan, S.E., Rea, I.M., Alexander, H.D., Morris, T.C. "Changes in natural killer cells, the CD57CD8 subset, and related cytokines in healthy aging." *J Clin Immunol* 1998; 18: 31–8.

Meites, D. "Role of the neuroendocrine system in aging." *Fiziol Zh* 1990; 36: 70–6.

Morley J.E., "Androgens and aging." *Maturitas* Feb 28 2001; 38(1): 61-71.

Morley J.E., "Testosterone replacement in older men and women." *J Gend Specif Med* 2001; 4(2): 49-53.

Murphy, C., Wetter, S., Morgan, C.D., Ellison, D.W., Geisler, M.W. "Age effects on central nervous system activity reflected in the olfactory event–related potential. Evidence for decline in middle age." *Ann NY Acad Sci* 1998; 855: 598–607.

National Institutes of Health, National Institute on Aging. *"Menopause"* (1992) available from World Wide Web: http://www.nih.gov/health/chip/nia/menop/men1.htm.

Neuhauser-Berthold, M., Herbert, B.M., Luhrmann, P.M., Sultemeier, A.A., Blum, W.F., Frey, J., Hebebrand, J. "Resting metabolic rate, body composition, and serum leptin concentrations in a free-living elderly population." *Eur J Endocrinol* 2000; 142: 486–92.

Nusbaum, N.J. "Aging and sensory senescence." *South Med J* 1999; 92: 267–75.

Paolisso, G., Tagliamonte, M.R., Rizzo, M.R., Carella, C., Gambardella, A., Barbieri, M., Varricchio, M. "Low plasma insulin-like growth factor-1 concentrations predict worsening of insulin-mediated glucose uptake in older people." *J Am Geriatr Soc* 1999; 47: 1312–8.

Paolisso, G., Tagliamonte, M.R., Rizzo, M.R., Giugliano, D. "Advancing age and insulin resistance: New facts about an ancient history." *Eur J Clin Invest* 1999; 29: 758–69.

Pfeilschifter J., "Hormone replacement and selective estrogen receptor modulators (SERMS) in the prevention and treatment of postmenopausal osteoporosis," *Orthopade* Jul 2001; 30(7): 462–72.

Piers, L.S., Soares, M.J., McCormack, L.M., O'Dea, K. "Is there evidence for an age-related reduction in metabolic rate?" *J Appl Physiol* 1998; 85: 2196–204.

Poehlman, E.T., Toth, M.J., Bunyard, L.B., Gardner, A.W., Donaldson, K.E., Colman, E., Fonong, T., Ades, P.A. "Physiological predictors of increasing total and central adiposity in aging men and women." *Arch Intern Med* 1995; 155: 2443–8.

Proctor, D.N., Balagopal, P., Nair, K.S. "Age-related sarcopenia in humans is associated with reduced synthetic rates of specific muscle proteins." *J Nutr* 1998; 128(2 Suppl): 351S–355S.

Roubenoff, R., Rall, L.C. "Humoral mediation of changing body composition during aging and chronic inflammation." *Nutr Rev* 1993; 51: 1–11.

Sanderson J.E., Haines C.J., Yeung L., Yip G.W., Tang K., Yim S.F., Jorgensen L.N., Woo J. "Anti-ischemic action of estrogen-progestogen continuous combined hormone replacement therapy in postmenopausal women with established angina pectoris: A randomized, placebo-controlled, double-blind, parallel-group trial." *J Cardiovasc Pharmacol* Sep 2001; 38(3): 372-83.

Shah M.G., Maibach HI, "Estrogen and skin: An overview." *Am J Clin Dermatol* 2001; 2(3): 143–50.

Shimokata, H., Kuzuya, F. "Two-point discrimination test of the skin as an index of sensory aging." *Gerontology* 1995; 41: 267–72.

Soares, M.J., Piers, L.S., O'Dea, K., Collier, G.R. "Plasma leptin concentrations, basal metabolic rates and respiratory quotients in young and older adults." *Int J Obes Relat Metab Disord* 2000; 24: 1592–9.

Stabler, S.P., Lindenbaum, J., Allen, R.H. "Vitamin B-12 deficiency in the elderly: current dilemmas." *Am J Clin Nutr* 1997; 66: 741–9.

Thomson, A.B., Keelan, M. "The aging gut." *Can J Physiol Pharmacol* 1986; 64: 30–8.

Thorner, M.O., Chapman, I.M., Gaylinn, B.D., Pezzoli, S.S., Hartman, M.L. "Growth hormone-releasing hormone and growth hormone-releasing peptide as therapeutic agents to enhance growth hormone secretion in disease and aging." *Recent Prog Horm Res* 1997; 52: 215–44; discussion 244–6.

Thornton, P.L., Ingram, R.L., Sonntag, W.E. "Chronic [D-Ala2]-growth hormone-releasing hormone administration attenuates age-related deficits in spatial memory." *J Gerontol A Biol Sci Med Sci* 2000; 55: B106–12.

van Boxtel, M.P., Buntinx, F., Houx, P.J., Metsemakers, J.F., Knottnerus, A., Jolles, J. "The relation between morbidity and cognitive performance in a normal aging population." *J Gerontol A Biol Sci Med Sci* 1998; 53: M147–54.

Verdu, E., Ceballos, D., Vilches, J.J., Navarro, X. "Influence of aging on peripheral nerve function and regeneration." *J Peripher Nerv Syst* 2000; 5: 191–208.

Wu, C.Y., Yu, T.J., Chen, M.J. "Age related testosterone level changes and male andropause syndrome." *Changgeng Yi Xue Za Zhi* 2000; 23: 348–53.

Yildirir A., Aybar F., Tokgozoglu L., Yarali H., Kabakci G., Bukulmez O. Sinici I., Oto A. "Effects of hormone replacement therapy on plasma homocysteine and C-reactive protein levels." *Gynecol Obstet Invest* 2002; 53(1): 54-8.

CHAPTER 4

"A Physician Gives His Opinion About the Entry of STH into the World of Bodybuilding." *Flex* June 1983; p. 76.

Abribat, T., et al. "Alteration of Growth Hormone Secretion in Aging: Peripheral Effects," in Bercu, B.B. & Walker, R. F. (eds), *Growth Hormone II, Basic and Clinical Aspects*. New York: Springer-Verlag, 1994.

American Diabetes Association, "Facts and Figures." (www.diabetes.org).

American Obesity Association, "AOA Fact Sheet." (http://www.obesity.org/subs/fastfacts/ obesity_US.shtm).

Angelin, B., Rudling, M. "Growth Hormone and Lipoprotein Metabolism." *Endocrinol and Metabolism* 1995; 2 (Suppl B): 25–28.

Ascoli, M., Segaloff, D.L. "Adenohypophyseal Hormones and Their Hypothalamic Releasing Factors," in Goodman & Gilman's (eds) *The Pharmacological Basis of Therapeutics* (9th ed.). New York: McGraw-Hill, 1996.

Ballesteros, M., Leung, K.C., Ross, R.J., Iismaa, T.P., Ho, K.K. "Distribution and Abundance of Messenger Ribonucleic Acid for Growth Hormone Receptor Isoforms in Human Tissues." *The Journal of Clinical Endocrinology & Metabolism* 2000; 85: 2865–2871.

Barbul. "Arginine and Immune Function." *Nutrition* 6(1): 53–60, (Update on Immunonutrition Symposium Supplement; Jan/Feb 1990).

Bauer, M.K., Harding, J.E., Breier, B.H., Gluckman, P.D. "Exogenous GH infusion to late-gestational fetal sheep does not alter fetal growth and metabolism." *J Endocrinol* 2001; 166: 591–7.

Baumbach, L., Schiavi, A., Bartlett, R., Perera, E., Day, J., Brown, M.R., Stein, S., Eidson, M., Parks, J.S., Cleveland, W. "Clinical, Biochemical, and Molecular Investigations of a Genetic Isolate of Growth Hormone Insensitivity (Laron's Syndrome)." *The Journal of Clinical Endocrinology & Metabolism* 1997; 82: 444–451.

Bengtsson, B.A. "Cardiovascular Risk Factors in Adults with Growth Hormone Deficiency." *Endocrinol and Metabolism* 1995; 2 (Suppl B): 29–35.

Bengtsson, B.A. *An Introduction to Growth Hormone Deficiency in Adults*. Oxford, UK: Oxford Clinical Communications, 1993.

Bengtsson, B.A., et al. "Treatment of Adults with Growth Hormone Deficiency with Recombinant Human Growth Hormone." *Journal of Clinical Endocrinology and Metabolism* 1993; 76: 309–17.

Berwaerts, J., Moorkens, G., Abs, R. "Secretion of growth hormone in patients with chronic fatigue syndrome." *Growth Horm IGF Res* 1998; 8 (Suppl B): 127–9.

Bjarnason, R., Wickelgren, R., Hermansson, M., Hammarqvist, F., Carlsson, B., Carlsson, L.M. "Growth Hormone Treatment Prevents the Decrease in Insulin-Like Growth Factor I Gene

Expression in Patients Undergoing Abdominal Surgery." *The Journal of Clinical Endocrinology & Metabolism* 1998; 83:1566–1572.

Blethen, S.L., Allen, D.B., Graves, D., August, G., Moshang, T., Rosenfeld, R. "Safety of recombinant deoxyribonucleic acid-derived growth hormone: The National Cooperative Growth Study experience." *The Journal of Clinical Endocrinology & Metabolism* 1996; 81: 1704–10.

Brevini, T.A., Bianchi, R., Motta, M. "Direct inhibitory effect of somatostatin on the growth of the human prostatic cancer cell line LNCaP: Possible mechanism of action." *The Journal of Clinical Endocrinology & Metabolism* 1993; 7: 7626–31.

Brixen, K, et al. "Growth Hormone (GH) and Adult Bone Remodeling: the Potential Use of GH in Treatment of Osteoporosis." *Journal of Pediatric Endocrinology (England)* 1993; 6: 65–71.

Caidahl, K., Eden, S., Bengtsson, B.A. "Cardiovascular and Renal Effects of Growth Hormone." *Clinical Endocrinolology (Oxford, England)* 1994; 40: 393–400.

Carroll, P.V., Christ, E.R., Bengtsson, B.A., Carlsson, L., Christiansen, J.S., Clemmons, D., Hintz, R., Ho, K., Laron, Z., Sizonenko, P., Sonksen, P.H., Tanaka, T., Thorne, M. "Growth hormone deficiency in adulthood and the effects of growth hormone replacement: A review. Growth Hormone Research Society Scientific Committee." *The Journal of Clinical Endocrinology & Metabolism* 1998; 83:382–395.

Cassoni, P., Papotti, M., Ghe, C., Catapano, F., Sapino, A., Graziani, A., Deghenghi, R., Reissmann, T., Ghigo, E., Muccioli, G. "Identification, characterization, and biological activity of specific receptors for natural (ghrelin) and synthetic growth hormone secretagogues and analogs in human breast carcinomas and cell lines." *The Journal of Clinical Endocrinology & Metabolism* 2001; 86: 1738–45.

Ceda, G., Valenti, G., Butterini, U., Hoffman, A.R. "Diminished Pituitary Response to Growth Hormone-Releasing Factor in Aging Male Rats." Endocrinology 1986; 118: 2109–14.

Chapman, I.M., Hartman, M.L., Pezzoli, S.S., Harrell, F.E. Jr., Hintz, R.L., Alberti, K.G., Thorner, M.O. "Effect of Aging on the Sensitivity of Growth Hormone Secretion to Insulin-Like Growth Factor-I Negative Feedback." *The Journal of Clinical Endocrinology & Metabolism* 1997; 82: 2996–3004.

Christiansen, J.S., et al. "Effects of Growth Hormone on Body Composition in Adults." *Hormone Research* 1990; 33 (suppl 4): 61–4.

Christopher, M., Hew, F.L., Oakley, M., Rantzau, C., Alford, F. "Defects of Insulin Action and Skeletal Muscle Glucose Metabolism in Growth Hormone-Deficient Adults Persist after 24 Months of Recombinant Human Growth Hormone Therapy." *The Journal of Clinical Endocrinology & Metabolism* 1998; 83: 1668–1681.

Cleare, A.J., Sookdeo, S.S., Jones, J., O'Keane, V., Miell, J.P. "Integrity of the growth hormone/insulin-like growth factor system is maintained in patients with chronic fatigue syndrome." *The Journal of Clinical Endocrinology & Metabolism* 2000; 85: 1433–9.

Clemmons, D.R. & Underwood, L. E. "Growth Hormone as a Potential Adjunctive Therapy for Weight Loss," in Underwood, L.E. (ed.) *Human Growth Hormone: Progresses and Challenges.* New York: Marcel Dekker, Inc., 1986.

Cohen, P., Clemmons, D.R., Rosenfeld R.G. "Does the GH–IGF axis play a role in cancer pathogenesis?" *Growth Horm IGF Res* 2000; 10: 297–305. (Review.)

Corpas, E. S., et al. "Human Growth Hormone and Human Aging." *Endocrine Reviews* 1993; 14: 20–39.

Crist, D.M., et al. "Exogenous Growth Hormone Treatment Alters Body Composition and Increases Natural Killer Cell Activity in Women with Impaired Endogenous Growth Hormone Secretion." *Metabolism* 1987; 36:1115–7.

Crist, D.M., Peake, G.T., Egan, P.A., Waters, D.L., "Body Composition Response to Exogenous GH during Training in Highly Conditioned Adults." *Journal of Applied Physiology* 1988; 65: 579–584.

Cuneo R.C., et al. "Cardiovascular Effects of Growth Hormone Treatment in Growth-Hormone-Deficient Adults: Stimulation of the Renin-Aldosterone System." *Clinical Science* 1991; 81: 587–92.

Davila, D.R., et al. "Role of Growth Hormone in Regulating T–Dependent Immune Events in Aged, Nude, and Transgenic Rodents." *Journal of neuroscience Research* 1987; 18:108–16.

de Zegher, F., Francois, I., van Helvoirt, M., Van den Berghe, G. "Clinical review 89: Small as fetus and short as child: from endogenous to exogenous growth hormone." *The Journal of Clinical Endocrinology & Metabolism* 1997; 82: 2021–2026.

Degerblad M., et al. "Reduced Bone Mineral Density in Adults with Growth Hormone Deficiency: Increased Bone Turnover During 12 Months of GH Substitution Therapy." *European Journal of Endocrinology* 1995; 133: 180–8.

Deijen, J.B., et al. "Cognitive Impairments and Mood Disturbances in Growth Hormone Deficient Men." *Psychoneuroendocrinology* 1996; 21: 313–22.

Donaldson, Thomas, Ph.D. *Life Extension Report* April 1991; vol. 11, no. 4, p. 32.

Dr. Julian Whitaker's Health & Healing, July 1995; vol. 5, no. 7, pp. 4–5.

Drake, W.M., Howell, S.J., Monson, J.P., Shalet, S.M. "Optimizing gh therapy in adults and children." *Endocrine Reviews* 2001; 22: 425–50. (Review.)

Edmondson, S.R., Russo, V.C., McFarlane, A.C., Wraight, C.J., Werther, G.A. "Interactions between Growth Hormone, Insulin-Like Growth Factor I, and Basic Fibroblast Growth Factor in Melanocyte Growth." *The Journal of Clinical Endocrinology & Metabolism* 1999; 84:1638–1644.

Eriksen E.F., et al. "Growth Hormone and Insulin-like Growth Factors as Anabolic Therapies for Osteoporosis." *Hormone Research (Switzerland)* 1993; 40: 95–8.

Ezzat, S., Fear, S., Gaillard, R.C., Gayle, C., Landy, H., Marcovitz, S., Mattioni, T., Nussey, S., Rees, A., Svanberg, E., "Gender-specific responses of lean body composition and non-gender-specific cardiac function improvement after GH replacement in GH-deficient adults," *J. Clin. Endocrinol. Metab.*, June 2002; 87(6): 2725–33.

Falanga, Vincent. "Growth Factors and Wound Healing." *Dermatologic Clinics* 1993; 11: 66.

Fazio, S. "Preliminary Study of Growth Hormone in the Treatment of Dilated Cardiomyopathy." *New England Journal of Medicine* 1996; 334: 809–814; comment: 856–7.

Fisker, S., Kristensen, K., Rosenfalck, A.M., Pedersen, S.B., Ebdrup, L., Richelsen, B., Hilsted, J., Sandahl, J., Christiansen, J.S., Jørgensen, J.O. "Gene Expression of a Truncated and the Full–Length Growth Hormone (GH) Receptor in Subcutaneous Fat and Skeletal Muscle in GH–Deficient Adults: Impact of GH Treatment." *The Journal of Clinical Endocrinology & Metabolism* 2001; 86: 792–796.

Frustaci, A., et al. "Reversible Dilated Cardiomyopathy Due to Growth Hormone Deficiency." *American Journal of Clinical Pathology* 1992; 97:503–511.

Fuh, V.L., Bach, M.A. "Growth hormone secretagogues: Mechanism of action and use in aging." *Growth Horm IGF Res* 1998; 8: 13–20.

Gibney, J., Wallace, J.D., Spinks, T., Schnorr, L., Ranicar, A., Cuneo, R.C., Lockhart, S., Burnand, K.G., Salomon, F., Sonksen, P.H., Russell-Jones, D. "The effects of 10 years of recombinant human growth hormone (GH) in adult GH-deficient patients." *The Journal of Clinical Endocrinology & Metabolism* 1999; 84: 2596–602.

Gusenoff, J.A., Harman, S.M., Veldhuis, J.D., Jayme, J.J., St Clair, C., Munzer, T., Christmas, C., O'Connor, K.G., Stevens, T.E., Bellantoni, M.F., Pabst, K., Blackman, M.R. "Cortisol and GH secretory dynamics, and their interrelationships, in healthy aged women and men." *Am J Physiol Endocrinol Metab* 2001; 280: E616–25.

Harvey, S., Scanes, C.G., and Daughaday, W.H. *Growth Hormone.* Boca Raton: CRC Press, 1995.

Hata, I., Shigematsu, Y., Ohshima, Y., Tsukahara, H., Fujisawa, K., Hiraoka, M., Nakamura, H., Masutani, H., Yodoi, J., Kotsuji, F., Sudo, M., Mayumi, M. "Involvement of thioredoxin in the regulation of growth hormone secretion in rat pituitary cell cultures." *Am J Physiol Endocrinol Metab* 2001; 281: E269–74.

Hataya, Y., Akamizu, T., Takaya, K., Kanamoto, N., Ariyasu, H., Saijo, M., Moriyama, K., Shimatsu, A., Kojima, M., Kangawa, K., Nakao, K. "A low dose of ghrelin stimulates growth hormone (GH) release synergistically with GH-releasing hormone in humans." *The Journal of Clinical Endocrinology & Metabolism* 2001; 86: 4552.

Hattori, N., Saito, T., Yagyu, T., Jiang, B.H., Kitagawa, K., Inagaki, C. "GH, GH Receptor, GH Secretagogue Receptor, and Ghrelin Expression in Human T Cells, B Cells, and Neutrophils." *The Journal of Clinical Endocrinology & Metabolism* 2001; 86: 4284–4291.

Hayes, V.Y., Urban, R.J., Jiang, J., Marcell, T.J., Helgeson, K., Mauras, N. "Recombinant Human Growth Hormone and Recombinant Human Insulin-like Growth Factor I Diminish the Catabolic Effects of Hypogonadism in Man: Metabolic and Molecular Effects." *The Journal of Clinical Endocrinology & Metabolism* 2001; 86: 2211–2219.

Hedin, L., Olsson, B., Diczfalusy, M., Flyg, C., Petersson, A.S., Rosberg, S., Albertsson-Wikland, K. "Intranasal administration of human growth hormone (hGH) in combination with a membrane permeation enhancer in patients with GH deficiency: A pharmacokinetic study." *J Clin Endocrinol Metab* 1993; 76: 962–7.

Heffernan, M.A., Jiang, W.J., Thorburn, A.W., Ng, F.M. "Effects of oral administration of a synthetic fragment of human growth hormone on lipid metabolism." *Am J Physiol Endocrinol Metab* 2000; 279: E501–7.

Hernberg-Stahl, E., Luger, A., Abs, R., Bengtsson, B.A., Feldt-Rasmussen, U., Wilton, P., Westberg, B., Monson, J.P.; KIMS International Board, KIMS Study Group, Pharmacia International Metabolic Database, "Healthcare consumption decreases in parallel with improvements in quality of life during GH replacement in hypopituitary adults with GH deficiency," *J. Clin. Endocrinol. Metab.*, November 2001; 86(11): 5277–81.

Ho, K.Y., Weussberger, A.J. "The Antinatriuretic Action of Biosynthetic Human Growth Hormone in Man Involves Activation of the Renin-Angiotensin System." *Metabolism* 1990; 39:133–7.

Howard, Ben. "Growing younger." *Longevity* October 1992; p. 41.

Hull, K.L., Harvey, S. "Growth hormone resistance: Clinical states and animal models." *Journal of Endocrinology* 1999; 163:165–72. (Review.)

Hull, K.L., Harvey, S. "Growth hormone: roles in female reproduction. *Journal of Endocrinology* 2001; 168: 1–23. (Review.)

Hymer, W.C., Kraemer, W.J., Nindl, B.C., Marx, J.O., Benson, D.E., Welsch, J.R., Mazzetti, S.A., Volek, J.S., Deaver, D.R. "Characteristics of circulating growth hormone in women after acute heavy resistance exercise." *Am J Physiol Endocrinol Metab* 2001; 281: E878–87.

Iida, K., Takahashi, Y., Kaji, H., Takahashi, M.O., Okimura, Y., Nose, O., Abe, H., Chihara, K. "Functional Characterization of Truncated Growth Hormone (GH) Receptor-(1–277) Causing Partial GH Insensitivity Syndrome with High GH-Binding Protein." *The Journal of Clinical Endocrinology & Metabolism* 1999; 84: 1011–1016.

Inzucchi, S.E., Robbins, R.J. "Effects of Growth Hormone on Human Bone Biology." *Journal of Clinical Endocrinology and Metabolism* 1994; 79: 691–94.

Ishikawa, M., Nimura, A., Horikawa, R., Katsumata, N., Arisaka, O., Wada, M., Honjo, M., Tanaka, T. "A Novel Specific Bioassay for Serum Human Growth Hormone." *The Journal of Clinical Endocrinology & Metabolism* 2000; 85: 4274–4279.

Janssen, Y.J., Hamdy, N.A., Frolich, M., Roelfsema, F. "Skeletal effects of two years of treatment with low physiological doses of recombinant human growth hormone (GH) in patients with adult–onset GH deficiency." *The Journal of Clinical Endocrinology & Metabolism* 1998; 83: 2143–8.

Jeanrenaud, B., Rohner-Jeanrenaud, F. "Effects of neuropeptides and leptin on nutrient partitioning: Dysregulations in obesity." *Annu Rev Med* 2001; 52:339–51. (Review.)

Joberg, M., Salazar, T., Espinosa, C., Dagnino, A., Avila, A., Eggers, M., Cassorla, F., Carvallo, P., Mericq, M.V. "Study of GH Sensitivity in Chilean Patients with Idiopathic Short Stature." *The Journal of Clinical Endocrinology & Metabolism* 2001; 86: 4375–4381

Johannsson, G., Svensson, J., Bengtsson, B.A. "Growth hormone and ageing." *Growth Horm IGF Res.* 2000; 10 (Suppl B): S25–30

Johannsson, G., et al. "Two Years of Growth Hormone (GH) Treatment Increase Isometric and Isokinetic Muscle Strength in GH–Deficient Adults." *Journal of Clinical Endocrinology and Metabolism* 1997; 82: 2877–84.

Johannsson, G., et al. "Growth Hormone Treatment of Abdominally Obese Men Reduces Abdominal Fat Mass, Improves Glucose and Lipoprotein Metabolism and Reduces Diastolic Blood Pressure." *Journal of Clinical Endocrinology and Metabolism* 1997; 82: 727–34.

Johannsson, G., et al. "Two Years of Growth Hormone Treatment Increases Bone Mineral Content and Density in Hypopituitary Patients with Adult-Onset Growth Hormone Deficiency." *J Clin Endocrinol Metab* Aug 1996; 81(8): 2865-73.

Johannsson, J.O., et al. "Treatment of Growth Hormone-Deficient Adults with Recombinant Human Growth hormone Increases the Concentration of Growth Hormone in the Cerebrospinal Fluids and Affects Neurotransmitters." *Neuroendocrinology* 1995; 61: 57–66.

Jorgensen, J.O.L. "Three Years of Growth Hormone Treatment in Growth Hormone-Deficient Adults: Near Normalization of Body Composition and Physical Performance." *European Journal of Endocrinology* 1994; 130: 224–8.

Jorgensen, J.O.L. "Adult Growth Hormone Deficiency." *Hormone Research* 1994; 42: 235–241.

Journal of the American Medical Association March 18, 1988; vol. 259, no. 11, p. 1703 (3).

Kahan, Z., Arencibia, J.M., Csernus, V.J., Groot, K., Kineman, R.D., Robinson, W.R., Schally, A.V. "Expression of growth hormone-releasing hormone (GHRH) messenger ribonucleic acid and the presence of biologically active GHRH in human breast, endometrial, and ovarian cancers." *The Journal of Clinical Endocrinology & Metabolism* 1999; 84: 582–9.

Kanaley, J.A., Weatherup-Dentes, M.M., Jaynes, E.B., Hartman, M.L. "Obesity attenuates the growth hormone response to exercise." *Journal of Clinical Endocrinology & Metabolism* 1999; 84: 3156–61.

Kelley, K., et al. "Gh3 Pituitary Adenoma Cells Can Reverse Thymic Aging in Rats." *Proceedings of the National Academy of Sciences* 1986; vol. 83, p. 5663, cited in "Longevity: A Fresh Shot of Life." *Omni* July 1987; vol. 1, no. 9, p. 85.

Khan, A.S., Lynch, C.D., Sane, D.C., Willingham, M.C., Sonntag, W.E. "Growth hormone increases regional coronary blood flow and capillary density in aged rats." *The Journals of Gerontology Series A: Biological Sciences and Medical Sciences* 2001; 56: B364–71.

Khansari, D.N., Gustad, T. "Effects of Long-Term, Low-Dose Growth Hormone Therapy on Immune Function and Life Expectancy of Mice." *Mechanisms of Ageing and Development* 1991; 57: 87–100.

Khorram, O., Garthwaite, M., Golos, T. "The influence of aging and sex hormones on expression of growth hormone–releasing hormone in the human immune system." *The Journal of Clinical Endocrinology & Metabolism* 2001; 86: 3157–61.

Khorram, O., Yeung, M., Vu, L., Yen, S.S. "Effects of [norleucine27] growth hormone-releasing hormone (GHRH) (1–29)- NH2 administration on the immune system of aging men and women." *The Journal of Clinical Endocrinology & Metabolism* 1997; 82: 3590–3596.

Kindblom, J.M., Göthe, S., Forrest, D., Törnell, J., Vennström, B., Ohlsson, C. "Growth hormone substitution reverses the growth phenotype but not the defective ossification in the thyroid hormone receptor a1–/–b–/– mice." *Journal of Endocrinology* 2001; 171: 15–22.

Klatz, R.M. (ed). *Anti-Aging Medical Therapeutics,* Vol 2. New York: Mary Ann Liebert Publishers, Inc., 1997.

Koller, E.A., Green, L., Gertner, J.M., Bost, M., Malozowski, S.N. "Retinal changes mimicking diabetic retinopathy in two nondiabetic, growth hormone-treated patients." *The Journal of Clinical Endocrinology & Metabolism* 1998; 83: 2380–3.

Korbonits, M., Kaltsas, G., Perry, L.A., Putignano, P., Grossman, A.B., Besser, G.M., Trainer, P.J. "The growth hormone secretagogue hexarelin stimulates the hypothalamo–pituitary–adrenal axis via arginine vasopressin." *Journal of Clinical Endocrinology and Metabolism* 1999; 84: 2489–95.

Lange, K.H., Isaksson, F., Juul, A., Rasmussen, M.H., Bulow, J., Kjaer, M. "Growth hormone enhances effects of endurance training on oxidative muscle metabolism in elderly women." *Am J Physiol Endocrinol Metab* 2000; 279: E989–96.

Lange, K.H., Lorentsen, J., Isaksson, F., Juul, A., Rasmussen, M.H., Christensen, N.J., Bulow, J.B., Kjaer, M. "Endurance training and GH administration in elderly women: effects on abdominal adipose tissue lipolysis." *Am J Physiol Endocrinol Metab* 2001; 280: E886–97.

Laursen, T., Gravholt, C.H., Heickendorff, L., Drustrup, J., Kappelgaard, A.M., Jorgensen, J.O., Christiansen, J.S. "Long-term effects of continuous subcutaneous infusion versus daily subcutaneous injections of growth hormone (GH) on the insulin-like growth factor system, insulin sensitivity, body composition, and bone and lipoprotein metabolism in GH–deficient adults." *The Journal of Clinical Endocrinology & Metabolism* 2001; 86: 1222–8.

Lawren, "The Hormone that Makes Your Body 20 Years Younger." *Longevity,* October 1990; p. 34.

Le Roith, D., Bondy, C., Yakar, S., Liu, J.L., Butler, A. "The somatomedin hypothesis: 2001." *Endocr Rev* 2001; 22: 53–74. (Review.)

Leal-Cerro, A., Povedano, J., Astorga, R., Gonzalez, M., Silva, H., Garcia-Pesquera, F., Casanueva, F.F., Dieguez, C. "The growth hormone (GH)-releasing hormone-GH-insulin-like growth factor-1 axis in patients with fibromyalgia syndrome." *The Journal of Clinical Endocrinology & Metabolism* 1999; 84: 3378–81.

Lehrman, Sally. "The Fountain of Youth?"*Harvard Health Letter* June 1992; vol. 17, no. 8, p. 1 (3).

Lewin, D.L. "Growth Hormone and Age: Something to Sleep on?" *Journal of NIH Research* 1993; 7:34–35.

Libby, R. "The Glow of Desire." *Journal of Longevity Research* 1996; 1.

Loh. E., Swain, J.L. "Growth Hormone for Heart Failure—Cause for Cautious Optimism." *New England Journal of Medicine* 1996; 334: 856–857.

Maccario, M., Tassone, F., Gianotti, L., Lanfranco, F., Grottoli, S., Arvat, E., Muller, E.E., Ghigo, E. "Effects of recombinant human insulin-like growth factor I administration on the growth hormone (gh) response to GH-releasing hormone in obesity." *The Journal of Clinical Endocrinology & Metabolism* 2001; 86: 167–71.

MacColl, G.S., Novo, F.J., Marshall, N.J., Waters, M., Goldspink, G., Bouloux, P.M. "Optimisation of growth hormone production by muscle cells using plasmid DNA." *Journal of Endocrinology* 2000; 165: 329–36.

Maheshwari, H., Sharma, L., Baumann, G. "Decline of plasma growth hormone binding protein in old age." *The Journal of Clinical Endocrinology & Metabolism* 1996; 81: 995–7.

Marcus R., Butterfield, G., Holloway, L., et al. "Effects of Short–Term Administration of Recombinant Human Growth Hormone to Elderly People." *J Clin Endocrinol Metab* 1990; 519–27.

Marcus, R., Hoffman, A.R. "Growth hormone as therapy for older men and women." *Annu Rev Pharmacol Toxicol* 1998; 38: 45–61. (Review.)

Merimee, et al. "Arginine Initiated Release of Growth Hormone: Factors Modifying the Response in Normal Men." *New England Journal of Medicine* 1969; 280 (26): 1434–38.

Mol, J.A., Henzen-Logmans, S.C., Hageman, P., Misdorp, W., Blankenstein, M.A., Rijnberk, A. "Expression of the gene encoding growth hormone in the human mammary gland." *The Journal of Clinical Endocrinology & Metabolism* 1995; 80: 3094–6.

Moussa, T.A., Youdim, B.H., Hochberg, Z. "Does Serum Growth Hormone (GH) Binding Protein Reflect Human GH Receptor Function?" *The Journal of Clinical Endocrinology & Metabolism* 2000; 85: 927–932.

Murray, R.D., Wieringa, G.E., Lissett, C.A., Darzy, K.H., Smethurst, L.E., Shalet, S.M., "Low-dose GH replacement improves the adverse lipid profile associated with the adult GH deficiency syndrome," *Clin. Endocrinol. (Oxf.)*, April 2002; 56(4):525–32.

Netter F. *Endocrine System,* The Ciba Collection, vol. 4.

Obuobie, K., Mullik, V., Jones, C., John, R., Rees, A.E., Davies, J.S., Scanlon, M.F., Lazarus, J.H. "McCune-Albright syndrome: Growth hormone dynamics in pregnancy." *The Journal of Clinical Endocrinology & Metabolism* 2001; 86: 2456–8.

Olivecrona, H., Ericsson, S., Angelin B. "Growth hormone treatment does not alter biliary lipid metabolism in healthy adult men." *The Journal of Clinical Endocrinology & Metabolism* 1995; 80: 1113–7.

Olivecrona, H., Hilding, A., Ekstrom, C., Barle, H., Nyberg, B., Moller, C., Delhanty, P.J., Baxter, R.C., Angelin, B., Ekstrom, T.J., Tally, M. "Acute and Short-Term Effects of Growth Hormone on Insulin-like Growth Factors and Their Binding Proteins: Serum Levels and Hepatic Messenger Ribonucleic Acid Responses in Humans." *The Journal of Clinical Endocrinology & Metabolism* 1999; 84: 553–560.

Orme, S.M. "Comparison of Measures of Body Composition in a Trial of Low Dose Growth Hormone Replacement Therapy." *Clinical Endocrinology* 1992; 37:453–9.

Ottosson, M., et al. "Growth Hormone Inhibits Lipoprotein Lipase Activity in Human Adipose Tissue." *Journal of Clinical Endocrinology and Metabolism* 1995; 80: 936–41.

Papotti, M., Ghe, C., Cassoni, P., Catapano, F., Deghenghi, R., Ghigo, E., Muccioli, G. "Growth hormone secretagogue binding sites in peripheral human tissues." *The Journal of Clinical Endocrinology & Metabolism* 2000; 85: 3803–7.

Pfeifer, M., Verhovec, R., Zizek, B., Prezelj, J., Poredos, P., Clayton, R.N. "Growth hormone (GH) treatment reverses early atherosclerotic changes in GH-deficient adults." *The Journal of Clinical Endocrinology & Metabolism* 1999; 84: 453–7.

Pollak, M. "The question of a link between insulin-like growth factor physiology and neoplasia." *Growth Horm IGF Res* 2000; 10 (Suppl B): S21–4.

Richesen, B., et al. "Growth Hormone Treatment of Obese Women for 5 Weeks: Effect on Body

Composition and Adipose Tissue LPL Activity." *American Journal of Physiology* 1994; 226 (2 Pt 1): E211–6.

Rosen, C.J., Conover, C. "Growth hormone/insulin-like growth factor–I axis in aging: a summary of a National Institutes of Aging-Sponsored Symposium." *The Journal of Clinical Endocrinology & Metabolism* 1997; 82: 3919–3922.

Rosen, T., Bengtsson, B.A. "Premature Mortality Due to Cardiovascular Disease in Hypopituitarism." *Lancet* 1990; 336: 285–8.

Rosen, T., et al. "Consequences of Growth Hormone Deficiency in Adults, and Effects of Growth Hormone Replacement Therapy." *Acta Paediatr* 1994; 399 (Suppl): 21–4.

Rosen, T., et al. "Decreased Psychological Well-being in Adult Patients with Growth Hormone Deficiency." *Clinical Endocrinology* 1994; 40: 111–6.

Rosen, T., et al. "Increased Body Fat Mass and Decreased Extracellular Fluid Vol. in Adults with Growth Hormone Deficiency." *Clinical Endocrinology* 1993; 38: 63–71.

Rosen. T., et al. "Cardiovascular Risk Factors in Adult Patients with Growth Hormone Deficiency." *Acta Endocrinologicat* 1993; 129: 195–200.

Rosenfalck, A.M., Maghsoudi, S., Fisker, S., Jorgensen, J.O., Christiansen, J.S., Hilsted, J., Volund, A.A., Madsbad, S. "The effect of 30 months of low-dose replacement therapy with recombinant human growth hormone (rhGH) on insulin and C-peptide kinetics, insulin secretion, insulin sensitivity, glucose effectiveness, and body composition in GH–deficient adults." *The Journal of Clinical Endocrinology & Metabolism* 2000; 85: 4173–81.

Rudling, M., et al. "Importance of Growth Hormone for the Induction of Hepatic Low Density Lipoprotein Receptors." *Proceedings of the National Academy of Sciences of the USA* 1992; 89: 6983–7.

Rudman, D. "Impaired Growth Hormone Secretion in the Adult Population: Relation to Age and Adiposity." *Journal of Clinical Investigation* 1981; 67:1361–9.

Rudman, D., et al. "Relations of Endogenous Anabolic Hormones and Physical Activity to Bone Mineral Density and Lean Body Mass in Elderly Men." *Clinical Endocrinology* 1994; 40: 653–61.

Rudman, D., *"Growth Hormone, Body Composition, and Aging."* *Journal of the American Geriatric Society* 1985; 33: 800–7.

Rudman, D., A.G. Feller, H.S. Nograj, et al. "Effects of Human Growth Hormone in Men Over 60 Years old." *New England Journal of Medicine* 1990; 323: 1–6.

Russell-Aulet, M., Jaffe, C.A., Demott-Friberg, R., Barkan, A.L. "In vivo semiquantification of hypothalamic growth hormone-releasing hormone (GHRH) output in humans: evidence for relative GHRH deficiency in aging." *Journal of Clinical Endocrinology and Metabolism* 1999; 84: 3490–7.

Russell-Jones, D.L. "The Effects of Growth Hormone on Protein Metabolism in Adult Growth Hormone Deficient Patients." *Clinical Endocrinology* 1993; 38: 427–31.

Salomon, F., R.C. Cuneo, R. Hesp, P.H. Sonksen, "The Effects of Treatment with Recombinant Human Growth Hormone on Body Composition and Metabolism in Adults with Growth Hormone Deficiency." *New England Journal of Medicine* 1989; 321: 1797–1803.

Sartorio, A., et al. "Growth Hormone Treatment in Adults with Childhood Onset Growth Hormone Deficiency: Effects on Psychological Capabilities." *Hormone Research* 1995; 44: 6–11.

Shalet, S.M., "Growth hormone therapy for adult growth hormone deficiency." *Int. J. Clin. Pract.*, March 1998; 52(2): 108–11.

Shetty. K.R., Duthie, E.H. "Anterior Pituitary Function and Growth Hormone Use in the Elderly." *Endocrine Aspects of Aging* 1995; 24: 213–231.

Simpson, H.L., Umpleby, A.M., Russell-Jones, D.L. "Insulin-like growth factor-I and diabetes." *Growth Horm IGF Res* 1998; 8: 83–95. (Review.)

Snyder, D., Underwood, L.D., Clemmons, D.R. "Persistent Lipolytic Effect of Exogenous Growth Hormone during Caloric Restriction." *American Journal of Medicine* 1995; 98: 129–34.

Sonksen, P.H. "Replacement Therapy in Hypothalamo-Pituitary Insufficiency After Childhood: Management in the Adult." *Hormone Research* 1990; 33 (Suppl. 4): 45–51.

Sonntag, W.E., et al. "Moderate Caloric Restriction Alters the Subcellular Distribution of Somatostatin mRNA and Increases Growth Hormone Pulse Amplitude in Aged Animals." *Neuroendocrinology* 1995; 61: 601–8.

Span, J.P., Pieters, G.F., Sweep, F.G., Hermus, A.R., Smals, A.G. "Gender Differences in rhGH–Induced Changes in Body Composition in GH-Deficient Adults." *The Journal of Clinical Endocrinology & Metabolism* 2001; 86: 4161–4165.

Stein, T.P., Schluter, M.D., Moldawer, L.L. "Endocrine relationships during human spaceflight." *Am J Physiol* 2001; 276: E155–62.

Suarez, M., et al., "Biometric analysis of controlled clinical study for growth factor formulation on multiple parameters of aging-related dysfunctions," High Tech Research Institute, 2002.

Sullivan, D.H., Carter, W.J., Warr, W.R., Williams, L.H. "Side effects resulting from the use of growth hormone and insulin-like growth factor-I as combined therapy to frail elderly patients." *The Journals of Gerontology Series A: Biological Sciences and Medical Sciences* 1998; 53: M183–7.

Terry, L.C., Chein, E. "Effects of Human Growth Hormone Administration (Low Dose–High Frequency) in 202 Patients." Personal communication to Dr. Ronald Klatz, January 1999.

Thompson, J.L., Butterfield, G.E., Gylfadottir, U.K., Yesavage, J., Marcus, R., Hintz, R.L., Pearman, A., Hoffman, A.R. "Effects of human growth hormone, insulin-like growth factor I, and diet and exercise on body composition of obese postmenopausal women." *The Journal of Clinical Endocrinology & Metabolism* 1998; 83: 1477–84.

Thorner, M.O. "The discovery of growth hormone-releasing hormone." *The Journal of Clinical Endocrinology & Metabolism* 1999; 84: 4671–6.

Thornton, P.L., Ingram, R.L., Sonntag, W.E. "Chronic [D–Ala2]-growth hormone-releasing hormone administration attenuates age-related deficits in spatial memory." *Journals of Gerontology Series A: Biological Sciences and Medical Sciences* 2000; 55: B106–12.

Tian, Z.G. "Recombinant Human Growth Hormone Promotes Hematopoietic Reconstitution After Syngeneic Bone Marrow Transplantation in Mice." *Stem Cells* 1998; 16: 193–199.

Toogood, A.A., O'Neill, P.A., Shalet, S.M. "Beyond the somatopause: growth hormone deficiency in adults over the age of 60 years." *The Journal of Clinical Endocrinology & Metabolism* 1996; 81: 460–5.

van Neck, J.W., Dits, N.F., Cingel, V., Hoppenbrouwers, I.A., Drop, S.L., Flyvbjerg, A. "Dose-response effects of a new growth hormone receptor antagonist (B2036–PEG) on circulating, hepatic and renal expression of the growth hormone/insulin-like growth factor system in adult mice." *Journal of Endocrinology* 2000; 167: 295–303.

Weindruch, R. "Caloric Restriction and Aging." *Scientific American* 1996; 274: 46–52.

Weiss, Rick, "A Shot at Youth," *Health* Nov–Dec 1993; vol. 7, no. 7, p. 38 (10).

Whitehead, H.M., et al. "Growth Hormone Treatment of Adults with Growth Hormone Deficiency: Results of a 13-month Placebo Controlled Cross-over Study." *Clinical Endocrinology* 1992; 36: 45–52.

Wolthers, T., Groftne, T., Moller, N., Christiansen, J.S., Orskov, H., Weeke, J., Jorgensen, J.O. "Calorigenic effects of growth hormone: the role of thyroid hormones." *The Journal of Clinical Endocrinology & Metabolism* 1996; 81: 1416–9.

Zarkesh–Esfahani, S.H., Kolstad, O., Metcalfe, R.A., Watson, P.F., Von Laue, S., Walters, S., Revhaug, A., Weetman, A.P., Ross, R.J.M. "High-Dose Growth Hormone Does Not Affect Proinflammatory Cytokine (Tumor Necrosis Factor, Interleukin-6, and Interferon) Release from Activated Peripheral Blood Mononuclear Cells or after Minimal to Moderate Surgical Stress." *The Journal of Clinical Endocrinology & Metabolism* 2000; 85: 3383–3390.

Zhang, X.J., Chinkes, D.L., Wolf, S.E., Wolfe, R.R. "Insulin but not growth hormone stimulates protein anabolism in skin wound and muscle." *Am J Physiol* 1999; 276:E712–20.

CHAPTER 5

Alberg, A.J., Gordon, G.B., Genkinger, J.M., Hoffman, S.C., Selvin, E., Comstock, G.W., Helzlsouer, K.J., "Serum dehydroepiandrosterone and dehydroepiandrosterone sulfate and risk of melanoma or squamous cell carcinoma of the skin," *Anticancer Res.*, November–December 2001; 21(6A): 4051–4.

Allen, J.D., McLung, J., Nelson, A.G., Welsch, M., "Ginseng supplementation does not enhance healthy young adults' peak aerobic exercise performance," *J. Am. Coll. Nutr.*, 1998; 17: 462–6.

Ben-Nathan, D., et al. "Protection by Dehydroepiandrosterone in Mice Infected with Viral Encephalitis." *Archives of Virology* 1991; 120: 263–271.

Brody, Jane. "Restoring Ebbing Hormones May Slow Aging." *New York Times* July 18, 1995; p. C3.

Coleman, D.L., et al. "Effect of Genetic Background on the Therapeutic Effects of Dehydroepiandrosterone (DHEA) in Diabetes-Obesity Mutants in Aged Normal Mice." *Diabetes* 1984; 33: 26.

Coleman, D.L., et al. "Therapeutic Effects of Dehydroepiandrosterone (DHEA) in Diabetic Mice." *Diabetes* 1982; 31: 830–833.

Cranton, Elmer, M.D., and James P. Frackelton, M.D., "Take Control of Your Aging." *Alternative Medicine Digest* Issue 8, pp. 23–28.

Cryer, Sibyl. "New Music and Stress Reduction Technique Increase Anti-Aging Hormone—DHEA—Study Says." Institute of Heartmath July 19, 1995; pp. 1–2.

"DHEA Replacement Therapy." *Life Extension Report* September 1993; vol. 13, no. 9, p. 67.

Fettner, Ann Giudici, "DHEA Gets Respect." *Harvard Health Letter* July 1994; vol. 19. no. 9.

Gaby, Alan R., M.D. "DHEA: The Hormone That Does It All." *Holistic Medicine* Spring 1993; pp. 19–23.

Green, J.E., Shibata, M.A., Shibata, E., Moon, R.C., Anver, M.R., Kelloff, G., Lubet, R., "2-difluoromethylornithine and dehydroepiandrosterone inhibit mammary tumor progression but not mammary or prostate tumor initiation in C3(1)/SV40 T/t-antigen transgenic mice," *Cancer Res.*, October 15, 2001; 61(20): 7449–55.

Life Extension Events. "DHEA Comes to the Mainstream." *Life Extension Magazine* September 1995; pp. 1–4.

Life Extension Events. "DHEA Replacement Therapy." *Life Extension Magazine* March 1, 1995; p. 4.

Life Extension Foundation. *The Physician's Guide to Life Extension Drugs* 1994 Edition; pp. 46–55.

Morales, A, J., et al. "Effects of Replacement Dose of Dehydroepiandrosterone in Men and Women of Advancing Age." *Journal of Clinical Endocrinology and Metabolism* 1994; 78: 1360-66.

Nasman, R., et al. "Serum dehydroepiandrosterone sulfate in Alzheimer's Disease and in Multi-Infarct Dementia." *Biological Psychiatry* 1991; 30:684–690.

Pawlikowski, M., Kolomecka, M., Wojtczak, A., Karasek, M., "Effects of six months melatonin treatment on sleep quality and serum concentrations of estradiol, cortisol, dehydroepiandrosterone sulfate, and somatomedin C in elderly women," *Neuroendocrinol. Lett.*, April 2002; 23 (suppl. 1): 17–9.

Pugh, T.D., Oberley, T.D., Weindruch, R., "Dietary intervention at middle age: caloric restriction but not dehydroepiandrosterone sulfate increases lifespan and lifetime cancer incidence in mice," *Cancer Res.*, April 1, 1999; 59(7): 1642–8.

Racchi, M., Govoni, S., Solerte, S.B., Galli, C.L., Corsini, E., "Dehydroepiandrosterone and the relationship with aging and memory: a possible link with protein kinase C functional machinery," *Brain Res. Rev.*, November 2001; 37(1–3): 287–93.

Rao, K.V., Johnson, W.D., Bosland, M.C., Lubet, R.A., Steele, V.E., Kelloff, G.J., McCormick, D.L., "Chemoprevention of rat prostate carcinogenesis by early and delayed administration of dehydroepiandrosterone," *Cancer Res.*, July 1, 1999; 59(13): 3084–9.

Regelson, W., and Kalimi, M. "Dehydroepiandrosterone (DHEA)—A Pleiotropic Steroid: How Can One Steroid Do So Much?" *Advances in Anti-Aging Medicine* (vol 1). New York: Mary Ann Liebert Publishers, Inc., 1996.

Regelson, W., et al. "Hormonal Intervention: 'Buffer Hormones' or 'State Dependency': The Role of Dehydroepiandrosterone (DHEA), Thyroid Hormone, Estrogen, and Hypophysectomy in Aging." Annals of the New York Academy of Science, 1988; 521: 260–273.

Reiter, W.J., Schatzl, G., Mark, I., Zeiner, A., Pycha, A., Marberger, M., "Dehydroepiandrosterone in the treatment of erectile dysfunction in patients with different organic etiologies," *Urol. Res.*, August 2001; 29(4): 278–81.

Roberts, E., et al. "Effects of Dehydroepiandrosterone and its Sulfate on Brain Tissue in Culture and on Memory in Mice." *Brain Research* 1987; 406: 357–362.

Sahelian, Ray, M.D., "The Fountain of Youth—The Never Ending Quest." *Muscular Development and Fitness* January 1996; p. 48.

Sunderland, T., et al. "Reduced Plasma Dehydroepiandrosterone Concentration in Alzheimer's Disease." *The Lancet* 1989; 2: 570.

Yen, S.S.C., Morales, A.J., Khorram, O. "Replacement of DHEA in Aging Men and Women, in Bellino, F. et al, (eds), Dehydroepiandrosterone (DHEA) and Aging." *Annals of the New York Academy of Sciences* 1995; 774: 128-142.

CHAPTER 6

Cowley, Geoffrey. "Melatonin." *Newsweek* August 7, 1995; pp. 46–49.

Hughes, Patrick. "The Hormone Whose Time Has Come." *Hippocrates* July-August 1994.

Kane, M.A., Johnson, A., and Robinson, W.A. "Serum Melatonin Levels in Melanoma Patients After Repeated Oral Administration." *Melanoma Research* 1994; 4: 59–65.

Kent, Saul, Life Extension Reports. "How Melatonin Combats Aging." *Life Extension Magazine* December 1995; pp. 10–27.

Lissoni, P., Meregalli, S., Barni, S., and Frigerio, F. "A Randomized Study of Immunotherapy with Low-Dose Subcutaneous Interleukin-2 Plus Melatonin vs. Chemotherapy with Cisplatin and Etoposide as First-Line Therapy for Advanced Non-Small Cell Lung Cancer." *Tumori* 1994; 80: 464–67.

McAuliffe, Kathleen. "Live 20 Years Longer, Look 20 Years Younger." *Longevity* October 1990.

Muller, J., Stone, P., and Braunwald, E. "Circadian Variation in the Frequency of Onset of Acute Myocardial Infarction." *New England Journal of Medicine* 1985; 313–21: 1315–22.

National Institute of Neurological Disorders and Stroke "Brain Basics: Understanding Sleep." http://www.ninds.nih.gov/health_and_medical/pubs/understanding_sleep_brain_ basic_.htm#Insomnia.

Pierpaoli, Walter, and William Regelson, with Carol Colman. *The Melatonin Miracle.* New York: Simon & Schuster, 1995; pp. 29–30.

Reiter, Russell J., Ph.D., and Jo Robinson. *Melatonin.* New York: Bantam Books, 1995; pp. 40–41,62–69; (9), 116–118.

Rozencwaig, R. et al. "The Role of Melatonin and Serotonin in Aging." *Medical Hypotheses* 1987; 23: 337.

Sahelian, Ray, M.D. "Melatonin: The Natural Sleep Medicine." *Total Health* August 1995; vol. 17, no. 4., p. 30 (3).

Sahelian, Ray, M.D. *Melatonin: Nature's Sleeping Pill.* California: Be Happier Press, 1995; pp. 39–48; 77–81; 83–85.

Zhdanova, I.V., Wurtman, R.J., and Schomer, D.L. "Sleep-inducing Effects of Low Doses of Melatonin Ingested in the Evening." *Clinical Pharmacology and Therapeutics* 1995; 57: 552–558.

CHAPTER 7

Asthana, S., Baker, L.D., Craft, S., Stanczyk, F.Z., Veith, R.C., Raskind, M.A., Plymate, S.R., "High-dose estradiol improves cognition for women with AD: results of a randomized study," *Neurology*, August 28, 2001; 57(4): 605–12.

Barrett-Connor E., Grady D., Sashegyi A., et al. "Raloxifene and Cardiovascular Events in Osteoporotic Postmenopausal Women: Four-Year Results From the MORE (Multiple Outcomes of Raloxifene Evaluation) Randomized Trial." *JAMA* 2002; 287(7): 847-857.

Cefalu, W.T., "The use of hormone replacement therapy in postmenopausal women with type 2 diabetes," *J. Womens Health Gend. Based Med.*, April 2001; 10(3): 241–55.

Genant, H.K., Baylink, D.J., and Gallagher, J. C. "Estrogens in the prevention of Osteoporosis in Postmenopausal Women." *American Journal of Obstetrics and Gynecology* 1989; vol. 161, no. 6, 1842, cited in *Office Nurse*, p. 8.

Keough, Carol (editor). "Breast Cancer," in *The Complete Book of Cancer Prevention.* Emmaus, PA: Rodale Press, 1988; pp. 7–15.

Keresztes, P.A. & Dan, A. J. "Estrogen and Cardiovascular Disease." *Cardiovascular Nursing* 1992; vol., 28, no. 1, p. 1, cited in *Office Nurse.*

National Institutes of Health, Osteoporosis and Related Diseases National Resource Center, "Fast Facts on Osteoporosis." (http://www.osteo.org/docs/90.553013828.html)

"NHLBI Stops Trial of Estrogen Plus Progestin Due to Increased Breast Cancer Risk," US Health and Human Services Press Release, July 9, 2002.

Notelovitz, M., "Estrogen Replacement Therapy: Indications, Contraindications, and Agent Selection." *American Journal of Obstetrics and Gynecology* 1989, 161 (6): 1832, cited in Rickert, Barbara, R.N., Ph.D., *Office Nurse,* June 1993; p. 9.

Shah, M.G., Maibach, H.I., "Estrogen and skin: an overview," *Am. J. Clin. Dermatol.,* 2001; 2(3): 143–50.

Stampfer, M.J., and Colditz, G.A., "Estrogen Replacement Thearpy and Coronary Heart Disease: A Quantitative Assessment of the Epidemiologic Evidence." *Preventive Medicine* 1991; vol. 20, no. 1, p. 47, cited in *Office Nurse,* p. 7.

Stampfer, M.J., Colditz, G.A., et al. "Postmenopausal Estrogen Therapy and Cardiovascular Disease: Ten-Year Follow-Up from the Nurses Health Study." *New England Journal of Medicine* 1991; vol. 325, no. 11, p. 756, cited in *Office Nurse,* p. 10.

Voigt, L.F., Weiss, N.S., et al. "Progestagen Supplementation of Exogenous Oestrogens and Risk of Endometrial Cancer." *Lancet* 1991; vol. 338, no. 8762, p. 274, cited in *Office Nurse,* p. 8.

Wallis, Claudia, "The Estrogen Dilemma." *Time* June 26, 1995; pp. 48–53.

Whitaker, Dr. Julian. *Dr. Julian Whitaker's Health & Healing* March 1993; vol. 3, no. 3, p. 3.

Williams, Dr. David G. "The Forgotten Hormone." *Alternatives for the Health Conscious Individual* December 1991; vol. 4, no. 6, pp. 42–51.

Yildirir, A., Aybar, F., Tokgozoglu, L., Yarali, H., Kabakci, G., Bukulmez, O., Sinici, I., Oto, A., "Effects of hormone replacement therapy on plasma homocysteine and C-reactive protein levels," *Gynecol. Obstet. Invest.,* 2002; 53(1): 54–8.

CHAPTER 8

Budenholzer, Brian R., M.D. "Prostate-Specific Antigen Testing to Screen for Prostate Cancer." *The Journal of Family Practice* September 1995; vol. 41, no. 13, pp. 270–76.

Fahim, M.S. "Effect of Panax Ginseng on Testosterone Level and Prostate in Male Rats." *Archives of Andrology* 1982; vol. 8, no. 4, pp. 261–263.

Horton, R. "Benign Prostatic Hyperplasia: A disorder of Androgen Metabolism in the Male." *Journal of the American Geriatrics Society* 1984; vol. 32, no. 5, pp. 380–385.

Keough, C. (ed). *The Complete Book of Cancer Prevention.* Emmaus, PA: Rodale Press, 1988; pp. 131–134.

Matsumoto, Alvin M., "Andropause—Are reduced androgen levels in aging men physiologically important?" *Western Journal of Medicine* November 1993; vol. 159, no. 5, p. 618–20.

Perry, P.J., Yates, W.R., Williams, R.D., Andersen, A.E., MacIndoe, J.H., Lund, B.C., Holman, T.L., "Testosterone therapy in late-life major depression in males," *J. Clin. Psychiatry,* December 2002; 63(12): 1096–101.

Rolf, C., von Eckardstein, S., Koken, U., Nieschlag, E., "Testosterone substitution of hypogonadal men prevents the age-dependent increases in body mass index, body fat and leptin seen in healthy ageing men: results of a cross-sectional study," *Eur. J. Endocrinol.,* April 2002; 146(4): 505–11.

Rudman, Daniel, Drinka, Paul J., Wilson, Charles R., Mattson, Dale E., Scherman, Francis, Cuisinier, Mary C., Schultz, Shiela. "Relations of Endogenous Anabolic Hormones and Physical Activity to Bone Density and Lean Body Mass in Elderly Men." *Clinical Endocrinology* 1994; 40, pp. 653–661.

Skerrett, P.J. "Interest in Growth Hormone May Be Shrinking." *Medical World News* December 1992; vol. 33, no. 12, p. 26.

Tan, R.S., Pu, S.J., "The andropause and memory loss: is there a link between androgen decline and dementia in the aging male?" *Asian J. Androl.*, September 2001; 3(3): 169–74.

Tenover, Joyce S., M.D., Ph.D., "Androgen Administration to Aging Men." *Clinical Andrology* December 1994; 23 (4): 877–87.

Thiebolt, L., Berthelay, S., Berthelay, J. "Preventive and Curative Action of a Bark Extract from an African Plant, Pygeum Africanum, on Experimental Prostatic Adenoma." *Therapie* 1971; vol. 26, no. 3, pp. 575–580.

CHAPTER 9

Balch, James F., M.D., and Balch, Phyllis A., C.N.C. *Prescription for Nutritional Healing.* Garden City Park, New York: Avery Publishing Group, 1990; p. 211.

Dilman, Vladimir, M.D., Ph.D., D.M.Sc., and Ward Dean M.D., et al. *The Neuroendocrine Theory of Aging and Degenerative Disease.* Florida: Center for Bio-gerontology, 1992; pp. 43–92.

Jennings, Isobel W. *Vitamins in Endocrine Metabolism.* Springfield, IL: Charles C Thomas, 1970; p. 80, cited in Langer, p. 33.

Langer, Stephen E., M.D., and James F. Scheer. *Solved: The Riddle of Illness,* 2nd edition. New Canaan, CT: Keats Publishing, Inc., 1995.

Pita, J.C., Jr., et al. "Dimunition of Large Pituitary Tumor After Replacement Therapy for Primary Hypothyroidism." *Neurology,* August 29, 1979; vol. 29, no. 8, pp. 1169–1172; and Guerrero, L.A. and R. Carnovale. "Regression of Pituitary Tumor After Thyroid Replacement in Primary Hypothyroidism." *Southern Medical Journal,* vol. 76, no. 4, April 1983; pp. 529–531, both cited in Langer, p. 141.

Spencer, J.G.C. "The Influence of the Thyroid in Malignant Disease." *British Journal of Cancer* 1954; vol. 8, no. 393, cited in Langer, p. 139.

Wild, Russell, Ed., et al. *The Complete Book of Natural and Medicinal Cures.* Emmaus, PA: Rodale Press, 1994; pp. 605–608.

Williams, Roger J., *Free and Unequal.* Austin, Texas: University of Texas Press, 1953; p. 19, cited in Langer, p. 11.

CHAPTERS 10, 11, 12, 13

American Botanical Council: http://www.herbalgram.org/index.html

Bath Information and Data Services (BIDS): http://www.bids.ac.uk

Drug Info.Net at www.druginfonet.com

Goldman, R., Klatz, R., *Human Growth Factors: Optimizing Your Peak Performance,* 2003. Contact A4M for availability of this title, tel: (773) 528-4333; email: a4m@worldhealth.net.

Goldman, R., Klatz, R., *Oligomeric Proanthocyanidins: Harvesting Nature's Anti-Aging Bounty, 2002.* Contact A4M for availability of this title, tel: (773) 528-4333; email: a4m@worldhealth.net.

Goldman, R., Klatz, R., *Sleep: Essential for Optimal Health,* 2003. Contact A4M for availability of this title, tel: (773) 528-4333; email: a4m@worldhealth.net.

Harvard Health Publications–Harvard Women's Health Watch http://www.health.harvard.edu/medline/Women/W1201b.html

Healthwell, http://www.healthwell.com

Integrated Pharmacology–Page, Curtis, Sutter, Walker, Hoffman. Published by Mosby, 1997

Intelihealth: http://www.intelihealth.com

Medscape: http://www.medscape.com

Medwatch–The FDA Safety Information and Adverse Event Reporting Program http://www.fda.gov/medwatch/index.html

MotherNature.com: http://www.mothernature.com

National Library of Medicine: http://www.nlm.nih.gov

Nutrition Focus: http://www.nutritionfocus.com

PDR Net: http://physician.pdr.net/physician

Phytochemical & Ethnobotanical Database: http://www.ars-grin.gov/duke

PSA Rising Magazine

RxList: http://www.rxlist.com

WholeHealthMd.com: http://www.wholehealthmd.com

CHAPTER 10

Ames, B.N., Elson Schwab, I., Silver, E.A., *Am. J. Clinical Nutrition,* April 2002; 75: 616–658.

"A vitamin a day," reported by Nutraingredients.com, April 3 2003.

Balch, James F., M.D., and Phyllis Balch, C.N.C. *Prescription for Nutritional Healing.* Garden City Park, NY: Avery Publishing Group, 1990; pp. 4–12.

Borek, Carmia, PhD. *Maximize Your Health-Span with Antioxidants.* CT: Keats Publishing, 1995; pp. 13–20.

Brody, J., "Nutrition a key to better health for elderly," *The New York Times,* August 21, 2001.

Cook, A., "Adults urged to take daily multivitamin," *Reuters Health,* June 19, 2002.

"Extra co-enzyme Q_{10} for statin-users?" *Treatmentupdate.* June 2001; 13(2): 4-7.

Coles, Stephen, M.D. "CoQ-10 and Life Span Extension." *Journal of Longevity Research* 1995; vol. 1, no. 5.

Davies, K.J., et al. *Biochemical Biophysical Research Communications* 1982; vol. 107, pp. 1198–1205; cited in Sharma, Hari, M.D., *Freedom from Disease,* Toronto: Veda Publishing, 1990; p. 126.

Dillard, C.J., et al. *Journal of Applied Physiology* 1978; vol. 45, pp. 927–932; cited in Sharma, Hari, M.D., *Freedom from Disease,* Toronto: Veda Publishing, 1990; p. 125.

Diplock, A.T. *American Journal of Clinical Nutrition,* vol. 53, 1991, pp. 189S–193S; cited in Sharma, Hari, M.D., *Freedom from Disease,* Toronto: Veda Publishing, 1990; p. 126.

DiMascio, P., et al. *American Journal of Clinical Nutrition,* 1991; vol. 53, pp. 194S–200S; cited in Sharma, Hari, M.D., *Freedom from Disease,* Toronto: Veda Publishing, 1990; p. 126.

Ebnother, Carl, M.D. "A New Theory of Heart Disease." *Journal of Longevity Research* vol. 1, no. 8, pp. 24–45.

Fletcher, B.L., and A.L. Tappel. *Environmental Research* 1973; vol. 6, pp. 165–175; cited in Sharma, Hari, M.D., *Freedom from Disease,* Toronto: Veda Publishing, 1990; p. 124.

Golden, F., "Day 3: Living to 1,000?" www.time.com.

Harris, R.W.C. *British Journal of Cancer* 1986; vol. 53, pp. 653–659; cited in Sharma, Hari, M.D., *Freedom from Disease,* Toronto: Veda Publishing, 1990; p. 126.

Hendler, S.S. *The Complete Guide to Anti–Aging Nutrients.* NY: Simon & Schuster, 1984; p. 88; cited in Sharma, Hari, M.D., *Freedom from Disease,* Toronto: Veda Publishing, 1990; p. 126.

Jaffe, S., "Scientists test theories on aging and their resolve," *The Plain Dealer,* December 16, 2002.

JAMA, 2002; 287: 3116–3126; 3127–3129.

Kamen, Betty, Ph.D. "Ester-C: The New Vitamin C Milestone." *Let's Live* October 1989.

"Life Extension Update: CoQ-10 Reduces Surgical Complications." *Life Extension Magazine* March 1, 1995; pp. 4–5.

"Megavitamins can fight disease: new evidence," www.new-nutrition.com/newspage/120402f.htm, accessed May 15, 2002.

Menkes, M.S., et al. *New England Journal of Medicine* 1986; vol. 315, 1250–1289, cited in Sharma, Hari, M.D., *Freedom from Disease,* Toronto: Veda Publishing, 1990; p. 126.

Moseley, Bill. "Interview with Linus Pauling." *Omni* December 1986; pp. 104, 106.

Mustafa, M.G. *Nutrition Reports International* 1975; vol. 11, pp. 475–481; cited in Sharma, Hari, M.D., *Freedom from Disease,* Toronto: Veda Publishing, 1990; p. 124.

Niki, E., et al. *American Journal of Clinical Nutrition,* vol. 53, 1991; pp. 201S–205S; cited in Sharma, Hari, M.D., *Freedom from Disease,* Toronto: Veda Publishing, 1990; p. 126.

Roehm, J. N., et al. *Archives of Environmental Health* 1972; vol. 24, pp. 237–242; cited in Sharma, Hari, M.D., *Freedom from Disease,* Toronto: Veda Publishing, 1990; p. 124.

Russell, Pauline. "Revolutionary New Form of Vitamin C." *Your Health* October 24, 1989.

Shekelle, R.B., et al. *Lancet,* vol. 2, 1981; pp. 1185–1190; cited in Sharma, Hari, M.D., *Freedom from Disease,* Toronto: Veda Publishing, 1990; p. 126.

Tappel, A.L. "Measurement of and Protection From in Vivo Lipid Peroxidation," in *Free Radicals in Biology,* vol. IV, ed., W.A. Pryor, New York: Academic Press, 1980; pp. 1–47; cited in Sharma, Hari, M.D., *Freedom from Disease,* Toronto: Veda Publishing, 1990; p. 125.

CHAPTER 11

Abraham, G.E. "Nutritional Factors in the Etiology of the Premenstrual Tension Syndromes." *Journal of Reproductive Medicine* 1983; 28: 446–464, cited in *Formulas for Life,* p. 168.

Anderson, R.A., et al. "Chromium Supplementation of Human Subjects: Effects on Glucose, Insulin, and Lipid Variables." *Metabolism* 1983; 32: 894–899, cited in Kronhausen, Eberhard, Ed.D., and Phyllis Kronhausen, Ed.D., with Harry B. Demopoulos, M.D., *Formulas for Life,* New York: William Morrow, 1989; p. 172.

Brooks J.D., Metter E.J., Chan D.W., Sokoll L.J., Landis P., Nelson W.G., Muller D., Andres R., Carter H.B. "Plasma selenium level before diagnosis and the risk of prostate cancer development." *J Urol* Dec 2001; 166(6): 2034-8.

Combs G.F. Jr, Clark L.C., Turnbull B.W. "An Analysis of Cancer Prevention by Selenium." *Biofactors* 2001; 14(1-4): 153-9.

Desowitz, R.S., and J.W. Barnwell. "Effect of Selenium and Dimethyl Dioctadecyl Ammonium Bromide on the Vaccine-Induced Immunity of Swiss–Webster Mice Against Malaria (Plasmodium Berghei)." *Infection and Immunity* 1980; 27: 87; cited in *Formulas for Life,* p. 154.

Dyckner, T., and P.O. Wester, "Effect of Magnesium on Blood Pressure." *British Medical Journal* 1983; 286: 1847, cited in *Formulas for Life,* p. 167.

Goei, G.S., and G.E. Abraham. "Effect of a Nutritional Supplement, Optivite, a Symptom of Premenstrual Tension." *Journal of Reproductive Medicine* 1983; 28: 527–531, cited in *Formulas for Life,* p. 168.

Iseri, L. T., et al. "Magnesium Therapy for Intractable Ventricular Tachyarrhythmias in Noromagnesemic Patients." *Western Journal of Medicine* 1983; 139: 823; cited in *Formulas for Life,* p. 167.

Mondrago, M.C., and W.G. Jaffe. "The Ingestion of Selenium in Caracas Compared with Some Other Cities of the World." *Archives of Latinoamerican Nutrition,* 1976; 26: 341–352; cited in *Formulas for Life,* pp. 152–153.

Riales, R. and M.J. Albrink. "Effect of Chromium Chloride Supplementation on Glucose Tolerance and Serum Lipids Including High-Density Lipoprotein of Adult Men." *American Journal of Clinical Nutrition* 1981; 34: 2670–2678, cited in *Formulas for Life,* p. 172.

Sakurai, H. and K. Tsuchiya. "A Tentative Recommendation for the Maximum Daily Intake of Selenium." *Environmental Physiological Biochemistry* 1975; 5:107–118; cited in *Formulas for Life,* pp. 152–153.

Salonen, J.T., et al. "Risk of Cancer in Relation to Serum Concentrations of Selenium and Vitamins A and E: Matched CSE Control Analysis of Prospective Data." *British Medical Journal* 1985; 290: 417, cited in *Formulas for Life,* p. 154.

Schrauzer, G.N., et al. "Selenium in Human Nutrition—Dietary Intakes and Effects of Supplementation." *Bioinorganic Chemistry,* 1978; 8:303–318; cited in *Formulas for Life,* pp. 152–153.

Shamberger, R.J., et al. "Antioxidants and cancer. Part VI. Selenium and Age-Adjusted Human Cancer Mortality." *Archives of Environmental Health* 1976; 31:231; cited in *Formulas for Life,* pp. 152–153.

Spallholz, J.E., et al. "Anti-Inflammatory, Immunologic, and Carcinostatic Attributes of Selenium in Experimental Animals," reviewed in *Advances in Experimental Medicines and Biology* 1981; 135: 43–62; cited in *Formulas for Life,* p. 154.

Turlapaty, P.D., and B.M. Altura. "Magnesium Deficiency Produces Spasms of Coronary Arteries: Relationship to Etiology of Sudden Death Ischemic Heart Disease." *Science* 1980; 208: 198; cited in *Formulas for Life,* p. 167.

CHAPTERS 12 AND 13

Adaikan, P.G., Gauthaman, K., Prasad, R.N., Ng, S.C. "Proerectile pharmacological effects of Tribulus terrestris extract on the rabbit corpus cavernosum." *Ann Acad Med Singapore* 2000; 29: 22–6.

Agarwal, K.C., Parks, R.E., Jr. "Forskolin: a potential antimetastatic agent." *Int J Cancer* 1983; 32: 801–4.

Ahmad, C.F., Khan, M.M., Rastogi, A.K., Kidwai, J.R. "Insulin and glucagon releasing activity of coleonol (forskolin) and its effect on blood glucose level in normal and alloxan diabetic rats." *Acta Diabetol Lat* 1991; 28: 71–7.

Amenta, F., Liu, A., Zeng, Y.C., Zaccheo, D. "Muscarinic cholinergic receptors in the hippocampus of aged rats: influence of choline alphoscerate treatment." *Mech Ageing Dev.* 1994; 76: 49–64.

Andres, E., Perrin, A.E., Kraemer, J.P., Goichot, B., Demengeat, C., Ruellan, A., Grunenberger, F., Constantinesco, A., Schlienger, J.L. "Anemia caused by vitamin B_{12} deficiency in subjects aged over 75 years: New hypotheses. A study of 20 cases." *Rev Med Interne* 2000; 21: 946–54.

Antonio, J., Street, C. "Glutamine: a potentially useful supplement for athletes." *Can J Appl Physiol* 1999; 24: 1–14.

Arcasoy, H.B., Erenmemisoglu, A., Tekol, Y., Kurucu, S., Kartal, M. "Effect of Tribulus terrestris L. saponin mixture on some smooth muscle preparations: a preliminary study." *Boll Chim Farm* 1998; 137: 473–5.

Arockia Rani, P.J., Panneerselvam, C. "Carnitine as a free radical scavenger in aging." *Exp Gerontol* 2001; 36: 1713–26.

Azzara, A., Carulli, G., Sbrana, S., Rizzuti-Gullaci, A., Minnucci, S., Natale, M., Ambrogi, F. "Effects of lysine–arginine association on immune functions in patients with recurrent infections." *Drugs Exp Clin Res* 1995; 21: 71–8.

Balch, J., and Balch, F. *Prescription for Nutritional Healing* (2nd ed). Garden City Park, NY: Avery Publishing Group, 1997; p.44.

Barbagallo, S.G., Barbagallo, M., Giodano, M., Meli, M., Panzarasa, R. "Alpha-Glycerophosphocholine in the mental recovery of cerebral ischemic attacks: An Italian multicenter clinical trial." *Ann NY Acad Sci.* 1994; 717: 253–269.

Barbul, A., Wasserkrug, H.L., Sisto, D.A., Seifter, E., Rettura, G., Levenson, S.M., Efron, G. "Thymic stimulatory actions of arginine." *JPEN J Parenter Enteral Nutr* 1980; 4: 446–9.

Bedir, E., Khan, I.A. "New steroidal glycosides from the fruits of Tribulus terrestris." *J Nat Prod* 2000; 63:1699–701.

Bellone, J., Bartolotta, E., Cardinale, G., Arvat, E., Cherubini, V., Aimaretti, G., Maccario, M., Mucci, M., Camanni, F., Ghigo, E. "Low dose orally administered arginine is able to enhance both basal and growth hormone-releasing hormone-induced growth hormone secretion in normal short children." *J Endocrinol Invest* 1993; 16: 521–5.

Biolo, G., Iscra, F., Bosutti, A., Toigo, G., Ciocchi, B., Geatti, O., Gullo, A., Guarnieri, G. "Growth hormone decreases muscle glutamine production and stimulates protein synthesis in hypercatabolic patients." *Am J Physiol Endocrinol Metab* 2000; 279: E323–32.

Birdsall, T.C. "5–Hydroxytryptophan: a clinically–effective serotonin precursor." *Altern Med Rev* 1998; 3: 271–80.

Cangiano, C., Ceci, F., Cairella, M., Cascino, A., Del Ben, M., Laviano, A., Muscaritoli, M., Rossi Fanelli, F. "Effects of 5–hydroxytryptophan on eating behavior and adherence to dietary prescriptions in obese adult subjects." *Adv Exp Med Biol* 1991; 294: 591–3.

Cangiano, C., Ceci, F., Cascino, A., Del Ben, M., Laviano, A., Muscaritoli, M., Antonucci, F., Rossi Fanelli, F. "Eating behavior and adherence to dietary prescriptions in obese adult subjects treated with 5–hydroxytryptophan." *American Journal of Clinical Nutrition (USA)* 1992; 56: 863–867.

Cangiano, C., Laviano, A., Del Ben, M., Preziosa, I., Angelico, F., Cascino, A., Rossi Fanelli, F. "Effects of oral 5-hydroxy-tryptophan on energy intake and macronutrient selection in non–insulin dependent diabetic patients." *Int J Obes Relat Metab Disord* 1998; 22: 648–54.

Cantorna, M.T., Nashold, F.E., Hayes, C.E. "Vitamin A deficiency results in a priming environment conducive for Th1 cell development." *Eur J Immunol* 1995; 25:1673–9.

Caprioli, J., Sears, M., Bausher, L., Gregory, D., Mead, A. "Forskolin lowers intraocular pressure by reducing aqueous inflow." *Invest Ophthalmol Vis Sci* 1984; 25: 268–77.

Caruso, I., Sarzi Puttini, P., Cazzola, M., Azzolini, V. "Double-blind study of 5-hydroxytryptophan versus placebo in the treatment of primary fibromyalgia syndrome." *J Int Med Res* 1990; 18:201–9.

Ceci, F., Cangiano, C., Cairella, M., Cascino, A., Del Ben, M., Muscaritoli, M., Sibilia, L., Rossi Fanelli, F. "The effects of oral 5–hydroxytryptophan administration on feeding behavior in obese adult female subjects." *J Neural Transm* 1989; 76:109–17.

Ceda, G.P., Ceresini, G., Denti, L., Marzani, G., Piovani, E., Banchini, A., Tarditi, E., Valenti, G. "Alpha-Glycerylphosphorylcholine administration increases the GH responses to GHRH of young and elderly subjects." *Horm Metab Res* 1992; 24:119–21.

Chiu, K.M., Schmidt, M.J., Havighurst, T.C., Shug, A.L., Daynes, R.A., Keller, E.T., Gravenstein, S. "Correlation of serum L-carnitine and dehydro-epiandrosterone sulphate levels with age and sex in healthy adults." *Age Ageing*. 1999; 28: 211–6.

Civitelli, R., Villareal, D.T., Agnusdei, D., Nardi, P., Avioli, L.V., Gennari, C. "Dietary L–lysine and calcium metabolism in humans." *Nutrition* 1992; 8: 400–5.

Cochard, A. Guilhermet, R., Bonneau, M. "Plasma growth hormone (GH), insulin and amino acid responses to arginine with or without aspartic acid in pigs. Effect of the dose." *Reprod Nutr Dev* 1998; 38: 331–43.

Costell, M., Grisolia, S. "Effect of carnitine feeding on the levels of heart and skeletal muscle carnitine of elderly mice." *FEBS Lett* 1993; 315: 43–6.

Costell, M., O'Connor, J.E., Grisolia, S. "Age-dependent decrease of carnitine content in muscle of mice and humans." *Biochem Biophys Res Commun* 1989; 161: 1135–43.

Coudray-Lucas, C., Le Bever, H., Cynober, L., De Bandt, J.P., Carsin, H. "Ornithine alpha-ketoglutarate improves wound healing in severe burn patients: a prospective randomized double-blind trial versus isonitrogenous controls." *Crit Care Med* 2000; 28: 1772–6.

Coutsoudis, A., Kiepiela, P., Coovadia, H.M., Broughton, M. "Vitamin A supplementation enhances specific IgG antibody levels and total lymphocyte numbers while improving morbidity in measles." *Pediatr Infect Dis J* 1992; 11: 203–9.

Cui, D., Moldoveanu, Z., Stephensen, C.B. "High–level dietary vitamin A enhances T–helper type 2 cytokine production and secretory immunoglobulin A response to influenza A virus infection in BALB/c mice." *J Nutr* 2000; 130: 1132–9.

Cynober, L. "Can arginine and ornithine support gut functions?" *Gut* 1994; 35 (Suppl 1): S42–5.

Daly, J.M., Reynolds, J., Thom, A., Kinsley, L., Dietrick–Gallagher, M., Shou, J., Ruggieri, B. "Immune and metabolic effects of arginine in the surgical patient." *Ann Surg* 1988; 208: 512–23.

Dawson, R. Jr., Pelleymounter, M.A., Cullen, N.J., Gollub, M., Liu, S. "An age-related decline in striatal taurine is correlated with a loss of dopaminergic markers." *Brain Res Bull* 1999; 48: 319–24.

De Bandt, J.P., Coudray-Lucas, C., Lioret, N., Lim, S.K., Saizy, R., Giboudeau, J., Cynober, L. "A randomized controlled trial of the influence of the mode of enteral ornithine alpha-ketoglutarate administration in burn patients." *J Nutr* 1998; 128: 563–9.

De Benedittis, G., Massei, R. "Serotonin precursors in chronic primary headache. A double-blind cross-over study with L-5-hydroxytryptophan vs. placebo." *J Neurosurg Sci* 1985; 29: 239–48.

De Giorgis, G., Miletto, R., Iannuccelli, M., Camuffo, M., Scerni, S. "Headache in association with sleep disorders in children: a psychodiagnostic evaluation and controlled clinical study— L-5-HTP versus placebo." *Drugs Exp Clin Res* 1987; 13: 425–33.

den Boer, J.A., Westenberg, H.G. "Behavioral, neuroendocrine, and biochemical effects of 5–hydroxytryptophan administration in panic disorder." *Psychiatry Res* 1990; 31: 267–78.

Devaux, Y., Grosjean, S., Seguin, C., David, C., Dousset, B., Zannad, F., Meistelman, C., De Talance, N., Mertes, P.M., Ungureanu–Longrois, D. "Retinoic acid and host-pathogen interactions: effects on inducible nitric oxide synthase in vivo." *Am J Physiol Endocrinol Metab* 2000; 279: E1045–53.

Ding, W., Li, D., Zhang, J. "Influences of taurine on thrombolysis." *Chung Hua Nei Ko Tsa Chih* 1996; 35: 378–81.

Djakoure, C., Guibourdenche, J., Porquet, D., Pagesy, P., Peillon, F., Li, J.Y., Evain–Brion, D. "Vitamin A and retinoic acid stimulate within minutes cAMP release and growth hormone secretion in human pituitary cells." *J Clin Endocrinol Metab* 1996; 81: 3123–6.

Duarte, J., Jimenez, R., Villar, I.C., Perez-Vizcaino, F., Jimenez, J., Tamargo, J. "Vasorelaxant effects of the bioflavonoid chrysin in isolated rat aorta." *Planta Med* 2001; 67: 567–9.

Evain–Brion, D., Porquet, D., Therond, P., Fjellestad–Paulsen, A., Greneche, M.O., Francois, L., Czernichow, P. "Vitamin A deficiency and nocturnal growth hormone secretion in short children." *Lancet* 1994; 343: 87–8.

Fabris, N., Mocchegiani, E. "Zinc, human diseases and aging." *Aging (Milano)* 1995; 7: 77–93.

Fabris, N., Mocchegiani, E., Provinciali, M. "Plasticity of neuroendocrine-thymus interactions during aging." *Exp Gerontol* 1997; 32: 415–29.

Fenech, M., Aitken, C., Rinaldi, J. "Folate, vitamin B_{12}, homocysteine status and DNA damage in young Australian adults." *Carcinogenesis* 1998; 19: 1163–71.

Florence, T.M. "The role of free radicals in disease." *Aust N Z J Ophthalmol* 1995; 23: 3–7.

Franceschi, C., Cossarizza, A., Troiano, L., Salati, R., Monti, D. "Immunological parameters in aging: Studies on natural immunomodulatory and immunoprotective substances." *Int J Clin Pharmacol Res* 1990; 10: 53–7.

Fregly, M.J., Lockley, O.E., Sumners, C. "Chronic treatment with L-5-hydroxytryptophan prevents the development of DOCA-salt-induced hypertension in rats." *J Hypertens* 1987; 5: 621–8.

Gaby, A. R. "DHEA: the Hormone That Does it All." *Holistic Medicine* Spring 1993; pp. 19–23.

Hankey, G.J., Eikelboom, J.W. "Homocysteine levels in patients with stroke: clinical relevance and therapeutic implications." *CNS Drugs* 2001; 15: 437–43.

Head, K.A. "Natural therapies for ocular disorders, part two: cataracts and glaucoma." *Altern Med Rev* 2001; 6: 141–66.

Henning, B.F., Tepel, M., Riezler, R., Naurath, H.J. "Long-term effects of vitamin B_{12}, folate, and vitamin B_6 supplements in elderly people with normal serum vitamin B_{12} concentrations." *Gerontology* 2001; 47: 30–5.

Hung, M.C., Shibasaki, K., Yoshida, R., Sato, M., Imaizumi, K. "Learning behaviour and cerebral protein kinase C, antioxidant status, lipid composition in senescence-accelerated mouse: influence of a phosphatidylcholine–vitamin B_{12} diet." *Br J Nutr* 2001; 86: 163–71.

Jeevanandam, M., Holaday, N.J., Petersen, S.R. "Ornithine-alpha-ketoglutarate (OKG) supplementation is more effective than its component salts in traumatized rats." *J Nutr* 1996; 126: 2141–50.

Juhl, J.H. "Fibromyalgia and the serotonin pathway." *Altern Med Rev* 1998; 3: 367–75.

Kamata, K., Sugiara, M., Kojima, S., Kasuya, Y. "Restoration of endothelium-dependent relaxation in both hypercholesterolemia and diabetes by chronic taurine." *Eur J Pharmacol* 1996; 303: 47–53.

Kapp, A., Zeck-Kapp, G. "Effect of Ca-panthotenate on human granulocyte oxidative metabolism." *Allerg Immunol (Leipz)* 1991; 37: 145–50.

Klatz, R.M. "The Clock Hormone." *Journal of Longevity Research* 1995; 1: 38–40.

Kruse, W., Raetzer, H., Heuck, C.C., Oster, P., Schellenberg, B., Schlierf, G. "Nocturnal inhibition of lipolysis in man by nicotinic acid and derivatives." *Eur J Clin Pharmacol* 1979; 16: 11–5.

Le Bricon, T., Cynober, L., Baracos, V.E. "Ornithine alpha-ketoglutarate limits muscle protein breakdown without stimulating tumor growth in rats bearing Yoshida ascites hepatoma." *Met Clin Exp* 1994; 43: 899–905.

Leung, L.H. "Pantothenic acid as a weight-reducing agent: fasting without hunger, weakness and ketosis." *Med Hypotheses* 1995; 44: 403–5.

Li, H., Xiong, S.T., Zhang, S.X., Liu, S.B., Luo, Y. "Immunological status of patients with obstructive jaundice and immunostimulatory effect of arginine." *J Tongji Med Univ* 1993; 13: 111–5.

Li, J.X., Shi, Q., Xiong, Q.B., Prasain, J.K., Tezuka, Y., Hareyama, T., Wang, Z.T., Tanaka, K., Namba, T., Kadota, S. "Tribulusamide A and B, new hepatoprotective lignanamides from the fruits of Tribulus terrestris: indications of cytoprotective activity in murine hepatocyte culture." *Planta Med* 1998; 64: 628–31.

Lim, E., Park, S., Kim, H. "Effect of taurine supplementation on the lipid peroxide formation and the activities of glutathione-related enzymes in the liver and islet of type I and II diabetic model mice." *Adv Exp Med Biol* 1998; 442: 99–103.

Liu, C., Wang, X.D., Bronson, R.T., Smith, D.E., Krinsky, N.I., Russell, R.M. "Effects of physiological versus pharmacological beta-carotene supplementation on cell proliferation and histopathological changes in the lungs of cigarette smoke-exposed ferrets." *Carcinogenesis* 2000; 21: 2245–53.

Lobley, G.E., Hoskin, S.O., McNeil, C.J. "Glutamine in animal science and production." *J Nutr* 2001; 131 (Suppl 9): 2525S–31S; discussion 2532S–4S.

Loche, S., Carta, D., Muntoni, A.C., Corda, R., Pintor, C. "Oral administration of arginine enhances the growth hormone response to growth hormone releasing hormone in short children." *Acta Paediatr* 1993; 82: 83–4.

Loew, D., Wanitschke, R., Schroedter, A. "Studies on vitamin B_{12} status in the elderly— prophylactic and therapeutic consequences." *Int J Vitam Nutr Res* 1999; 69: 228–33.

Lohninger, S., Strasser, A., Bubna-Littitz, H. "The effect of L-carnitine on T-maze learning ability in aged rats." *Arch Gerontol Geriatr* 2001; 32: 245–253.

Marconi, C., Sassi, G., Carpinelli, A., Cerretelli, P. "Effects of L-carnitine loading on the aerobic and anaerobic performance of endurance athletes." *Eur J Appl Physiol* 1985; 54: 131–5.

Mayeux, R., Stern, Y., Sano, M., Williams, J.B., Cote, L.J. "The relationship of serotonin to depression in Parkinson's disease." *Mov Disord* 1988; 3: 237–44.

McCarty, M.F. "Exploiting complementary therapeutic strategies for the treatment of type II diabetes and prevention of its complicaitons." *Med Hypotheses* 1997; 49: 143–52.

McCarty, M.F. "Vascular nitric oxide may lessen Alzheimer's risk." *Med Hypotheses* 1998; 51: 465–76.

Medawar, P.B., Hunt, R. "Anti-cancer action of retinoids." *Immunology* 1981; 42: 349–53.

Medina, J.H., Paladini, A.C., Wolfman, C., Levi de Stein, M., Calvo, D., Diaz, L.E., Pena, C. "Chrysin (5,7–di–OH–flavone), a naturally occurring ligand for benzodiazepine receptors, with anticonvulsant properties." *Biochem Pharmacol* 1990; 40: 2227–31.

Mero, A., Miikkulainen, H., Riski, J., Pakkanen, R., Aalto, J., Takala, T. "Effects of bovine colostrum supplementation on serum IGF-I, IgG, hormone, and saliva IgA during training." *J Appl Physiol* 1997; 83: 1144–51.

Metzger, H., Lindner, E. "The positive inotropic-acting forskolin, a potent adenylate cyclase activator." *Arzneimittelforschung* 1981; 31: 1248–50.

Mocchegiani, E., Giacconi, R., Muzzioli, M., Cipriano, C. "Zinc, infections and immunosenescence." *Mech Ageing Dev* 2000; 121: 21–35. (Review.)

Mocchegiani, E., Muzzioli, M., Giacconi, R. "Zinc and immunoresistance to infection in aging: new biological tools." *Trends Pharmacol Sci* 2000; 21: 205–8.

Mokshagundam, S.P., Barzel, U. "Thyroid Disease in the Elderly." *Journal of the American Geriatrics Society* 1993; 41:1361–69.

Morales, A.J., et al. "Effects of Replacement Dose of Dehydroepiandrosterone in Men and Women of Advancing Age." *Journal of Clinical Endocrinology and Metabolism* 1994; 78: 1360–66.

Morley, J.E., Melmed, S., Reed, A., Kasson, B.G., Levin, S.R., Pekary, A.E., Hershman, J.M. "Effect of vitamin A on the hypothalamo-pituitary-thyroid axis." *Am J Physiol* 1980; 238: E174–9.

Muccioli, G., Raso, G.M., Ghe, C., Di Carlo, R. "Effect of L-alpha glycerylphosphorylcholine on muscarinic receptors and membrane microviscosity of aged rat brain." *Prog Neuropsychopharmacol Biol Psychiatry* 1996; 20: 323–39.

Nicolodi, M., Sicuteri, F. "5-hydroxytryptophan can prevent nociceptive disorders in man." *Adv Exp Med Biol* 1999; 467: 177–82.

Nicolodi, M., Sicuteri, F. "Fibromyalgia and migraine, two faces of the same mechanism. Serotonin as the common clue for pathogenesis and therapy." *Adv Exp Med Biol* 1996; 398: 373–9.

Nikawa, T., Odahara, K., Koizumi, H., Kido, Y., Teshima, S., Rokutan, K., Kishi, K. "Vitamin A prevents the decline in immunoglobulin A and Th2 cytokine levels in small intestinal mucosa of protein–malnourished mice." *J Nutr* 1999; 129: 934–41.

Nilsson, K., Gustafson, L., Hultberg, B. "Improvement of cognitive functions after cobalamin/folate supplementation in elderly patients with dementia and elevated plasma homocysteine." *Int J Geriatr Psychiatry* 2001; 16: 609–14.

Nilsson-Ehle, H. "Age-related changes in cobalamin (vitamin B_{12}) handling. Implications for therapy." *Drugs Aging* 1998; 12: 277–92.

Offenbacher, E.G. "Chromium in the elderly." *Biol Trace Elem Res* 1992; 32: 123–31.

Parry-Billings M., Dimitriadis G.D., Leighton B., Dunger D.B., Newsholme E.A. "The Effects of Growth Hormone Administration in Vivo on Skeletal Muscle Glutamine Metabolism of the Rat." *Horm Metab Res.* Jun 1993; 25(6): 292-3.

Peat, R. "Thyroid: Misconceptions." *Townsend Letter for Doctors* Nov 1993; 1120–22.

Pierpaoli, W., Regelson, W., and Colman, C. *The Melatonin Miracle.* New York: Simon & Schuster, 1995.

Playford, R.J., MacDonald, C.E., Calnan, D.P., Floyd, D.N., Podas, T., Johnson, W., Wicks, A.C., Bashir, O., Marchbank, T. "Co-administration of the health food supplement, bovine colostrum, reduces the acute non-steroidal anti-inflammatory drug-induced increase in intestinal permeability." *Clin Sci (Lond)* 2001; 100: 627–33.

Podlepa, E.M., Liudkovskaia, I.V., Dmitrovskii, A.A., Bykhovskii, V.I. "Effect of vitamin B_{12} on carnitine synthesis in the body of rats." *Nauchnye Doki Vyss Shkoly Biol Nauki* 1988; 5: 20–3.

Potter, J.F., Levin, P., Anderson, R.A., Freiberg, J.M., Andres, R., Elahi, D. "Glucose metabolism in glucose-intolerant older people during chromium supplementation." *Metabolism* 1985; 34: 199–204.

Prasad, A.S., Fitzgerald, J.T., Hess, J.W., Kaplan, J., Pelen, F., Dardenne, M. "Zinc deficiency in elderly patients." *Nutrition* 1993; 9: 218–24.

Preuss, H.G., Anderson, R.A. "Chromium update: Examining recent literature 1997–1998." *Curr Opin Clin Nutr Metab Care* 1998; 1: 509–12.

Puttini, P.S., Caruso, I. "Primary fibromyalgia syndrome and 5-hydroxy-L-tryptophan: a 90-day open study." *J Int Med Res* 1992; 20: 182–9.

Raifen, R., Altman, Y., Zadik, Z. "Vitamin A levels and growth hormone axis." *Hormone Res* 1996; 46: 279–81.

Rani, P.J., Panneerselvam, C. "Protective efficacy of L-carnitine on acetylcholinesterase activity in aged rat brain." *J Gerontol A Biol Sci Med Sci* 2001; 56: B140–1.

Raschke, P., Massoudy, P., Becker, B.F. "Taurine protects the heart from neutrophil-induced reperfusion injury." *Free Radic Biol Med* 1995; 19: 461–71.

Ratloff, J. "Drug of Darkness: Can a Pineal Hormone Head Off Everything from Breast Cancer to Aging?" *Science News* 1995; 147: 300–1.

Rebouche. C.J. "Carnitine function and requirements during the life cycle." *FASEB J* 1992; 6: 3379–86.

Regelson, W., and Kalimi, M. "Dehydroepiandrosterone (DHEA)—A Pleiotropic Steroid: How Can One Steroid Do So Much?" in Klatz, R.M., (ed.) *Advances in Anti-Aging Medicine* (vol 1). New York: Mary Ann Liebert Publishers, Inc., 1996.

Reiter, R., and Robinson, J. *Melatonin.* New York: Bantam Books, 1995.

Ribeiro, C.A. "5-Hydroxytryptophan in the prophylaxis of chronic tension-type headache: A double-blind, randomized, placebo-controlled study. For the Portuguese Head Society." *Headache* 2000; 40: 451–6.

Rizzon, P., Biasco, G., DiBase, M. "High doses of L–carnitine in acute myocardial infarction: Metabolic and antiarrhythmic effects." *Eur Heart J* 1989; 10: 502–8.

Rohde, T., Krzywkowski, K., Pedersen, B.K. "Glutamine, exercise, and the immune system—Is there a link?" *Exerc Immunol Rev* 1998; 4: 49–63.

Rokitzki, L., Sagredos, A., Reuss, F., Petersen, G., Keul, J. "Pantothenic acid levels in blood of athletes at rest and after aerobic exercise." *Z Ernahrungswiss* 1993; 32: 282–8.

Rozencwaig, R., et al. "The Role of Melatonin and Serotonin in Aging." *Medical Hypotheses* 1987; 23: 337.

Schlegel, L., Coudray–Lucas, C., Barbut, F., Le Boucher, J., Jardel, A., Zarrabian, S., Cynober, L. "Bacterial dissemination and metabolic changes in rats induced by endotoxemia following intestinal E. coli overgrowth are reduced by ornithine alpha-ketoglutarate administration." *J Nutr* 2000; 130: 2897–902.

Shin, J.S., Kim, K.S., Kim, M.B., Jeong, J.H., Kim, B.K. "Synthesis and hypoglycemic effect of chrysin derivatives." *Bioorg Med Chem Lett* 1999; 9: 869–74.

Siani, A., Pagano, E., Iacone, R., Iacoviello, L., Scopacasa, F., Strazzullo, P. "Blood pressure and metabolic changes during dietary L–arginine supplementation in humans." *Am J Hypertens* 2000; 13(5 Pt 1): 547–51.

Singh, R.B., Niaz, M.A., Agarwal, P., Beegum, R., Sachan, D.S. "A randomised double–blind, placebo-controlled study of L-carnitine in suspected acute myocardial infarction." *Postgrad Med J* 1996; 72: 45–50.

Slyshenkov, V.S., Omelyanchik, S.N., Moiseenok, A.G., Petushok, N.E., Wojtczak, L. "Protection by pantothenol and beta–carotene against liver damage produced by low-dose gamma radiation." *Acta Biochim Pol* 1999; 46: 239–48.

Suleiman, M.S., Moffatt, A.C., Dihmis, W.C., Caputo, M., Hutter, J.A., Angelini, G.D., Bryan, A.J. "Effect of ischaemia and reperfusion on the intracellular concentration of taurine and glutamine in the hearts of patients undergoing coronary artery surgery." *Biochim Biophys Acta* 1997; 1324: 223–31.

Suzuki, Y., Kawikawa, T., Kobayashi, A. "Effects of L-carnitine on tissue levels of acyl carnitine, acylcoenzyme A and high energy phosphate in ischemic dog hearts." *Jpn Circ J* 1981; 45: 687–690.

Suzuki, Y., Kawikawa, T., Yamazaki, N. "Effects of L-carnitine on cardiac hemodynamics." *Jpn Heart J* 1981; 22: 219–25.

Trachtman, H., Futterweit, S., Maesaka, J., Ma, C., Valderrama, E., Fuchs, A., Tarectecan, A.A., Rao, P.S., Sturman, J.A., Boles, T.H., et al. "Taurine ameliorates chronic streptozocin–induced diabetic nephropathy in rats." *Am J Physiol* 1995; 269 (3 Pt 2): F429–38.

Tsukawaki, M., Suzuki, K., Suzuki, R., Takagi, K., Satake, T. "Relaxant effects of forskolin on guinea pig tracheal smooth muscle." *Lung* 1987; 165: 225–37.

van Praag, H.M. "Serotonin precursors in the treatment of depression." *Adv Biochem Psychopharmacol* 1982; 34: 259–86.

Vaxman, F., Olender, S., Lambert, A., Nisand, G., Aprahamian, M., Bruch, J.F., Didier, E., Volkmar, P., Grenier, J.F. "Effect of pantothenic acid and ascorbic acid supplementation on human skin wound healing process. A double-blind, prospective and randomized trial." *Eur Surg Res* 1995; 27: 158–66.

Vaxman, F., Olender, S., Lambert, A., Nisand, G., Grenier, J.F. "Can the wound healing process be improved by vitamin supplementation? Experimental study on humans." *Eur Surg Res* 1996; 28: 306–14.

Wallach, S. "Clinical and biochemical aspects of chromium deficiency." *J Am Coll Nutr.* 1985; 4: 107–20.

Walsh, D.E., Griffith, R.S., Behforooz, A. "Subjective response to lysine in the therapy of herpes simplex." *J Antimicrob Chemother.* 1983; 12: 489–96.

Wang, B., Ma, L., Liu, T. "406 cases of angina pectoris in coronary heart disease treated with saponin of Tribulus terrestris." *hong Xi Yi Jie He Za Zhi* 1990; 10: 85–7, 68.

Weir, D.G., Scott, J.M. "Brain function in the elderly: role of vitamin B_{12} and folate." *Br Med Bull* 1999; 55: 669–82.

Wellbourne, T.C. "Increased plasma bicarbonate and growth hormone after an oral glutamine load." *Am J Clin Nutr* 1995; 61:1058–61.

Wernerman, J., Hammarkvist, F., Ali, M.R., Vinnars, E. "Glutamine and ornithine-alpha-ketoglutarate but not branched-chain amino acids reduce the loss of muscle glutamine after surgical trauma." *Metabolism* 1989; 38 (8 Suppl 1): 63–6.

Yamauchi, T.K., Azuma, J., Hishimoto, S. "Taurine protection against experimental arterial calcinosis in mice." *Biochem Biophys Res Commun* 1986; 140: 579–83.

Yen, S.S.C., Morales, A.J., Khorram, O. "Replacement of DHEA in Aging Men and Women," in Bellino, F., et al., eds, "Dehydroepiandrosterone (DHEA) and Aging." *Annals of the New York Academy of Sciences* 1995; 774: 128–142.

Yoshida, S., Kaibara, A., Ishibashi, N., Shirouzu, K. "Glutamine supplementation in cancer patients." *Nutrition* 2001; 17: 766–8.

You, H.S., Chang, K.J. "Effects of taurine supplementation on lipid peroxidation, blood glucose and blood lipid metabolism in streptozotocin–induced diabetic rats." *Adv Exp Med Biol* 1998; 442: 163–68.

CHAPTER 14

"Aim for a healthy weight," National Heart, Lung, and Blood Institute, www.nhlbi.nih.gov/health/public/heart/obesity/lose_wt/risk.htm, accessed March 18, 2003.

Borek, Carmia, Ph.D. *Maximize Your Health Span with Antioxidants.* New Canaan, CT: Keats Publishing, 1995; p. 63.

Buzina-Suboticanec, K., Buzina, R., Stavljenic, A., Farley, T.M., Haller, J., Bergman-Markovic, B., Gorajscan, M. "Ageing, nutritional status and immune response." *Int J Vitam Nutr Res* 1998; 68: 133–41.

"Calculate your body mass index," National Heart, Lung, and Blood Institute, www.nhlbisupport.com/bmi/, accessed March 18, 2003.

"Consumption of Food Group Servings: People's Perceptions vs. Reality." *Nutrition Insights,* No. 20 October 2000; (http://www.usda.gov/cnpp/Insights/Insight20.PDF)

"Do you know the health risks of being overweight?" National Institute of Diabetes and Digestive and Kidney Diseases, www.niddk.nih.gov/health/nutrit/pubs/health.htm, accessed March 17, 2003.

Elias, M., et al., *Intl. J. Obesity,* February 2003.

Ford, Norman. *Lifestyle for Longevity.* Gloucester, MA: Para Research, 1984; pp. 82–83.

Fox, M., "US military losing war against fat, expert says," *Reuters,* November 11, 2001.

Kaufman, Dr. Richard Clark. *The Age Reduction System.* NY: Rawson Associates, 1986; p. 125.

Krause, D., Mastro, A.M., Handte, G., Smiciklas-Wright, H., Miles, M.P., Ahluwalia, N. "Immune function did not decline with aging in apparently healthy, well-nourished women." *Mech Ageing Dev* 1999; 112: 43–57.

Lesourd, B., Mazari, L. "Nutrition and immunity in the elderly." *Proc Nutr Soc* 1999; 58: 685–95.

Lipschitz, D.A. "Nutrition, aging, and the immunohematopoietic system." *Clin Geriatr Med* 1987; 3: 319–28.

Mattson, M.P. "Existing data suggest that Alzheimer's disease is preventable." *Ann N Y Acad Sci* 2000; 924: 153–9.

"Middle-age fat as bad as smoking, study says," *Chicago Tribune,* January 7, 2003.

National Heart, Lung, and Blood Institute, *Obesity Research.* 1998; 6 (suppl. 2): 51S–210S.

"New state data show obesity and diabetes still on the rise," *CDC Press Release,* December 31, 2002.

"1.7 billion—the numbers of obese worldwide," NutraIngredients.com, March 17, 2003.

Reaney, P., "Obesity threatens to reverse gains in longevity," *Reuters,* October 30, 2002.

Seidell, J.C., et al., *Am. J. Pub. Health,* 1986; 76: 264–69.

Sinatra, Stephen T., M.D. *Optimum Health* Tennesee: Lincoln Bradley Publishing Group, 1996, pp. 206–208.

Solfrizzi, V., Panza, F., Torres, F., Mastroianni, F., Del Parigi, A., Venezia, A., Capurso, A. "High monounsaturated fatty acids intake protects against age-related cognitive decline." *Neurology* 1999; 52: 1563–9.

Sonntag, W.E., Lynch, C.D., Cefalu, W.T., Ingram, R.L., Bennett, S.A., Thornton, P.L., Khan, A.S. "Pleiotropic effects of growth hormone and insulin-like growth factor (IGF)-1 on biological aging: inferences from moderate caloric-restricted animals." *J Gerontol A Biol Sci Med Sci* 1999; 54: B521–38.

Sultenfuss, Sherry, Wilson M.S., and Thomas J. Sultenfuss, M.D. *A Women's Guide to Vitamins and Minerals.* New York: Contemporary Books, 1995; pp. 173–174.

Tanner, L., "Study: 47 million adults have obesity-related syndrome," *Chicago Tribune,* January 15, 2002.

Wild, Russell, Ed., et al. *The Complete Book of Natural and Medicinal Cures.* Emmaus, PA: Rodale Press, 1994; pp. 28–32.

CHAPTER 15

Balch, J.F., Balch, P.A., Prescription for Nutritional Healing, 2nd edition. Avery Publishing, 1997.

Golan, R., Optimal Wellness. Ballantine Books, 1995.

CHAPTER 16

Beere, P.A., Russell, S.D., Morey, M.C., Kitzman, D.W., Higginbotham, M.B. "Aerobic exercise training can reverse age-related peripheral circulatory changes in healthy older men." *Circulation* 1999; 100: 1085–94.

Birge, S.J., Dalsky, G. "The role of exercise in preventing osteoporosis." *Public Health Rep* 1989; 104 (Suppl): 54–8.

Blain, H., Vuillemin, A., Blain, A., Jeandel, C. "The preventive effects of physical activity in the elderly." *Presse Med* 2000; 29: 1240–8.

Cooper, Kenneth, M.D. *It's Better to Believe.* Nashville, TN: Thomas Nelson Publishers Inc., 1995.

Coudert, J., Van Praagh, E. "Endurance exercise training in the elderly: Effects on cardiovascular function." *Curr Opin Clin Nutr Metab Care* 2000; 3: 479–83.

DeSouza, C.A., Shapiro, L.F., Clevenger, C.M., Dinenno, F.A., Monahan, K.D., Tanaka, H., Seals, D.R. "Regular aerobic exercise prevents and restores age-related declines in endothelium-dependent vasodilation in healthy men." *Circulation* 2000; 102: 1351–7.

Evans, W.J. "Exercise and nutritional needs of elderly people: effects on muscle and bone." *Gerodontology* 1998; 15:15–24.

Kaufman, Dr. Richard Clark. *The Age Reduction System.* New York: Rawson Associates, 1986; p. 209–210.

Klatz, Ronald, D.O., and Alan Hirsch, M.D. "The Ageless Athlete." *Sports Clinic, The Professional's Journal of Sports Fitness* Spring 1992.

Kressig, R., Proust, J. "Physical activity and aging." *Schweiz Med Wochenschr* 1998; 128: 1181–6.

Mazzeo, R.S. "Aging, immune function, and exercise: Hormonal regulation." *Int J Sports Med* 2000; 21 (Suppl 1): S10–3.

McGuire, D.K., Levine, B.D., Williamson, J.W., Snell, P.G., Blomqvist, C.G., Saltin, B., Mitchell, J.H. "A 30-year follow-up of the Dallas Bedrest and Training Study: II. Effect of age on cardiovascular adaptation to exercise training." *Circulation* 2001; 104: 1358–66.

Rogers, M.A., Evans, W.J. "Changes in skeletal muscle with aging: effects of exercise training." *Exerc Sport Sci Rev* 1993; 21: 65–102.

Schilke, J.M. "Slowing the aging process with physical activity." *J Gerontol Nurs* 1991; 17: 4–8.

Spirduso, Waneen, W., Ed.D. *Physical Dimensions of Aging* Champaign, IL: Human Kinetics, 1995; p. 147.

Starling, R.D., Ades, P.A., Poehlman, E.T. "Physical activity, protein intake, and appendicular skeletal muscle mass in older men." *Am J Clin Nutr* 1999; 70: 91–6.

Venjatraman, J.T., Fernandes, G. "Exercise, immunity and aging." *Aging (Milano)* 1997; 9: 42–56.

CHAPTER 17

Clark, Etta. *Growing Old Is Not for Sissies: Portraits of Senior Athletes.* Corte Madera, CA: Pomegranate Calendars and Books, 1986.

Gallagher, Marty. "Ageless Muscle." *Muscle and Fitness* January 1996; pp. 162–165.

Interview February 1, 1996: Bob Delmonteque.

Interview January 16, 1996; Richard Orenstein (associate and colleague of Jack La Lanne).

Moore, K. "The Times of Their Lives." *Runner's World* 1992; vol. 20, 44–47, p. 44;

Norris, Rebecca, "Heels Over Head." *American Health* September 1995; p. 108.

CHAPTER 18

Goldman, R., Klatz, R., *Sleep: Essential for Optimum Health*, 2003.

"Sleep Council suggests siestas" October 27, 2001; CNN.com. http://cnn.com/health

Van Cauter, E., Leproult, R., Plat, L. "Age-related changes in slow wave sleep and REM sleep and relationship with growth hormone and cortisol levels in healthy men." *JAMA* 2000; 284: 861–8.

CHAPTER 19

Adapted from Eliot, Robert S., M.D., "The Do-It-Yourself Stress Clinic Test." *Longevity* January 1994; pp. 45–47, 71–74.

Balch, James F., M.D., and Phyllis A. Balch, C.N.C., *Prescription for Nutritional Healing.* Garden City Park: Avery Publishing Group, 1990; p. 298.

Cohen, Jessica. "The Healing Touch." *Longevity* January 1994; pp. 26, 64, 66.

Eppley, K., et al. *Journal of Clinical Psychology*, vol. 45, 1989; pp. 957–974, cited in Sharma, p. 183.

Jevning, R., *The Physiologist*, vol. 21, 1978; p. 60, cited in Sharma, pp. 179, 182.

Levine, S.A., and P.M. Kidd. "Antioxidant Adaptation: Its Role in Free Radical Pathology, Biocurrents Division." Allergy Research Group, San Leandro, 1986; pp. 241–242, cited in Hari Sharma, M.D., *Freedom from Disease*, Toronto: Veda Publishing, 1993; pp. 173–174.

Sapse AT. "Stress, cortisol, interferon, and 'stress' diseases I. Cortisol as the cause of 'stress' diseases," *Med Hypothesis*, 1984 Jan; 13(1):31–44.

Wallace, R.K., et al. *International Journal of Neuroscience* 1982; 16, pp. 53–58, cited in Sharma, p. 189.

Williams, Gurney, "Mind, Body, Spirit: Portable Meditation, Stress Relief for Those on the Go." *Longevity* May 1993; p. 72.

CHAPTER 20

"Beauty Flash," *Self,* May 2003, p. 60.

Begoun, P., Don't Go to the Cosmetics Counter Without Me. Beginning Press, 2003.

Chung, J.H., Kang, S., Varani, J., Lin, J., Fisher, G.J., Voorhees, J.J., "Decreased extracellular-signal-regulated kinase and increased stress-activated MAP kinase activities in aged human skin *in vivo*," *J. Invest. Dermatol.*, 2000; 115: 177–182.

"Clinical Update: Skin aging on the cellular level," *Anti-Aging Medical News,* Spring–Summer 2001.

Evans, R., "Skin Lies," *Allure,* April 2002.

Giacomoni, P.U., Declercq, L., Hellemans, L., Maes, D., "Aging of human skin: review of a mechanistic model and first experimental data," *IUBMB Life,* April 2000; 49(4): 259–63.

Gieske, K., "Spot Check," *Self,* November 2002; 62–64.

Gordon, M., Fugate, A.E., The Complete Idiot's Guide to Beautiful Skin. Alpha Books, 1998.

Hamanaka, S., Hara, M., Nishio, H., Otsuka, F., Suzuki, A., Uchida, Y., "Human epidermal glucosylceramides are major precursors of stratum corneum ceramides," *Journal of Investigative Dermatology,* August 2002; 119(2): 416.

Kohen, R., Gati, I., "Skin low molecular weight: antioxidants and their role in aging and in oxidative stress," *Toxicology,* 2000; 148: 149–157.

Lee, L.H., "Clear, healthy skin today," *Self,* October 2002; 201.

Leyden, J., "What is photo-aged skin?" *Eur. J. Dermatol.,* March 2001; 11(2): 165–7.

Kucharekova, M., Schalkwijk, Van De Kerkhof, J.P.C.M., Van De Valk, P.G.M., "Effect of a lipid-rich emollient containing ceramide 3 in experimentally induced skin barrier dysfunction," *Contact Dermatitis,* June 2002; 46(6): 331.

"Mature Skin," *American Academy of Dermatology,* www.aad.org/pamphlets/agingskin/html.

Michalun, N., Michalun, M.V., Milady's Skin Care & Cosmetic Ingredients Dictionary, 2nd edition, Delmar/Thompson Learning, 2001.

"New wrinkle on a bad habit," *Popular Science,* September 2001; 41.

"The Clear-Skin Diet," *Men's Health,* April 2003; 44.

Varani, J., Warner, R.L., Gharaee-Kermani, M., et al., "Vitamin A antagonizes decreased cell growth and elevated collagen-degrading matrix metalloproteinases and stimulates collagen accumulation in naturally aged human skin," *J. Invest. Dermatol.,* 2000; 114: 480–486.

Verzijl, N., DeGroot, J., Oldehinkel, E., Bank, R.A., Thorpe, S.R., Baynes, J.W., Bayliss, M.T., Bijlsma, J.W., Lafeber, F.P., Tekoppele, J.M.. "Age-related accumulation of Maillard reaction products in human articular cartilage collagen," *Biochem. J.,* September 1, 2000; 350 (Pt 2): 381–7.

CHAPTER 21

Goldman, R., Klatz, R., *Cellular Phone/RF Radiation: Medical Menaces of a Modern-Day Medical Convenience,* 2002.

CHAPTER 23

Board of Editors, "The Future of Human Evolution," *Scientific American,* March 2001.

"Communication and education: Converging technologies for improving human performance," US Commerce Dept. /National Science Foundation, November 2002.

"Frequently asked questions about genetics," National Human Genome Institute, at http://www.genome.gov/10001191.

Huang G.T., "Mind-Machine Merger," *Technology Review,* May 2000.

"International consortium completes human genome project," National Human Genome Institute, at http://www.genome.gov/11006929, April 14, 2003.

"Methods for discovering and scoring single nucleotide polymorphisms," National Human Genome Institute, at http://www.genome.gov/10001029.

Minsky, M., "Will robots inherit the earth?" *Scientific American,* October 1994.

Raeburn, R., "Oh, so you have a pig's heart too," *Business Week,* March 27, 2000.

Schwartz, P., "Wanna bet?" *Wired,* May 2002; 131.

Stover, D., "Growing hearts from scratch," at www.popsci.com.

"The human genome project," *Anti-Aging Medical News,* Spring 2002; 13.

Index

About the Authors

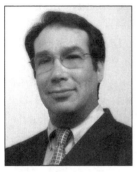

Dr. Ronald Klatz, who coined the term "anti-aging medicine," is recognized as a leading authority in the new clinical science of anti-aging medicine. Since 1981, Dr. Klatz has been integral in the pioneering exploration of new therapies for the treatment and prevention of age-related degenerative diseases. He is the physician founder and president of the American Academy of Anti-Aging Medicine Inc. (A4M), a nonprofit medical organization dedicated to the advancement of technology to detect, prevent, and treat age-related disease and to promote research into methods to retard and optimize the human aging process. As a world-renowned expert in anti-aging medicine, Dr. Klatz is a popular lecturer at A4M sponsored/ co-supported events in anti-aging medicine. He is instrumental in the continuing development of A4M's educational website, www. worldhealth.net, with an Internet audience exceeding 500,000 viewers, for which he serves as Senior Medical Editor.

Dr. Klatz oversees continuing medical education programs co-sponsored by A4M that are AMA/ACCME approved, for more than 50,000 physicians, health practitioners, and scientists from over 100 countries worldwide each year. In addition, Dr. Klatz is Professor, Department of Internal Medicine at the University of Central America Health Sciences. Dr. Klatz is board certified in the specialties of family practice, sports medicine, and anti-aging medicine.

Dr. Klatz co-founded the National Academy of Sports Medicine, which provides medical specialty training in musculoskeletal rehabilitation, conditioning, physical fitness, and exercise to 35,000 healthcare professionals internationally. He was a founder and key patent developer for Organ Recovery Systems, a biomedical research company focusing on technologies for brain resuscitation, trauma and emergency medicine, organ transplant, and blood preservation.

Dr. Klatz is the inventor, developer, or administrator of numerous medical and scientific patents. In recognition of his pioneering medical breakthroughs, he was awarded the Gold Medal in Science for Brain Resuscitation Technology (1993) and the Grand Prize in Medicine for Brain Cooling Technology (1994). In addition, Dr.

Klatz has been named as a Top 10 Medical Innovator in Biomedical Technology (1997) by the National Institute of Electromedical Information, and received the Ground Breaker Award in Health Care (1999) with Presidential Acknowledgment by William Jefferson Clinton from Transitional Services of New York.

The author of several nonfiction bestsellers, including *Grow Young with HGH* (HarperCollins, 1997), Dr. Klatz also has co-authored *The New Anti-Aging Revolution* (Basic Health Publications, 2003), *Infection Protection* (Harper Resource, 2002), *Ten Weeks to a Younger You* (Sports Tech Labs, 1999), *New Anti-Aging Secrets for Maximum Lifespan* (Sports Tech Labs, 1999), *Brain Fitness* (Bantam Doubleday Dell, 1999), *Hormones of Youth* (Sports Tech Labs, 1998), *Seven Anti-Aging Secrets* (Elite Sports Medicine, 1996), *Death in the Locker Room: Drugs & Sports* (Elite Sports Medicine, 1992), and *The E Factor* (William Morrow & Co., 1988).

Dr. Klatz has served as a contributor, editor, reviewer, and advisor to *Archives of Gerontology and Geriatrics, Journal of Gerontology, Osteopathic Annals Medical Journal, Patient Care Medical Journal, Total Health for Longevity,* and *50+ Plus* magazine. His columns on wellness and longevity have appeared in *Pioneer Press* (a division of Time-Life Inc.), *Townsend Letter for Doctors and Patients, Spa Management Journal, The Wellness Channel, Fitness & Longevity Digest, Alternative Medicine Digest, Nutritional Science News, Healing Retreats & Spas, Skin Inc.,* and *Longevity SA* (for which he had served as Senior Medical Editor).

Dr. Klatz has co-hosted the national Fox Network television series *Anti-Aging Update* and served as national advisor for Physician's Radio Network. He has appeared in interviews on *CNN, USA Today TV, ABC News, NBC News, CBS News, Good Morning America, The Today Show, the Oprah Winfrey Show, Extra Daily TV News* (partial list). Dr. Klatz has participated in articles appearing in *The New York Times, USA Today, Chicago Tribune, Newsweek, Harper's Bazaar, MacLean's* (Canada), *Forbes Magazine,* and *Investor's Business Daily* (partial list).

Dr. Klatz is highly regarded by scientific and academic colleagues for his continuing medical education lectures on the demographics of aging and the impact of biomedical technologies on longevity. His scientific articles have been published in *Resident and Staff Physician, British Journal of Sports Medicine, Medical Times/The Journal of Family Medicine, Osteopathic Annals,* and *American Medical Association News* (partial list).

Dr. Klatz is a graduate of Florida Technological University. He received the Doctor of Medicine (M.D.) Degree from the Central America Health Sciences University, School of Medicine, a government-sanctioned, Ministry of Health-approved, and World Health Organization–listed medical university. Dr. Klatz received his Doctor of Osteopathic Medicine and Surgery (D.O.) degree from the College of Osteopathic Medicine and Surgery (Des Moines, Iowa).

Dr. Klatz has held several distinguished teaching or research positions, at Tufts University, the University of Oklahoma School of Osteopathic Medicine, Des Moines University School of Medicine, and the Chicago College of Osteopathic Medicine.

A consultant to the biotechnology industry and a respected advisor to several members of the U.S. Congress and others on Capitol Hill, Dr. Klatz devotes much of his time to research and to the development of advanced biosciences for the benefit of humanity.

Medical Patents Awarded to Dr. Klatz (partial list):

Brain Resuscitation Device and Method
U.S. Patent #5,149,321 (Method); Australian Patent #637,964; U.S. Patent #5,234,405 (Device); Patents Pending in Canada, Japan, Europe, Hong Kong, Singapore

Brain Cooling Device and Method
U.S. Patent #5,261,399; Australian Patent #666,314; Patents Pending in Canada, Japan. Europe, Hong Kong. Singapore; Docket #WPB 36622B

Brain Resuscitation and Organ Preservation Device/Method
Docket #WPB 36622C; U.S. Patent #5,395,314; U.S. Patent #5,234,405; U.S. Patent #5,584,804; Patents Pending in Australia, Canada, Japan, South Korea, Hong Kong, Europe, Malaysia, Indonesia, Singapore

Method for Treating the Brain & Associated Nervous Tissue
U.S. Patent #5,584,804 (CIP)

Apparatus for Cooling Living Tissue
U.S. Patent #5,584,804 (CIP) ; U.S. Patent #5,709,634; Patents Pending in China, Indonesia, Israel, India, South Korea, Malaysia, Philippines, Singapore, Taiwan

Method for Preserving Organs other than the Brain
U.S. Patent #5,395,314 (CIP)

Circulation Device and Method for Preserving Organs other than the Brain
U.S. Patent #5,584,804 (CIP); Total Body Cooling System; Docket #WPB 38615; Patents Pending in Thailand. Malaysia, India, Taiwan, Indonesia

Combined Liquid Ventilation and Cardiopulmonary Resuscitation Method
U.S. Patent #5,927,273

Method of Providing Circulation via Lung Expansion and Deflation
U.S. Patent RE 36,460

Apparatus and Method for Cooling the Brain, Brain Stem, and Associated Neurologic Tissues
U.S. Patent 6,030,412

Balloon Bladder Catheter for Urology
Docket #WPB 39273

Quick Access Interathoracic Balloon Pumping/Cooling System
Docket #WPB 39229

Hyper-Augmentative Immune Therapy
Docket #WPB 36210

Organ Resuscitation Catheter
Docket #WPB 39274

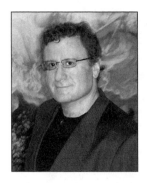 **Dr. Robert Goldman** has spearheaded the development of numerous international medical organizations and corporations. Dr. Goldman has served as a Senior Fellow at the Lincoln Filene Center, Tufts University, and as an Affiliate at the Philosophy of Education Research Center, Graduate School of Education, Harvard University. Dr. Goldman is Professor; Graduate School of Medicine, Swinburne University, Australia, and Clinical Consultant, Department of Obstetrics and Gynecology, Korea Medical University. He is also Professor, Department of Internal Medicine at the University of Central America Health Sciences, Department of Internal Medicine. Dr. Goldman is a Fellow of the American Academy of Sports Physicians and a Board Diplomat in Sports Medicine and Board Certified in Anti-Aging Medicine.

Dr. Goldman received his Bachelor of Science Degree (B.S.) from Brooklyn College in New York, then conducted three years of independent research in steroid biochemistry and attended the State University of New York. He received the Doctor of Medicine (M.D.) Degree from the Central America Health Sciences University, School of Medicine in Belize, a government-sanctioned, Ministry of Health-approved, and World Health Organization–listed medical university. He received his Doctor of Osteopathic Medicine and Surgery (D.O.) degree from Chicago College of Osteopathic Medicine at Midwestern University. His Ph.D. work was in the field of androgenic anabolic steroid biochemistry.

He co-founded and serves as Chairman of the Board of Life Science Holdings, a biomedical research company which has had more than 150 medical patents under development in the areas of brain resuscitation, trauma and emergency medicine, organ transplant, and blood preservation technologies. He has overseen cooperative research agreement development programs in conjunction with such prominent institutions as the American National Red Cross, the U.S. National Aeronautics and Space Administration (NASA), the Department of Defense, and the FDA's Center for Devices & Radiological Health.

Dr. Goldman is the recipient of the Gold Medal for Science (1993), the Grand Prize for Medicine (1994), the Humanitarian Award (1995), and the Business Development Award (1996).

During the late 1990s, Dr. Goldman received honors from Minister of Sports and government health officials of numerous nations. In 2001, Excellency Juan Antonio Samaranch awarded Dr. Goldman the International Olympic Committee Tribute Diploma for contributions to the development of sport and Olympism.

In addition, Dr. Goldman is a black belt in karate, Chinese weapons expert, and world champion athlete with over twenty world strength records. He has also been listed in the *Guinness Book of World Records*. Some of his past performance records include 13,500 consecutive sit-ups and 321 consecutive handstand pushups.

Dr. Goldman was an All-College athlete in four sports, a three-time winner of the John F. Kennedy (JFK) Physical Fitness Award, was voted Athlete of the Year, was the recipient of the Champions Award, and was inducted into the World Hall of Fame of Physical Fitness. In 1995, Dr. Goldman was awarded the Healthy American Fitness Leader Award from the President's Council on Physical Fitness & Sports and U.S. Chamber of Commerce.

Dr. Goldman is Chairman of the International Medical Commission overseeing sports medicine committees in more than 176 nations. He has served as a Special Advisor to the President's Council on Physical Fitness & Sports. He is founder and international President Emeritus of the National Academy of Sports Medicine and the cofounder and chairman of the American Academy of Anti-Aging Medicine (A4M). Dr. Goldman visits an average of twenty countries annually to promote brain research and sports medicine programs.

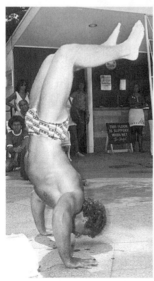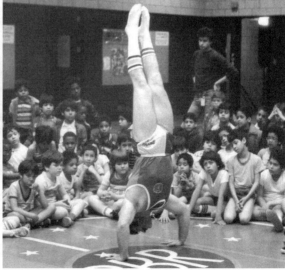

Dr. Bob Goldman setting the world record in handstand pushups with 321 repetitions.

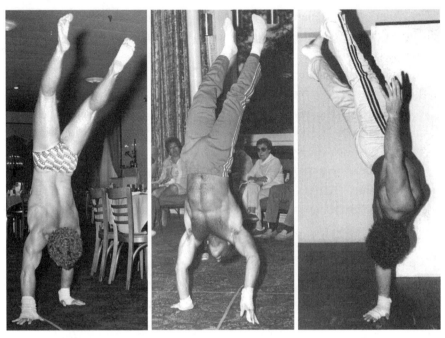

Dr. Bob Goldman during the world record 50 yard handstand sprint trials.

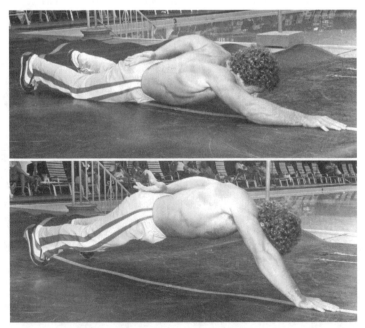

Dr. Bob Goldman setting the world record for 161 consecutive
overhead straight one-arm extension pushups.

Dr. Goldman, President's Council on Physical Fitness & Sports

Dr. Goldman served as Special Advisor to the President's Council on Physical Fitness & Sports under Governor Schwarzenegger's Chairmanship of the Council.

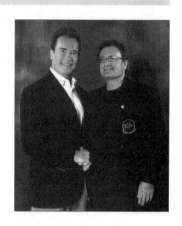

Dr. Goldman (right) with friend Gov. Arnold Schwarzenegger.

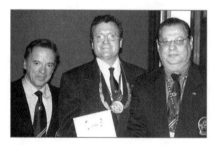

Dr. Goldman (center), shown here with Dr. Rafael Santonja (Spain), past President of the Olympic Weight Lifting Federation of Spain, and Professor Dr. Eduardo H. De Rose (Brazil), of the International Olympic Medical Commission.

Dr. Goldman, Recipient of the Gold Order of the International Federation of Body Builders (IFBB)

Dr. Robert Goldman, World Chairman IFBB Medical Commission, receives the IFBB's highest award—the IFBB Gold Order—at the World Championships in Shanghai, China, in 2005.

A4M MEMBERSHIP BENEFITS

Becoming a member of A4M gains you access to over a decade of established anti-aging expertise. Position yourself as being the first to learn of the latest breakthroughs in preventive and interventive techniques that help your patients achieve their personal best in wellness, maximum longevity and a fulfilling quality of life.

Join now, increase your practice income and take advantage of the following membership benefits:

- **Physician Referral Service:** A4M fields approximately 2,000 inquires monthly from the public, interested in finding a qualified anti-aging medical specialist, groups and other services. A4M will direct patient inquiries in your area to your practice. Your placement at www.worldhealth.net will strategically position your product/service at buyer's fingertips around the world, day and night. Ask about our online marketing opportunities:

- **Anti-Aging Physicians and Health Practitioners Directory:** Hundreds of listings of physicians, searchable by name and location

- **Anti-Aging Clinics and Spas Directory**

- **Anti-Aging Products and Services Directory**

- **American Board Certification Programs:** A4M membership makes you eligible to take the written and oral exam to become board-certified. ABAAM offers medical professionals recognition of specialty knowledge and clinical practice of anti-aging medical care. The following are the available certifications:

- **The American Board of Anti-Aging Medicine (ABAAM) for Physician Members only:** issues Board Certification to individuals with M.D. (Doctor of Medicine), D.O. (Doctor of Osteopathic Medicine), and M.B.B.S. (Bachelor of Medicine/Bachelor of Science) degrees.

- **The American Board of Anti-Aging Health Practitioners (ABAAHP) for Scientific Healthcare Members only:** Issues Diplomate Certificate to Doctors of Chiropractic (DC), Doctors of Dentistry (DDS), Naturopathic Doctors (ND), Doctors of Podiatric Medicine (DPM), Registered Pharmacists (RPh), scientists (PhD and similar), Registered Nurses, Nurse Practitioners, and Physician Assistants.

- **Advertising opportunities:** Receive special discounts on print advertising, online advertising and conference booths and reach out to your prospective customers. Maximize your advertising visibility worldwide, with a minimum exposure to 100,000-plus decision-making buyers of leading-edge healthcare products and services.

- **Complimentary subscription to our award-winning journal, Anti-Aging Medical News:** This trendsetting industry publication for the field of anti-aging healthcare serves as a forum of exchange between physicians and professionals delivering clinical healthcare, scientists, researchers, government and private institutions and commercial entities.

- **Discounts on all A4M-sponsored events:** The Accreditation Council for Continuing Medical Education (ACCME) recognizes the educational programs sponsored by A4M. Members receive discounts to these events including our Annual World Congresses on Anti-Aging Medicine & Regenerative Biomedical Technologies. As members, you will receive special incentive DISCOUNTS (up to nearly 50% discounts on the actual on-site value of the registration). You will get the opportunity to meet thousands of doctors, guest speakers, exhibitors and key members of the industry and media.

- **Discounts on A4M Educational Materials:** Learn anti-aging from the organization that created the anti-aging specialty with our library of. State-of-the-Science educational books, videos, tapes, and CDROMs.

- **Complimentary Electronic Biotech Newsletters:** E-Biotech Newsletter (EBN) is a service of the American Academy of Anti-Aging Medicine, a non-profit society of physicians and scientists focused on clinical answers to ageing related disorders leading to a longer and healthier lifespan. Along with reports from our medical correspondents at 26 universities and medical research centers EBN scans over 100 scientific publications and news services each week to extract and digest the latest and most promising advances in medicine that relate to the early detection treatment prevention and reversal of aging related conditions including topics such as: cancer, heart attack, obesity, chronic fatigue, memory disorders, arthritis, prostate disease, sexual dysfunction, brain implant stimulations, stem cell research, cloning, genetic engineering, anti-aging medicine, human augmentation , medical robotics and more. If its hot, new, and it will improve your life, your abilities, or your lifespan then you'll find it at EBN, the official newsletter of A4M's WorldHealth.net

AMERICAN ACADEMY OF ANTI-AGING MEDICINE (A4M)
NEW MEMBERSHIP / RENEWAL APPLICATION FORM

Name: _____

Degrees: ☐ MD ☐ DO ☐ MBBS ☐ DC ☐ DDS ☐ ND ☐ PhD
☐ RPh ☐ RN ☐ NP ☐ PA ☐ Other: _____

Title: _____

Practice/Company: _____

Mailing Address: _____

City, State, Zip, Country: _____

Phone: _____ Fax: _____

Email: _____ Website: _____

MEMBERSHIP CATEGORY

	1 YEAR	2 YEARS	5 YEARS
☐ Physician Membership (MD, DO, MBBS)	$150.00	$250.00	$500.00
☐ Scientific/Healthcare (DC, DDS, ND, DPM, R.Ph, PhD, RN, NP, PA)	$ 95.00	$150.00	—
☐ Preferred General Public	$ 89.95	—	—

I wish to be accepted as a member of the American Academy of Anti-Aging Medicine and agree to abide by its By Laws and Code of Ethics:

Signed: _____ Date: _____

Please Select a Voluntary Contribution Level (optional):
☐ US$50 ☐ US$100 ☐ US$150 ☐ (Other) US$_____

Payment in the amount of US$_____ is enclosed (membership dues + contribution)

PAYMENT INFORMATION

Your membership will not be processed without full payment or if your credit card is declined.

☐ Check #: _____ payable to A4M ☐ Credit Card ☐ MC ☐ Visa ☐ AMEX

Name on CC: _____ CC#: _____

Security #: _____ Expires: _____

Signature: _____ Date: _____

Remit completed form to: **Academy of Anti-Aging Medicine**
1510 West Montana Street
Chicago, IL 60614 USA
Ph: 773-528-1000 • Fax: 773-528-5390
Tracking Group #_____

An Organizational Membership affords you extended benefits. Contact the A4M Membership Department for details. Allow 6–8 weeks for processing new membership applications and receipt of Welcoming Kit and Member Certificate.

Membership Return Policy: Applicants wishing to return their A4M membership are required to comply with A4M's Membership Return Policy. Instructions are available on the Membership page at www.worldhealth.net and from the A4M Membership Department. For inquiries, contact Customer Services at: 773-528-1000 or e-mail membership@worldhealth.net.

121 WAYS TO LIVE 121 YEARS ... AND MORE!

Prescriptions for Longevity

Ronald Klatz and Robert Goldman

Nobody wants to get old. And why would they? The aging process eventually affects every one of our body systems—from mental function and sexual performance to physical appearance, ability, and strength. But chronological age has little to do with a person's biological age: Some people are old at fifty, while others are still sharp and spry at ninety.

Today's scientists know quite a bit about what causes a person to grow old. The things we've always considered "normal aging" are actually caused by physiological problems that, in many cases, respond to medical treatment and healthy lifestyle habits. As a result, the human life span can be significantly increased while maintaining or even improving quality of life!

This contemporary approach to aging—known as anti-aging medicine—is a clinical specialty practiced by more than 20,000 physicians worldwide. It applies advanced scientific and medical technologies for the early detection, prevention, treatment, and reversal of age-related dysfunctions, disorders, and diseases.

Soon we will all be able to look forward to a future of boundless health and vitality by implementing anti-aging approaches to help us feel, look, and perform better today. Readers can start by enjoying *121 Ways to Live 121 Years . . . and More!*—a handbook for living a long and healthy life. This book provides hundreds of practical tips readers can implement today to help them live a satisfying and productive life.

$9.95 • 160 PAGES • TRADE PAPERBACK • ISBN: 978-1-59120-197-7